Basic Principles and Operative Management of the Rotator Cuff

EDITED BY

C. BENJAMIN MA, MD
CHIEF OF SPORTS MEDICINE
ASSOCIATE PROFESSOR
SPORTS MEDICINE AND SHOULDER SURGERY
ORTHOPAEDIC INSTITUTE
UNIVERSITY OF CALIFORNIA, SAN FRANCISCO
SAN FRANCISCO, CALIFORNIA

BRIAN T. FEELEY, MD
ASSISTANT PROFESSOR
SPORTS MEDICINE AND SHOULDER SURGERY
ORTHOPAEDIC INSTITUTE
UNIVERSITY OF CALIFORNIA, SAN FRANCISCO
SAN FRANCISCO, CALIFORNIA

SLACK
INCORPORATED

www.slackbooks.com

ISBN: 978-1-61711-004-7

Published by: SLACK Incorporated
                6900 Grove Road
                Thorofare, NJ 08086 USA
                Telephone: 856-848-1000
                Fax: 856-848-6091
                www.slackbooks.com

Contact SLACK Incorporated for more information about other books in this field or about the availability of our books from distributors outside the United States.

Library of Congress Cataloging-in-Publication Data

Ma, C. B. (C. Benjamin), -
    Basic principles and operative management of the rotator cuff / edited by C.B. Ma, Brian T. Feeley.
        p. ; cm.
    Includes bibliographical references and index.
    ISBN 978-1-61711-004-7 (alk. paper)
    I. Feeley, Brian T., - II. Title.
    [DNLM: 1. Rotator Cuff--surgery. 2. Orthopedic Procedures--methods. 3. Rotator Cuff--injuries. 4. Rotator Cuff--physiopathology. 5. Shoulder Impingement Syndrome--surgery. WE 810]
    LC classification not assigned
    617.9--dc23
                            2011052580

Printed in the United States of America.

Last digit is print number: 10 9 8 7 6 5 4 3 2 1

DEDICATION

We would like to dedicate this textbook on the rotator cuff to our mentor, Russell Warren, MD. We are often told that no one can truly be a "triple threat" in academic medicine—someone who can be a skilled physician surgeon, an inspiring teacher, and an astute researcher. During our time in fellowship and beyond, Dr. Warren has served as a mentor and role model of how truly to be great at all things. It is the energy, enthusiasm, and devotion that he displays to all aspects of his life that makes us push ourselves to be better surgeons, researchers, and teachers.

We would also like to dedicate this book to the residents at UCSF. It brings us great pleasure and truly a privilege to teach an outstanding group of people. We do hope that this book will help in your pursuit of all your orthopedic careers.

CONTENTS

ACKNOWLEDGMENTS

We are most grateful for the tremendous time and effort put into this project by the collaborating authors. Without them, this book would not have been possible. Their expertise in the subject of rotator cuff tears and their time spent sharing their thoughts and surgical techniques are greatly appreciated.

We would also like to thank our families for their support during this endeavor as well as the many other times they have supported our time away from them.

To Sarina, Sonali, and Leena: thank you for listening to all my talk about shoulders and rotator cuff tears.

Brian T. Feeley, MD

To my wife, Anita, and children, Gabrielle and Conrad: thank you for all your support and making it fun for me to come home everyday. Daddy is also writing essays with you all.

C. Benjamin Ma, MD

ABOUT THE EDITORS

Brian T. Feeley, MD grew up in the San Francisco Bay Area. He attended Stanford University in California for his undergraduate degree, where he developed a passion for translational research. He continued at Stanford for medical school, and after almost embarking on a career in cardiothoracic surgery, he ultimately decided on orthopedic surgery.

Dr. Feeley served his orthopedic residency at the University of California, Los Angeles (UCLA) and his sports medicine and shoulder fellowship at the Hospital for Special Surgery, New York, NY. Since completing training, he has been on staff at the University of California, San Francisco (UCSF).

Dr. Feeley's clinical focus is on athletic injuries of the shoulder, knee, and hip. He has a special interest in the management of rotator cuff tears and reverse shoulder arthroplasty. His primary research interest is the basic science behind the muscle atrophy and fatty infiltration seen in rotator cuff tears.

Dr. Feeley currently lives in San Francisco with his wife, Sarina, and his two children, Sonali and Leena. He enjoys surfing as much as possible to keep his rotator cuffs in shape.

C. Benjamin Ma, MD was born and raised in Hong Kong, China. He came to the United States to attend Brown University in Providence, RI and majored in bioelectrical engineering. He attended medical school at Johns Hopkins University School of Medicine in Baltimore, MD, where he started his research interest in orthopedics and soft tissue healing. He went to the University of Pittsburgh Medical Center in Pennsylvania for his orthopedic surgery training, where he studied under Dr. Freddie Fu and Dr. Savio Woo. He then spent a year at the Hospital for Special Surgery for his Sports Medicine and Shoulder Fellowship. He has been on staff at UCSF since 2003 and is now Chief of the Sports Medicine and Shoulder Service. His clinical interest is in shoulder and knee surgeries and his research activities have been on improving the outcomes on the management of shoulder rotator cuff problems and advanced imaging on cartilage and rotator cuff muscles.

Contributing Authors

Christina Allen, MD *(Chapter 5)*
Associate Clinical Professor
Orthopedic Surgery
Division of Sports Medicine
Orthopaedic Institute
University of California, San Francisco
San Francisco, California

Asheesh Bedi, MD *(Chapter 3)*
Assistant Professor
Sports Medicine & Shoulder Surgery
MedSport, Department of Orthopedic Surgery
University of Michigan
Ann Arbor, Michigan

Fernando Contreras, MD *(Chapter 14)*
Fellow, Sports Medicine and Shoulder Service
Hospital for Special Surgery
New York, New York

Edward V. Craig, MD *(Chapter 17)*
Attending Surgeon
Hospital for Special Surgery
Professor, Clinical Orthopedic Surgery
Cornell Medical School
New York, New York

Ryan Dellamaggiora, MD *(Chapter 1)*
Fellow, Sports Medicine
Department of Orthopedic Surgery
University of California, San Francisco
San Francisco, California

Demetris Delos, MD *(Chapter 21)*
Chief Resident
Department of Orthopedic Surgery
Hospital for Special Surgery
New York, New York

Jonathan F. Dickens, MD, CPT, USA *(Chapter 16)*
Resident
Department of Orthopedics
Walter Reed National Military Medical Center
Bethesda, Maryland

William H. Dunbar V, MD *(Chapter 10)*
Attending Surgeon
The Ryu Hurvitz Orthopedic Clinic
Santa Barbara, California

Warren R. Dunn, MD, MPH *(Chapter 8)*
Assistant Professor
Team Physician
Division of General Internal Medicine and
    Public Health
Center for Health Services Research
Vanderbilt University Medical Center
Nashville, Tennessee

Neal S. ElAttrache, MD *(Chapter 13)*
Fellowship Director
Kerlan-Jobe Orthopaedic Clinic
Los Angeles, California

Robert A. Gallo, MD *(Chapter 9)*
Assistant Professor, Orthopedic Surgery
Department of Orthopedics
Penn State Hershey College of Medicine
Milton S. Hershey Medical Center
Hershey, Pennsylvania

Seth C. Gamradt, MD *(Chapter 19)*
Assistant Professor
Orthopedic Surgery and Sports Medicine
Department of Orthopedic Surgery
Orthopaedic Hospital
University of California, Los Angeles
Los Angeles, California

Jonathan Gelber, MD *(Chapter 19)*
Resident Physician
Department of Orthopedic Surgery
Harbor-UCLA Medical Center
Torrance, California

Carolyn M. Hettrich, MD, MPH *(Chapter 22)*
Assistant Professor
Department of Orthopedic Surgery
University of Iowa Carver College of Medicine
Iowa City, Iowa

Stephanie H. Hsu, MD *(Chapter 20)*
Clinical Fellow
Center for Shoulder, Elbow and Sports Medicine
NewYork-Presbyterian/Columbia   University
    Medical Center
New York, New York

Jaicharan J. Iyengar, MD (Chapter 15)
Assistant Professor
Sports Medicine and Shoulder Surgery
Orthopaedic Institute
University of California, San Francisco
San Francisco, California

James D. Kelly II, MD (Chapter 24)
San Francisco Shoulder, Elbow and Hand Clinic
San Francisco, California

Kelly G. Kilcoyne, MD, CPT, USA (Chapter 16)
Resident
Department of Orthopedics
Walter Reed National Military Medical Center
Bethesda, Maryland

Zakary A. Knutson, MD (Chapter 17)
Oklahoma Sports and Orthopedics Institute
Oklahoma City, Oklahoma
Professor
Department of Orthopedic Surgery and
    Rehabilitation
University of Oklahoma
Norman, Oklahoma

Abbas Kothari, BS (Chapter 12)
Department of Orthopedic Surgery
University of California, San Francisco
San Francisco, California

John E. Kuhn, MD (Chapter 22)
Associate Professor
Chief of Shoulder Surgery
Vanderbilt University School of Medicine
Nashville, Tennessee

Drew Lansdown, MD (Chapter 12)
Resident
Department of Orthopedic Surgery
University of California, San Francisco
San Francisco, California

Dominique Laron, MD (Chapter 4)
Department of Orthopedic Surgery
Sports Medicine Center
University of California, San Francisco
San Francisco Veterans Affairs Medical Center
San Francisco, California

Thay Q. Lee, PhD (Chapter 2)
Orthopaedic Biomechanics Laboratory
Senior Research Career Scientist, VA Long
    Beach Healthcare System
Professor and Vice Chairman for Research,
    Department of Orthopedic Surgery
Professor, Department of Biomedical
    Engineering
University of California, Irvine Medical Center
Orange, California

William N. Levine, MD (Chapters 11, 20)
Vice Chairman and Professor
Department of Orthopedic Surgery
Co-Director, Center for Shoulder, Elbow and
    Sports Medicine
NewYork-Presbyterian/Columbia University
    Medical Center
New York, New York

Thomas M. Link, MD (Chapter 6)
Professor, Radiology
Department of Radiology and Biomedical
    Imaging
University of California, San Francisco
San Francisco, California

Xuhui Liu, MD (Chapter 4)
Department of Orthopedic Surgery
University of California, San Francisco
San Francisco Veterans Affairs Medical Center
San Francisco, California

Anthony Luke, MD, MPH (Chapter 7)
Associate Professor and Director
Primary Care Sports Medicine
Department of Orthopedics
Department of Family and Community Medicine
University of California, San Francisco
San Francisco, California

Michelle H. McGarry, MS (Chapter 2)
Biomedical Engineer
Orthopaedic Biomechanics Laboratory
Long Beach, California

Todd C. Moen, MD (Chapter 11)
Carrell Clinic
Dallas, Texas

Lee Jae Morse, MD (Chapter 5)
Orthopedic Resident
Department of Orthopedic Surgery
University of California, San Francisco
San Francisco, California

Lorenzo Nardo, MD (Chapter 6)
Musculoskeletal and Quantitative Imaging
    Research
Department of Radiology and Biomedical
    Imaging
University of California, San Francisco
San Francisco, California

Michael L. Nguyen, MD (Chapter 2)
Resident
Department of Orthopedic Surgery
University of California, Irvine Medical Center
Orange, California

Maxwell C. Park, MD (Chapter 13)
Southern California Permanente Medical Group
Clinical Faculty, Orthopaedic Biomechanics
    Laboratory
VA Long Beach Healthcare System
Department of Orthopedic Surgery
Kaiser Foundation Hospital
Woodland Hills Medical Center
Los Angeles, California

Frank A. Petrigliano, MD (Chapter 19)
Assistant Professor-in-Residence
Department of Orthopedic Surgery
Orthopaedic Hospital
University of California, Los Angeles
Los Angeles, California

Paul J. Pursley, PT, SCS, CSCS (Chapter 18)
Senior Physical Therapist
Department of Rehabilitation Therapies
Institute for Orthopaedics, Sports Medicine and
    Rehabilitation
University of Iowa Hospitals and Clinics
Iowa City, Iowa

Ryan J. Quigley, BS (Chapter 2)
MD/PhD Candidate
Orthopaedic Biomechanics Laboratory
University of California, Irvine School of
    Medicine
Irvine, California

Scott A. Rodeo, MD (Chapter 14)
Co-Chief, Sports Medicine and Shoulder Service
Attending Orthopedic Surgeon
Hospital for Special Surgery
Professor, Orthopedic Surgery
Weill Cornell Medical College
New York, New York

John-Paul H. Rue, MD, CDR, USN (Chapter 16)
Department of Orthopedic Surgery and Sports
    Medicine
Naval Health Clinic Annapolis
United States Naval Academy
Annapolis, Maryland
Assistant Professor of Surgery
Department of Surgery
Uniformed Services
University of the Health Sciences
Bethesda, Maryland

Richard K. N. Ryu, MD (Chapter 10)
Senior Attending Surgeon
The Ryu Hurvitz Orthopedic Clinic
Santa Barbara, California

William Schairer, BA (Chapter 1)
Sports Medicine and Shoulder Surgery
Department of Orthopedic Surgery
University of California, San Francisco
San Francisco, California

Michael A. Shaffer, PT, ATC, OCS (Chapter 18)
Coordinator for Sports Rehabilitation
Sports Medicine
University of Iowa
Clinical Supervisor
Department of Rehabilitation Therapies
Institute for Orthopaedics, Sports Medicine and
    Rehabilitation
University of Iowa Hospitals and Clinics
Iowa City, Iowa

Jack G. Skendzel, MD (Chapter 3)
House Officer
Department of Orthopedic Surgery
University of Michigan
Ann Arbor, Michigan

Alison R. I. Spouge, MD, FRCPC (Chapter 7)
Associate Professor
Western University
Director of Musculoskeletal Imaging
Department of Medical Imaging
University Hospital
London Health Sciences Centre
London, Ontario, Canada

Ehsan Tabaraee, MD (Chapter 23)
Resident Physician
Department of Orthopedic Surgery
University of California, San Francisco
San Francisco, California

Suketu Vaishnav, MD (Chapter 24)
San Francisco Shoulder, Elbow and Hand Clinic
San Francisco, California

Russell F. Warren, MD (Chapter 21)
Professor of Orthopedic Surgery
Weill Cornell Medical College
NewYork-Presbyterian Hospital
Hospital for Special Surgery
New York, New York

Brian R. Wolf, MD, MS (Chapter 18)
Associate Professor
Department of Orthopedics
University of Iowa Hospitals and Clinics
Head Team Physician
Sports Medicine
University of Iowa
Institute for Orthopaedics, Sports Medicine and
    Rehabilitation
Iowa City, Iowa

Bob Yin, MD (Chapter 20)
Resident
Center for Shoulder, Elbow and Sports Medicine
NewYork-Presbyterian/Columbia   University
    Medical Center
New York, New York

FOREWORD

Basic Principles and Operative Management of the Rotator Cuff edited by Benjamin Ma and Brian Feeley is a well done review of the multiple issues affecting the rotator cuff. The editors have organized an excellent group of authors who have brought us up to date on multiple types of cuff disease. In particular, in the past decade, we have witnessed a resurgence of interest in cuff disease with considerable research on the biology of cuff failure and methods for fixation.

In addition, the development of the reverse prosthesis from Grammont's original design has lead to multiple variations that have offered an alternative to the painful patient with pseudoparalysis. Cuff tear arthropathy is well described, and while there is some overlap in the chapters, the pathophysiology and clinical treatments are well integrated.

Cuff repair, which has seen a plethora of anchors, sutures, and their configurations discussed in the literature, is illustrated and reviewed. A transosseous-equivalent appears to provide a better contact area but is time dependent. A double-row technique is used to provide a better contact area and ultimate failure load over a single row, but the clinical difference appears to be small.

The section on muscle physiology and the alterations that occur with a rotator cuff tear such as fatty infiltration, atrophy, and fibrosis is noted with an excellent description of the alternations and their etiology. This raises the question of an earlier repair of a torn cuff, rather than watchful waiting in younger patients. The diagnostic and imaging sections are nicely illustrated and clinical correlations referenced. The ultrasound section in particular will help in improving the surgeon's use of diagnostic imaging. The chapter on impingement does not solve the controversy of an acromioplasty or not but gives a good perspective on its use. Partial tears of the cuff are noted and their management nicely illustrated. The natural history of partial tears is well referenced. The surgical approaches are well presented.

Rotator cuff tears and the technique of both open and arthroscopic repair with a "Pearls and Pitfalls" section will greatly aid the surgeon. The biology of tendon healing and the causes of failure are clearly stated and its pathophysiology updated. Revision rotator cuff repair and surgical options including biologic augmentation are classified. Massive cuff tears and the arthroscopic treatment, particularly the releases required, are presented nicely. In dealing with massive tears, the reader is walked through a series of surgical options including arthroscopic or open repair biologic augmentation and tendon transfers. The outcome of tendon transfers is difficult to predict but can be useful in some patients.

The reverse prosthesis had been a significant development in the world of shoulder surgery. Its mechanics and techniques for insertion are well done. The indications section covers the changing opinion on its uses as its utilization has increased significantly. Over all, this is a thoughtful book that accomplishes its main goals. The student of shoulder disease at all levels should find this book to be well referenced and provide superb research for improving the care of our patients.

Russell F. Warren, MD
Professor of Orthopedic Surgery
Weill Cornell Medical College
NewYork-Presbyterian Hospital
Hospital for Special Surgery
New York, New York

INTRODUCTION

The treatment of rotator cuff tears continues to be a challenge for orthopedic surgeons, therapists, and trainers. Rotator cuff tears are an extremely common injury—one that is almost ubiquitous with advancing age. However, despite the fact that it is a common injury, the natural history of rotator cuff tears is not well understood and the basic biology of the tendon and muscle has only recently been explored.

When deciding to write this book, we were surprised to find that there was no "go-to" source for orthopedic surgeons to learn about the rotator cuff. For that reason, we sought to prepare more than just a general textbook or a "how-to" surgical technique book. We wanted to write a comprehensive book on the rotator cuff so that clinicians could understand the basic biology, natural history, and treatment principles of rotator cuff tears. We also wanted to provide detailed information on surgical techniques that the experienced shoulder surgeon could employ of the complicated massive or revision cuff tears. We have included chapters on reconstructive options for patients with irreparable rotator cuff injuries. Our goal is to have a comprehensive text that is a resource for the management of any type of rotator cuff injury.

CHAPTER 1

Anatomy of the Rotator Cuff

Ryan Dellamaggiora, MD; William Schairer, BA; and Brian T. Feeley, MD

The shoulder is a complex joint that allows for a large range of motion in multiple planes. In order to achieve this, the shoulder relies on an extremely shallow socket in the glenoid and motion that occurs both at the glenohumeral joint and the scapulothoracic joint. The rotator cuff muscles, as well as the larger muscles in the shoulder girdle, provide the dynamic stability and control over the shoulder that allow for this impressive range of motion and function. Understanding the bony and soft tissue anatomy is important in understanding the pathology and surgical treatment options for rotator cuff tears. This chapter will summarize the anatomy of the shoulder that is relevant to the rotator cuff function.

Scapula

The scapula is a thin bone that sits on the posterior thoracic wall and serves as the support strut of the shoulder, the articular surface for the glenohumeral joint, and the origin for the muscles of the rotator cuff. It is a thin and flat triangle-shaped bone that is thicker at the edges than the body. The scapula sits 30 to 40 degrees anterior to the coronal plane on the thorax, and motion in this plane is referred to as *scaption* (Figure 1-1).[1]

The lateral aspect of the scapula broadens to form the glenoid vault and the glenoid, the articular surface for the glenohumeral joint. The glenoid articular surface is congruent with the articular surface of the humerus head[2] and covers approximately 35% of the humeral articular surface.[3,4] The glenoid socket depth is only 9 mm in the superoinferior axis and 5 mm in the anteroposterior (AP) axis.[5] The glenoid is covered with more cartilage on the edges than in the center.[2,6] The center of the glenoid has the least cartilage and is called the *bare area*.[6] The glenoid has 5 degrees of superior tilt and 7 degrees of retroversion relative to the main body of the scapula; however, in the resting position, the glenoid has a slight downward tilt due to the pull of the muscles.[7]

Ma CB, Feeley BT, eds.
Basic Principles and Operative Management
of the Rotator Cuff (pp 1-14)
© 2012 SLACK Incorporated

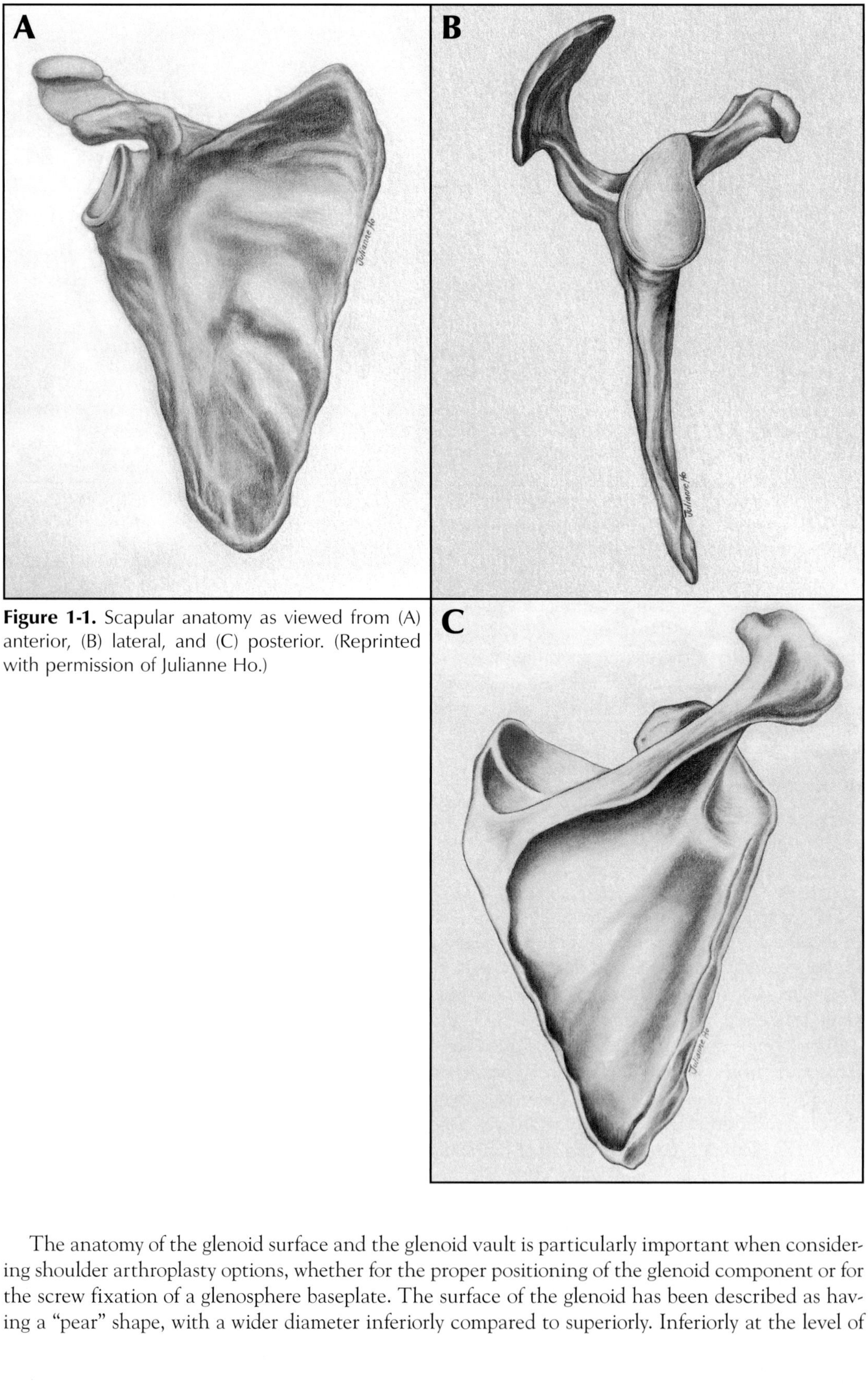

Figure 1-1. Scapular anatomy as viewed from (A) anterior, (B) lateral, and (C) posterior. (Reprinted with permission of Julianne Ho.)

The anatomy of the glenoid surface and the glenoid vault is particularly important when considering shoulder arthroplasty options, whether for the proper positioning of the glenoid component or for the screw fixation of a glenosphere baseplate. The surface of the glenoid has been described as having a "pear" shape, with a wider diameter inferiorly compared to superiorly. Inferiorly at the level of

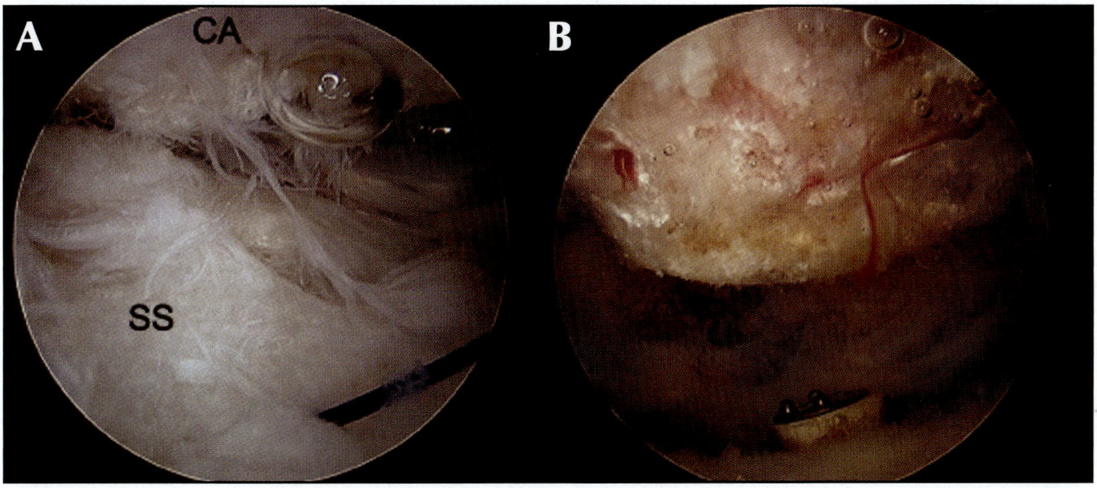

Figure 1-2. (A) Arthroscopic image of the CA ligament attached to the undersurface of the acromion. The ligament is frayed in the setting of a supraspinatus (SS) degenerative tear. (B) Acromial spur after débridement of the CA ligament.

the bare area, the glenoid has an average AP diameter of 26 to 32 mm.[8-11] The average AP diameter is significantly smaller in women than in men by 4 to 5 mm.[8,10] Average version was 1.23 degrees (±3.5 degrees) of anteversion from the transverse axis, but this was highly variable.[8] The glenoid vault depth averages 41.0 mm ±6.1 mm.[11] In cases with bone loss, screw fixation can be difficult but may be acquired medially in the base of the coracoid, the scapular spine, and the lateral column.[12]

From the anterolateral surface of the scapula, the coracoid process projects anterior, superior, and laterally. The coracoacromial (CA) ligament attaches from the superolateral aspect of the coracoid and runs superiorly, fanning out to attach on the undersurface of the acromion. The CA ligament is often frayed in impingement, partial-thickness, and full-thickness rotator cuff tears. In the setting of a massive rotator cuff tear, the CA ligament can be the final structure preventing anterosuperior escape of the humeral head (Figure 1-2). Bony spurs can develop within the body of the CA ligament, which can lead to partial- and full-thickness rotator cuff tears.

The acromion is an anterior extension of the scapular spine and acts as the superior portion of the supraspinatus arch. The acromion develops from 3 separate ossification centers—the mesoacromion, meta-acromion, and preacromion. Failure of these to fully fuse is common, occurring in up to 15% of the population, and is usually asymptomatic.[13] However, some patients can develop os acromiale that remain mobile, resulting in shoulder pain and impingement-like symptoms.[13]

The scapular spine is a bony ridge that runs medial to lateral in a slightly superior direction. It divides the top third from the lower two-thirds, creating the supraspinatus and infraspinatus fossae, respectively. The spine continues past the lateral border of the scapula to become the acromion.[14]

HUMERAL HEAD ANATOMY

The humerus articulates with the glenoid to form the glenohumeral joint and also serves as the site of attachment for the muscles of the rotator cuff. The articular surface of the humeral head is approximately one-third of a sphere[15] with a radius of curvature of about 2.35 cm.[16] The head is retroverted 25 to 35 degrees with a 45-degree neck shaft angle.[17] This geometry positions the articular surface of the humerus in line with the glenoid. The greater tuberosity projects laterally off the humeral head while the lesser tuberosity projects anteriorly. Each tuberosity has distinct flat surfaces termed *facets*. The greater tuberosity is divided into superior, middle, and inferior facets, while the lesser tuberosity is divided into superior and inferior facets; the inferior facets are triangular while the others are quadrangular.[16] The greater and lesser tuberosities are separated by the bicipital groove, in which the long head of the biceps tendon and the anterolateral branch of the anterior circumflex artery are found. The bicipital groove extends distally approximately 8 cm, or one-quarter the length of the humerus.[18]

MUSCULATURE

The majority of the scapula serves as an origin for the rotator cuff muscles, as well as shoulder stabilizing muscles—17 muscles attach to the scapula and help guide glenohumeral motion. The primary elevator of the shoulder is the anterior, middle, and posterior deltoid muscle. The superior vector of the deltoid contraction is counteracted by the rotator cuff musculature that acts to compress and depress the glenohumeral joint. The force couples of the shoulder are discussed in Chapter 2. The other scapular muscles act to stabilize and position the scapula to enable more motion and to maximize forces across the glenohumeral joint (Table 1-1). The focus of our discussion will be the rotator cuff musculature.

Supraspinatus

The supraspinatus muscle originates in the supraspinatus fossa on the superior and posterior surface of the scapula. The muscle belly can be divided into an anterior region and a smaller posterior region; the larger anterior region fills approximately 75% of the fossa. These 2 regions come together as the muscles move laterally, and a common muscle and tendon unit is formed. Distally, the anterior tendon inserts onto the anterosuperior aspect of the greater facet, while the posterior tendon inserts onto the posterosuperior aspect of the greater tuberosity. Anteriorly, the fibers of the supraspinatus tendon are enveloped in the coracohumeral (CH) ligament, and together they cross over the top of the bicipital groove, forming a roof for the long head of the biceps tendon. Posteriorly, the supraspinatus and infraspinatus tendons have some shared fibers. The supraspinatus functions as an abductor of the shoulder and humeral head depressor, providing a downward force to counteract the superior vector created by the deltoid. The supraspinatus has a central role in the motion of the shoulder as it has been shown to be active in any motion involving "elevation."[19,20] The deltoid is a larger, stronger muscle, but the shoulder loses 50% of its lifting strength when supraspinatus and the other rotator cuff muscles are inhibited using ultrasound-guided nerve block[21] or in the setting of a large rotator cuff tear.

Infraspinatus

The infraspinatus is responsible for the majority of the external rotation of the proximal humerus.[19] It is a pennate muscle with a median raphe that originates from the infraspinatus fossa of the scapula and the scapular spine and inserts into the greater tuberosity. The infraspinatus blends with the supraspinatus anteriorly and the teres minor inferiorly. In addition to active external rotation of the shoulder, the infraspinatus acts as a humeral head depressor and stabilizes the shoulder to prevent anterior subluxation.

Teres Minor

The teres minor originates from the inferolateral border of the scapula and the fascia of the infraspinatus. An alternate origin has been described where the teres minor originates from the medial border of the scapula, overlying a portion of the infraspinatus.[22] The inferior edge of the teres minor forms the superior border of the quadrilateral space laterally and the triangular space medially. It inserts into the lower portion of the posterior greater tuberosity. Along with the infraspinatus,

TABLE 1-1. MUSCLE ATTACHMENTS TO THE SCAPULA

MUSCLE	ORIGIN	INSERTION	INNERVATION	FUNCTION
Deltoid	Anterior clavicle, acromion process, spine of scapula	Deltoid tuberosity	Axillary	Abduction
Supraspinatus	Supraspinatus fossa	Greater tuberosity	Suprascapular	Compression, abduction
Infraspinatus	Infraspinatus fossa	Greater tuberosity	Suprascapular	Compression, external rotation
Teres minor	Inferolateral border of scapula	Greater tuberosity	Axillary	Compression, external rotation
Subscapularis	Subscapularis fossa	Lesser tuberosity	Upper and lower subscapular	Compression, internal rotation
Levator scapulae	Transverse processes C1-C4	Medial border of scapula	Dorsal scapular	Scapular elevation, abduction
Rhomboids	Spinous processes C7-T5	Medial border of scapula	Dorsal scapular	Scapular elevation, adduction
Trapezius	Spinous processes C7-T12	Spine of scapula	Spinal accessory	Scapular rotation, adduction
Latissimus dorsi	Spinous processes T7-L5, posterior sacrum, posterior ileum, lower 3-4 ribs, tip of the scapula	Floor of bicipital groove of humerus	Thoracodorsal	Adduction, extension, and internal rotation of humerus
Teres major	Lateral border of scapula	Medial side of bicipital groove of humerus	Lower subscapular	Adduction, internal rotation
Serratus anterior	Superior lateral surfaces of ribs 1-9	Medial border and inferior angle of scapula	Long thoracic	Scapular abduction, stabilization on thoracic cage
Coracobrachialis	Coracoid	Middle humerus	Musculocutaneous	Flexion, adduction of humerus
Biceps brachii (long head)	Supraglenoid tuberosity	Radial tuberosity	Musculocutaneous	Compression, elbow flexion, forearm supination
Biceps brachii (short head)	Coracoid	Radial tuberosity	Musculocutaneous	Compression, elbow flexion, forearm supination
Triceps (long head)	Infraglenoid tubercle	Olecranon process of ulna	Axillary	Adduction
Pectoralis minor	Ribs 3-5	Coracoid	Medial pectoral	Stabilizes scapula against thoracic wall
Omohyoid	Superior border of scapula	Hyoid	Ansa cervicalis	Depresses larynx and hyoid bone

the teres minor is an external rotator of the humerus. Multiple studies have demonstrated that it provides up to 45% of the external rotation force[19,23] and acts as an active stabilizer against anterior subluxation.

Subscapularis

The subscapularis is the largest and strongest muscle in the rotator cuff.[24] It is a multipennate muscle that originates from the subscapularis fossa on the anterior surface of the scapula. The upper two-thirds of the muscle have multiple tendinous bands that converge to insert into the lesser tuberosity, the bicipital groove, and the greater tuberosity. Its fibers also extend from the lesser tuberosity across the bicipital groove to create a sling that envelops the long head of the biceps tendon. It is often these fibers that appear intact in a patient with a subscapularis rupture, causing the treating surgeon to miss the diagnosis on magnetic resonance imaging (MRI) and during arthroscopic visualization. The lower third of the muscle inserts into the inferior aspect of the lesser tuberosity. The primary function of subscapularis is internal rotation of the humerus, but it also has a significant role in glenohumeral compression and preventing posterior subluxation.[25]

INNERVATION OF THE ROTATOR CUFF

The supraspinatus is innervated by the suprascapular nerve (SSN) with contributions from C5 and C6. The nerve enters near the midpoint of the muscle after it passes through the suprascapular notch, a recess in the superior border of the scapula just medial to the base of the coracoid process. The transverse scapular ligament forms the roof of the suprascapular notch, which can be a cause of compression. Tears of the superior or posterior rotator cuff tendons lead to atrophy of the muscle as well as muscle retraction. It is suspected that retraction of the supraspinatus can cause increased tension on the SSN as the nerve is tethered in the suprascapular notch, leading to progressive atrophy and fatty infiltration.[26] As mentioned previously, the notch can also be a point of compression by cysts from superior labral tears[27] as well as compression from masses or vascular abnormalities.[17,27,28]

The infraspinatus is innervated by the SSN after it has given its branches to the supraspinatus. The SSN passes through the spinoglenoid notch, which, unlike the suprascapular notch, is not spanned by a ligament. This is also an area of possible compression from labral cysts or from vascular anomalies that leads to isolated infraspinatus pathology, such as weakness, atrophy, and fatty infiltration (Figure 1-3).

The teres minor is innervated by the posterior branch of the axillary nerve (C5 and C6).

The subscapularis is innervated by the upper (C5) and lower (C5 and C6) subscapular nerves that are branches of the posterior cord of the brachial plexus. There are usually 2 upper subscapular nerves that are shorter in length. There are also usually 2 lower subscapular nerves that tend to be longer in length, corresponding with the longer excursion needed for the motion of the shoulder.[28]

VASCULATURE OF THE ROTATOR CUFF

The primary blood supply of the rotator cuff muscles are branches of the axillary artery. The blood supply of the supraspinatus is the suprascapular artery, which is a branch of the axillary artery. It crosses near the SSN, but it courses over the transverse scapular ligament and gives off branches into the supraspinatus muscle. This artery is able to supply a majority of the muscle and proximal tendon, but there is a "watershed" area approximately 8 to 12 mm from the insertion onto the greater tuberosity where the blood supply is decreased. It is this area that is felt to be at a higher risk for tendon degeneration and tears due to its poor blood supply. Interestingly, no studies to our knowledge have evaluated the blood flow to the rotator cuff muscle following a large rotator cuff tear. Fealy

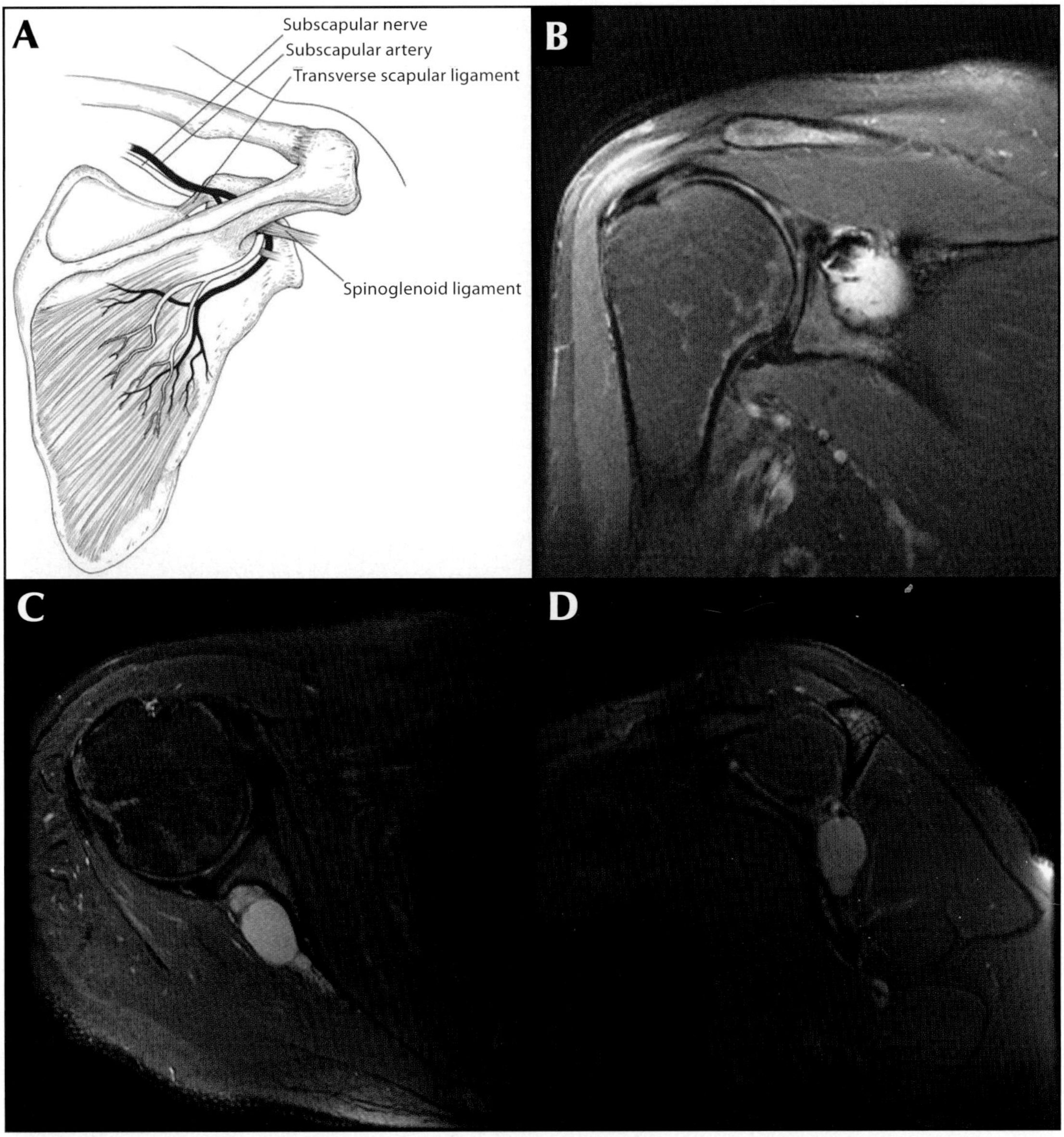

Figure 1-3. (A) Illustration of suprascapular anatomy as it relates to the scapula. The suprascapular notch is roofed by the transverse scapular ligament, and the spinoglenoid notch is covered by the spinoglenoid ligament; both structures have the potential to compress the nerve. The SSN passes through the suprascapular notch, across the floor of the supraspinatus fossa, and past the spinoglenoid notch. The artery passes above the transverse scapular ligament. (Safran MR, Nerve injury about the shoulder in athletes: part 1. Suprascapular nerve and axillary nerve, *Am J Sports Med*, volume 32, issue 3, pp 803-819, copyright © 2004 by Sage Publications. Reprinted by Permission of SAGE Publications.) (B) T2-weighted coronal oblique MRI of a large cyst that is compressing the SSN in the spinoglenoid notch. (C) Axial and (D) sagittal images of the same cyst. The patient required open decompression of the cyst.

and colleagues have shown altered vascular patterns in the rotator cuff tendon following rotator cuff repair using high-power ultrasound,[29] but changes in the vascular supply to the muscle itself after a cuff tear have not been evaluated.

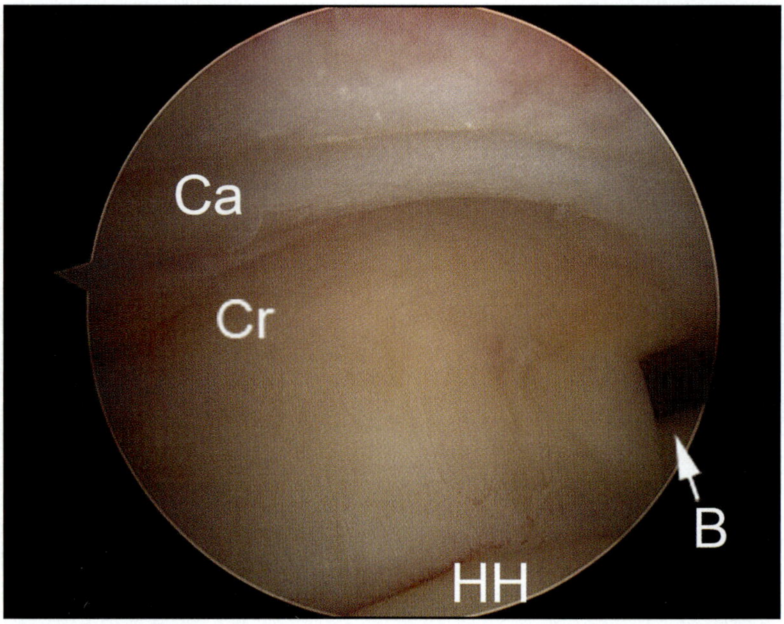

Figure 1-4. Arthroscopic view of the rotator cable (Ca) and crescent (Cr). The humeral head (HH) and biceps (B) tendon are identified.

The blood supply of the infraspinatus consists of 2 branches off of the suprascapular artery.[30] Some studies have described an alternative blood supply from the dorsal or circumflex scapular branch in up to two-thirds of cases.[31] The blood supply of teres minor originates from several vessels in the area, but most commonly from the posterior humeral scapular circumflex artery.[31]

The subscapularis blood supply is derived from an anastomotic loop. The posterior scapular artery, a branch of the transverse cervical artery, travels down the medial border of the scapula to anastomose with the subscapular artery, a branch of the axillary artery. Additionally, the suprahumeral artery and posterior circumflex humeral artery have been found to supply the subscapularis.[32]

TENDON ANATOMY AND HISTOLOGY

Rotator Cable/Crescent

The rotator cable is a rope-like fibrous structure near the distal cuff that runs perpendicular to the supraspinatus and infraspinatus tendons just medial to the greater tuberosity. The anterior and posterior ends of the cable are attached to the humerus. The rotator crescent is a relatively avascular, fan-like fibrous structure that runs parallel to the supraspinatus and infraspinatus tendons. The crescent connects the middle of the cable to the humerus. The rotator cable and crescent together have been described as a suspension bridge, with the cable distributing forces from the supraspinatus and infraspinatus, potentially minimizing consequences of a tear in the crescent (Figure 1-4).[33,34]

The rotator cable originates from the greater and lesser tuberosities. In the anterior part of the cable, the CH ligament fuses with the cable, and they are indistinguishable. Superficial fibers of the rotator cable insert on the lesser tuberosity, while deep fibers blend and insert with the supraspinatus tendon at its point of insertion on the superior facet of the greater tuberosity. Posteriorly, the cable lies deep to the infraspinatus tendon as it inserts in between the infraspinatus and teres minor tendons on the posterior side of the greater tuberosity.[35] The rotator cable and associated anatomy are able to be visualized both on ultrasound[24] and MRI.[35,36] The average rotator crescent was 1.82 mm, while the rotator cable was found to be 4.72 mm.[37] The thicker rotator cable is hypothesized to provide stress shielding from tears in the thinner crescent.

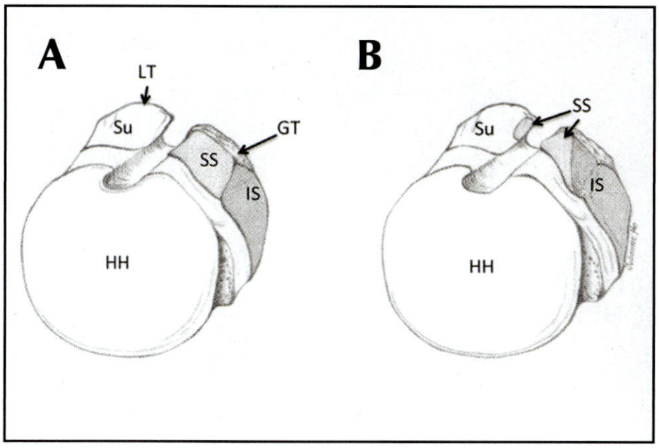

Figure 1-5. Insertions of the rotator cuff on the greater and lesser tuberosity. The figure illustrates the right humeral head. (A) The traditional insertions of the subscapularis (Su), supraspinatus (SS), and infraspinatus (IS) onto the greater tuberosity (GT) and lesser tuberosity (LT). (B) Alternative insertions as described by Mochizuki et al. (Adapted from Mochizuki T, Sugaya H, Uomizu M, et al. Humeral insertion of the supraspinatus and infraspinatus. New anatomical findings regarding the footprint of the rotator cuff. *J Bone Joint Surg.* 2008;90(5):962-969. Reprinted with permission of Julianne Ho.)

Insertional Anatomy

The humeral insertions of the rotator cuff muscles are critical to understanding the nature of rotator cuff tears and how to repair them. The subscapularis footprint is the largest of the 4 rotator cuff muscles with an average maximum medial to lateral width of 12.5 to 20 mm, with the largest portion of the footprint found inferiorly. Studies have found that subscapularis fibers extend beyond the lesser tuberosity, but there is some controversy as to whether they attach to the greater tuberosity.[38,39] The supraspinatus, infraspinatus, and teres minor attach to the greater tuberosity. Grossly, the supraspinatus and infraspinatus tendons blend with the fibrous layer of the joint capsule 15 mm proximal to insertion on the humerus. The fibers of the supraspinatus tendon insert into the anteromedial region of the superior facet of the greater tuberosity, with the anterior and posterior tendon portions inserting into the anterosuperior and posterosuperior aspect of the greater facet, respectively.[37] Measurements of the footprint area of the supraspinatus demonstrated an average medial to lateral dimension of 12.7 and 12.3 mm, while the average anterior to posterior length ranged from 24.3 to 40.7 mm.[38,39] More recently, the supraspinatus footprint has been described as smaller and the infraspinatus footprint much larger than previously reported (Figure 1-5).[40] In this study, the supraspinatus footprint is described as being more triangular and the infraspinatus more trapezoidal. The authors found that the insertion of the supraspinatus extended to the lesser tuberosity in 21% of specimens.[41]

The supraspinatus tendon also has fibers that fuse with the subscapularis tendon, forming a sheath around the biceps tendon in the bicipital groove. Supraspinatus tendon fibers project from the greater tuberosity to the lesser tuberosity, forming the roof of this sheath.[42] The details of the supraspinatus and subscapularis tendons and their function in stabilizing the long head of the biceps tendon has negated the previous notion of a separate transverse humeral ligament, which has been found not to exist.[43]

The attachment of the rotator cuff tendons to the greater and lesser tuberosities is formed by an enthesis. The transition from rotator cuff tendon to bone is separated into 4 zones: the tendon, uncalcified fibrocartilage, calcified fibrocartilage, and bone.[44] The tendon zone is composed predominantly of dense cartilage bundles and extracellular matrix. Collagen type 1 is abundant in the tendon zone but is replaced by collagen type 2 in the fibrocartilage zone. The calcified fibrocartilage zone is clearly delineated from uncalcified fibrocartilage by a continuous tidemark seen under light microscope. In the bone zone, collagen fibers directly enter the bone matrix.[45]

Histology of the supraspinatus and infraspinatus tendons at their distal insertion point reveals 5 separate layers (Figure 1-6).[42] The most superficial layer is 1-mm thick and contains CH ligament fibers oriented oblique to the fibers of the rotator cuff tendons, as well as large arterioles. The second layer is about 4-mm thick and contains groups of tightly packed longitudinal tendon fibers,

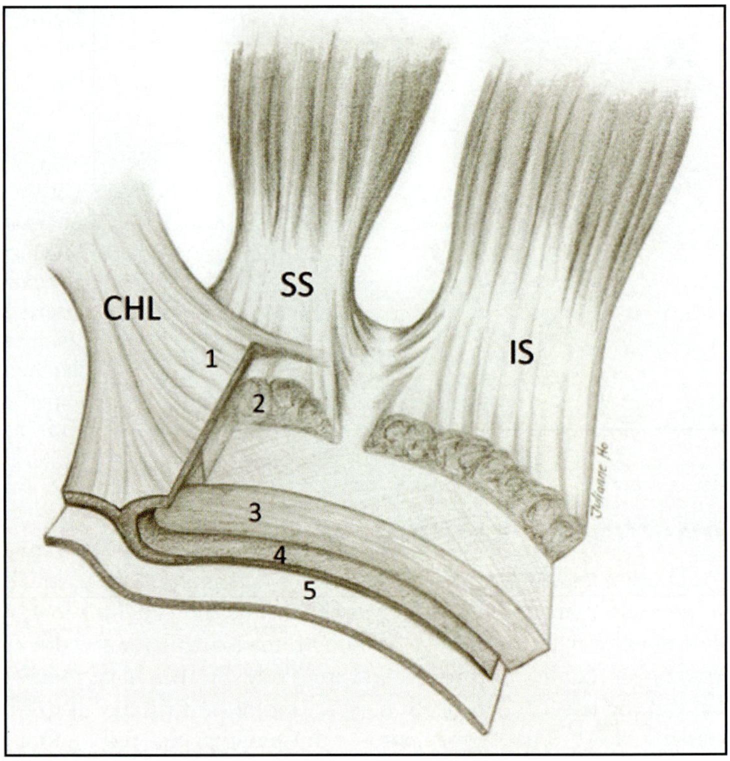

Figure 1-6. Five layers of the supraspinatus (SS) and infraspinatus (IS) tendon. The most superficial layer (1) is the superficial CH ligament (CHL). Layer 2 contains the main oriented fascicles; layer 3 consists of the smaller less oriented fascicles; layer 4 is the deep CHL; and layer 5 is the joint capsule. (Adapted from Clark JM, Harryman DT II. Tendons, ligaments, and capsule of the rotator cuff. Gross and microscopic anatomy. *J Bone Joint Surg Am.* 1992;(75)5:713-725. Reprinted with permission of Julianne Ho.)

which extend from the muscle bellies to their insertions into the proximal humerus. Large arterioles continue through this layer. The third layer is 3-mm thick and contains crossing, loosely packed groups of tendon fibers that are intertwining from the supraspinatus and infraspinatus tendons. Smaller blood vessels are seen in this layer compared to previous layers. The fourth layer contains thick bands of collagen fibers and small capillaries embedded in loose connective tissue that arise from the CH ligament. The fifth layer is a thin sheet of collagen fibrils in an amorphous layer of Sharpey fibers that forms the shoulder capsule. The mixing of these layers is most intricate around the bicipital groove. The fibers of supraspinatus tendon cross over the top of the groove to form a roof over the tendon of the long head of the biceps. The fibers of the subscapularis cross under the long head of the biceps to form the floor. Together, they form a stabilizing sling for the long head of the biceps tendon.

THE ROTATOR INTERVAL

The rotator interval is the triangular space defined by the superior border of the subscapularis tendon and the anterior border of the supraspinatus (Figure 1-7). The coracoid process marks the medial base of the triangle, while the lateral ridge of the bicipital groove marks the apex. This area consists of relatively little musculature, but contains ligamentous structures and parts of the joint capsule. It offers a safe entry point into the anterior aspect of the shoulder for arthroscopic and some open procedures.

The most superficial structure of the rotator interval is the superficial fibers of the CH ligament. The CH ligament originates at the proximal third of the lateral surface of the coracoid process and inserts directly into the rotator cable, close to the greater and lesser tuberosities.[35,46] It is

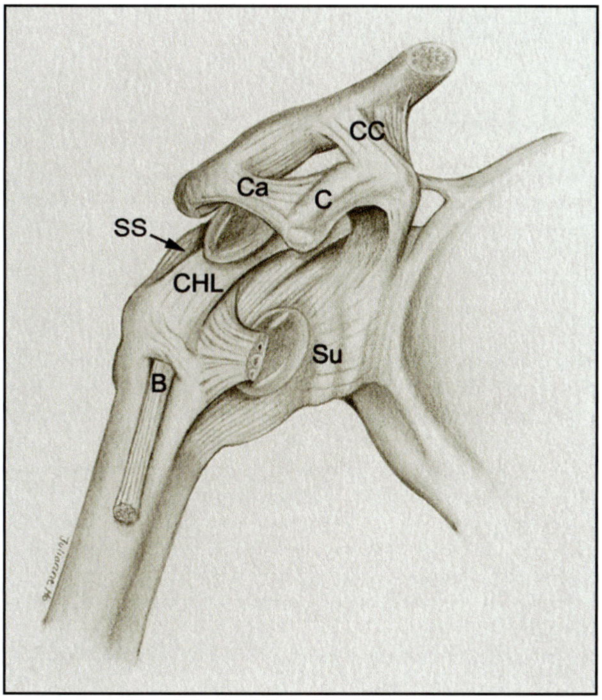

Figure 1-7. Schematic drawing of the anterior shoulder and rotator interval. The CH ligament (CHL) runs from the coracoid (C) to the humerus, overlying the biceps (B) tendon. The subscapularis (Su) forms the inferior border of the rotator interval, and the supraspinatus (SS) the superior border. The coracoacromial ligament (Ca) and coracoclavicular (CC) ligaments are identified. (Reprinted with permission of Julianne Ho.)

centrally located in the rotator interval and increases shoulder stability in the anterior portion of the capsule.[47] Below these superficial CH ligament fibers are supraspinatus and subscapularis tendons, which, as discussed earlier, insert on the greater and lesser tuberosities and also form a fibrous sheath around the biceps tendon. Additionally, these tendons blend with CH ligament fibers at their points of insertion. A third layer consists of deep fibers of the CH ligament, which insert mostly to the greater tuberosity, as well as the lesser tuberosity. The fibers directed toward the lesser tuberosity also make part of the sheath covering the biceps tendon. The deepest layer of the rotator interval consists of the superior glenohumeral ligament and the joint capsule. The superior glenohumeral ligament originates with the long head of the biceps tendon at the supraglenoid tuberosity. It inserts laterally to the lesser tuberosity and forms part of the anterior sheath around the biceps tendon.[48]

CONCLUSION

The glenohumeral joint allows for extensive motion through the limited bony contact between the glenoid and proximal humerus. The stability of this joint is maintained through the surrounding soft tissues. Important in dynamic stability of the glenohumeral joint are the muscles of the rotator cuff. Not only do they provide stability, but they also allow for the motion of the glenohumeral joint. The 4 muscles of the rotator cuff—supraspinatus, infraspinatus, teres minor, and subscapularis—originate from the scapula and insert into the proximal humerus, allowing their diverse and important actions at the shoulder. Microscopic examination of these tendon attachments reveals possible etiologies of injury. The supraspinatus and infraspinatus insert to the humerus through the rotator cable and crescent and distribute forces across the greater tuberosity, which may be protective. The supraspinatus and subscapularis tendons interact at the bicipital groove to form a fibrous sheath surrounding the long head of the biceps tendon. In the subsequent chapters, the biomechanics, pathology, and treatment options of the rotator cuff will be illustrated and discussed.

REFERENCES

1. Canale ST, Beaty JH. *Campbell's Operative Orthopaedics*. 11th ed. St. Louis, MO: Mosby; 2007.

2. Soslowsky LJ, Flatow EL, Bigliani LU, Mow VC. Articular geometry of the glenohumeral joint. *Clin Orthop Relat Res*. 1992;285:181-190.

3. Saha AK. Mechanics of elevation of glenohumeral joint. Its application in rehabilitation of flail shoulder in upper brachial plexus injuries and poliomyelitis and in replacement of the upper humerus by prosthesis. *Acta Orthop Scand*. 1973;44(6):668-678.

4. Bechtol CO. Biomechanics of the shoulder. *Clin Orthop Relat Res*. 1980;146:37-41.

5. Hata Y. Anatomic study of the glenoid labrum. *J Shoulder Elbow Surg*. 1992;1(4):207-214.

6. Burkhart SS, Debeer JF, Tehrany AM, Parten PM. Quantifying glenoid bone loss arthroscopically in shoulder instability. *Arthroscopy*. 2002;18(5):488-491.

7. Freedman L, Munro RR. Abduction of the arm in the scapular plane: scapular and glenohumeral movements. A roentgenographic study. *J Bone Joint Surg Am*. 1966;48(8):1503-1510.

8. Churchill RS, Brems JJ, Kotschi H. Glenoid size, inclination, and version: an anatomic study. *J Shoulder Elbow Surg*. 2001;10(4):327-332.

9. Codsi MJ, Bennetts C, Powell K, Iannotti JP. Locations for screw fixation beyond the glenoid vault for fixation of glenoid implants into the scapula: an anatomic study. *J Shoulder Elbow Surg*. 2007;16(3 Suppl):S84-S89.

10. von Schroeder HP, Kuiper SD, Botte MJ. Osseous anatomy of the scapula. *Clin Orthop Relat Res*. 2001;383:131-139.

11. Bicknell RT, Patterson SD, King GJ, Chess DG, Johnson JA. Glenoid vault endosteal dimensions: an anthropometric study with special interest in implant design. *J Shoulder Elbow Surg*. 2007;16(3 Suppl):S96-S101.

12. Humphrey C. Optimizing glenosphere position and fixation in reverse shoulder arthroplasty, part two: the three-column concept. *J Shoulder Elbow Surg*. 2008;17(4):595-601.

13. Sammarco V. Os acromiale: frequency, anatomy, and clinical implications. *J Bone Joint Surg Am*. 2000;82(3):394-400.

14. Lapner PC, Uhthoff HK, Papp S. Scapula fractures. *Orthop Clin North Am*. 2008;39(4):459-474, vi.

15. Bost FC IV. The pathological changes in recurrent dislocation of the shoulder: a report of Bankart's operative procedure. *J Bone Joint Surg Am*. 1942;24:595-613.

16. Berghs BM, Derveaux T, Speeckaert W, Vanslambrouck K, De Wilde LF. Three-dimensional analysis of the orientation and the inclination of the rotator cuff footprint. *J Shoulder Elbow Surg*. 2011;20(4):637-645.

17. Sarrafian SK. Gross and functional anatomy of the shoulder. *Clin Orthop Relat Res*. 1983;173:11-19.

18. Wafae N, Atencio Santamaria LE, Vitor L, Pereira LA, Ruiz CR, Wafae GC. Morphometry of the human bicipital groove (sulcus intertubercularis). *J Shoulder Elbow Surg*. 2010;19(1):65-68.

19. Colachis SC Jr, Strohm BR, Brechner VL. Effects of axillary nerve block on muscle force in the upper extremity. *Arch Phys Med Rehabil*. 1969;50(11):647-654.

20. Howell SM, Imobersteg AM, Seger DH, Marone PJ. Clarification of the role of the supraspinatus muscle in shoulder function. *J Bone Joint Surg Am*. 1986;68(3):398-404.

21. Colachis SC Jr., Strohm BR. Effect of suprascapular and axillary nerve blocks on muscle force in upper extremity. *Arch Phys Med Rehabil*. 1971;52(1):22-29.

22. Waterston D. Variations in the teres minor muscle. *Anat Anz*. 1908;32:331-333.

23. Cain PR, Mutschler TA, Fu FH, Lee SK. Anterior stability of the glenohumeral joint. A dynamic model. *Am J Sports Med*. 1987;15(2):144-148.

24. Morag Y, Jacobson JA, Lucas D, Miller B, Brigido MK, Jamadar DA. US appearance of the rotator cable with histologic correlation: preliminary results. *Radiology*. 2006;241(2):485-491.

25. Symeonides PP. The significance of the subscapularis muscle in the pathogenesis of recurrent anterior dislocation of the shoulder. *J Bone Joint Surg Br*. 1972;54(3):476-483.

26. Vad VB, Southern D, Warren RF, Altchek DW, Dines D. Prevalence of peripheral neurologic injuries in rotator cuff tears with atrophy. *J Shoulder Elbow Surg*. 2003;12(4):333-336.

27. Chen AL, Ong BC, Rose DJ. Arthroscopic management of spinoglenoid cysts associated with SLAP lesions and suprascapular neuropathy. *Arthroscopy*. 2003;19(6):E15-E21.

28. McCann PD, Cordasco FA, Ticker JB, et al. An anatomic study of the subscapular nerves: a guide for EMG analysis of the subscapularis muscle. *J Shoulder Elbow Surg*. 1994;3(2):94-99.

29. Fealy S, Adler RS, Drakos MC, et al. Patterns of vascular and anatomical response after rotator cuff repair. *Am J Sports Med*. 2006;34(1):120-127.

30. Hollinshead W, ed. *Anatomy for Surgeons*. 3rd ed. New York, NY: Harper & Row; 1982.

31. Salmon M. *Arteries of the Muscles of the Extremities and the Trunk and Arterial Anastomotic Pathways of the Extremities*. St. Louis, MO: Quality Medical Publishing; 1994.

32. Determe D, Rongieres M, Kany J, et al. Anatomic study of the tendinous rotator cuff of the shoulder. *Surg Radiol Anat*. 1996;18(3):195-200.

33. Burkhart SS, Esch JC, Jolson RS. The rotator crescent and rotator cable: an anatomic description of the shoulder's "suspension bridge." *Arthroscopy*. 1993;9(6):611-616.

34. Halder AM, O'Driscoll SW, Heers G, et al. Biomechanical comparison of effects of supraspinatus tendon detachments, tendon defects, and muscle retractions. *J Bone Joint Surg Am.* 2002;84-A(5):780-785.

35. Kask K, Kolts I, Lubienski A, Russlies M, Leibecke T, Busch LC. Magnetic resonance imaging and correlative gross anatomy of the ligamentum semicirculare humeri (rotator cable). *Clin Anat.* 2008;21(5):420-426.

36. Sheah K, Bredella MA, Warner JJ, Halpern EF, Palmer WE. Transverse thickening along the articular surface of the rotator cuff consistent with the rotator cable: identification with MR arthrography and relevance in rotator cuff evaluation. *AJR Am J Roentgenol.* 2009;193(3):679-686.

37. Kim SY, Boynton EL, Ravichandiran K, Fung LY, Bleakney R, Aqur AM. Three-dimensional study of the musculo-tendinous architecture of supraspinatus and its functional correlations. *Clin Anat.* 2007;20(6):648-655.

38. Dugas JR, Campbell DA, Warren RF, Robie BH, Millett PJ. Anatomy and dimensions of rotator cuff insertions. *J Shoulder Elbow Surg.* 2002;11(5):498-503.

39. Ruotolo C, Fow JE, Nottage WM. The supraspinatus footprint: an anatomic study of the supraspinatus insertion. *Arthroscopy.* 2004;20(3):246-249.

40. Mochizuki T, Sugaya H, Uomizu M, et al. Humeral insertion of the supraspinatus and infraspinatus. New anatomical findings regarding the footprint of the rotator cuff. *J Bone Joint Surg Am.* 2008;90(5):962-969.

41. Mochizuki T, Sugaya H, Uomizu M, et al. Humeral insertion of the supraspinatus and infraspinatus. New anatomical findings regarding the footprint of the rotator cuff. Surgical technique. *J Bone Joint Surg Am.* 2009;91(Suppl 2 Pt 1):1-7.

42. Clark JM, Harryman DT, 2nd. Tendons, ligaments, and capsule of the rotator cuff. Gross and microscopic anatomy. *J Bone Joint Surg Am.* 1992;74(5):713-725.

43. MacDonald K, Bridger J, Cash C, Parkin I. Transverse humeral ligament: does it exist? *Clin Anat.* 2007;20(6):663-667.

44. Benjamin M, Evans EJ, Copp L. The histology of tendon attachments to bone in man. *J Anat.* 1986;149:89-100.

45. Maffulli N, Renstrom P, Leadbetter WB. *Tendon Injuries: Basic Science and Clinical Medicine.* New York, NY: Springer; 2005.

46. Kolts I, Busch LC, Tomusk H, et al. Anatomy of the coracohumeral and coracoglenoidal ligaments. *Ann Anat.* 2000;182(6):563-566.

47. Plancher KD, Johnston JC, Peterson RK, Hawkins RJ. The dimensions of the rotator interval. *J Shoulder Elbow Surg.* 2005;14(6):620-625.

48. Jost B, Koch PP, Gerber C. Anatomy and functional aspects of the rotator interval. *J Shoulder Elbow Surg.* 2000;9(4):336-341.

CHAPTER 2

BIOMECHANICS OF THE ROTATOR CUFF

Michael L. Nguyen, MD; Ryan J. Quigley, BS;
Michelle H. McGarry, MS; and Thay Q. Lee, PhD

The shoulder is an incredibly complex joint due to its multiple passive and active structures working together for stability and joint motion. Not the least of these structures is the rotator cuff, a group of muscles surrounding the glenohumeral joint that act as both passive and active stabilizers and help to provide concavity compression as well as the torque needed for motion in multiple planes. The biomechanics of the shoulder are intimately associated with the rotator cuff, as altered biomechanics are often the result of rotator cuff pathology and vice versa. Rotator cuff tears often result in loss of strength and stability. In this chapter, the shoulder motion, rotator cuff pathology, and the biomechanical basis behind different rotator cuff repair strategies are discussed in depth.

SHOULDER MOTION

Shoulder motion is composed of many joints, primarily the glenohumeral and scapulothoracic joints. Abduction in the scapular plane is created by both joints in a movement termed *scapulo-humeral rhythm*. In Freedman and Munro's[1] classic article, they describe shoulder abduction in the scapular plane as a 3:2 ratio between glenohumeral and scapulothoracic motion. Further studies have described a 2:1 ratio,[2,3] but there is variation, especially in the first 30 degrees of abduction.[1,2,4] Most biomechanical studies performed today use an overall glenohumeral to scapulothoracic ratio of 2:1. The sternoclavicular and acromioclavicular joints move at the extremes of motion. Generally, shoulder motion is broken down into 3 planes of motion: abduction and adduction in the coronal plane, flexion and extension in the sagittal plane, and rotation about the long axis of the humerus. Arm abduction has an arc of motion of approximately 0 to 180 degrees, flexion and extension is approximately 180 degrees, and internal and external rotation is approximately 150 degrees. There are 3 possible glenohumeral motions: spinning, sliding, and rolling. During spinning, the contact point on the glenoid remains constant, but there is change in the humeral contact point. The opposite is sliding, where the contact point on the humerus remains the same but changes on the

Ma CB, Feeley BT, eds.
Basic Principles and Operative Management
of the Rotator Cuff (pp 15-32)
© 2012 SLACK Incorporated

glenoid. This is seen in pure translation of the humeral head. Rolling is a combination of spinning and sliding, where the contact point changes on both surfaces (Figure 2-1).

Many biomechanical tests have been performed to try and elucidate the role of the rotator cuff in glenohumeral motion.[2,5-30] The subscapularis has been shown to internally rotate and adduct the humerus. The supraspinatus is known as a shoulder abductor, but its role in humeral rotation is dependent on the initial position of the humerus. A study by Gates and colleagues[9] characterized the effect of the anterior and posterior subregions of the supraspinatus on humeral rotation. Using different angles of glenohumeral abduction and differential loading of the anterior and posterior subregions, the authors concluded that, in the scapular plane, the anterior subregion of the supraspinatus acts as both an internal and external rotator depending on the initial humeral position. On the other hand, the posterior subregion acts only as an external rotator. The infraspinatus and teres minor work as humeral external rotators and are most active with the humerus adducted.

Force Couples About the Glenohumeral Joint

A force couple is defined as 2 forces that act on an object to cause rotation. In order to reach a state of equilibrium, the sum of forces on an object must be equal in magnitude and opposite in direction. Two major force couples act synergistically on the glenohumeral joint: one in the coronal plane and the other in the transverse plane.

Inman and colleagues[2] first described the force couple acting in the coronal plane between the deltoid and inferior rotator cuff (infraspinatus, teres minor, and subscapularis; Figure 2-2). The deltoid moment lies above the center of rotation, while the inferior cuff moment acts parallel to the lateral border of the scapular below the center of rotation. This force couple is important in producing stable glenohumeral abduction. More recently, the pectoralis major and latissimus dorsi have been included in this force couple. The depressor moment produced by the inferior rotator cuff may be too weak to counterbalance the strong deltoid moment. However, the pectoralis major and latissimus dorsi have similar depressor moments as the deltoid[31] and, therefore, are now thought to work along with the inferior rotator cuff in the coronal plane force couple.[32] Recent biomechanics studies have replicated the moments produced by the pectoralis major and latissimus dorsi in order to create a more anatomic shoulder construct.[31-37]

The transverse force couple is composed of moments produced by the subscapularis anteriorly and infraspinatus and teres minor posteriorly (Figure 2-3). Inability to maintain a balanced transverse force couple can lead to anterior or posterior translation of the humeral head. For example, in the setting of a massive rotator cuff tear involving the infraspinatus and teres minor (or posterior moment), the larger moment produced by the subscapularis can lead to anterior translation of the humeral head. This uncoupling between forces leads to an unstable fulcrum for glenohumeral motion.

A cadaveric study by Mihata and colleagues[38] looked at the effects of a simulated weakened subscapularis as seen in overhand throwers on glenohumeral kinematics and contact pressures. In their model, they used a custom shoulder testing system that replicated multiple lines of pull for the rotator cuff, deltoid, pectoralis major, and latissimus dorsi. Therefore, the authors used all muscles in the transverse and coronal force couples. They found that less force on the subscapularis led to a significant increase in external rotation and posterosuperior glenohumeral contact pressure. This is likely due to the disrupted transverse force couple leading to an imbalance between anterior and posterior forces. The strong moment arm of the infraspinatus, usually restrained by the subscapularis, now has a stronger moment arm relative to the subscapularis moment arm on the humerus, leading to posterosuperior translation. These results give insight to the pathophysiology behind internal impingement and partial-thickness articular-sided rotator cuff tears seen in throwing athletes.

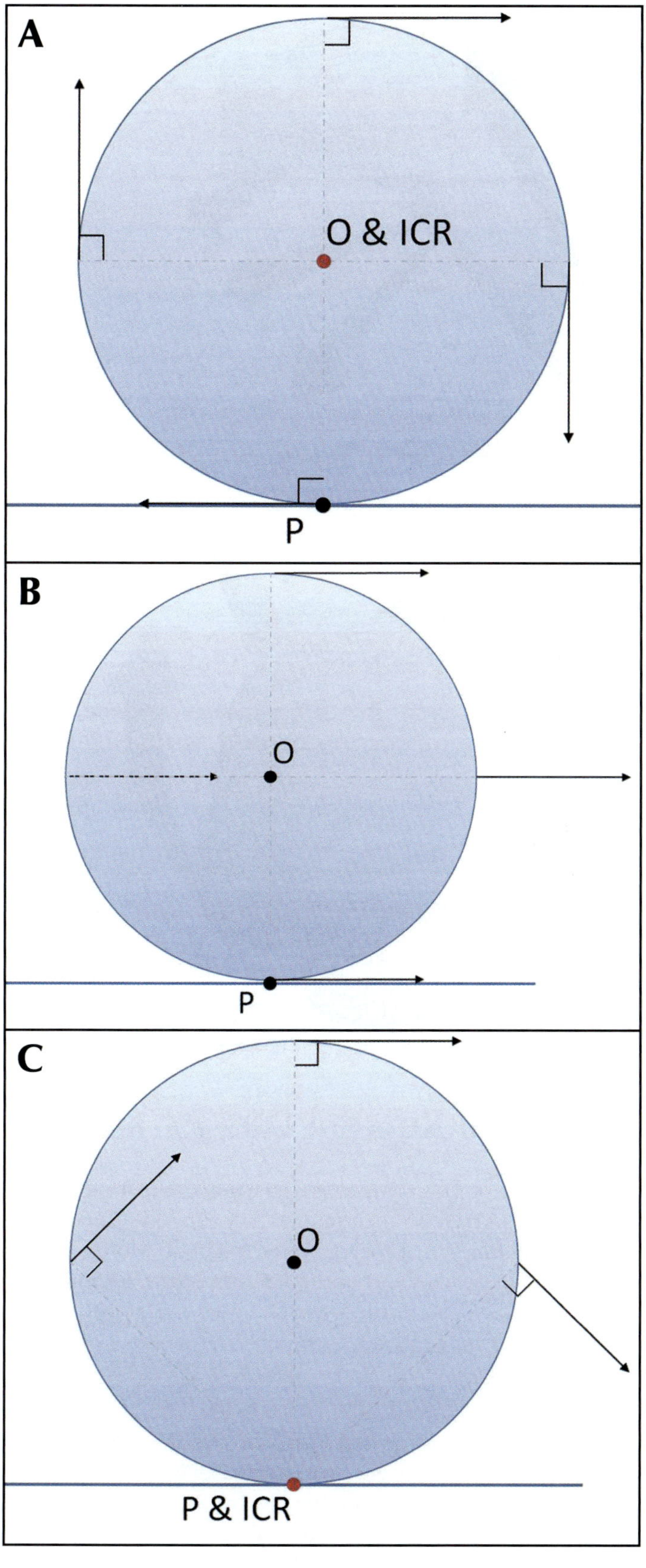

Figure 2-1. Three types of gleno-humeral motion: (A) spinning, (B) sliding, and (C) rolling (O, geometric center; P, point of contact; ICR, instantaneous center of rotation).

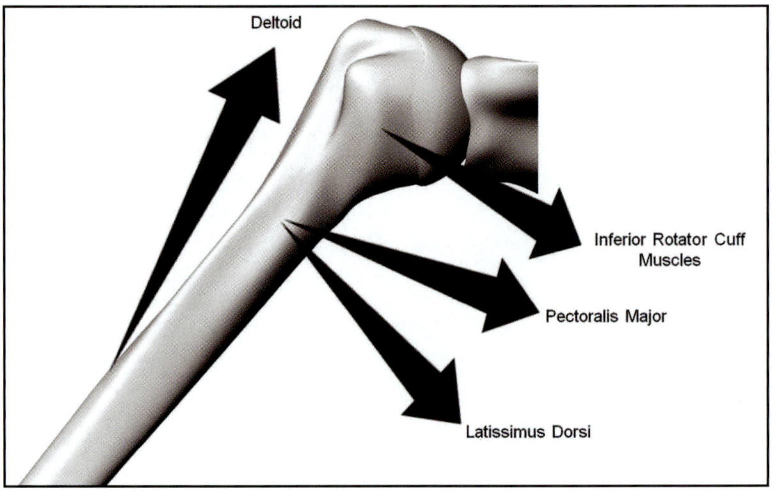

Figure 2-2. The coronal plane force couple with the deltoid acting superiorly and the inferior rotator cuff (subscapularis, infraspinatus, teres minor), pectoralis major, and latissimus dorsi acting inferiorly.

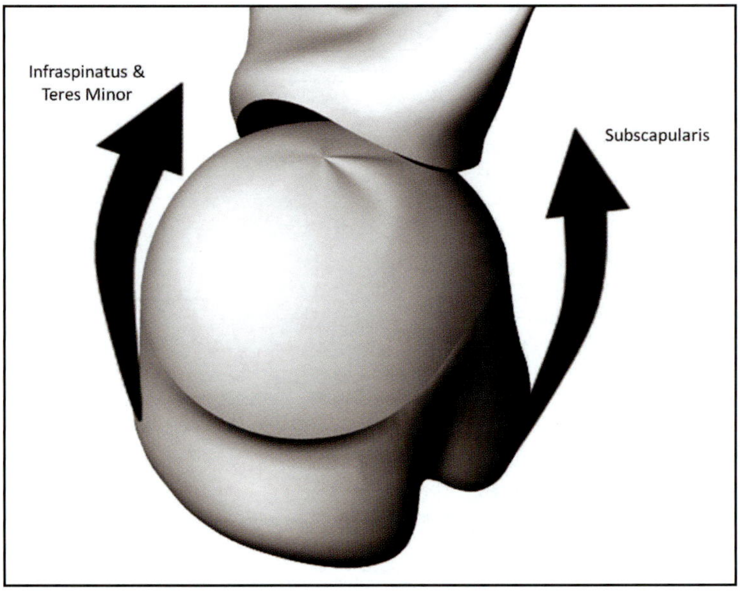

Deltoid

Inferior Rotator Cuff
Muscles

Pectoralis Major

Latissimus Dorsi

Figure 2-3. The transverse plane force couple composed of the infraspinatus and teres minor acting posteriorly and the subscapularis acting anteriorly.

Infraspinatus &
Teres Minor

Subscapularis

CHANGES IN BIOMECHANICS WITH ROTATOR CUFF PATHOLOGY

The maximum contractile force of a muscle is based on many factors, including sarcomere length, cross-sectional area, and initial position. Most muscles have their maximum contractile force in the mid-range of muscle length, and their force is diminished at the extremes of length. Muscle force is based on strong bony connections in order to produce a strong fulcrum for movement. Patients with rotator cuff tears frequently complain of loss of active motion and strength of the shoulder. Tendon defects change the amount of torque able to be generated by the rotator cuff for motion.

Partial-Thickness Rotator Cuff Tears

Partial-thickness rotator cuff tears are a common cause of shoulder pain and are more common than full-thickness rotator cuff tears. Cadaveric shoulders have shown the incidence of partial-thickness rotator cuff tears to be between 13% and 32%.[39-41] They typically involve younger patients and they most commonly involve the supraspinatus tendon.[42,43] Articular-sided partial-thickness rotator cuff tears are 2 to 3 times more common than bursal-sided tears.[42,44-50]

Biomechanical studies have shown that a partial-thickness rotator cuff tear increases the strain distribution on the intact rotator cuff. Mazzocca and colleagues[51] showed there is an increase in strain with greater than 50% involvement of the supraspinatus in partial-thickness rotator cuff tears. They also showed that the strain returned to the intact state after repair. The depth of a supraspinatus partial-thickness rotator cuff tear has been shown to be directly associated with strain in the intact tendon. Yang and colleagues[52] showed that, as the depth of an anterior supraspinatus partial-thickness rotator cuff tear approached 50%, there is a nonlinear relationship between strain and thickness. This implied that partial-thickness rotator cuff tears greater than 50% should warrant greater concern for the surgeon, and the chance for tear propagation was greater. Bey and colleagues[53] used magnetic resonance imaging (MRI) to assess intratendinous strains in cadaveric shoulders in different angles of glenohumeral abduction. An articular-sided partial-thickness rotator cuff tear was created in each specimen, and results showed that the tear increased intratendinous strain at all abduction angles above 15 degrees. With the articular side of the cuff and humeral head in contact with each other at lower abduction angles, the authors postulate that this contact could play a role in load sharing between the two.

Using a finite element analysis model, Sano and colleagues[54] showed that all types of partial-thickness rotator cuff tears (bursal-sided, articular-sided, and intrasubstance) increased stress concentration on the articular surface around the tear. An increased abduction angle also produced increased stress concentration around the tear site. In the intact tendon model, as well as all 3 tear models, there was an increase in stress seen on the articular side compared to the bursal side.

While the surgical principles of repair of partial-thickness rotator cuff tears are still debated, there is no doubt that a partial-thickness rotator cuff tear increases the strain around the surrounding intact cuff. Whether the increase in strain is enough to cause further tear propagation is dependent on the size and location of the tear. The findings from these studies led the authors to conclude that many partial-thickness rotator cuff tears may eventually lead to a full-thickness tear, which is consistent with other clinical studies.[55,56]

Full-Thickness Rotator Cuff Tears

Full-thickness rotator cuff tears are less frequent than partial-thickness rotator cuff tears and usually occur in an older population. In a cadaveric study by Fukuda and colleagues,[57] there was a prevalence of 7% for full-thickness tears and 13% for partial-thickness tears. Other studies have reported a prevalence of full-thickness tears ranging from 8% to 26%.[58,59] Patients often complain of shoulder pain and weakness.

The location, size, and shape of the rotator cuff tear ultimately define the biomechanical changes that occur. A cadaveric study by Andarawis-Puri and colleagues[60] showed that increasing the width of a full-thickness supraspinatus tear beyond 33% caused an increase in maximum and a decrease in minimum strain in the infraspinatus tendon. There was no difference in strain in the infraspinatus between an intact supraspinatus tendon and a tear with a width below 33%. This implies a strain-shielding effect of the infraspinatus tendon, which may prevent tear propagation in the supraspinatus, likely due to overlapping tendinous insertions. These results also show a reciprocal strain-shielding effect of the supraspinatus on the infraspinatus. They also found that anterior one-third tears of the supraspinatus do not affect the strain pattern of the infraspinatus. Mura and colleagues[61] showed that the infraspinatus is an important producer of abduction torque, and rotator cuff tears that extend into the infraspinatus significantly decrease abduction torque. These tears were also shown to lead to superior migration of the humeral head.

Rotator cuff tears commonly propagate from anterior to posterior; however, it is unknown when the biomechanical environment is altered. In a recent study by Oh and colleagues,[34] it was shown that a tear of the entire supraspinatus significantly increased rotational range of motion and decreased abduction capability. Further tear progression to the infraspinatus significantly shifted the humeral head posteriorly at the mid-range of rotation and superiorly at maximum internal rotation. This study also evaluated the effects of pectoralis major and latissimus dorsi muscle loading and concluded that the pectoralis major and latissimus dorsi played an important role to depress and

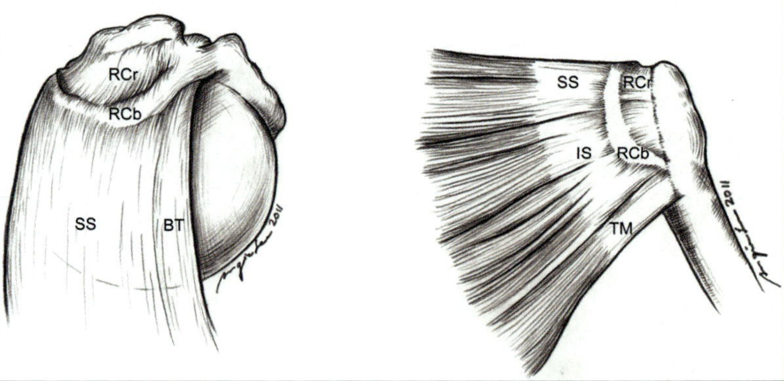

Figure 2-4. The anatomy of the rotator cable (RCb). As seen, it is a thickened band that inserts posteriorly at the inferior edge of the infraspinatus tendon and inserts anteriorly just posterior to the bicipital groove. It encloses the thinner region of the rotator cuff known as the rotator crescent (RCr) (SS, supraspinatus; BT, biceps tendon; IS, infraspinatus; TM, teres minor). (Reprinted with permission of Angie Lee.)

stabilize humeral head migration. This is in agreement with previous studies showing the importance of the pectoralis major and latissimus dorsi in the coronal plane force couple to stabilize the glenohumeral joint.[31,32] These findings suggest that once a rotator cuff tear has progressed to include the entire supraspinatus, surgical intervention may be necessary to restore normal glenohumeral joint biomechanics and prevent further tear progression. Also, in order to stabilize the glenohumeral joint with a rotator cuff tear, exercises should emphasize strengthening the remaining intact musculature including the pectoralis major and latissimus dorsi.

Rotator Cable and Crescent

Burkhart and colleagues[62] first coined the terms *rotator crescent* and *rotator cable* after repeatedly noticing a thick bundle of fibers on the articular surface of the rotator cuff on arthroscopy. They called the thick cable-like structure the *rotator cable*, and the thinner tissue from the cable to the enthesis was named the *rotator crescent*. Multiple radiographic, anatomic, and histologic studies have confirmed the presence of the rotator cable and crescent.[63-69] The rotator cable is an extension of the coracohumeral ligament that runs perpendicular to the supraspinatus from just posterior to the bicipital groove to the posterior border of the infraspinatus (Figure 2-4). It is thought that the rotator cable protects the thinner, avascular rotator crescent.[70] Clinically, a study by Kim and colleagues[71] showed that rotator cuff tears involving the anterior attachment of the rotator cable have a higher incidence of fatty degeneration, and Nguyen and colleagues[72] showed that, in massive rotator cuff tears involving this anterior attachment, reconstruction using a suture anchor decreases gap formation throughout the entire repair. They named this surgical technique the "margin convergence to bone," and it uses a suture anchor just posterior to the bicipital groove to reconstruct the anterior attachment. One limb of the double-loaded suture is placed in the anterior supraspinatus and the other through the rotator interval to provide both footprint reconstruction and margin convergence (Figure 2-5). This technique significantly decreased gap formation throughout the entire repair when compared to soft-tissue margin convergence. This study highlighted the importance of anatomic repair of the rotator cuff and the role of the rotator cable to stress-shield the rotator crescent.

DIFFERENT ROTATOR CUFF REPAIRS AND THEIR BIOMECHANICAL EFFECTS

Shoulder arthroscopy has opened a world of rotator cuff pathology that was once deemed "unfixable." Mechanical and technical advancements in rotator cuff repair are evolving at a rapid pace, and biomechanical studies are keeping pace to try and find the best repair strategies. While no one

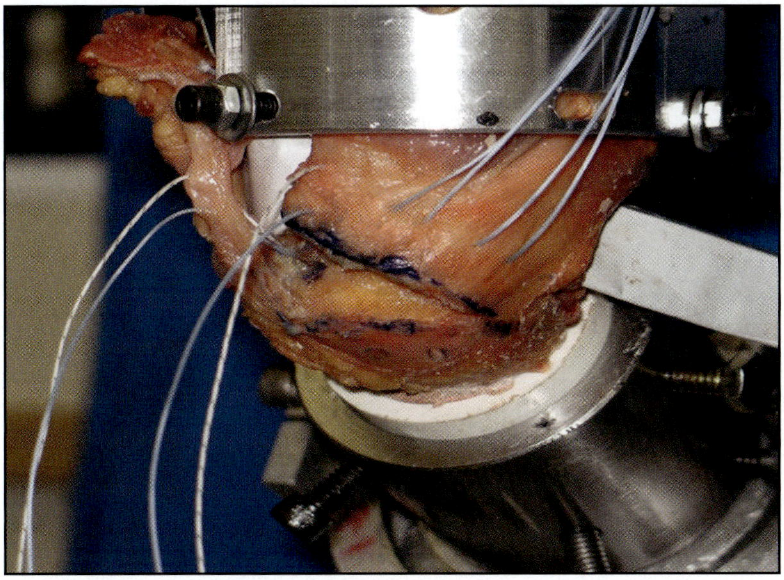

Figure 2-5. Margin convergence to bone technique that uses a suture anchor placed just posterior to the bicipital groove to reconstruct the anterior attachment of the rotator cable.

repair is sufficient for all tears, there are trends in the literature that show better biomechanical characteristics of newer-generation repairs. Gerber and colleagues[73] state the ideal rotator cuff repair would initially minimize gap formation and provide high fixation strength. An optimal repair would also restore as much of the original contact area as possible. Many different repair techniques and constructs have been developed to provide this ideal construct.

Biomechanical Testing Methods

To evaluate and compare the biomechanical characteristics of repaired tissues, materials testing systems are used where the construct undergoes both cyclic loading and loading to failure (Figure 2-6). For each cycle of the cyclic loading, 2 important biomechanical parameters are typically determined. The first is the linear stiffness of the construct, which is defined as the slope of the linear portion of the load-elongation curve with units of N/mm. Intuitively, the construct's stiffness is its resistance to deformation. The second is the hysteresis of the construct, which is defined as the area between the loading and unloading curves on the load-elongation curve. Hysteresis represents energy dissipated throughout the construct during each loading cycle. This energy can be dissipated in many ways, including suture anchor-bone slippage, knot slippage, tissue fiber alignment, etc. Hysteresis will usually decrease with each cycle during cyclic loading as well as with increasing stiffness of a construct.

When the construct is loaded to failure, 4 important biomechanical parameters are determined. The first is the linear stiffness of the construct, which is determined in the same fashion as described for cyclic loading. The next parameter is yield load, which is the load at which the load/elongation curve deviates from linearity (ie, when the stiffness begins to decrease). The yield load represents the transition point between elastic and plastic deformation of the construct. Prior to reaching yield load, the construct is in the elastic deformation range where all deformation is reversible; however, after surpassing the yield load, permanent plastic deformation occurs. The next parameter is the ultimate load, which represents the maximum load sustained by the construct prior to failure. Last, the energy absorbed by the construct can be calculated at both yield load and ultimate load by calculating the area under the load-elongation curve.

The last biomechanical parameter commonly used is gap formation. Gap formation is the migration of the tendon edge away from the footprint with loading. It is commonly measured using video digitizing software to track the movement of the tendon edge as the construct is loaded, whether it be cyclic loading or load to failure.

Figure 2-6. A typical materials testing load deformation curve for (A) cyclic loading and (B) load to failure with relevant parameters (Stiffness, red in A and B; hysteresis, teal shaded area in A; energy absorbed to yield, purple shaded area in B; energy absorbed to ultimate load, teal shaded area in B).

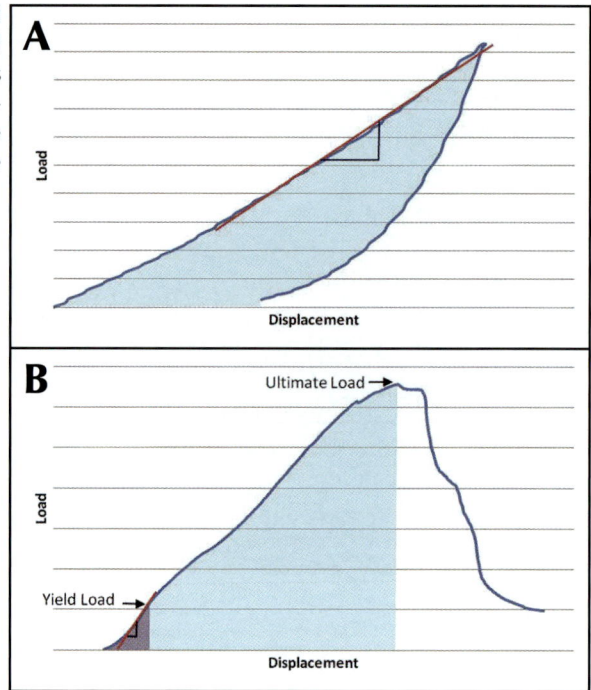

Single-Row Repair of the Rotator Cuff

In the 1980s, the treatment of rotator cuff disease took a major turn toward arthroscopic treatment. Ellman's[74] classic paper in 1985 was the first to describe arthroscopic subacromial decompression and acromioplasty for chronic external shoulder impingement. However, in order to repair the rotator cuff, an open approach implementing a transosseous repair construct was still considered the gold standard. The development of high-quality suture anchors with high pullout strengths and better arthroscopic instrumentation led to surgeons attempting more arthroscopic rotator cuff repairs. The first-generation repair techniques involved a single row of suture anchors placed at the lateral footprint. The suture was then passed through the torn tendon edge, and the tendon was tied down to the anchor (Figure 2-7). A limitation of this repair is that it relies on the lateral tendon edge for fixation, which can be compromised in chronic tears. Also, a single-row repair only allows for footprint reconstruction and contact pressure at the insertion point of the suture anchor. There is concern about the inability to establish the medial-to-lateral footprint with a single-row construct, which may account for the suboptimal healing rates and high retear rates.[75] This is especially evident with the arm in abduction where one can have lift-off of the medial aspect of the tendon (Figure 2-8).

A study by Apreleva and colleagues[76] looked at 4 different repair constructs and the contact area characteristics. The authors found that while no repair method completely restored the area of the original supraspinatus insertion, the transosseous repair restored 20% more area than any of the other repair types. They concluded that a transosseous repair provides better potential for healing. This is consistent with a study by Park and colleagues,[77] in which a bovine model and pressure-sensitive film were used to assess contact characteristics of a transosseous repair versus single-row mattress configuration and single-row simple suture configuration. Once again, the mean contact area and interface pressure were significantly larger in the transosseous repair than either of the single-row constructs.

A study by Yu and colleagues[37] looked at cadaveric specimens already with full-thickness, U-shaped supraspinatus tears to determine the biomechanical characteristics before repair, after

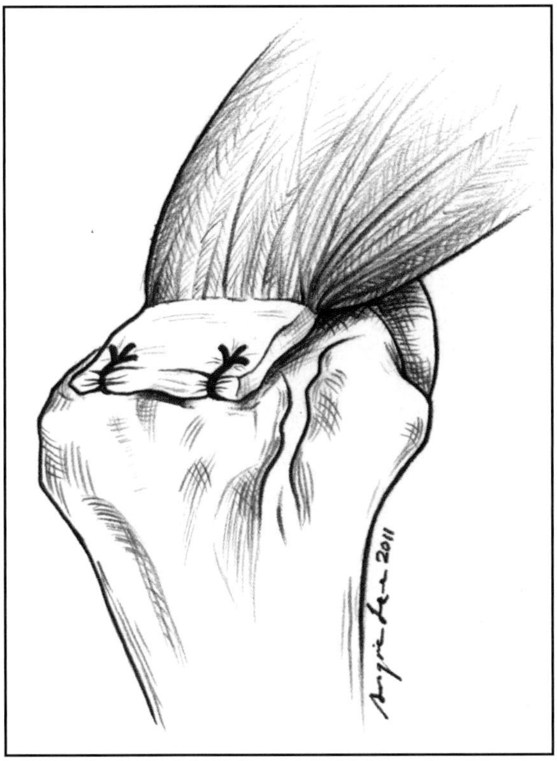

Figure 2-7. The single-row rotator cuff repair with 2 anchors placed at the lateral edge of the tendon footprint and simple sutures passed through the torn tendon edge. (Reprinted with permission of Angie Lee.)

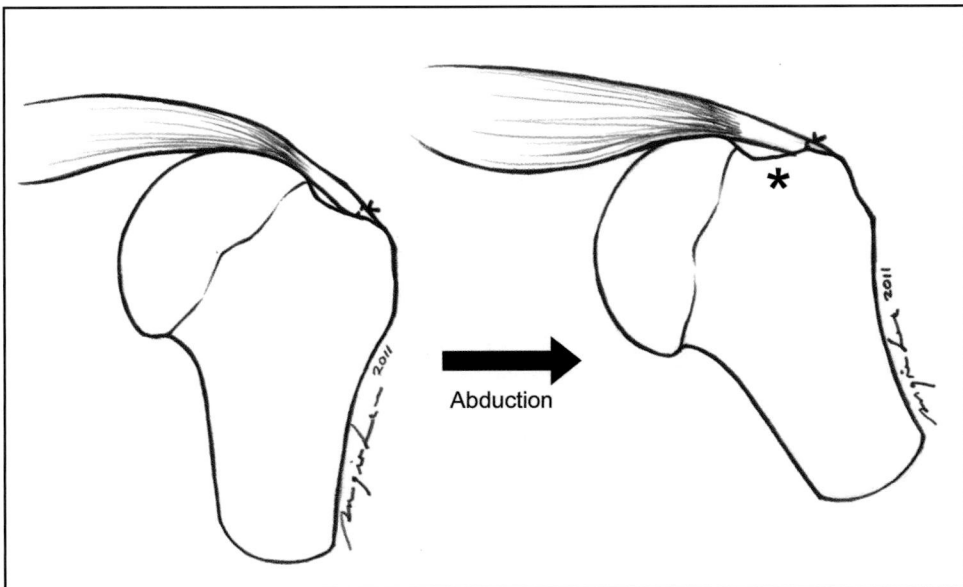

Figure 2-8. Lift-off of the medial portion of the tendon over the footprint (*) in a single row repair with the arm in abduction. (Reprinted with permission of Angie Lee.)

transosseous repair, and then after creating a complete supraspinatus tear. They used a 3-dimensional digitizing system to detect any changes in humeral position, and they used pressure-sensitive film to assess any change in contact characteristics. With a simulated complete rotator cuff tear, they found that the humerus shifted inferiorly compared to the repaired supraspinatus tear.

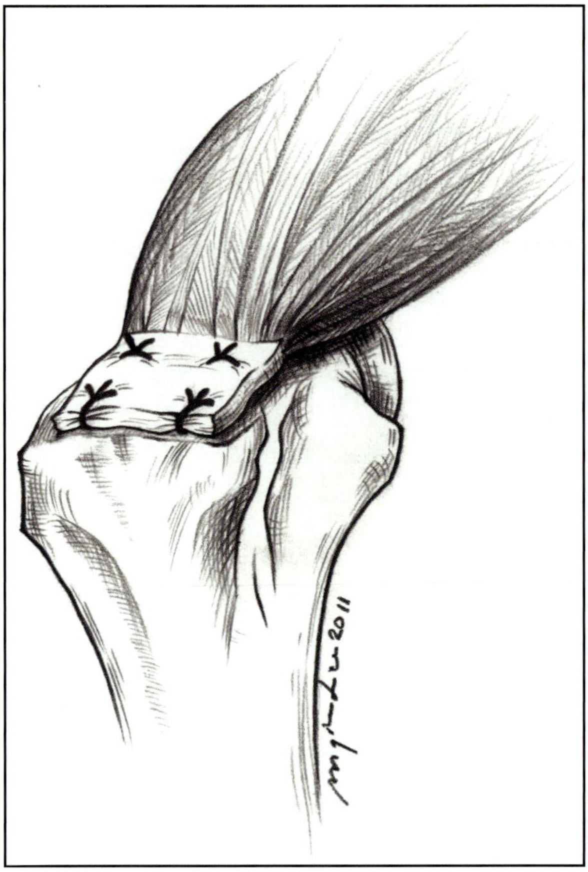

Figure 2-9. The original double-row repair with a medial row of suture anchors placed just lateral to the articular margin and the lateral row of suture anchors placed just medial to the "drop off" of the greater tuberosity. (Reprinted with permission of Angie Lee.)

Interestingly, there was no increase in glenohumeral contact pressure in the repair group compared to either of the tear groups. The only measurable effect that supraspinatus repair provided was an increase in percent inferior force at 10 degrees abduction and 60 N of load on all muscles. This increase may represent a greater concavity-compression effect, which would provide increased stability of the glenohumeral joint.

Ahmad and colleagues[78] attempted to quantify the amount of motion between the repaired tendon and bone in a transosseous repair versus a single-row construct. This is important, as the ideal repair construct would minimize motion in the immediate postoperative setting in order to allow healing of the tendon to bone. They found that the transosseous suture repair allowed less motion in internal and external rotation compared to the single-row construct.

Original Double-Row Repair

Fealy and colleagues[79] originally described a double-row rotator cuff repair using a mini-open approach. They described a repair with one row of suture anchors medially and another laterally in order to increase the repair's surface area to increase healing potential and distribute stress over a larger area. Lo and Burkhart then described their arthroscopic technique for a double-row repair.[80] The first row is placed just lateral to the articular margin. Then, the lateral anchors are inserted just medial to the "drop-off" point of the greater tuberosity. The medial sutures are passed through the medial aspect of the tendon in a mattress fashion and tied down. These sutures are then cut. The lateral sutures are then passed through the tendon in a simple suture formation and are tied down. This gives medial row and lateral row fixation to increase the contact area of the repair (Figure 2-9).

Multiple basic science studies have shown the superiority of double-row fixation compared with single-row. A study by Mazzocca and colleagues[81] tested a single-row construct versus 3 different double-row constructs. While there was no difference in load to failure and displacement with cyclic loading between any of the groups, a significantly larger footprint width was seen in the double-row constructs compared to the single-row construct. The results of this study differed from the results of other studies[82,83] that showed improved biomechanical characteristics of a double-row repair compared with a single-row repair. There was significantly decreased gap formation at the first and last cycle, decreased initial strain throughout the entire footprint, as well as increased stiffness and load to failure in the double-row group.

In a chronic rotator cuff tear, the lateral tendon edge is often retracted and immobile. In this situation, Snyder has promoted a medialized single-row repair in order to reduce tension on the repair and promote healing.[84] A study by Domb and colleagues[85] compared high-tension double-row and medialized single-row constructs. They found that the high-tension double-row repair fared better than the medialized single-row construct. There was significantly decreased displacement at first cycle, stiffness in the final cycle, and ultimate load to failure. The authors concluded that, when possible, a retracted tear should be repaired with a double-row construct.

A study by Ma and colleagues[86] tested a standard double-row repair with 3 different single-row repairs: the Mason-Allen stitch, massive cuff stitch, and 2 simple sutures. The massive cuff stitch, first described by Ma and colleagues,[87] uses a horizontal loop as a stop-stitch to prevent pullout. The double-row construct was as good as or better than all single-row repair constructs in all parameters tested.

Waltrip and colleagues[88] developed a novel double-row technique that used a transosseous lateral row along with a medial row of anchors. They dubbed this the "double-layer" rotator cuff repair and tested it against a single-row construct and a traditional transosseous construct. Instead of load to failure, they used cyclic loading to test the constructs and defined failure as a 1-cm gap at the repair site. The double-layer technique required significantly more cycles to fail, but there was no significant difference between the traditional transosseous construct and the single-row construct. This study was consistent with the results of Meier and Meier,[89] which compared transosseous, single-row, and double-row repairs. Once again using cyclic loading and failure defined as 1 cm of gap formation, the double-row construct showed improved biomechanical characteristics compared to the other groups.

The same authors also used 3-dimensional mapping to analyze the footprint area restored in single-row, double-row, and transosseous constructs.[90] They found that a double-row repair consistently repaired 100% of the area of the footprint, while a single-row construct only restored 46% and a transosseous repair restored only 71% of the footprint.

A study by Sano and colleagues[91] used 3 finite element models to characterize stress concentration at the repair site in a single-row, double-row, and transosseous repair. In the single-row and double-row models, there was a high stress concentration on the bursal surface of the tendon and at the site of the anchors. With simulated muscle contraction, the stress moved proximally along the bursal surface of the tendon. In the double-row construct, there was more stress in the medial row of anchors than in the lateral row. In the transosseous model, the highest stress concentration was seen at the cortex of the greater tuberosity and at the surface of the bony trough. With simulated muscle contraction, the highest stress stayed in the bony trough, and there was no significant concentration inside the tendon. This is advantageous for chronic rotator cuff tears with a degenerated tendon where the tendon cannot tolerate large amounts of strain.

Transosseous-Equivalent Rotator Cuff Repair

The transosseous-equivalent (TOE) or "suture-bridge" configuration was developed by Park and colleagues[92] in order to optimize contact area and pressure to increase healing. The medial row of anchors is placed at the articular margin, and the sutures are passed in a mattress fashion, ideally 10 to 12 mm medial to the lateral edge of the tear. The sutures are then tied but not cut. Instead,

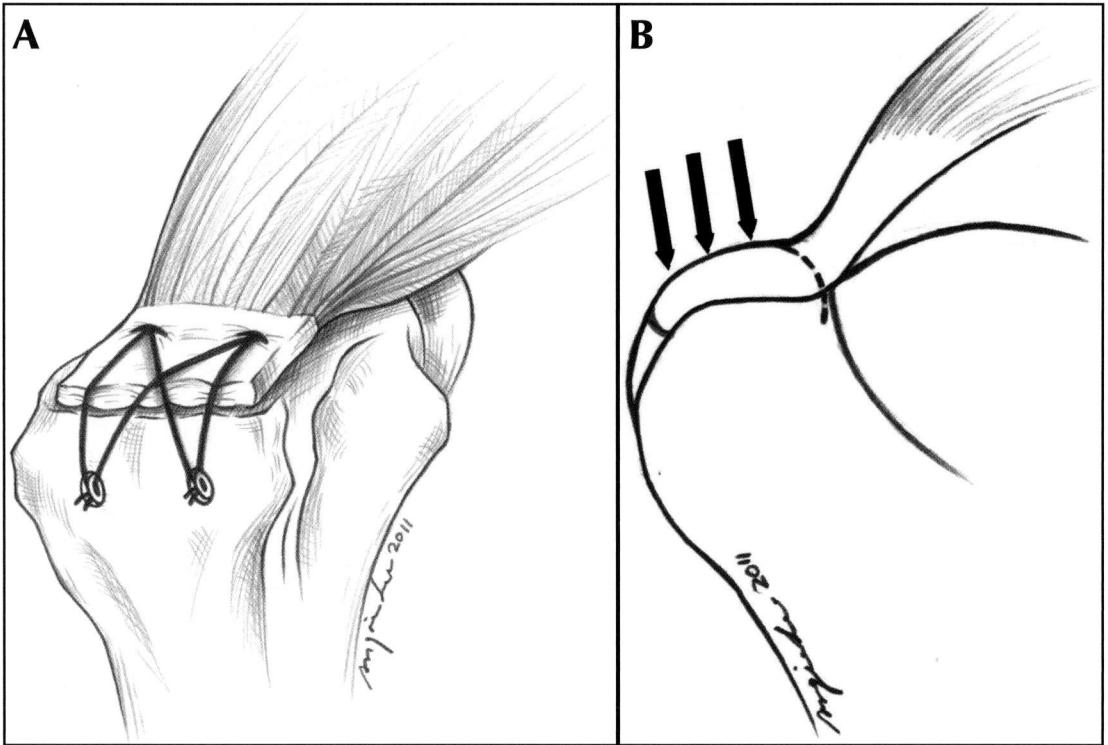

Figure 2-10. (A) The TOE repair developed by Park and colleagues.[92] Compared to the original double-row repair, the lateral row of anchors is placed distally. (B) This more distal placement allows tensioning of the suture bridge, which provides compression between the tendon and bone. (Reprinted with permission of Angie Lee.)

a suture limb from each anchor is brought laterally over the "tendon bridge" and fixed using a Bio-Tenodesis screwdriver (Arthrex, Naples, FL). One or two anchors can be used laterally depending on the size of the tear. The lateral fixation points are 1 cm distal to the lateral edge of the tuberosity (Figure 2-10A). Multiple different knotless suture anchors have been developed for lateral row fixation instead of the Bio-Tenodesis screwdriver.

The major differences between the TOE and initial double-row fixation techniques are the suture bridge over the tendon and the more distal fixation points for the lateral row. The suture bridge connects the medial and lateral rows, as well as the anteroposterior rows, allowing compression throughout the entire footprint. This highlights the difference between footprint coverage and contact pressure. While a standard double-row repair may allow the same amount of the footprint to be covered, a TOE differs from an unlinked double-row construct in that compression is throughout the entire repair instead of only at the anchor insertion points. By placing the lateral row of anchors orthogonal from the rotator cuff-loading vector, a compression vector over the tendon is created to increase pressure at the footprint (Figure 2-10B). This greatly increases the contact pressure along the repaired tendon in the TOE repair compared to the double-row repair.

In biomechanical studies by Park and colleagues,[93,94] the TOE and first-generation double-row techniques were compared. Using a materials testing machine and video digitizing system, they found that ultimate load to failure was significantly increased in the TOE group compared to the double-row group. Gap formation and stiffness were not found to be statistically different, although there was a trend toward decreased gap formation in the TOE group. They also looked at the contact characteristics of a 4-strand suture bridge versus a standard double-row repair using pressure-sensitive film. There was a significant increase in mean pressurized contact area and mean contact pressure in the TOE group (Figure 2-11).

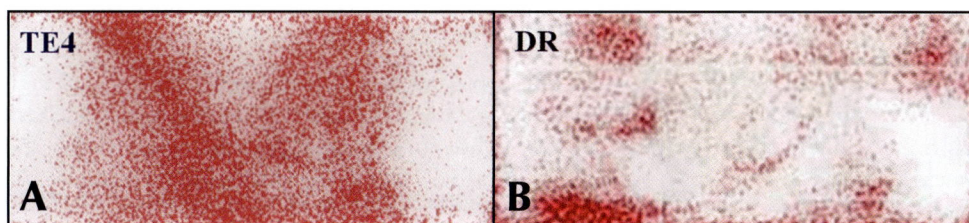

Figure 2-11. Contact pressure measurements using Fujifilm on (A) TOE and (B) double-row repairs showed the TOE repair increased contact area and contact pressure compared to the double-row repair. (Reprinted from *J Shoulder Elbow Surg*, vol 16, iss 4, Park MC, ElAttrache NS, Tibone JE, Ahmad CS, Jun BJ, Lee TQ, Part I: footprint contact characteristics for a TOE rotator cuff repair technique compared with a double-row repair technique, pp 461-468, Copyright 2007, with permission from Elsevier.)

In all of these biomechanical studies, the humerus was held in a fixed position, not allowing for rotation. However, it has been shown that the supraspinatus can act as an internal or external rotator based on the position of the humerus.[9,95] Park and colleagues[96] have shown that allowing for dynamic external rotation of the humerus with loading changes the gap formation and strain compared to the humerus fixed. As expected, external rotation produces higher gap formation and tendon strain anteriorly than posteriorly. A subsequent study by Park and colleagues[97] tested a standard double-row construct with the TOE allowing for dynamic external rotation. They found that the TOE had a significantly higher yield load than the double-row construct, but there was no difference in gap formation, stiffness, ultimate load to failure, and energy absorbed to failure. In the TOE construct, they found significantly greater gap formation anteriorly than posteriorly, but this was not seen in the double-row group. The authors state that this is likely due to anchor placement; in the double-row construct, there is an anchor placed directly at the anterolateral edge of the tear while the anterolateral anchor for the TOE is placed further distal-lateral. This study also highlights the possible need for stronger anterior fixation with the TOE in order to prevent gap formation.

A novel study by Mazzocca and colleagues[98] used a pressure-sensitive sensor to look at different repair constructs over time. They tested a single-row, double-row, TOE, and suture-chain TOE. The suture-chain TOE uses FiberChain (Arthrex) to connect the medial and lateral rows, but, unlike the TOE, the anterior and posterior anchors are not connected. They then looked at the pressure force and contact area immediately after repair, every minute for the first 10 minutes, every 3 minutes for the next 30 minutes, and then every 30 minutes until a total of 160 minutes have passed. All repair techniques had decreased contact force, pressure, and area at 160 minutes compared with immediately after repair, but the TOE had the highest contact pressure and force at all time points. The TOE was the only repair with a statistically significant increase in pressure and force when compared with the single-row construct at all time points; however, the TOE also had the greatest loss of force after 160 minutes. The contact pressure in all groups dropped at least 32% after 160 minutes. This study emphasizes the importance of a strong, stable rotator cuff repair in the immediate postoperative period, and it shows that a TOE provides the strongest initial construct in order to optimize the potential for healing.

Busfield and colleagues[99] looked at the importance of the medial row knots in a TOE configuration. In both groups with supraspinatus tears, a TOE configuration was used, but in one, the medial row was fixed with a knotless suture anchor while a standard anchor with knots was used in the other group. Biomechanical testing showed greater gap formation during cyclic loading and yield load in the knotless group as well as a decreased ultimate load. Therefore, the authors concluded that a medial row of knots provides a biomechanically stronger construct compared with knotless fixation.

Clinical Studies

The goal of creating a better biomechanical construct is to try and optimize the chances of the rotator cuff healing. However, there are conflicting data in the literature concerning healed rotator cuff tears and clinical outcomes. A review of the literature by Slabaugh and colleagues[100] showed that there is no general consensus to this question no matter what radiographic study or clinical outcome score is used.

A systematic review of the literature by Nho and colleagues[101] showed no difference in clinical outcomes between single-row and double-row repair; however, they also reported that a double-row construct increased healing rates in 2 of the 3 studies with radiographic analysis, which would imply a better biomechanical construct. Two of the studies that compose this review were Level I randomized studies,[102,103] and both showed no clinical difference between single-row and double-row repair. However, neither of these studies implemented a TOE repair, and in both studies, the configuration of their double-row repair has come into question.[104]

CONCLUSION

The rotator cuff plays an integral part in glenohumeral stability and motion. Tears of the rotator cuff alter the biomechanics, including the strain patterns of the intact cuff, which can lead to tear propagation. While there is sure to be further evolution of repair constructs, currently, the TOE repair developed by Park and colleagues[92] consistently provides the best biomechanical characteristics. However, it is important to note that the ideal healing environment for these cuff repairs is still unknown.

REFERENCES

1. Freedman L, Munro RR. Abduction of the arm in the scapular plane: scapular and glenohumeral movements. A roentgenographic study. *J Bone Joint Surg Am*. 1966;48(8):1503-1510.
2. Inman VT, Saunders JB, Abbott LC. Observations of the function of the shoulder joint. *Clin Orthop Relat Res*. 1996;330:3-12.
3. Laumann U. Kinesiology of the shoulder joint. In: Kouelbel R, Helbig B, Blauth W, eds. *Shoulder Replacement*. Berlin, Germany: Springer-Verlag; 1987:23-31.
4. Doody SG, Freedman L, Waterland JC. Shoulder movements during abduction in the scapular plane. *Arch Phys Med Rehabil*. 1970;51(10):595-604.
5. An KN, Browne AO, Korinek S, Tanaka S, Morrey BF. Three-dimensional kinematics of glenohumeral elevation. *J Orthop Res*. 1991;9(1):143-149.
6. De Duca CJ, Forrest WJ. Force analysis of individual muscles acting simultaneously on the shoulder joint during isometric abduction. *J Biomech*. 1973;6(4):385-393.
7. DiGiovine NM, Jobe FW, Pink M, Perry J. An electromyographic analysis of the upper extremity in pitching. *J Shoulder Elbow Surg*. 1992;1(1):15-25.
8. Ekholm J, Arborelius UP, Hillered L, Ortqvist A. Shoulder muscle EMG and resisting moment during diagonal exercise movements resisted by weight-and-pulley-circuit. *Scand J Rehabil Med*. 1978;10(4):179-185.
9. Gates JJ, Gilliland J, McGarry MH, et al. Influence of distinct anatomic subregions of the supraspinatus on humeral rotation. *J Orthop Res*. 2010;28(1):12-17.
10. Glousman R. Electromyographic analysis and its role in the athletic shoulder. *Clin Orthop Relat Res*. 1993;288:27-34.
11. Glousman R, Jobe F, Tibone J, Moynes D, Antonelli D, Perry J. Dynamic electromyographic analysis of the throwing shoulder with glenohumeral instability. *J Bone Joint Surg Am*. 1988;70(2):220-226.
12. Gowan ID, Jobe FW, Tibone JE, Perry J, Moynes DR. A comparative electromyographic analysis of the shoulder during pitching. Professional versus amateur pitchers. *Am J Sports Med*. 1987;15(6):586-590.
13. Hughes RE, An KN. Force analysis of rotator cuff muscles. *Clin Orthop Relat Res*. 1996;330:75-83.
14. Jobe FW, Moynes DR, Tibone JE, Perry J. An EMG analysis of the shoulder in pitching. A second report. *Am J Sports Med*. 1984;12(3):218-220.
15. Jobe FW, Tibone JE, Perry J, Moynes D. An EMG analysis of the shoulder in throwing and pitching. A preliminary report. *Am J Sports Med*. 1983;11(1):3-5.

16. Juul-Kristensen B, Bojsen-Moller F, Finsen L, et al. Muscle sizes and moment arms of rotator cuff muscles determined by magnetic resonance imaging. *Cells Tissues Organs.* 2000;167(2-3):214-222.

17. Karlsson D, Peterson B. Towards a model for force predictions in the human shoulder. *J Biomech.* 1992;25(2):189-199.

18. Kronberg M, Nemeth G, Brostrom LA. Muscle activity and coordination in the normal shoulder. An electromyographic study. *Clin Orthop Relat Res.* 1990;257:76-85.

19. McCann PD, Wootten ME, Kadaba MP, Bigliani LU. A kinematic and electromyographic study of shoulder rehabilitation exercises. *Clin Orthop Relat Res.* 1993;288:179-188.

20. McMahon PJ, Jobe FW, Pink MM, Brault JR, Perry J. Comparative electromyographic analysis of shoulder muscles during planar motions: anterior glenohumeral instability versus normal. *J Shoulder Elbow Surg.* 1996;5(2 Pt 1):118-123.

21. Morris AD, Kemp GJ, Frostick SP. Shoulder electromyography in multidirectional instability. *J Shoulder Elbow Surg.* 2004;13(1):24-29.

22. Pande P, Hawkins R, Peat M. Electromyography in voluntary posterior instability of the shoulder. *Am J Sports Med.* 1989;17(5):644-648.

23. Poppen NK, Walker PS. Forces at the glenohumeral joint in abduction. *Clin Orthop Relat Res.* 1978;135:165-170.

24. Ringelberg JA. EMG and force production of some human shoulder muscles during isometric abduction. *J Biomech.* 1985;18(12):939-947.

25. Sigholm G, Herberts P, Almstrom C, Kadefors R. Electromyographic analysis of shoulder muscle load. *J Orthop Res.* 1984;1(4):379-386.

26. Townsend H, Jobe FW, Pink M, Perry J. Electromyographic analysis of the glenohumeral muscles during a baseball rehabilitation program. *Am J Sports Med.* 1991;19(3):264-272.

27. van der Helm FC. A finite element musculoskeletal model of the shoulder mechanism. *J Biomech.* 1994;27(5):551-569.

28. van der Helm FC. Analysis of the kinematic and dynamic behavior of the shoulder mechanism. *J Biomech.* 1994;27(5):527-550.

29. Veeger HE, Van der Helm FC, Van der Woude LH, Pronk GM, Rozendal RH. Inertia and muscle contraction parameters for musculoskeletal modelling of the shoulder mechanism. *J Biomech.* 1991;24(7):615-629.

30. Wakabayashi I, Itoi E, Sano H, et al. Mechanical environment of the supraspinatus tendon: a two-dimensional finite element model analysis. *J Shoulder Elbow Surg.* 2003;12(6):612-617.

31. Kuechle DK, Newman SR, Itoi E, Morrey BF, An KN. Shoulder muscle moment arms during horizontal flexion and elevation. *J Shoulder Elbow Surg.* 1997;6(5):429-439.

32. Halder AM, Zhao KD, O'Driscoll SW, Morrey BF, An KN. Dynamic contributions to superior shoulder stability. *J Orthop Res.* 2001;19(2):206-212.

33. Huffman GR, Tibone JE, McGarry MH, Phipps BM, Lee YS, Lee TQ. Path of glenohumeral articulation throughout the rotational range of motion in a thrower's shoulder model. *Am J Sports Med.* 2006;34(10):1662-1669.

34. Oh JH, Jun BJ, McGarry MH, Lee TQ. Does a critical rotator cuff tear stage exist? A biomechanical study of rotator cuff tear progression in human cadaver shoulders. *J Bone Joint Surg Am.* 2011;93:2100-2109.

35. Schamblin M, Gupta R, Yang BY, McGarry MH, McMaster WC, Lee TQ. In vitro quantitative assessment of total and bipolar shoulder arthroplasties: a biomechanical study using human cadaver shoulders. *Clin Biomech (Bristol, Avon).* 2009;24(8):626-631.

36. Shapiro TA, McGarry MH, Gupta R, Lee YS, Lee TQ. Biomechanical effects of glenoid retroversion in total shoulder arthroplasty. *J Shoulder Elbow Surg.* 2007;16(3 Suppl):S90-S95.

37. Yu J, McGarry MH, Lee YS, Duong LV, Lee TQ. Biomechanical effects of supraspinatus repair on the glenohumeral joint. *J Shoulder Elbow Surg.* 2005;14(1 Suppl S):65S-71S.

38. Mihata T, Gates J, McGarry MH, Lee J, Kinoshita M, Lee TQ. Effect of rotator cuff muscle imbalance on forceful internal impingement and peel-back of the superior labrum: a cadaveric study. *Am J Sports Med.* 2009;37(11):2222-2227.

39. Lohr JF, Uhthoff HK. [Epidemiology and pathophysiology of rotator cuff tears]. *Orthopade.* 2007;36(9):788-795.

40. Sano H, Ishii H, Trudel G, Uhthoff HK. Histologic evidence of degeneration at the insertion of 3 rotator cuff tendons: a comparative study with human cadaveric shoulders. *J Shoulder Elbow Surg.* 1999;8(6):574-579.

41. Yamanaka K, Fukuda H. Pathologic studies of the supraspinatus tendon with reference to incomplete partial thickness tear. In: Takagishi N, ed. *The Shoulder.* Tokyo, Japan: Professional Postgraduate Services; 1987:220-224.

42. Gartsman GM. Arthroscopic acromioplasty for lesions of the rotator cuff. *J Bone Joint Surg Am.* 1990;72(2):169-180.

43. Gartsman GM, Milne JC. Articular surface partial-thickness rotator cuff tears. *J Shoulder Elbow Surg.* 1995;4(6):409-415.

44. Andrews JR, Broussard TS, Carson WG. Arthroscopy of the shoulder in the management of partial tears of the rotator cuff: a preliminary report. *Arthroscopy.* 1985;1(2):117-122.

45. Ellman H. Diagnosis and treatment of incomplete rotator cuff tears. *Clin Orthop Relat Res.* 1990;254:64-74.

46. Gartsman GM. Arthroscopic treatment of rotator cuff disease. *J Shoulder Elbow Surg.* 1995;4(3):228-241.

47. Itoi E, Tabata S. Incomplete rotator cuff tears. Results of operative treatment. *Clin Orthop Relat Res.* 1992;284:128-135.

48. Olsewski JM, Depew AD. Arthroscopic subacromial decompression and rotator cuff debridement for stage II and stage III impingement. *Arthroscopy*. 1994;10(1):61-68.

49. Ryu RK. Arthroscopic subacromial decompression: a clinical review. *Arthroscopy*. 1992;8(2):141-147.

50. Weber SC. Arthroscopic debridement and acromioplasty versus mini-open repair in the management of significant partial-thickness tears of the rotator cuff. *Orthop Clin North Am*. 1997;28(1):79-82.

51. Mazzocca AD, Rincon LM, O'Connor RW, et al. Intra-articular partial-thickness rotator cuff tears: analysis of injured and repaired strain behavior. *Am J Sports Med*. 2008;36(1):110-116.

52. Yang S, Park HS, Flores S, et al. Biomechanical analysis of bursal-sided partial thickness rotator cuff tears. *J Shoulder Elbow Surg*. 2009;18(3):379-385.

53. Bey MJ, Ramsey ML, Soslowsky LJ. Intratendinous strain fields of the supraspinatus tendon: effect of a surgically created articular-surface rotator cuff tear. *J Shoulder Elbow Surg*. 2002;11(6):562-569.

54. Sano H, Wakabayashi I, Itoi E. Stress distribution in the supraspinatus tendon with partial-thickness tears: an analysis using two-dimensional finite element model. *J Shoulder Elbow Surg*. 2006;15(1):100-105.

55. Kartus J, Kartus C, Rostgard-Christensen L, Sernert N, Read J, Perko M. Long-term clinical and ultrasound evaluation after arthroscopic acromioplasty in patients with partial rotator cuff tears. *Arthroscopy*. 2006;22(1):44-49.

56. Yamanaka K, Matsumoto T. The joint side tear of the rotator cuff. A followup study by arthrography. *Clin Orthop Relat Res*. 1994;304:68-73.

57. Fukuda H, Mikasa M, Yamanaka K. Incomplete thickness rotator cuff tears diagnosed by subacromial bursography. *Clin Orthop Relat Res*. 1987;223:51-58.

58. Cotton RE, Rideout DF. Tears of the humeral rotator cuff; a radiological and pathological necropsy survey. *J Bone Joint Surg Br*. 1964;46:314-328.

59. Tempelhof S, Rupp S, Seil R. Age-related prevalence of rotator cuff tears in asymptomatic shoulders. *J Shoulder Elbow Surg*. 1999;8(4):296-299.

60. Andarawis-Puri N, Ricchetti ET, Soslowsky LJ. Interaction between the supraspinatus and infraspinatus tendons: effect of anterior supraspinatus tendon full-thickness tears on infraspinatus tendon strain. *Am J Sports Med*. 2009;37(9):1831-1839.

61. Mura N, O'Driscoll SW, Zobitz ME, et al. The effect of infraspinatus disruption on glenohumeral torque and superior migration of the humeral head: a biomechanical study. *J Shoulder Elbow Surg*. 2003;12(2):179-184.

62. Burkhart SS, Esch JC, Jolson RS. The rotator crescent and rotator cable: an anatomic description of the shoulder's "suspension bridge." *Arthroscopy*. 1993;9(6):611-616.

63. Clark J, Sidles JA, Matsen FA. The relationship of the glenohumeral joint capsule to the rotator cuff. *Clin Orthop Relat Res*. 1990;254:29-34.

64. Clark JM, Harryman DT 2nd. Tendons, ligaments, and capsule of the rotator cuff. Gross and microscopic anatomy. *J Bone Joint Surg Am*. 1992;74(5):713-725.

65. Fallon J, Blevins FT, Vogel K, Trotter J. Functional morphology of the supraspinatus tendon. *J Orthop Res*. 2002;20(5):920-926.

66. Kask K, Kolts I, Lubienski A, Russlies M, Leibecke T, Busch LC. Magnetic resonance imaging and correlative gross anatomy of the ligamentum semicirculare humeri (rotator cable). *Clin Anat*. 2008;21(5):420-426.

67. Kolts I, Busch LC, Tomusk H, et al. Macroscopical anatomy of the so-called "rotator interval." A cadaver study on 19 shoulder joints. *Ann Anat*. 2002;184(1):9-14.

68. Morag Y, Jacobson JA, Lucas D, Miller B, Brigido MK, Jamadar DA. US appearance of the rotator cable with histologic correlation: preliminary results. *Radiology*. 2006;241(2):485-491.

69. Sheah K, Bredella MA, Warner JJ, Halpern EF, Palmer WE. Transverse thickening along the articular surface of the rotator cuff consistent with the rotator cable: identification with MR arthrography and relevance in rotator cuff evaluation. *AJR Am J Roentgenol*. 2009;193(3):679-686.

70. Burkhart SS. Fluoroscopic comparison of kinematic patterns in massive rotator cuff tears. A suspension bridge model. *Clin Orthop Relat Res*. 1992;284:144-152.

71. Kim HM, Dahiya N, Teefey SA, Keener JD, Galatz LM, Yamaguchi K. Relationship of tear size and location to fatty degeneration of the rotator cuff. *J Bone Joint Surg Am*. 2010;92(4):829-839.

72. Nguyen ML, Quigley RJ, McGarry MH, et al. Margin convergence to bone for reconstruction of the anterior attachment of the rotator cable in massive rotator cuff tears. Paper presented at: American Shoulder and Elbow Surgeons 2010 Closed Meeting; October 20-23, 2010; Scottsdale, AZ.

73. Gerber C, Schneeberger AG, Beck M, Schlegel U. Mechanical strength of repairs of the rotator cuff. *J Bone Joint Surg Br*. 1994;76(3):371-380.

74. Ellman H. Arthroscopic subacromial decompression: a prelim report. *Orthop Trans*. 1985;9:49.

75. Galatz LM, Ball CM, Teefey SA, Middleton WD, Yamaguchi K. The outcome and repair integrity of completely arthroscopically repaired large and massive rotator cuff tears. *J Bone Joint Surg Am*. 2004;86-A(2):219-224.

76. Apreleva M, Ozbaydar M, Fitzgibbons PG, Warner JJ. Rotator cuff tears: the effect of the reconstruction method on three-dimensional repair site area. *Arthroscopy*. 2002;18(5):519-526.

77. Park MC, Cadet ER, Levine WN, Bigliani LU, Ahmad CS. Tendon-to-bone pressure distributions at a repaired rotator cuff footprint using transosseous suture and suture anchor fixation techniques. *Am J Sports Med*. 2005;33(8):1154-1159.

78. Ahmad CS, Stewart AM, Izquierdo R, Bigliani LU. Tendon-bone interface motion in transosseous suture and suture anchor rotator cuff repair techniques. *Am J Sports Med.* 2005;33(11):1667-1671.

79. Fealy S, Kingham TP, Altchek DW. Mini-open rotator cuff repair using a two-row fixation technique: outcomes analysis in patients with small, moderate, and large rotator cuff tears. *Arthroscopy.* 2002;18(6):665-670.

80. Lo IK, Burkhart SS. Double-row arthroscopic rotator cuff repair: re-establishing the footprint of the rotator cuff. *Arthroscopy.* 2003;19(9):1035-1042.

81. Mazzocca AD, Millett PJ, Guanche CA, Santangelo SA, Arciero RA. Arthroscopic single-row versus double-row suture anchor rotator cuff repair. *Am J Sports Med.* 2005;33(12):1861-1868.

82. Kim DH, ElAttrache NS, Tibone JE, et al. Biomechanical comparison of a single-row versus double-row suture anchor technique for rotator cuff repair. *Am J Sports Med.* 2006;34(3):407-414.

83. Smith CD, Alexander S, Hill AM, et al. A biomechanical comparison of single and double-row fixation in arthroscopic rotator cuff repair. *J Bone Joint Surg Am.* 2006;88(11):2425-2431.

84. Snyder SJ. Single vs. double row suture anchor fixation rotator cuff repair. Paper presented at: American Orthopaedic Society of Sports Medicine Specialty Day at the 75th Annual Meeting of the American Academy of Orthopaedic Surgeons; March 5-9, 2008; San Francisco, CA.

85. Domb BG, Glousman RE, Brooks A, Hansen M, Lee TQ, ElAttrache NS. High-tension double-row footprint repair compared with reduced-tension single-row repair for massive rotator cuff tears. *J Bone Joint Surg Am.* 2008;90(Suppl 4):35-39.

86. Ma CB, Comerford L, Wilson J, Puttlitz CM. Biomechanical evaluation of arthroscopic rotator cuff repairs: double-row compared with single-row fixation. *J Bone Joint Surg Am.* 2006;88(2):403-410.

87. Ma CB, MacGillivray JD, Clabeaux J, Lee S, Otis JC. Biomechanical evaluation of arthroscopic rotator cuff stitches. *J Bone Joint Surg Am.* 2004;86-A(6):1211-1216.

88. Waltrip RL, Zheng N, Dugas JR, Andrews JR. Rotator cuff repair. A biomechanical comparison of three techniques. *Am J Sports Med.* 2003;31(4):493-497.

89. Meier SW, Meier JD. The effect of double-row fixation on initial repair strength in rotator cuff repair: a biomechanical study. *Arthroscopy.* 2006;22(11):1168-1173.

90. Meier SW, Meier JD. Rotator cuff repair: the effect of double-row fixation on three-dimensional repair site. *J Shoulder Elbow Surg.* 2006;15(6):691-696.

91. Sano H, Yamashita T, Wakabayashi I, Itoi E. Stress distribution in the supraspinatus tendon after tendon repair: suture anchors versus transosseous suture fixation. *Am J Sports Med.* 2007;35(4):542-546.

92. Park MC, ElAttrache NS, Ahmad CS, Tibone JE. "Transosseous-equivalent" rotator cuff repair technique. *Arthroscopy.* 2006;22(12):1360 e1-5.

93. Park MC, ElAttrache NS, Tibone JE, Ahmad CS, Jun BJ, Lee TQ. Part I: footprint contact characteristics for a transosseous-equivalent rotator cuff repair technique compared with a double-row repair technique. *J Shoulder Elbow Surg.* 2007;16(4):461-468.

94. Park MC, Tibone JE, ElAttrache NS, Ahmad CS, Jun BJ, Lee TQ. Part II: biomechanical assessment for a footprint-restoring transosseous-equivalent rotator cuff repair technique compared with a double-row repair technique. *J Shoulder Elbow Surg.* 2007;16(4):469-476.

95. Ihashi K, Matsushita N, Yagi R, Handa Y. Rotational action of the supraspinatus muscle on the shoulder joint. *J Electromyogr Kinesiol.* 1998;8(5):337-346.

96. Park MC, Jun BJ, Park CJ, Ahmad CS, ElAttrache NS, Lee TQ. The biomechanical effects of dynamic external rotation on rotator cuff repair compared to testing with the humerus fixed. *Am J Sports Med.* 2007;35(11):1931-1939.

97. Park MC, Idjadi JA, ElAttrache NS, Tibone JE, McGarry MH, Lee TQ. The effect of dynamic external rotation comparing 2 footprint-restoring rotator cuff repair techniques. *Am J Sports Med.* 2008;36(5):893-900.

98. Mazzocca AD, Bollier MJ, Ciminiello AM, et al. Biomechanical evaluation of arthroscopic rotator cuff repairs over time. *Arthroscopy.* 2010;26(5):592-599.

99. Busfield BT, Glousman RE, McGarry MH, Tibone JE, Lee TQ. A biomechanical comparison of 2 technical variations of double-row rotator cuff fixation: the importance of medial row knots. *Am J Sports Med.* 2008;36(5):901-906.

100. Slabaugh MA, Nho SJ, Grumet RC, et al. Does the literature confirm superior clinical results in radiographically healed rotator cuffs after rotator cuff repair? *Arthroscopy.* 2010;26(3):393-403.

101. Nho SJ, Slabaugh MA, Seroyer ST, et al. Does the literature support double-row suture anchor fixation for arthroscopic rotator cuff repair? A systematic review comparing double-row and single-row suture anchor configuration. *Arthroscopy.* 2009;25(11):1319-1328.

102. Burks RT, Crim J, Brown N, Fink B, Greis PE. A prospective randomized clinical trial comparing arthroscopic single- and double-row rotator cuff repair: magnetic resonance imaging and early clinical evaluation. *Am J Sports Med.* 2009;37(4):674-682.

103. Franceschi F, Ruzzini L, Longo UG, et al. Equivalent clinical results of arthroscopic single-row and double-row suture anchor repair for rotator cuff tears: a randomized controlled trial. *Am J Sports Med.* 2007;35(8):1254-1260.

104. Burkhart SS, Cole BJ. Bridging self-reinforcing double-row rotator cuff repair: we really are doing better. *Arthroscopy.* 2010;26(5):677-680.

CHAPTER 3

TENDON DEGENERATION IN THE ROTATOR CUFF

Jack G. Skendzel, MD and Asheesh Bedi, MD

Overuse injuries of the rotator cuff are a significant source of pain and morbidity.[1] Despite an aging population and documented associations between rotator cuff tears and increasing age, the pathogenesis of rotator cuff tendinopathy remains poorly understood.[1-9] The natural history of rotator cuff tears is unfavorable, as these lesions fail to spontaneously heal and progress in size over time.[10,11] This progression in tear size is accompanied by fatty infiltration and atrophy of the rotator cuff musculature and no evidence of reversal or repair of the degeneration process.[12-14] Furthermore, recurrent tears after surgical repair remain a significant issue for large and massive tears, with documented failure rates ranging from 11% to 94%.[15-19] While arthroscopic surgical techniques have considerably evolved, including the use of double-row repair to improve time-zero biomechanics, our understanding and ability to improve the biologic milieu for tendon-to-bone healing has lagged behind. This chapter reviews the current understanding of the pathogenesis and biology of rotator cuff tendinopathy and outlines various treatment modalities and future directions for research into biologic augmentation of tendon-to-bone healing after rotator cuff repair.

PATHOGENESIS

Tendinopathy is a term that describes a continuum of specific histopathologic changes that occur to tendons as a result of overuse.[20] Historically, the term *tendinitis* was used to describe pain from symptomatic tendons; however, this nomenclature implied an inflammatory process despite histologic studies demonstrating minimal or absent inflammatory changes.[21,22] Overall, tendinitis treatment modalities that target the inflammatory process have shown limited efficacy.[6,14] Nonetheless, several recent studies have demonstrated altered gene expression related to an inflammatory response as well as an increased infiltration of mast cells and macrophages in early mild to moderate tendinopathy.[6,23,24] While not all cases of rotator cuff tendinosis progress to a frank tear, the process of tendon degeneration does not regress over time and is not reversible.[25] Tendinosis is a

Ma CB, Feeley BT, eds.
*Basic Principles and Operative Management
of the Rotator Cuff (pp 33-48)*
© 2012 SLACK Incorporated

common phenomenon and is not isolated only to the rotator cuff; it is a frequent source of pain in other anatomic areas, including the patellar tendon, the origin of the forearm extensor tendons, and the Achilles tendon.[20,24,26]

ANATOMY AND HISTOLOGY

Tendons are composed of dense, highly organized bundles of collagen fibrils designed to transmit forces from muscle to bone through a highly organized enthesis, allowing for joint movement.[24] Macroscopically, normal tendons are usually brilliant white in color with a firm texture, while microscopic examination reveals collagen bundles arranged in a dense, parallel, slightly wavy configuration.[24] In contrast, degenerative tendons appear gray or brown in color and are soft and fragile.[8] Microscopically, there is disorganization of the collagen bundles and increased mucoid ground substance, as well as the infiltration of small blood vessels, fibrinoid and hypoxic degeneration, and fibrocartilaginous metaplasia often with calcium deposition.[3,24,27-29] Rotator cuff tears are a result of a degenerative process that occurs at the insertion of the tendon to bone, known as the enthesis.[30] Degenerative changes at the rotator cuff insertion may predispose the tendon to failure and development of a full-thickness rotator cuff tear.[31] Although the exact etiology of tendon degeneration is unknown, its pathogenesis is likely multifactorial and includes mechanical, biological, and patient-specific factors. During the degenerative process, the normal biologic process of remodeling is disrupted, leading to a loss of tissue or replacement of normal tissue with poorer quality tendon. Several authors have proposed a continuum of pathology, progressing from asymptomatic degeneration to full-thickness tears.[7,32] Broadly, the mechanisms responsible for rotator cuff degeneration and tendinopathy are categorized as either extrinsic or intrinsic factors.

Extrinsic Factors

In 1972, Neer hypothesized that anatomic variations in the shape of the acromion and osteophyte formation at the acromial attachment of the coracoacromial (CA) ligament caused repetitive trauma to a critical portion of the supraspinatus tendon.[33] Neer attributed 95% of all rotator cuff tears to impingement.[33] Several anatomic factors have been described that can predispose a shoulder to subacromial impingement, including the morphology of the acromion, the presence of an os acromiale, acromioclavicular (AC) joint degenerative disease with osteophyte formation, as well as a narrow subacromial space.[34-38] Glenohumeral instability is also an important factor predisposing to rotator cuff degeneration and tearing.[39]

Surgical acromioplasty of the anterior one-third of the acromion was developed by Neer in an attempt to prevent impingement and temper the pathologic process of tendon degeneration and rotator cuff tearing. Later, Bigliani and colleagues[38] described a classification system for anterior acromion morphology and its relationship to rotator cuff tears, with a type III (hooked) acromion present in the majority of cases. Whether acromion shape is congenital or is an acquired deformity as a result of secondary intrinsic factors remains a controversial topic.[40,41] A predisposition to rotator cuff tearing in patients with an unfused epiphysis of the anterior acromion (os acromiale) has been suggested in the literature, despite a paucity of literature to support a causal relationship.[35,42,43] In a retrospective cadaveric analysis, Oeullette and colleagues[43] concluded that there was no statistically significant difference in the prevalence of rotator cuff tears between individuals with an os acromiale when compared to control subjects. There was, however, a significant increase in the prevalence of rotator cuff tears when a step-off deformity was between the os acromiale and acromion, suggesting tendon injury through mechanical abrasion.

AC joint arthritis with osteophyte formation and joint hypertrophy may also contribute to mechanical impingement of the rotator cuff, owing to its location directly above the subacromial space and rotator cuff tendons.[37,44,45] The development of osteophytes that project from the AC joint in a caudal direction can injure the rotator cuff tendons.[37] Nyffeler and colleagues[46] also reported on a statistically significant association between a large lateral extension of the acromion and full-thickness rotator cuff tears. In addition, abnormal glenoid morphology is associated with rotator cuff disease. In a cadaveric study using soft x-rays and visual inspection for rotator cuff pathology, Konno and colleagues[47] demonstrated that the presence of a hooked osteophyte in the anterior and inferior portions of the glenoid was commonly observed with a full-thickness rotator cuff tear in 43% of shoulders. While this study did not prove a causative relationship between glenoid osteophyte formation and rotator cuff tears, the authors did suggest that the radiographic presence of an osteophyte may be used as an indicator of rotator cuff pathology.

Abnormal contact between the rotator cuff and glenoid rim has also been implicated in partial-thickness rotator cuff tearing. The term *internal impingement* describes a pinching of the postero-superior supraspinatus and anterior infraspinatus between the posterosuperior aspect of the glenoid rim and the humerus with the arm in a position of 90-degree abduction and maximal external rotation.[39,48] Several authors have suggested that repetitive contact between the glenoid rim and rotator cuff tendons may contribute to tendon degeneration and subsequent partial-thickness articular-sided rotator cuff tears, particularly in overhead athletes.[39] Other authors have called into question, however, the assumption that internal impingement is a process exclusive to throwing athletes and that the presence of partial-thickness rotator cuff tearing with superior labral abnormalities in a nonathletic population may point to a separate cause, such as tensile overload instead of mechanical impingement.[49-52] Multiple different theories have been proposed to explain internal impingement. Some authors believe that the primary pathology involves anterior glenohumeral laxity and subtle instability with anterosuperior translation of the humeral head,[53-55] while others have postulated that a posterior capsular contracture with decreased internal rotation and resultant posterosuperior translation of the humeral head is responsible.[56,57] Impingement and potential injury to the rotator cuff tendons can also occur as a result of bony contact between the coracoid process and lesser tuberosity, termed *subcoracoid impingement*.[58,59] In addition, dynamic factors such as changes in scapular position can alter the space available for the rotator cuff in the subacromial space. In a magnetic resonance imaging study performed by Solem-Bertoft and colleagues,[36] there was a significant narrowing of the anterior opening of the subacromial space when moving from a retracted to a protracted shoulder position. While the clinical significance is uncertain, the effects of posture and scapular position and the dynamic nature of the subacromial space may contribute to the development of extrinsic impingement.

Medical Factors

Patient-specific extrinsic factors, such as diabetes mellitus, the effects of smoking (nicotine), and the use of nonsteroidal anti-inflammatory drugs (NSAIDs) also impact rotator cuff degeneration and healing. In a study of rotator cuff healing in a diabetic rat model, Bedi and colleagues[60] demonstrated that sustained hyperglycemia impaired tendon-to-bone healing after rotator cuff repair and reduced collagen fiber organization and fibrocartilage formation at the healing enthesis. In addition, biomechanical parameters, including ultimate strength and stiffness of the repair construct, were reduced overall. Fox and colleagues have shown that the metabolic condition of poorly controlled diabetes negatively affects the mechanical properties of the native tendon as well and that these altered structural properties may predispose diabetic patients to a greater risk of tendinopathy and/or traumatic rupture.[61] Clinical studies have associated diabetes mellitus with decreased postoperative range of motion and to be at higher risk for complications, such as wound infection.[62,63]

Several authors have also shown nicotine to impair rotator cuff healing. In a rat shoulder model, Galatz and colleagues[64] demonstrated that nicotine caused decreased cellular proliferation and decreased type I collagen expression 28 days after rotator cuff repair. In addition, the nicotine group showed delayed matrix remodeling and an overall delay in tendon-to-bone healing. Although no studies exist regarding the specific biologic alterations on the rotator cuff tendons, the effects of nicotine on biologic systems elsewhere in the body is well reported.[65,66] In a clinical study, Baumgarten and colleagues[67] showed a dose- and time-dependent relationship between tobacco use and rotator cuff tears that was independent of patient age, suggesting a causative effect. Future research is needed to investigate the significant biochemical alterations in smokers with rotator cuff tears.

Nonsteroidal Anti-Inflammatory Drugs and Corticosteroids

NSAIDs also affect tendon-to-bone healing and rotator cuff disease. Cohen and colleagues[68] reported inhibition of bone-to-tendon healing in a rat rotator cuff tear model after administration of either celecoxib (a COX-2 selective inhibitor) or indomethacin (a nonselective COX inhibitor). Load-to-failure was significantly lower in all animals receiving celecoxib or indomethacin at all time points (2, 4, and 8 weeks after repair), and there was no consistent reformation of the fibrocartilage zone with less robust and less organized collagen at 4 and 8 weeks after repair. These results have questioned the routine use of NSAIDs in the early postoperative period after rotator cuff repair.

Corticosteroid use may also have deleterious effects on rotator cuff tendon and tendon-to-bone healing. The effect of corticosteroids on normal, healthy rotator cuff tendons has been demonstrated in several animal studies. Haraldsson and colleagues[69] studied the effects of corticosteroids on tensile strength of isolated collagen fascicles in an adult rat tail incubated in either high- or low-dose methylprednisolone. Their data show a decrease in the tensile strength after 3- and 7-day incubations with both high and low doses of corticosteroid. Although cross-linking remained unaffected, the results suggest that weakening of individual collagen fascicles may contribute to decreased mechanical properties and predispose the tendon to rupture. Tillander and colleagues[70] investigated the effects of repeated triamcinolone injections into the subacromial space on the supraspinatus and infraspinatus tendons in a rat model. After 5 subacromial injections, microscopic evaluation demonstrated changes to the tendon structure, including necrosis and fragmentation of the collagen bundles with increased inflammatory cells between bundles. The authors urged the cautious use of repeated subacromial corticosteroid injections. Animal studies have also investigated the effect of corticosteroids on injured tendons. In a rat model, Mikolyzk and colleagues[71] created a full-thickness infraspinatus defect 2 mm medial to its humeral insertion and subjected test animals to a single dose of methylprednisolone injected into the subacromial space. At 1 week, there was a significant decrease in the mechanical properties of both intact and injured rotator cuff tissue, which returned to control levels by 3 weeks. The authors concluded that even a single dose of corticosteroid causes a significant but transient reduction in the strength of the rotator cuff, suggesting that the effects of a single subacromial corticosteroid injection must be weighed against any potential benefit.

Deleterious effects of corticosteroid use have been shown in human studies. In an in vitro experiment, Wong and colleagues[72] prepared primary human tenocyte cultures obtained from healthy patellar tendons in donors after anterior cruciate ligament (ACL) reconstruction with bone-patellar tendon-bone autografts. The effects of various concentrations of triamcinolone were then studied, including adverse effects to human tenocytes with a dose-dependent reduction in cell viability, an overall decrease in cell proliferation, and a decrease in collagen synthesis. All of these changes may predispose the tendon to rupture. In another study, Wong and colleagues also demonstrated a reversal in the detrimental effects of glucocorticoids on human tenocytes after the administration of platelet-derived growth factor BB (PDGF-BB).[73]

Overall, there is limited evidence to support significant benefits of corticosteroid use. Koester and colleagues conducted a systematic review of randomized controlled trials to investigate the effects of subacromial corticosteroid injections in the management of rotator cuff disease.[74] Nine articles that met inclusion criteria were included in the analysis; these randomized controlled trials focused specifically on rotator cuff disease and not other pathologic conditions of the shoulder, although most studies had significant limitations in terms of methodology and statistical analysis with a lack of validated, patient-oriented outcome measures. For these reasons, it was difficult for the authors to draw concrete conclusions from the analyzed body of literature regarding the efficacy, safety, and clinical outcomes related to subacromial injection. The authors concluded that there is no evidence to support the efficacy of subacromial corticosteroid injection in individuals with subacromial impingement. The effects of NSAID or corticosteroid use in the nonoperative management of impingement was the focus of a double-blind, randomized controlled trial performed by Karthikeyan and colleagues[75] to compare the efficacy of a single subacromial injection of an NSAID (tenoxicam) with methylprednisolone in patients with clinical evidence of subacromial impingement. The methylprednisolone group showed significant improvements in the Constant-Murley score at 6 weeks when compared to the tenoxicam group, and the improvement in the DASH score was significantly increased in the methylprednisolone group at the 2-, 4-, and 6-week periods. The authors concluded that a single subacromial corticosteroid injection led to improved patient outcomes and shoulder function when compared to tenoxicam.

Fluoroquinolones

Fluoroquinolones are a widely used group of broad-spectrum antibiotics that have been implicated in tendon rupture, particularly the Achilles tendon. There are reports of spontaneous rotator cuff tendon rupture in patients undergoing treatment with a fluoroquinolone.[76,77] The exact mechanism of injury remains unknown and is likely multifactorial. Histologic evaluation in human studies has revealed hyaline and mucoid degeneration, chondroid metaplasia, and changes in collagen fiber arrangement.[78] Sendzik and colleagues[79] showed alterations at the cellular level, including less matrix production and apoptosis even at low levels of plasma quinolone concentration. Corps and colleagues[80] incubated human tendon-derived cells with fluoroquinolones and measured the expression of matrix metalloproteinases (MMPs), showing reduced MMP-13 levels and increased MMP-1, demonstrating changes on the molecular level that may play significant roles in the development of quinolone-dependent tendon degeneration and tearing.

Clinical Studies

There is limited evidence to support extrinsic factors as the major cause of rotator cuff degeneration and subsequent tearing. Fukuda and colleagues[3] performed a histologic analysis of rotator cuff tendons with bursal-sided tears in patients with clinical symptoms of subacromial impingement, showing disruption of the tendon enthesis in all specimens in addition to chondrocyte metaplasia and hypervascularity in the distal stump. The authors concluded that bursal-sided rotator cuff tears are related to multiple factors, including subacromial impingement from repeated arm use above the horizontal level. However, not all cases of impingement may be deleterious to the structural integrity of the rotator cuff. In a cadaveric model, Yamamoto and colleagues[81] demonstrated a normal contact phenomenon between the rotator cuff and acromion and CA ligament in all cadavers despite a lack of gross pathologic changes. Their study suggests that nonpathologic subacromial contact may be present in normal shoulders and that not all cases of "impingement" are pathologic. In addition, the authors postulate that bursal-sided rotator cuff tears may be secondary to increased contact pressure due to an age-related increase in stiffness of the CA ligament and its contact with the rotator cuff tendons. Furthermore, in an ultrasonographic study of living patients with rotator cuff tears, Kim and colleagues concluded that most degenerative rotator cuff tears occur more posteriorly than previously thought, near the junction of the supraspinatus and infraspinatus.[82] One explanation for these findings is an age-related degeneration and weakening of the rotator crescent, as described by Burkhart and colleagues,[83] making it more susceptible to tearing. In their study, the center point of the rotator crescent corresponds to the most common location of tearing, approximately 15 to 16 mm posterior to the biceps tendon and not in close proximity to the CA ligament or anterior acromial dysmorphology.[82]

Several authors have called into question the importance of external impingement as the primary pathologic factor in the development of tendinopathy and tearing, focusing instead on intrinsic causes. Ozaki and colleagues[84] and Ogata and Uhthoff[85] conclude that the majority of rotator cuff tears are not a result of subacromial impingement but rather are the result of an intrinsic degenerative tendinopathy, supporting Codman's original theory.[86] Furthermore, these same authors have contradicted Neer's description of subacromial spur formation as a causative factor in rotator cuff tears, instead supporting a reverse effect; that is, the change in acromion morphology and the formation of CA spurs occurs in a response to intrinsic tendon degeneration and rotator cuff tearing.[84]

Intrinsic Factors

Intrinsic degeneration of the rotator cuff refers to biologic and structural changes within the tendon itself. A variety of causes are implicated, including repetitive microtrauma, tendon hypovascularity, oxidative stress and apoptosis, as well as age-related tendon changes. The presence of a significant inflammatory response in rotator cuff degeneration and healing remains controversial. Multiple studies[9,27,31,85-88] have attempted to define the biochemical alterations and traumatic factors responsible for intrinsic causes of rotator cuff tendinopathy, but further investigation is needed to improve the understanding of rotator cuff degeneration.

Microtrauma of the rotator cuff may trigger cellular damage and decreased mechanical properties of the tendons, thereby predisposing them to rupture. Hashimoto and colleagues[87] demonstrated disorientation of collagen fibers with myxoid degeneration and chondroid metaplasia with calcification in a series of 80 torn rotator cuff tendons. Kannus and Jozsa[27] showed characteristic histologic changes, including mucoid tendinopathy, hypoxic degeneration, and the presence of calcifications in biopsy specimens of 891 consecutive patients with a spontaneous rotator cuff tear. Additionally, Longo and colleagues[89] reported on histopathologic changes in supraspinatus tendons from patients with rotator cuff tears, demonstrating that tendon degeneration occurs not only at the site of rupture, but through the remainder of the macroscopically intact tendon. All of these studies support a primary degenerative process in addition to microtrauma as the primary cause of rotator cuff tearing. The location of initial tendon degeneration and microtrauma further supports an intrinsic etiology of rotator cuff disease. Most degeneration occurs on the articular side of the tendon, leading to a significant reduction in tensile strength.[9,31] Codman described these defects as so-called "rim rents."[86] While the etiology remains multifactorial, the overall result of these intrinsic degenerative changes at the tendon insertion is weakening of the tissue without complete repair, increasing the likelihood of clinically significant rotator cuff tendinopathy and subsequent tears.[9,27,84,85]

Likely, rotator cuff degeneration is a multifactorial process with both extrinsic and intrinsic contributing factors. Anatomic factors such as outlet impingement, shoulder instability, and trauma play a role in tendon degeneration and may be implicated in the development of rotator cuff tearing. While CA arch morphology has been strongly associated with rotator cuff tears, some degree of subacromial contact may be present in normal shoulders. Environmental factors such as smoking and corticosteroid use, as well as systemic illness such as diabetes mellitus, play important but not clearly defined roles in rotator cuff tendinopathy.

BIOLOGY OF ROTATOR CUFF DEGENERATION

The biologic changes responsible for rotator cuff tendon repair, remodeling, and healing involve changes in gene expression, variable expression of growth factors and cytokines, and alterations in the extracellular matrix (ECM). The process of tendon and tendon-to-bone healing is a complicated, highly coordinated event involving multiple factors. When tendon damage occurs, degeneration as well as repair occurs during 3 stages: (1) inflammatory phase, (2) repair phase, and (3) remodeling phase.[90] The inflammatory phase begins within the first week. During this period, infiltrating macrophages release transforming growth factor-beta-1 (TGF-β1), which increases collagen production, contributing to the formation of a fibrovascular scar.[91] As normal bone-to-tendon healing progresses, there is an abundant cellular response with the production of numerous cytokines, including increased production of key ECM proteins (type III collagen) that bear little resemblance to the native insertion.[92] The role of genetic and molecular factors, including those in the interleukin (IL) family, MMPs and their inhibitors (tissue inhibitor of metalloproteinases, or TIMPs), as well as tumor necrosis factor-alpha (TNF-α) and TGF-β1 and -β3, has been clearly documented during this phase of rotator cuff healing.[92-94] Understanding the biologic factors important for rotator cuff healing is important to reliably treat these injuries, as favorable long-term outcomes are predicated upon a structurally intact repair.[95]

Bone Morphogenic Proteins

Bone morphogenic proteins (BMPs) are a group of growth factors that are involved in a large variety of cell processes. Several growth factors, including BMP-2 and BMP-7, are already widely used in clinical applications to enhance bone regeneration.[96] The use of BMPs in rotator cuff repair has shown promise to improve healing in several animal studies. Rodeo and colleagues demonstrated the possibility of increased tissue formation in the gap between tendon and bone of a rotator cuff model using osteoinductive proteins.[97] The authors tested an osteoinductive protein mixture containing BMP-2 to -7, TGF-β1-3, and fibroblast growth factors (FGFs) in a sheep infraspinatus repair model. The group receiving the mixture demonstrated a significant increase in bone and tissue formation in the tendon-to-bone gap, corresponding to greater load-to-failure at both 6 and 12 weeks postoperatively. Other studies have also shown improved tendon-to-bone healing through administration of BMPs, a part of the TGF-β superfamily. In another sheep rotator cuff repair model, Seeherman and colleagues[98] delivered recombinant human BMP-12 via a hyaluronan paste of sponge carrier applied locally to acute rotator cuff repairs and demonstrated significantly increased load-to-failure and stiffness in the experimental group when compared to the control group. Histologically, there was an improved orientation of the collagen fibers at the repair site, suggesting that the experimental group exhibited accelerated healing. Nonetheless, the appearance of the enthesis in both groups did not demonstrate the organization of the normal tendon-to-bone attachment or normal tendon.[98] In a rat rotator cuff repair model, cartilage-derived morphogenetic protein 2 growth factor (also known as BMP-13) was shown to increase healing rates, collagen formation, and repair strength at 4 and 6 weeks when compared to control animals.[99] Other agents such as BMP-12 have been shown to increase type I collagen synthesis and improve the tensile strength and stiffness of repaired tendons in an in vitro gene transfer model in chicken tendon cells.[100] Although animal studies of BMPs in tendon healing have shown improved strength and speed of healing, future studies are required to delineate the response of human rotator cuff tendon to these various growth factors.

Proinflammatory Cytokines

There are alterations in many growth factor pathways during all phases of rotator cuff pathology, and the balance between pro- and anti-inflammatory cytokines may play an integral role in early tendon healing. IL-4 is an anti-inflammatory cytokine that stimulates fibroblasts, while IL-6 is proinflammatory and an inhibitor of fibroblast activity.[101] Lin and colleagues[101] created full-thickness partial patellar transections in IL-4 and IL-6 knockout mice. Their results showed inferior mechanical properties in the IL-6 knockout mice when compared to the IL-4 knockout and control mice, despite an upregulation of TNF-α in the IL-6-deficient animals. Perry and colleagues[102] used a rat supraspinatus tendon overuse model to determine the roles of inflammatory and angiogenic markers by measuring messenger ribonucleic acid (mRNA) expression levels of COX-2, 5-lipoxygenase activating protein (FLAP), vascular endothelial growth factor (VEGF), and von Willebrand factor (vWF) through polymerase chain reaction. FLAP expression increased at 3 days, then decreased by 1 week, only to increase again with peak levels demonstrated at 8 weeks of overuse. VEGF and vWF levels were increased at 3 days and generally remained higher throughout the study, supporting a role for increased angiogenesis very early in the overuse process that persists along the course of injury. The results of these studies suggest a critical role for cytokines in tendon healing and that some mounting of an inflammatory response is required.

Matrix Metalloproteinases

MMPs are a family of zinc-dependent endopeptidases that participate in maintenance of the ECM. TIMPs are natural inhibitors of MMPs and work by modulating the reparative and degradative pathways involved in homeostasis of the ECM.[103] In tendinopathy, an increased rate of matrix remodeling may alter the tendon biomechanical properties and predispose to tearing. Lo and colleagues have shown that a disruption of this homeostasis and increased MMP activity may be associated with rotator cuff tendinopathy.[104] Comparative biopsies of rotator cuff tendon from individuals with rotator cuff tears and control specimens from cadavers demonstrated significant alterations in mRNA expression of both MMPs and TIMPs in those samples with a rotator cuff tear.[104] In addition, Bedi and colleagues[94] inhibited MMP expression in a rat supraspinatus repair model with recombinant alpha-2-macroglobulin protein, a universal MMP inhibitor, documenting a significant decrease in collagen degradation and improved collagen organization at 4 weeks when compared to controls. There was, however, no significant difference between the experimental and control groups in terms of ultimate load-to-failure or stiffness. In a separate study, the use of doxycycline to inhibit MMPs (specifically MMP-13) improved collagen organization and mechanical strength with improved load-to-failure in a rat rotator cuff repair model.[105] Thornton and colleagues investigated the response of several MMPs and TIMPs, including MMP-13, MMP-3, and TIMP-2, in a rat model with altered tendon mechanical loading.[106] Their results showed an increase in expression of all factors in response to tendon detachment (stress deprivation). In addition, the authors subjected the tendons to intermittent cyclic hydrostatic compression, thereby simulating the effects of impingement, finding an increased expression of MMP-13. This suggests that the mechanical effects of impingement under the CA arch on rotator cuff tendons may precipitate altered tendon biology, supporting an extrinsic cause in the pathogenesis of rotator cuff tearing. These results indicate that MMPs and TIMPs play an important role in the pathophysiology of rotator cuff tendinopathy, and future studies are required to further explore their role in clinical applications.

Tissue Hypoxia

Hypoxia within the rotator cuff has been suggested to play a role in degeneration and tearing. The first detailed description of intratendinous arterial patterns was provided by Brockis.[107] Subsequently, several authors studied the vascularity of the rotator cuff. Moseley and Goldie[108] researched the arterial pattern in 72 patients, concluding that while there was no evidence to support decreased vascularization in areas of the rotator cuff prone to degenerative changes, there was a "critical zone" corresponding to the region of anastomoses between the osseous and tendinous vessels. Rothman[109] and Lohr and Uhthoff[110] confirmed an area of hypovascularity most commonly involving the supraspinatus tendon, in a distal portion of the tendon just proximal to its insertion, concluding that areas of decreased blood flow may be important in the development of degenerative rotator cuff lesions and may be associated with advancing age. In contrast, Levy and colleagues[111] used laser Doppler flowmetry in patients during arthroscopic surgery and were unable to find an area of hypoperfusion in the normal rotator cuff. Fealy and colleagues[112] performed power Doppler sonography analysis in patients who underwent rotator cuff repair to examine the vascular patterns after repair. This study demonstrated a robust vascular response, greatest in the peritendinous region, which consistently and predictably decreased over time after rotator cuff repair. Interestingly, the site of suture anchor placement and decortication of the rotator cuff footprint on the humerus consistently delivered the lowest amount of blood flow postoperatively, calling into question the need for decortication to create a healthy bed of bleeding bone at the footprint.[112]

Vascular Factors

Neovascularity is a critical component of proper tendon healing. VEGF, TGF-β1, and bFGF (FGF-2) have been shown to modulate a vascular response during tendon healing, although no studies have clearly defined their expression in a rotator cuff tear model.[113-116] Benson and colleagues[117] studied tissue from 24 patients with impingement and rotator cuff tears, comparing the expression of hypoxia inducible factor-1-α, BNip3 (proapoptotic member of the Bcl-2 family), and terminal deoxynucleotidyl transferase dUTP nick end labeling to 3 controls, concluding that hypoxic damage was present in tears of various magnitudes (small, medium, and large) and may contribute to cell loss through apoptosis. FGFs, namely FGF-1 and FGF-2 (bFGF), play an important role in angiogenesis and tendon healing, as shown by Ide and colleagues[118] in a rat model of supraspinatus tendon repair. In specimens treated with FGF, there were improved biomechanical properties and significantly increased bone ingrowth at the healing enthesis at 2 weeks when compared to control samples. At 4 and 6 weeks postoperatively, there was no difference between operated FGF-treated and control specimens in terms of histologic tendon-to-bone insertion maturity and strength. While further research is needed, the theoretic ability to manipulate the angiogenic and apoptotic responses during rotator cuff degeneration and healing may offer significant therapeutic benefit.

Identification of the specific genetic pathways may contribute to the pathogenesis of rotator cuff degeneration and may lead to novel therapies to prevent progression of the disease process. Molloy and colleagues[23] used microarray analysis in a rat overuse model to investigate gene expression in supraspinatus tendinopathy, showing upregulation of glutamate-signaling proteins previously thought to exist only in the central nervous system. These data suggest an "excitotoxic" mechanism where overactive glutamine signaling leads to increased cell apoptosis, thereby causing structural changes to the tissue that may contribute to tendinopathy. Based on these pilot studies, glutamate antagonists may offer future promise in the treatment of tendinopathy.

TREATMENT MODALITIES

Numerous biologic and mechanical treatment approaches have been developed based on the principles and known pathogenesis of the rotator cuff. The goal of all surgical and biological interventions is to alter the unfavorable natural history of tendon degeneration and tear progression, as well as to improve the rate of structural healing after surgical repair of large and massive tears. Novel treatment modalities are being investigated in the treatment of tendon degeneration and tearing, including the use of biological factors, cytokines, and cell-based treatments. These therapies have the potential to induce a robust healing response and regenerate tendons with relatively low morbidity. Technological advances allow for the harvesting of cells and specific tissues and provide the ability to culture these cells and implant them at the site of disease by way of carrier materials.

Preliminary animal studies have shown promising results in the application of bone marrow-derived mesenchymal stem cells (MSCs) for rotator cuff tears. Gulotta and colleagues[119] demonstrated that the addition of bone-marrow derived MSCs to a rat rotator cuff healing model did not improve the composition or strength of the healing insertion site. However, supraspinatus tendon defects treated with MSCs that were genetically modified to overexpress MT1-MMP, a metalloproteinase involved in endochondral ossification and promotion of the formation of mineralized cartilage, showed more fibrocartilage and improved mechanical properties, including higher ultimate stress-to-failure and higher stiffness at 4 weeks.[120] Seeherman and colleagues[98] showed improved strength and rigidity in a sheep rotator cuff tear model treated with recombinant BMP-12. Uggen and colleagues[121] investigated the effect of recombinant human PDGF BB (rhPDGF-BB)-coated sutures on rotator cuff healing in a sheep model. The histologic examination showed improved organization of gap tissue and extensive cartilage formation at the tendon-to-bone interface. At 6 weeks, however, there was no significant difference in ultimate load-to-failure.

Obaid and Connell[122] performed a systematic review of the literature to define the current levels of evidence regarding cell therapy for treatment of tendinopathy and tendon repair. The authors concluded that, while much progress has been made regarding the use of cell therapy for tendinopathy and tendon repair, overall, the evidence in human studies is limited, and there is a need for further clinical trials. Commonly used cell types include MSCs, fibroblasts, and tendon progenitor/stem cells; each has unique advantages and disadvantages.[122-127] Mesenchymal stem cells derived from bone marrow have been shown to increase the rate of tendon healing and maturation, in addition to improving the histologic properties of injured tendon. A drawback, however, is a limited ability to prevent these cells from differentiating into unwanted lineages such as cartilage, bone, and muscle. MSCs from other sources, such as those derived from adipose tissue or synovium and muscle, have shown potential to improve tendon-to-bone healing and are readily available, although further investigations are required to define their role in tendon healing and in the degenerative process of the rotator cuff. Fibroblasts harvested from skin also represent a widely available source of cells and can be harvested in noninvasive methods with low donor-site morbidity. Their efficacy has been demonstrated in the treatment of chronic lateral epicondylitis, but further trials are needed.[128] Autologous tenocytes implanted into massive rotator cuff defects have shown promising results in a rabbit model, as shown by Chen and colleagues.[129] After introduction of these cells by either porcine-derived collagen scaffolds or small intestine submucosa, there was similar quality tissue as in the control group at 8 weeks. Dines and colleagues also demonstrated improved histology scores and increased load-to-failure in a rat rotator cuff tear model treated with tenocytes transduced with PDGF-β and insulin-like growth factor-1 via a retroviral vector and seeded onto polyglycolic acid scaffolds.[130]

Biologic agents such as MSCs can improve the osseointegration between tendon and bone. Lim and colleagues[131] performed ACL reconstruction in adult rabbits using hamstring tendon autografts coated with MSCs in a fibrin glue carrier. At 8 weeks, the reconstructions with MSC enhancement demonstrated a significantly higher load-to-failure and stiffness when compared to the control group, with the development of an intervening zone of cartilage that resembled the chondral enthesis of a normal ACL insertion. Similarly, Ouyang and colleagues[132] performed hallucis longus transfer into calcaneal bone tunnels in a rabbit model, and the tunnel was then injected with bone marrow MSCs in a fibrin glue. Histologic analysis of the experimental group showed an accelerated healing process with the formation of fibrocartilage-like tissue and a more perpendicular orientation of the collagen fibers between tendon and bone. Although this fibrocartilage-like tissue only formed at about one-half of the tendon-bone interface, this was attributed to a nonuniform distribution of the MSCs at the interface and the lack of certain transduction signals necessary to induce MSC differentiation. Overall, there is immense potential for treatment approaches that alter the biologic environment in tendinopathy and tendon tearing. The ability to deliver multipotent cells and chemical factors to the site of injury may improve the rate of healing and improve clinical results. Further studies are required to define the role of these novel treatments in humans.

Conclusion

The etiology of rotator cuff tendinopathy and degeneration is multifactorial and reflects extrinsic, intrinsic, and patient-specific factors. Despite improved surgical techniques, our understanding of tendon-to-bone healing remains incomplete, and the development of recurrent tears is a significant problem after repair of large rotator cuff tears. Extrinsic causes of tendinopathy include subacromial impingement, os acromiale and degenerative changes about the AC joint, glenohumeral instability, and trauma; however, intrinsic causes and repetitive microtrauma are believed to be the predominant factors responsible for tendon degeneration. Inflammatory factors are released during tendon degeneration, beginning the important process of healing that takes place via a complex cellular and growth factor-mediated response. Several treatment strategies that alter the balance between pro- and anti-inflammatory mediators, as well as those that deliver specific factors or pluripotent stem cells to the site of injury may evolve to change the way in which rotator cuff tendinopathy and tears are managed.

References

1. Almekinders LC, Almekinders SV. Outcome in the treatment of chronic overuse sports injuries—a retrospective study. *J Orthop Sports Phys Ther.* 1994;19:157-161.
2. Yamaguchi K, Ditsios K, Middleton WD, Hildebolt CF, Galatz LM, Teefey SA. The demographic and morphological features of rotator cuff disease—a comparison of asymptomatic and symptomatic shoulders. *J Bone Joint Surg Am.* 2006;88A:1699-1704.

3. Fukuda H, Hamada K, Yamanaka K. Pathology and pathogenesis of bursal-side rotator cuff tears viewed from en bloc histologic sections. *Clin Orthop Rel Res.* 1990;(254):75-80.

4. Nho SJ, Yadav H, Shindle MK, MacGillivray JD. Rotator cuff degeneration—etiology and pathogenesis. *Am J Sports Med.* 2008;36:987-993.

5. Abate M, Silbernagel KG, Siljeholm C, et al. Pathogenesis of tendinopathies: inflammation or degeneration? *Arthritis Res Ther.* 2009;11:15.

6. Millar NL, Hueber AJ, Reilly JH, et al. Inflammation is present in early human tendinopathy. *Am J Sports Med.* 2010;38:2085-2091.

7. Lewis JS. Rotator cuff tendinopathy: a model for the continuum of pathology and related management. *Br J Sports Med.* 2010;44:918-923.

8. Xu YH, Murrell GAC. The basic science of tendinopathy. *Clin Orthop Rel Res.* 2008;466:1528-1538.

9. Sano H, Ishii H, Trudel G, Uhthoff HK. Histologic evidence of degeneration at the insertion of 3 rotator cuff tendons: a comparative study with human cadaveric shoulders. *J Shoulder Elbow Surg.* 1999;8:574-579.

10. Yamaguchi K, Tetro AM, Blam O, Evanoff BA, Teefey SA, Middleton WD. Natural history of asymptomatic rotator cuff tears: a longitudinal analysis of asymptomatic tears detected sonographically. *J Shoulder Elbow Surg.* 2001;10:199-203.

11. Weber SC. Arthroscopic debridement and acromioplasty versus mini-open repair in the treatment of significant partial-thickness rotator cuff tears. *Arthroscopy.* 1999;15:126-131.

12. Almekinders LC, Temple JD. Etiology, diagnosis, and treatment of tendonitis: an analysis of the literature. *Med Sci Sports Exerc.* 1998;30:1183-1190.

13. Andres BM, Murrell GAC. Treatment of tendinopathy: what works, what does not, and what is on the horizon. *Clin Orthop Rel Res.* 2008;466:1539-1554.

14. Bisset L, Beller E, Jull G, Brooks P, Darnell R, Vicenzino B. Mobilisation with movement and exercise, corticosteroid injection, or wait and see for tennis elbow: randomised trial. *Br Med J.* 2006;333:939-941.

15. Bishop J, Klepps S, Lo IK, Bird J, Gladstone JN, Flatow EL. Cuff integrity after arthroscopic versus open rotator cuff repair: a prospective study. *J Shoulder Elbow Surg.* 2006;15:290-299.

16. Boileau P, Brassart N, Watkinson DJ, Carles M, Hatzidakis AM, Krishnan SG. Arthroscopic repair of full-thickness tears of the supraspinatus: does the tendon really heal? *J Bone Joint Surg Am.* 2005;87A:1229-1240.

17. Galatz LM, Ball CM, Teefey SA, Middleton WD, Yamaguchi K. The outcome and repair integrity of completely arthroscopically repaired large and massive rotator cuff tears. *J Bone Joint Surg Am.* 2004;86A:219-224.

18. Gerber C, Fuchs B, Hodler J. The results of repair of massive tears of the rotator cuff. *J Bone Joint Surg Am.* 2000;82A:505-515.

19. Lafosse L, Brozska R, Toussaint B, Gobezie R. The outcome and structural integrity of arthroscopic rotator cuff repair with use of the double-row suture anchor technique. *J Bone Joint Surg Am.* 2007;89A:1533-1541.

20. Maffulli N, Khan KM, Puddu G. Overuse tendon conditions: time to change a confusing terminology. *Arthroscopy.* 1998;14:840-843.

21. Uhthoff HK, Sano H. Pathology of failure of the rotator cuff tendon. *Orthop Clin North Am.* 1997;28:31-41.

22. Chard MD, Cawston TE, Riley GP, Gresham GA, Hazleman BL. Rotator cuff degeneration and lateral epicondylitis—a comparative histological study. *Ann Rheum Dis.* 1994;53:30-34.

23. Molloy TJ, Kemp MW, Wang Y, Murrell GAC. Microarray analysis of the tendinopathic rat supraspinatus tendon: glutamate signaling and its potential role in tendon degeneration. *J Appl Physiol.* 2006;101:1702-1709.

24. Khan KM, Cook JL, Bonar F, Harcourt P, Astrom M. Histopathology of common tendinopathies—update and implications for clinical management. *Sports Med.* 1999;27:393-408.

25. Uhthoff HK, Matsumoto F. Rotator cuff tendinopathy. *Sports Med Arthrosc.* 2000;8:56-68.

26. Nirschl RP, Pettrone FA. Tennis elbow—surgical treatment of lateral epicondylitis. *J Bone Joint Surg Am.* 1979;61:832-839.

27. Kannus P, Jozsa L. Histopathological changes preceding spontaneous rupture of a tendon—a controlled-study of 891 patients. *J Bone Joint Surg Am.* 1991;73A:1507-1525.

28. Riley GP, Goddard MJ, Hazleman BL. Histopathological assessment and pathological significance of matrix degeneration in supraspinatus tendons. *Rheumatology.* 2001;40:229-230.

29. Longo UG, Franceschi F, Ruzzini L, et al. Light microscopic histology of supraspinatus tendon ruptures. *Knee Surg Sports Traumatol Arthrosc.* 2007;15:1390-1394.

30. Uhthoff HK, Trudel G, Himori K. Relevance of pathology and basic research to the surgeon treating rotator cuff disease. *J Orthop Sci.* 2003;8:449-456.

31. Sano H, Ishii H, Yeadon A, Backman DS, Brunet JA, Uhthoff HK. Degeneration at the insertion weakens the tensile strength of the supraspinatus tendon: a comparative mechanical and histologic study of the bone-tendon complex. *J Orthop Res.* 1997;15:719-726.

32. Cook JL, Purdam CR. Is tendon pathology a continuum? A pathology model to explain the clinical presentation of load-induced tendinopathy. *Br J Sports Med.* 2009;43:409-416.

33. Neer CS. Anterior acromioplasty for chronic impingement syndrome in shoulder—a preliminary report. *J Bone Joint Surg Am.* 1972;A54:41-50.

34. MacGillvray JD, Fealy S, Potter HG, O'Brien SJ. Multiplanar analysis of acromion morphology. *Am J Sports Med.* 1998;26:836-840.

35. Sammarco VJ. Os acromiale: frequency, anatomy, and clinical implications. *J Bone Joint Surg Am.* 2000;82A:394-400.

36. Solem-Bertoft E, Thuomas KA, Westerberg CE. The influence of scapular retraction and protraction on the width of the subacromial space—an MRI study. *Clin Orthop Rel Res.* 1993:99-103.

37. Prescher A. Anatomical basics, variations, and degenerative changes of the shoulder joint and shoulder girdle. *Eur J Radiol.* 2000;35:88-102.

38. Bigliani LU, Morrison DS, April EW. The morphology of the acromion and rotator cuff impingement. *Orthop Trans.* 1986;10:228.

39. Walch G, Boileau P, Noel E, Donell ST. Impingement of the deep surface of the supraspinatus tendon on the posterosuperior glenoid rim: an arthroscopic study. *J Shoulder Elbow Surg.* 1992;1:238-245.

40. Nicholson GP, Goodman DA, Flatow EL, Bigliani LU. The acromion: morphologic condition and age-related changes. A study of 420 scapulas. *J Shoulder Elbow Surg.* 1996;5:1-11.

41. Shah NN, Bayliss NC, Malcolm A. Shape of the acromion: congenital or acquired—a macroscopic, radiographic, and microscopic study of acromion. *J Shoulder Elbow Surg.* 2001;10:309-316.

42. Swain RA, Wilson FD, Harsha DM. The os acromiale: another cause of impingement. *Med Sci Sports Exerc.* 1996;28:1459-1462.

43. Ouellette H, Thomas BJ, Kassarjian A, et al. Re-examining the association of os acromiale with supraspinatus and infraspinatus tears. *Skeletal Radiol.* 2007;36:835-839.

44. Hawkins RJ, Kennedy JC. Impingement syndrome in athletes. *Am J Sports Med.* 1980;8:151-158.

45. Shaffer BS. Painful conditions of the acromioclavicular joint. *J Am Acad Orthop Surg.* 1999;7:176-188.

46. Nyffeler RW, Werner CNL, Sukthankar A, Schmid MR, Gerber C. Association of a large lateral extension of the acromion with rotator cuff tears. *J Bone Joint Surg Am.* 2006;88A:800-805.

47. Konno N, Itoi E, Kido T, Sano A, Urayama M, Sato K. Glenoid osteophyte and rotator cuff tears: an anatomic study. *J Shoulder Elbow Surg.* 2002;11:72-79.

48. Davidson PA, ElAttrache NS, Jobe CM, Jobe FW. Rotator cuff and posterior-superior glenoid labrum injury associated with increased glenohumeral motion: a new site of impingement. *J Shoulder Elbow Surg.* 1995;4:384-390.

49. Budoff JE, Nirschl RP, Ilahi OA, Rodin DM. Internal impingement in the etiology of rotator cuff tendinosis revisited. *Arthroscopy.* 2003;19:810-814.

50. Jobe CM. Posterior superior glenoid impingement—expanded spectrum. *Arthroscopy.* 1995;11:530-536.

51. Garofalo R, Karlsson J, Nordenson U, Cesari E, Conti M, Castagna A. Anterior-superior internal impingement of the shoulder: an evidence-based review. *Knee Surg Sports Traumatol Arthrosc.* 2010;18:1688-1693.

52. Meister K. Injuries to the shoulder in the throwing athlete. Part one: biomechanics/pathophysiology/classification of injury. *Am J Sports Med.* 2000;28:265-275.

53. Jobe FW, Giangarra CE, Kvitne RS, Glousman RE. Anterior capsulolabral reconstruction of the shoulder in athletes in overhand sports. *Am J Sports Med.* 1991;19:428-434.

54. Mihata T, Lee YS, McGarry MH, Abe M, Lee TQ. Excessive humeral external rotation results in increased shoulder laxity. *Am J Sports Med.* 2004;32:1278-1285.

55. Paley KJ, Jobe FW, Pink MM, Kvitne RS, ElAttrache NS. Arthroscopic findings in the overhand throwing athlete: evidence for posterior internal impingement of the rotator cuff. *Arthroscopy.* 2000;16:35-40.

56. Grossman MG, Tibone JE, McGarry MH, Schneider DJ, Veneziani S, Lee TQ. A cadaveric model of the throwing shoulder: a possible etiology of superior labrum anterior-to-posterior lesions. *J Bone Joint Surg Am.* 2005;87A:824-831.

57. Burkhart SS, Morgan CD, Ben Kibler W. The disabled throwing shoulder: spectrum of pathology. Part 1: pathoanatomy and biomechanics. *Arthroscopy.* 2003;19:404-420.

58. Bhatia DN, de Beer JF, du Toit DF. Coracoid process anatomy: implications in radiographic imaging and surgery. *Clin Anat.* 2007;20:774-784.

59. Schulz CU, Anetzberger H, Glaser C. Coracoid tip position on frontal radiographs of the shoulder: a predictor of common shoulder pathologies? *Br J Radiol.* 2005;78:1005-1008.

60. Bedi A, Fox AJS, Harris PE, et al. Diabetes mellitus impairs tendon-bone healing after rotator cuff repair. *J Shoulder Elbow Surg.* 2010;19:978-988.

61. Fox AJS, Bedi A, Deng XH, et al. Diabetes mellitus alters the mechanical properties of the native tendon in an experimental rat model. *J Orthop Res.* 2011; in press.

62. Chen AL, Shapiro JA, Ahn AK, Zuckerman JD, Cuomo F. Rotator cuff repair in patients with type I diabetes mellitus. *J Shoulder Elbow Surg.* 2003;12:416-421.

63. Namdari S, Green A. Range of motion limitation after rotator cuff repair. *J Shoulder Elbow Surg.* 2010;19:290-296.

64. Galatz LM, Silva MJ, Rothermich SY, Zaegel MA, Havlioglu N, Thomopoulos S. Nicotine delays tendon-to-bone healing in a rat shoulder model. *J Bone Joint Surg Am.* 2006;88A:2027-2034.

65. Leow YH, Maibach HI. Cigarette smoking, cutaneous vasculature, and tissue oxygen. *Clin Dermatol.* 1998;16:579-584.

66. Sloan A, Hussain I, Maqsood M, Eremin O, El-Sheemy M. The effects of smoking on fracture healing. *Surg J R Coll Surg Edinb Irel*. 2010;8:111-116.

67. Baumgarten KM, Gerlach D, Galatz LM, et al. Cigarette smoking increases the risk for rotator cuff tears. *Clin Orthop Rel Res*. 2010;468:1534-1541.

68. Cohen DB, Kawamura S, Ehteshami JR, Rodeo SA. Indomethacin and celecoxib impair rotator cuff tendon-to-bone healing. *Am J Sports Med*. 2006;34:362-369.

69. Haraldsson BT, Langberg H, Aagaard P, et al. Corticosteroids reduce the tensile strength of isolated collagen fascicles. *Am J Sports Med*. 2006;34:1992-1997.

70. Tillander B, Franzen LE, Karlsson MH, Norlin R. Effect of steroid injections on the rotator cuff: an experimental study in rats. *J Shoulder Elbow Surg*. 1999;8:271-274.

71. Mikolyzk DK, Wei AS, Tonino P, et al. Effect of corticosteroids on the biomechanical strength of rat rotator cuff tendon. *J Bone Joint Surg Am*. 2009;91A:1172-1180.

72. Wong MWN, Tang YN, Fu SC, Lee KM, Chan KM. Triamcinolone suppresses human tenocyte cellular activity and collagen synthesis. *Clin Orthop Rel Res*. 2004:277-281.

73. Wong MWN, Tang YYN, Lee SKM, Fu BSC, Chan BP, Chan CKM. Effect of dexamethasone on cultured human tenocytes and its reversibility by platelet-derived growth factor. *J Bone Joint Surg Am*. 2003;85A:1914-1920.

74. Koester MC, Dunn WR, Kuhn JE, Spindler KP. The efficacy of subacromial corticosteroid injection in the treatment of rotator cuff disease: a systematic review. *J Am Acad Orthop Surg*. 2007;15:3-11.

75. Karthikeyan S, Kwong HT, Upadhyay PK, Parsons N, Drew SJ, Griffin D. A double-blind randomised controlled study comparing subacromial injection of tenoxicam or methylprednisolone in patients with subacromial impingement. *J Bone Joint Surg Br*. 2010;92B:77-82.

76. Borderie P, Marcelli C, Herisson C, Simon L. Spontaneous rotator cuff tear during fluoroquinolone antibiotics treatment—a report of 2 cases. *Arthritis Rheum*. 1993;36:S163.

77. Khaliq Y, Zhanel GG. Fluoroquinolone-associated tendinopathy: a critical review of the literature. *Clin Infect Dis*. 2003;36:1404-1410.

78. Movin T, Gad A, Guntner P, Foldhazy Z, Rolf C. Pathology of the Achilles tendon in association with ciprofloxacin treatment. *Foot Ankle Int*. 1997;18:297-299.

79. Sendzik J, Shakibaei M, Schafer-Korting M, Stahlmann R. Fluoroquinolones cause changes in extracellular matrix, signalling proteins, metalloproteinases and caspase-3 in cultured human tendon cells. *Toxicology*. 2005;212:24-36.

80. Corps AN, Harrall RL, Curry VA, Hazleman BL, Riley GP. Contrasting effects of fluoroquinolone antibiotics on the expression of the collagenases, matrix metalloproteinases (MMP)-1 and-13, in human tendon-derived cells. *Rheumatology*. 2005;44:1514-1517.

81. Yamamoto N, Muraki T, Sperling JW, et al. Contact between the coracoacromial arch and the rotator cuff tendons in nonpathologic situations: a cadaveric study. *J Shoulder Elbow Surg*. 2010;19:681-687.

82. Kim HM, Dahiya N, Teefey SA, et al. Location and initiation of degenerative rotator cuff tears. An analysis of three hundred and sixty shoulders. *J Bone Joint Surg Am*. 2010;92A:1088-1096.

83. Burkhart SS, Esch JC, Jolson RS. The rotator crescent and rotator cable—an anatomic description of the shoulders suspension bridge. *Arthroscopy*. 1993;9:611-616.

84. Ozaki J, Fujimoto S, Nakagawa Y, Masuhara K, Tamai S. Tears of the rotator cuff of the shoulder associated with pathological changes in the acromion—a study in cadavers. *J Bone Joint Surg Am*. 1988;70A:1224-1230.

85. Ogata S, Uhthoff HK. Acromial enthesopathy and rotator cuff tear—a radiologic and histologic postmortem investigation of the coracoacromial arch. *Clin Orthop Rel Res*. 1990;(254):39-48.

86. Codman EA. *The Shoulder: Rupture of the Supraspinatus Tendon and Other Lesions in or About the Subacromial Bursa*. Boston, MA: Thomas Todd; 1934.

87. Hashimoto T, Nobuhara K, Hamada T. Pathologic evidence of degeneration as a primary cause of rotator cuff tear. *Clin Orthop Rel Res*. 2003;(415):111-120.

88. Gotoh M, Hamada K, Yamakawa H, Tomonaga A, Inoue A, Fukuda HO. Significance of granulation tissue in torn supraspinatus insertions: an immunohistochemical study with antibodies against interleukin-1 beta, cathepsin D, and matrix metalloprotease-1. *J Orthop Res*. 1997;15:33-39.

89. Longo UG, Franceschi F, Ruzzini L, et al. Histopathology of the supraspinatus tendon in rotator cuff tears. *Am J Sports Med*. 2008;36:533-538.

90. Carpenter JE, Thomopoulos S, Flanagan CL, DeBano CM, Soslowsky LJ. Rotator cuff defect healing: a biomechanical and histologic analysis in an animal model. *J Shoulder Elbow Surg*. 1998;7:599-605.

91. Hays PL, Kawamura S, Deng XH, et al. The role of macrophages in early healing of a tendon graft in a bone tunnel. *J Bone Joint Surg Am*. 2008;90A:565-579.

92. Galatz LM, Sandell LJ, Rothermich SY, et al. Characteristics of the rat supraspinatus tendon during tendon-to-bone healing after acute injury. *J Orthop Res*. 2006;24:541-550.

93. Choi HR, Kondo S, Hirose K, Ishiguro N, Hasegawa Y, Iwata H. Expression and enzymatic activity of MMP-2 during healing process of the acute supraspinatus tendon tear in rabbits. *J Orthop Res*. 2002;20:927-933.

94. Bedi A, Kovacevic D, Hettrich C, et al. The effect of matrix metalloproteinase inhibition on tendon-to-bone healing in a rotator cuff repair model. *J Shoulder Elbow Surg*. 2010;19:384-391.

95. Rodeo SA, Arnoczky SP, Torzilli PA, Hidaka C, Warren RF. Tendon-healing in a bone tunnel—a biomechanical and histological study in the dog. *J Bone Joint Surg Am.* 1993;75A:1795-1803.

96. Axelrad TW, Einhorn TA. Bone morphogenetic proteins in orthopaedic surgery. *Cytokine Growth Factor Rev.* 2009;20:481-488.

97. Rodeo SA, Potter HG, Kawamura S, Turner AS, Kim HJ, Atkinson BL. Biologic augmentation of rotator cuff tendon-healing with use of a mixture of osteoinductive growth factors. *J Bone Joint Surg Am.* 2007;89A:2485-2497.

98. Seeherman HJ, Archambault JM, Rodeo SA, et al. rhBMP-12 accelerates healing of rotator cuff repairs in a sheep model. *J Bone Joint Surg Am.* 2008;90A:2206-2219.

99. Murray DH, Kubiak EN, Jazrawi LM, et al. The effect of cartilage-derived morphogenetic protein 2 on initial healing of a rotator cuff defect in a rat model. *J Shoulder Elbow Surg.* 2007;16:251-254.

100. Lou JR, Tu YZ, Burns M, Silva MJ, Manske P. BMP-12 gene transfer augmentation of lacerated tendon repair. *J Orthop Res.* 2001;19:1199-1202.

101. Lin TW, Cardenas L, Glaser DL, Soslowsky LJ. Tendon healing in interleukin-4 and interleukin-6 knockout mice. *J Biomech.* 2006;39:61-69.

102. Perry SM, McIlhenny SE, Hoffman MC, Soslowsky LJ. Inflammatory and angiogenic mRNA levels are altered in a supraspinatus tendon overuse animal model. *J Shoulder Elbow Surg.* 2005;14:79S-83S.

103. Magra M, Maffulli N. Matrix metalloproteases: a role in overuse tendinopathies. *Br J Sports Med.* 2005;39:789-791.

104. Lo IKY, Marchuk LL, Hollinshead R, Hart DA, Frank CB. Matrix metalloproteinase and tissue inhibitor of matrix metalloproteinase mRNA levels are specifically altered in torn rotator cuff tendons. *Am J Sports Med.* 2004;32:1223-1229.

105. Bedi A, Fox AJS, Kovacevic D, Deng XH, Warren RF, Rodeo SA. Doxycycline-mediated inhibition of matrix metalloproteinases improves healing after rotator cuff repair. *Am J Sports Med.* 2010;38:308-317.

106. Thornton GM, Shao X, Chung M, et al. Changes in mechanical loading lead to tendon-specific alterations in MMP and TIMP expression: Influence of stress deprivation and intermittent cyclic hydrostatic compression on rat supraspinatus and Achilles tendons. *Br J Sports Med.* 2010;44:698-703.

107. Brockis JG. The blood supply of the flexor and extensor tendons of the fingers in man. *J Bone Joint Surg Br.* 1953;35:131-138.

108. Moseley HF, Goldie I. The arterial pattern of the rotator cuff of the shoulder. *J Bone Joint Surg Br.* 1963;45:780-789.

109. Rothman R. Vascular anatomy of human rotator cuff. *Anat Rec.* 1964;148:329.

110. Lohr JF, Uhthoff HK. The microvascular pattern of the supraspinatus tendon. *Clin Orthop Rel Res.* 1990:35-38.

111. Levy O, Relwani J, Zaman T, Even T, Venkateswaran B, Copeland S. Measurement of blood flow in the rotator cuff using laser Doppler flowmetry. *J Bone Joint Surg Br.* 2008;90B:893-898.

112. Fealy S, Adler RS, Drakos MC, et al. Patterns of vascular and anatomical response after rotator cuff repair. *Am J Sports Med.* 2006;34:120-127.

113. Hou Y, Mao ZB, Wei XL, et al. Effects of transforming growth factor-beta 1 and vascular endothelial growth factor 165 gene transfer on Achilles tendon healing. *Matrix Biol.* 2009;28:324-335.

114. Zhang F, Liu H, Stile F, et al. Effect of vascular endothelial growth factor on rat Achilles tendon healing. *Plast Reconstr Surg.* 2003;112:1613-1619.

115. Hamada Y, Katoh S, Hibino N, Kosaka H, Hamada D, Yasui N. Effects of monofilament nylon coated with basic fibroblast growth factor on endogenous intrasynovial flexor tendon healing. *J Hand Surg [Am].* 2006;31A:530-540.

116. Dahlgren LA, Mohammed HO, Nixon AJ. Temporal expression of growth factors and matrix molecules in healing tendon lesions. *J Orthop Res.* 2005;23:84-92.

117. Benson RT, McDonnell SM, Knowles HJ, Rees JL, Carr AJ, Hulley PA. Tendinopathy and tears of the rotator cuff are associated with hypoxia and apoptosis. *J Bone Joint Surg Br.* 2010;92B:448-453.

118. Ide J, Kikukawa K, Hirose J, et al. The effect of a local application of fibroblast growth factor-2 on tendon-to-bone remodeling in rats with acute injury and repair of the supraspinatus tendon. *J Shoulder Elbow Surg.* 2009;18:391-398.

119. Gulotta LV, Kovacevic D, Ehteshami JR, Dagher E, Packer JD, Rodeo SA. Application of bone marrow-derived mesenchymal stem cells in a rotator cuff repair model. *Am J Sports Med.* 2009;37:2126-2133.

120. Gulotta LV, Kovacevic D, Montgomery S, Ehteshami JR, Packer JD, Rodeo SA. Stem cells genetically modified with the developmental gene MT1-MMP improve regeneration of the supraspinatus tendon-to-bone insertion site. *Am J Sports Med.* 2010;38:1429-1437.

121. Uggen C, Dines J, McGarry M, Grande D, Lee T, Limpisvasti O. The effect of recombinant human platelet-derived growth factor BB-coated sutures on rotator cuff healing in a sheep model. *Arthroscopy.* 2010;26:1456-1462.

122. Obaid H, Connell D. Cell therapy in tendon disorders. What is the current evidence? *Am J Sports Med.* 2010;38:2123-2132.

123. De Bari C, Dell'Accio F, Tylzanowski P, Luyten FP. Multipotent mesenchymal stem cells from adult human synovial membrane. *Arthritis Rheum.* 2001;44:1928-1942.

124. Fan JB, Varshney RR, Ren L, Cai DZ, Wang DA. Synovium-derived mesenchymal stem cells: a new cell source for musculoskeletal regeneration. *Tissue Eng Part B-Rev.* 2009;15:75-86.

125. Williams JT, Southerland SS, Souza J, Calcutt AF, Cartledge RG. Cells isolated from adult human skeletal muscle capable of differentiating into multiple mesodermal phenotypes. *Am Surg.* 1999;65:22-26.

126. Awad HA, Butler DL, Boivin GP, et al. Autologous mesenchymal stem cell-mediated repair of tendon. *Tissue Eng.* 1999;5:267-277.

127. Hankemeier S, van Griensven M, Ezechieli M, et al. Tissue engineering of tendons and ligaments by human bone marrow stromal cells in a liquid fibrin matrix in immunodeficient rats: results of a histologic study. *Arch Orthop Trauma Surg.* 2007;127:815-821.

128. Connell D, Datir A, Alyas F, Curtis M. Treatment of lateral epicondylitis using skin-derived tenocyte-like cells. *Br J Sports Med.* 2009;43:293-298.

129. Chen JM, Willers C, Xu JK, Wang A, Zheng MH. Autologous tenocyte therapy using porcine-derived bioscaffolds for massive rotator cuff defect in rabbits. *Tissue Eng.* 2007;13:1479-1491.

130. Dines JS, Grande DA, Dines DM. Tissue engineering and rotator cuff tendon healing. *J Shoulder Elbow Surg.* 2007;16:204S-207S.

131. Lim JK, Hui J, Li L, Thambyah A, Goh J, Lee EH. Enhancement of tendon graft osteointegration using mesenchymal stem cells in a rabbit model of anterior cruciate ligament reconstruction. *Arthroscopy.* 2004;20:899-910.

132. Ouyang HW, Goh JCH, Lee EH. Use of bone marrow stromal cells for tendon graft-to-bone healing—histological and immunohistochemical studies in a rabbit model. *Am J Sports Med.* 2004;32:321-327.

CHAPTER 4

MUSCLE DEGENERATION IN ROTATOR CUFF TEARS

Xuhui Liu, MD; Dominique Laron, MD; and Brian T. Feeley, MD

Central to understanding the pathophysiology of rotator cuff disease is developing an understanding of the changes that occur in the muscle itself following a rotator cuff tear. Unlike tendon degeneration, which has been a focus of study for many years, relatively few studies have evaluated the processes that occur in the muscle following a rotator cuff tear. However, it has recently been shown that the characteristic changes that occur—muscle atrophy and fatty infiltration—are independent predictors of poor function and high retear rates following rotator cuff repair. This chapter will review the basic science and clinical relevance of muscle atrophy and fatty infiltration in the setting of rotator cuff tears.

MUSCLE STRUCTURE AND REGULATION OF MUSCLE SIZE AND ATROPHY

Myocytes and Extracellular Matrix

Although a thorough description of muscle structure and function is beyond the scope of this chapter, a basic understanding of muscle cell structure and function is important when discussing the harmful changes that occur after a rotator cuff tear. Muscle is a unique and dynamic organ that is able to regulate its size based on a diverse set of signals including growth hormones, signal transduction pathways, and mechanical signals. Muscles respond to growth stimuli by increasing protein synthesis to develop larger mass without an increase in myocyte number. The myocyte itself is a unique cell that enables the function of muscle to occur.

Different from most other cells in the human body, the myocyte is a multinucleate cell with a mature myocyte often containing more than 100 nuclei. The intracellular matrix of myocytes are made of myofibrils, which are long chains of sarcomeres—the contractile units of the myocytes (Figure 4-1). In addition to myocytes, there are a number of other types of cells, including

Ma CB, Feeley BT, eds.
*Basic Principles and Operative Management
of the Rotator Cuff (pp 49-60)*
© 2012 SLACK Incorporated

Figure 4-1. Diagram of a muscle unit. A muscle cell is composed of multiple nuclei with myofibrils that are the contractile units of the muscle. Actin makes up the thin filament, and myosin makes up the thick filament. The sarcomere contracts as the muscle fires due to the actions of the myosin and actin. (Reprinted with permission of Julianne Ho.)

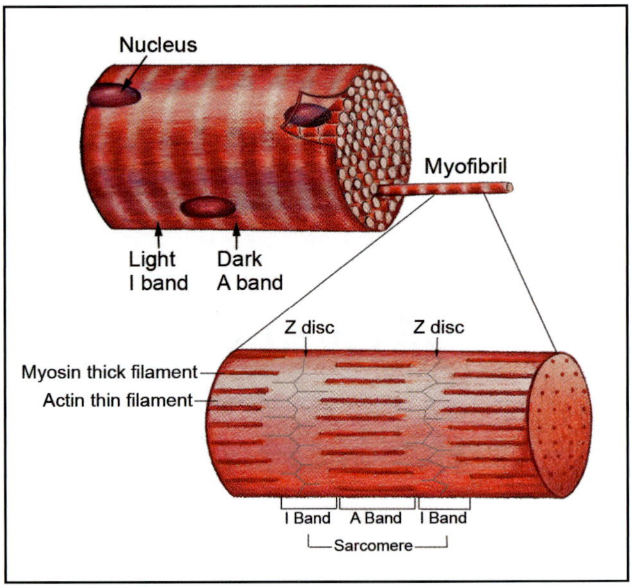

fibroblasts, blood vessel endothelium cells, and muscle progenitor or stem cells (satellite cells and muscle special cells). Muscle satellite cells are thought to be primary progenitor cells in skeletal muscle and are responsible for replacing dying myocyte nuclei by merging into adjacent myocytes.[1] Satellite cells can also form new myocytes, a process that is mainly seen in muscle development and regeneration.[2]

Myofibers are connected to each other through the extracellular matrix (ECM). Muscle ECM has a central role in cell communication and transduction of mechanical force signals. The ECM also is important in regulating muscle differentiation, growth, repair, and remodeling. It stores various growth factors and other bioactive molecules, including active and inactive proteases, which can be released and activated based on appropriate signals. Significant remodeling of ECM, including increased collagenous connective tissue (fibrosis) and adipose tissue (fatty infiltration), occurs during muscle atrophy. A group of zinc or calcium-dependent proteinases, called matrix metalloproteinases (MMPs), is believed to play an important role in ECM remodeling in skeletal muscle.[3] Recent studies, including our own work, have revealed significantly increased expression of important members of MMPs, including MMP-2, MMP-9, and MMP-13 in muscle atrophy.[4] These factors likely result in increased breakdown of the ECM in muscle atrophy states. MMPs have also been implicated in tendon degeneration (see Chapter 2 for a full discussion) and degradation in other disease states as well.[5]

Molecular Regulation of Muscle Size and Protein Synthesis

Although new mature myocytes are rarely added to the muscle itself, muscle is a dynamic structure that must respond to changes in demand throughout daily activity and life. Regulation of muscle size is based on the control of protein synthesis at a cellular level. These pathways are complex and are likely intertwined to control protein synthesis and breakdown. Many factors, including mechanical signals, growth hormones, insulin-like growth factor (IGF), and nuclear factor-kappa-B (NF-κB), have been implicated in regulating muscle size.[6] Alterations in these signals can cause an increase in muscle size or a decrease in muscle size, usually through protein degradation pathways.

The majority of the studies using animal models to evaluate muscle atrophy in a rotator cuff tear model have focused on the expression of muscle atrophy genes that alter the expression of ubiquitin ligases that increase protein degradation. It is hypothesized through other models of muscle atrophy that NF-κB has a central role in the development of muscle atrophy through 3 principal pathways[7]:

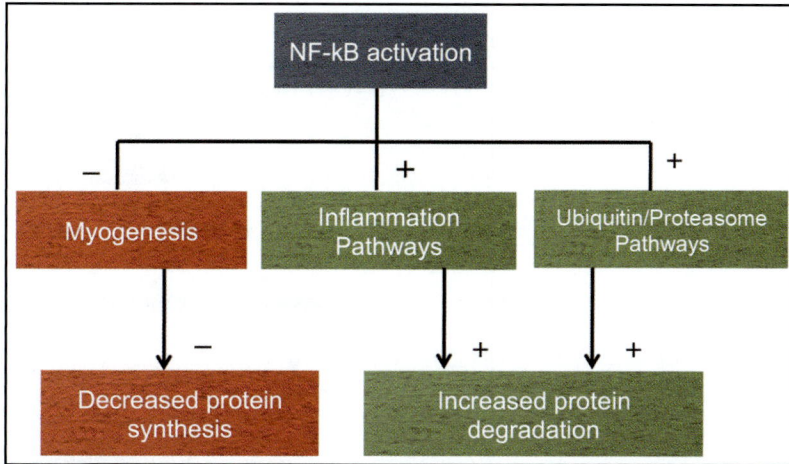

Figure 4-2. NF-κB has a central role in the development of muscle atrophy through 3 principal pathways: 1) it can augment the expression of several proteins of the ubiquitin-proteasome system that are involved in the degradation of specific muscle proteins; 2) NF-κB may increase the expression of inflammation-related molecules, which directly or indirectly promote muscle wasting; 3) NF-κB can interfere with the process of myogenic differentiation that may be required for regeneration of atrophied skeletal muscles.

1. It can augment the expression of several proteins of the ubiquitin-proteasome system that are involved in the degradation of specific muscle proteins.

2. NF-κB may increase the expression of inflammation-related molecules, which directly or indirectly promote muscle wasting.

3. NF-κB can interfere with the process of myogenic differentiation that may be required for regeneration of atrophied skeletal muscles (Figure 4-2).[8]

The ubiquitin-proteasome system is the primary regulator of protein breakdown, which provides a mechanism for selective degradation of regulatory and structural proteins. The key enzymes in this system are ubiquitin ligases.[9] NF-kB and forkhead transcription factor (FOXO) are responsible for increased expression of these proteins.[10,11] Two inducible E3 ubiquitin ligases, atrogin-1 (also known as MAFbx) and muscle ring finger protein 1 (MuRF1), have been identified as responsible for the degradation of the bulk of skeletal muscle in multiple different atrophying conditions.[12-14] In addition, it has been shown that these factors are upregulated in patients with chronic supraspinatus tears. Targeted deletion of MuRF1 and atrogin-1 resulted in reduced muscle atrophy in response to denervation and hindlimb suspension models. It has been shown that NF-κB acts as an inducible regulator of MURF1 and atrogin-1, thus supporting a central role for NF-κB, MuRF1, and atrogin-1 in the protein degradation found in the development of muscle atrophy.[7]

Given that muscle must respond to mechanical loading, it makes sense that muscle can alter its protein regulation based on mechanical signaling. Recent studies during the past 10 years have focused on how muscle is able to transfer the signal of mechanical load to the upregulation of muscle protein synthesis. Multiple studies have suggested that Akt/mammalian target of rapamycin (mTOR) pathway plays a central role in signal transduction pathway network in muscle size regulation.[15-20] mTOR serves as a downstream effector in the IGF pathway, insulin pathway, testosterone pathway, and mechanical pathways in regulating muscle protein synthesis. It is also involved in muscle protein degradation by interfering with major muscle protein degradation pathways, including autophagy and ubiquitin-proteasome pathways (Figure 4-3). These factors increase protein synthesis. Interestingly, phosphorylation of Akt also inhibits FOXO translocation, thereby inhibiting activation

Figure 4-3. Schematic of the role of the Akt/mTOR pathway in the regulation of muscle atrophy.

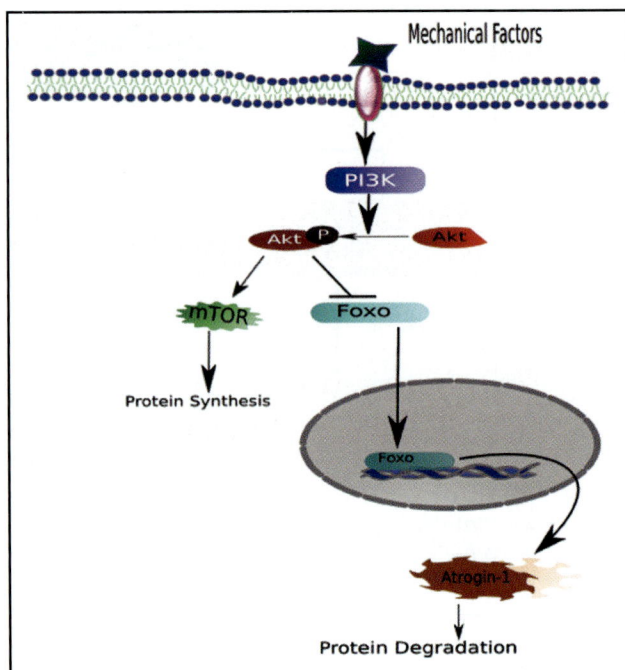

of atrogin-1 and MuRF and protein degradation.[21,22] In the setting of mechanical unloading, growth factors such as IGF-1 and mechanical growth factor are decreased, and there is marked downregulation of this pathway, leading to protein degradation and muscle atrophy.[23] These studies have been performed in hindlimb suspension and other typical models of muscle atrophy but only recently have been studied in a rotator cuff model. In our laboratory, we have demonstrated that this pathway demonstrates altered expression in a rat model of massive rotator cuff tears.[24] Given its ability to be regulated by pharmacologic inhibition, this pathway represents an interesting potential target for modulating the atrophy after a rotator cuff repair.

FATTY INFILTRATION AND MUSCLE INJURY

It has been widely observed that the rupture of the rotator cuff tendons often results in the degeneration of the cuff muscles with an increase in the degree of fatty infiltration that is roughly proportional to the size of the tear. Especially in elderly populations and following massive tears, cuff muscles often demonstrate marked muscle atrophy and fatty infiltration as seen by both computed tomography and magnetic resonance imaging (MRI) and on a gross level at the time of surgical intervention (Figure 4-4). Histological evidence of fatty infiltration has been further confirmed through muscle biopsies at the time of surgical intervention and in multiple animal studies. Stains of muscle following chronic and massive rotator cuff tears have demonstrated high amounts of fat that correlate with levels of fatty infiltration seen on radiologic imaging. Goutallier and colleagues proposed grading fatty infiltration based on the ratio of fat to muscle.[25] Stage 0 corresponds to normal-appearing muscle; Stage 1 demonstrates muscle with fatty streaking; in Stage 2, there are higher levels of fatty infiltration but muscle is still the dominant feature; Stage 3 exhibits equal levels of fat and muscle; and in Stage 4, fat is the predominant feature. Stage 2 is considered pathologic and major, as Stage 0 and 1 may be observed in otherwise normal rotator cuffs. This grading system is important, as the level of fatty infiltration has been shown to be significantly increased along with tear severity. This system also correlates the decrease in muscle function seen following massive tears with the levels of fatty infiltration at time of repair. The quantities of fatty infiltration are not only

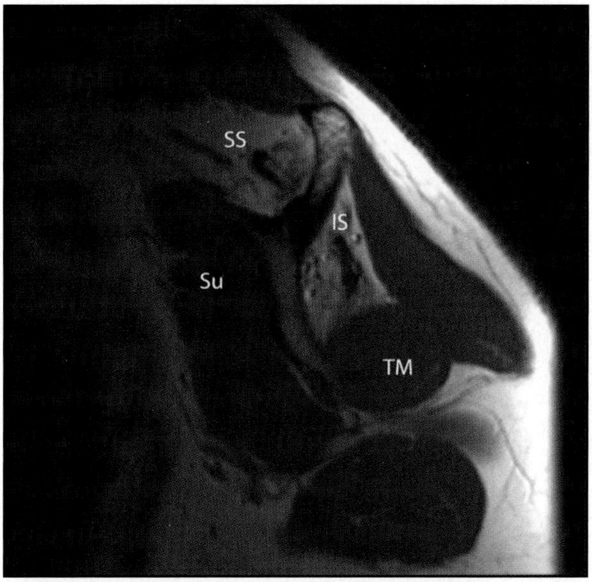

Figure 4-4. MRI T1 sagittal demonstrating marked muscle atrophy in the supraspinatus (SS) and infraspinatus (IS), with normal muscle in the subscapularis (Su) and teres minor (TM).

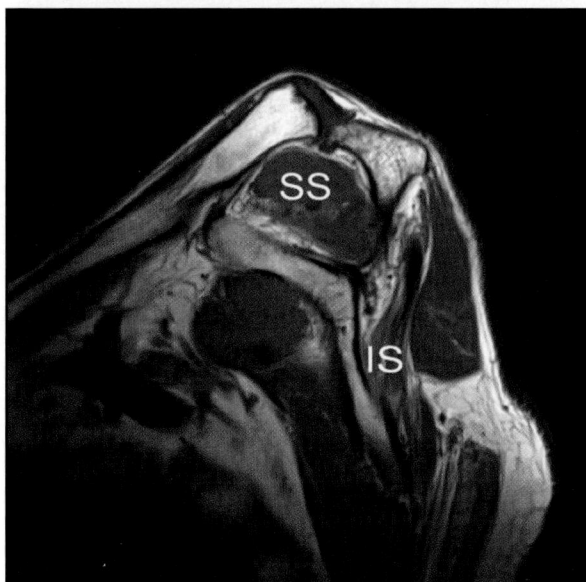

Figure 4-5. Example of a patient with increased muscle atrophy and fatty infiltration in the setting of an isolated supraspinatus tear. On MRI evaluation, there is normal muscle bulk and minimal atrophy in the supraspinatus (SS), but marked atrophy and fatty infiltration of the infraspinatus (IS). On arthroscopic evaluation, there was a moderate-sized tear of the supraspinatus, but the infraspinatus was intact.

important due to their effects on decreased muscle function, but there is a level of fatty infiltration that is irreversible, even following repair. Patients graded with pathologic levels of fatty infiltration exhibit limited range of active external rotation compared to those graded 2 or less. Fatty infiltration is an important predictor of disease progression and may potentially predict surgical outcome. Thus, the gross and radiologic appearance of fatty infiltration may serve as a basis to guide treatment and intervention.

Despite the importance of fatty infiltration in the outcomes of rotator cuff repair, little is known about the underlying etiology of this process. It has been postulated that denervation of the supraspinatus causes fatty changes within the muscle, but even in the setting of an intact nerve, it has been found that the supraspinatus and infraspinatus can undergo fatty infiltration. In a recent study, Cheung and colleagues found that substantial fatty infiltration of the infraspinatus can be seen even in the absence of an infraspinatus tear if there is a supraspinatus tear present (Figure 4-5).[26] In addition, it is not clear what cells are responsible for the increase in fat in the muscle following the formation of a rotator cuff tear. It is hypothesized that one of the stem cell populations that reside in adult skeletal muscle, such as satellite cells, muscle-derived stem cells, or muscle side population cells, is responsible for adipogenic differentiation, but this has not been proven. There are many factors that have been found to induce adipogenic differentiation of muscle stem cells including oxidative stress,[27] aging,[28] and muscle degeneration.[29] Finally, the role of denervation on adipogenic differentiation has not been determined.

Understanding the molecular pathways responsible for fatty infiltration will allow further research to determine potential pharmacologic interventions that can reverse this process following rotator cuff repair. One of the central regulators of adipogenesis is peroxisome proliferator-activated receptor γ (PPARγ). The nuclear receptor PPARγ is a ligand-activated transcription factor that plays an important role in the control of gene expression in multiple physiologic processes.[30] It was initially characterized as a central regulator of the development of adipose cells. PPARγ signaling has also been implicated in the control of cell proliferation, macrophage function, and immunity.[31] PPARγ is the dominant or "master" regulator of adipogenesis. It is induced during the differentiation of preadipocytes into adipocytes and is highly expressed in both brown and white adipose tissue. It functions in a transcriptional cascade that involves activation by Wnt, KLF2, CAAT/enhancer binding protein (C/EBP), and Add1/SREBP1c.[32,33] These proteins bind directly to the PPARγ promoter and induce many target genes involved in adipogenesis. It has been demonstrated that PPARγ is both sufficient and necessary for fat cell differentiation.[34]

Despite the increasing knowledge regarding the physiology of PPARγ in regard to adipogenesis, few studies have investigated the role of PPARγ in the development of skeletal muscle changes. It is known that, during muscle injury, C/EBP is activated in response to muscle injury and has a dual role in activating NF-κB activity as well as stimulating the development of PPARγ.[33] One recent study in a sheep model found that C/EBP and PPARγ expression was increased following transection of the rotator cuff.[35] Although this was promising, it is clearly difficult to use large animal studies to evaluate pharmacologic interventions on the PPARγ pathway. Interestingly, C/EBP also increases FOXO expression, which may enhance muscle atrophy.[31,35,36] In a mouse model of rotator cuff tears, Itoigawa and colleagues recently found increased expression of PPARγ and C/EBP from 7 to 28 days after creation of a rotator cuff tear, with concomitant increase in fat staining within the muscle.[37] The authors also found a decrease in the expression of Wnt10b, which may lead to adipogenic differentiation of myogenic stem cells.

In addition to the molecular changes that occur in the rotator cuff muscle following rotator cuff tears, there are morphologic changes that may account for some of the characteristic pathophysiologic changes that are found in the rotator cuff muscle. Meyer and colleagues demonstrated that changes in the pennate angle were found following rotator cuff tears in a sheep model.[38] Using electron microscopy, the authors found normal muscle fibers with unaltered myofibrillar structure, while interstitial fat and fibrous tissue had increased from 3.9% to 45.9% (p<0.0001) of the muscle volume. Geometric modeling showed that the increase of the pennation angle separated the muscle fiber bundles, and infiltrating fat cells filled the created space between the reoriented muscle fibers. The authors concluded that fatty infiltration is therefore not seen as a degenerative process but a necessary rearrangement of the tissue after macroarchitectural changes caused by musculotendinous retraction. Importantly, the authors found that these changes can be reversible with tension returned to the muscle-tendon unit, suggesting that repair may improve the outcomes by decreasing the degree of atrophy and fatty infiltration through mechanical and geometric means.[39]

MUSCLE FIBROSIS IN THE SETTING OF MUSCLE ATROPHY

Skeletal muscle fibrosis is a major pathologic hallmark of chronic myopathies in which myofibers are replaced by progressive deposition of ECM proteins. This muscle fibrosis is found in many of the muscular dystrophies as well as following injury and denervation. Progressive muscle fibrosis leads to smaller muscle fibers with concomitant decreased contractility and function. A major role in the

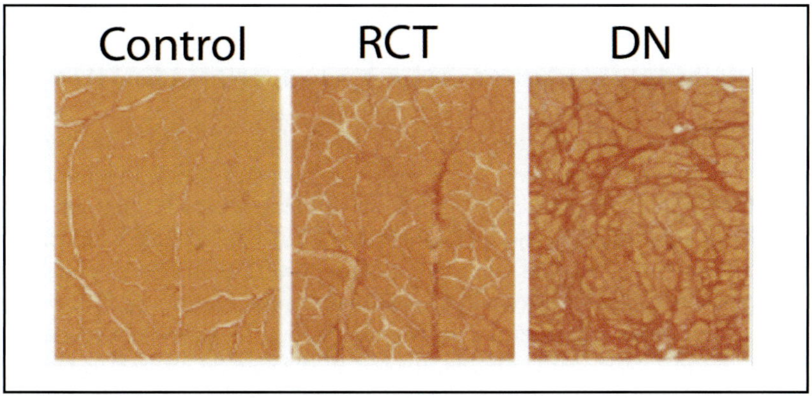

Figure 4-6. Histologic evaluation of rat rotator cuff muscle 6 weeks after the creation of a rotator cuff tear (RCT) or denervation of the muscle (DN). Control muscle is seen in the first panel. This is a picric acid stain that stains the collagen red as a marker for increased muscle fibrosis. In the rotator cuff tear group and denervation group, significantly more muscle fibrosis is seen.

onset of fibrosis is exerted by myofibroblasts that result from transdifferentiation of muscle progenitor cells during the regenerative process. In our previous studies, we have found increased muscle fibrosis following creation of a rotator cuff tear.[40]

Transforming growth factor-beta (TGF-β) is a pleiotropic cytokine that has a central role in many different processes. It has been found to promote myofibroblast differentiation and plays a major role in both wound healing and fibrosis. Binding of active TGF-β to its receptor triggers several signaling pathways including the PI3K/Akt pathway (as described above) and the well-characterized Smad pathway.[41,42] TGF-β has been found to be a critical regulator of the development of fibrosis across many different organ systems.[43] TGF-β induces normal scar formation but is also important in the development of pulmonary and renal fibrosis and has been found to regulate gene expression in muscle fibrosis.[44-48] The cytokine signal is transduced via a heteromeric complex of 2 types of transmembrane serine/threonine kinase receptors that phosphorylate receptor-activated Smad proteins. Subsequently, the translocation into the nucleus of Smad complex and its association with additional transcriptional factors determines the transcriptional regulation of target genes. Recently, it has been found that the transformation of myoblasts into myofibroblasts occurs via up-regulation of the sphingosine Kinase-1/S1p3 axis.[49] Interestingly, recent studies have found that there is crosstalk between the Akt-mTOR pathways in the development of muscle atrophy. Sartori and colleagues found that TGF-β activation induces muscle atrophy that is independent from MuRF1 upregulation but partially dependent on the Akt-mTOR pathway.[50] The Smad2 and Smad3 transcription factors were found to be the dominant transcription factors downstream of Akt, and thus these 2 pathways may enhance the degree of atrophy seen.[50] No studies to date have evaluated the role of TGF-β in rotator cuff muscle atrophy. In a rat model of massive cuff tears, there was a significant increase in the amount of fibrosis seen following creation of a rotator cuff tear (Figure 4-6).[51] This was accentuated with denervation of the rotator cuff muscle, suggesting that denervation may also enhance the development of muscle fibrosis. Previous studies in other animal models have also demonstrated increased muscle fibrosis in the setting of rotator cuff tears. Gerber and colleagues demonstrated an increase of connective tissue in a sheep model of chronic rotator cuff tears.[52] Similarly, Fabis and colleagues demonstrated an increase in interstitial volume in a rabbit supraspinatus tendon detachment model at 6 and 12 weeks following tendon detachment.[53] Based on these studies, it appears clear that fibrosis develops in the setting of rotator cuff tears, but the clinical consequences of this fibrosis are uncertain. Further study evaluating the specific pathways that contribute to this fibrosis and investigation toward the clinical relevance of this finding are important to understand the muscle changes seen following rotator cuff tears.

CLINICAL CONSEQUENCES OF MUSCLE ATROPHY AND FATTY INFILTRATION

Rotator cuff tears are an extremely common cause of shoulder pain and disability.[54,55] Up to 20% of patients older than 50 years of age have evidence of a rotator cuff tear.[56] In addition, patients with asymptomatic cuff tears tend to progress to larger, symptomatic tears.[57] The outcomes of surgical repair of small rotator cuff tears are good, but there has been limited success in the surgical treatment of massive rotator cuff tears. Cofield and colleagues found that 94% of patients with a small rotator cuff tear repair had a good or excellent outcome, compared to only 27% of patients with a massive rotator cuff tear.[58] Massive rotator cuff tears have been found to be associated with atrophy of the supraspinatus and infraspinatus muscle, fibrosis of the muscle, as well as fatty infiltration of the muscles.[59,60] It also appears that there is a component of denervation of the rotator cuff in these massive rotator cuff tears, which may have an important role in the advanced atrophy, fibrosis, and fatty infiltration seen in these injuries.[61]

Both atrophy and fatty infiltration have been correlated with poor functional outcome following rotator cuff tear repair, and atrophy and fatty infiltration have been shown to be irreversible even following successful repair.[61] Importantly, patients with large rotator cuff tears with atrophy and fatty infiltration have poorer clinical outcomes than those who do not have these changes. Gladstone and colleagues evaluated 38 patients prospectively in order to evaluate the effect of muscle atrophy and fatty infiltration on the clinical outcomes following rotator cuff repair.[62] The authors found that, although clinical outcome scores improved considerably, there is a strong negative correlation between muscle quality and outcomes in most cases. Muscle atrophy and fatty infiltration were independent predictors of American Shoulder and Elbow Surgeons and Constant scores, and both atrophy and fatty infiltration can progress even in the case of a successful repair. Thus, it appears that the natural history of large tears is the development of atrophy and fatty infiltration leading to poorer outcomes, likely due to the inelasticity and poor function of the muscle-tendon unit. This provides a solid rationale to fix rotator cuff tears before advanced muscle atrophy and fatty infiltration occur. Despite most studies showing that muscle atrophy and fatty infiltration are irreversible following rotator cuff repair, Burkhart and colleagues found that repair in the setting of even Grade 3 or 4 fatty degeneration can lead to improvement in clinical function as well as an improvement in the amount of atrophy and fat present in the muscle in select cases.[63,64]

ROLE OF DENERVATION OF THE ROTATOR CUFF

It is theorized that retraction of the supraspinatus muscle after a large rotator cuff tear changes the course of the suprascapular nerve (SSN) through the suprascapular notch, potentially creating increased tension on the nerve and placing the nerve at risk for injury.[65] Studies in patients with massive rotator cuff tears have found altered electromyography (EMG) findings consistent with an SSN neuropathy. Costouros and colleagues evaluated 26 patients with massive rotator cuff tears with EMG/Nerve Conduction Study to evaluate for the presence of peripheral neuropathy.[66] Fourteen of the 26 patients had evidence of a peripheral nerve injury, with 7 having an isolated SSN injury. Interestingly, 6 of the 7 patients who underwent repair of the rotator cuff demonstrated partial or full recovery of the SSN palsy, suggesting that traction indeed causes injury to the nerve. Importantly, the nerve appears to have the ability to recover following repair. Patients with an isolated SSN neuropathy develop changes that mimic the atrophy and fatty infiltration seen in the setting of a massive rotator cuff tear. SSN neuropathy is considered a rare condition, but, in patients with a massive rotator cuff tear, this finding actually might be quite common. In a recently published study, Boykin and colleagues found that 42% of patients with a massive rotator cuff tear demonstrated changes on EMG that were consistent with a SSN injury.[67] Most commonly, there were abnormal motor unit action potentials (seen in 88% of these patients) with 33% of patients demonstrating evidence of denervation. Thus, denervation is likely more prevalent than clinically recognized, and consideration should be made to perform electrodiagnostic studies in the preoperative period. It is unclear at this time if these changes are reversible, but at least one study suggests that denervation can be reversed following surgery.

On a molecular level, denervation of skeletal muscle leads to increased muscle atrophy with increased expression of NF-kB, FOXO1, and atrogin-1.[21] Dreyer and colleagues have found that denervation through spinal cord injury resulted in a reduction in phosphorylation of mTOR, S6K1, and eIF4G.[68] The authors concluded that paraplegia-induced muscle atrophy in rats is associated with a general downregulation of the mTOR signaling pathway. Similarly, Agata and colleagues found that there was altered expression of mTOR and Akt in denervated soleus muscles, a change that could be decreased with mechanical stretch.[69] These studies suggest that denervation influences several of the same pathways that have been found to have altered regulation with muscle atrophy, and thus the combination of mechanical unloading and denervation significantly influences the development of the changes seen following rotator cuff tears.

CONCLUSION/FUTURE DIRECTIONS

Despite the important clinical consequences of muscle atrophy and fatty infiltration in the outcomes of rotator cuff repair, we are still in our infancy in understanding the underlying pathophysiology involved in the characteristic changes seen. Future studies will need to be focused on understanding the cellular and molecular regulation of muscle atrophy, fibrosis, and fatty infiltration in order to develop pharmacologic and other novel treatment modalities to improve the clinical outcomes following rotator cuff repair even in the setting of massive cuff tears. Although a majority of basic science studies involving the rotator cuff have focused on the tendon and improving tendon-to-bone healing, the next step in improving our understanding and clinical outcomes will come from understanding and altering the changes seen within the muscle following rotator cuff tears.

REFERENCES

1. Shi X, Garry DJ. Muscle stem cells in development, regeneration, and disease. *Genes Dev.* 2006;1:1692-1708.
2. Buckingham M, Montarras D. Skeletal muscle stem cells. *Curr Opin Genet Dev.* 2008;18:330-336.
3. Aitken KJ, Block G, Lorenzo A, et al. Mechanotransduction of extracellular signal-regulated kinases 1 and 2 mitogen-activated protein kinase activity in smooth muscle is dependent on the extracellular matrix and regulated by matrix metalloproteinases. *Am J Pathol.* 2006;169:459-470.
4. Skittone LK, Liu X, Tseng A, Kim HT. Matrix metalloproteinase-2 expression and promoter/enhancer activity in skeletal muscle atrophy. *J Ortho Res.* 2008;26:357-363.
5. Lakemeier S, Braun J, Efe T, et al. Expression of matrix metalloproteinases 1, 3, and 9 in differing extents of tendon retraction in the torn rotator cuff. *Knee Surg Sports Traumatol Arthrosc.* 2011;19(10):1760-1765.
6. Kwon O, Tranter M, Jones WK, Sankovic JM, Banerjee RK. Differential translocation of nuclear factor-kappaB in a cardiac muscle cell line under gravitational changes. *J Biomech Eng.* 2009;131:064503.
7. Li H, Malhotra S, Kumar A. Nuclear factor-kappa B signaling in skeletal muscle atrophy. *J Mol Med.* 2008;86:1113-1126.
8. Dogra C, Changotra H, Wergedal JE, Kumar A. Regulation of phosphatidylinositol 3-kinase (PI3K)/Akt and nuclear factor-kappa B signaling pathways in dystrophin-deficient skeletal muscle in response to mechanical stretch. *J Cell Physiol.* 2006;208:575-585.
9. Kimura N, Kumamoto T, Oniki T, et al. Role of ubiquitin-proteasome proteolysis in muscle fiber destruction in experimental chloroquine-induced myopathy. *Muscle Nerve.* 2009;39:521-528.
10. Senf SM, Dodd SL, Judge AR. FOXO signaling is required for disuse muscle atrophy and is directly regulated by Hsp70. *Am J Physiol Cell Physiol.* 2010;298:C38-C45.
11. Senf SM, Dodd SL, McClung JM, Judge AR. Hsp70 overexpression inhibits NF-kappaB and Foxo3a transcriptional activities and prevents skeletal muscle atrophy. *Faseb J.* 2008;22:3836-3845.

12. Shi H, Scheffler JM, Zeng C, et al. Mitogen-activated protein kinase signaling is necessary for the maintenance of skeletal muscle mass. *Am J Physiol Cell Physiol*. 2009;296:C1040-1048.

13. Edstrom E, Altun M, Hagglund M, Ulfhake B. Atrogin-1/MAFbx and MuRF1 are downregulated in aging-related loss of skeletal muscle. *J Gerontol A Biol Sci Med Sci*. 2006;61:663-674.

14. Foletta VC, White LJ, Larsen AE, Leger B, Russell AP. The role and regulation of MAFbx/atrogin-1 and MuRF1 in skeletal muscle atrophy. *Eur J Physiol*. 2011;461:325-335.

15. Miyazaki M, Noguchi M, Takemasa T. Intermittent reloading attenuates muscle atrophy through modulating Akt/mTOR pathway. *Med Sci Sports Exercise*. 2008;40:848-855.

16. Mammucari C, Schiaffino S, Sandri M. Downstream of Akt: FoxO3 and mTOR in the regulation of autophagy in skeletal muscle. *Autophagy*. 2008;4:524-526.

17. Southgate RJ, Neill B, Prelovsek O, et al. FOXO1 regulates the expression of 4E-BP1 and inhibits mTOR signaling in mammalian skeletal muscle. *J Biol Chemistry*. 2007;282:21176-21186.

18. Bodine SC. mTOR signaling and the molecular adaptation to resistance exercise. *Med Sci Sports Exercise*. 2006;38:1950-1957.

19. Leger B, Cartoni R, Praz M, et al. Akt signalling through GSK-3beta, mTOR and Foxo1 is involved in human skeletal muscle hypertrophy and atrophy. *J Physiol*. 2006;576:923-933.

20. Bodine SC, Stitt TN, Gonzalez M, et al. Akt/mTOR pathway is a crucial regulator of skeletal muscle hypertrophy and can prevent muscle atrophy in vivo. *Nature Cell Biol*. 2001;3:1014-1019.

21. Leger B, Senese R, Al-Khodairy AW, et al. Atrogin-1, MuRF1, and FoXO, as well as phosphorylated GSK-3beta and 4E-BP1 are reduced in skeletal muscle of chronic spinal cord-injured patients. *Muscle Nerve*. 2009;40:69-78.

22. Zheng B, Ohkawa S, Li H, Roberts-Wilson TK, Price SR. FOXO3a mediates signaling crosstalk that coordinates ubiquitin and atrogin-1/MAFbx expression during glucocorticoid-induced skeletal muscle atrophy. *FASEB Journal*. 2010;24:2660-2669.

23. Latres E, Amini AR, Amini AA, et al. Insulin-like growth factor-1 (IGF-1) inversely regulates atrophy-induced genes via the phosphatidylinositol 3-kinase/Akt/mammalian target of rapamycin (PI3K/Akt/mTOR) pathway. *J Biol Chemistry*. 2005;280:2737-2744.

24. Liu X, Manzano G, Kim HT, Feeley BT. The role of mTOR in the development of muscle atrophy in a rat model of rotator cuff tears. Presented at the ISAKOS Annual Meeting, Rio De Janero, Brazil; 2011.

25. Goutallier D, Postel JM, Bernageau J, Lavau L, Voisin MC. Fatty muscle degeneration in cuff ruptures. Pre- and postoperative evaluation by CT scan. *Clin Orthop Relat Res*. 1994:78-83.

26. Cheung S, Dillon E, Tham SC, et al. The presence of fatty infiltration in the infraspinatus: its relation with the condition of the supraspinatus tendon. *Arthroscopy*. 2011;27:463-470.

27. Csete M, Walikonis J, Slawny N, et al. Oxygen-mediated regulation of skeletal muscle satellite cell proliferation and adipogenesis in culture. *J Cell Physiol*. 2001;189:189-196.

28. Brack AS, Conboy MJ, Roy S, et al. Increased Wnt signaling during aging alters muscle stem cell fate and increases fibrosis. *Science*. 2007;317:807-810.

29. Hosoyama T, Ishiguro N, Yamanouchi K, Nishihara M. Degenerative muscle fiber accelerates adipogenesis of intra-muscular cells via RhoA signaling pathway. *Differentiation*. 2009;77:350-359.

30. Rosen ED. The transcriptional basis of adipocyte development. *Prostaglandins Leukot Essent Fatty Acids*. 2005;73:31-34.

31. Tontonoz P, Spiegelman BM. Fat and beyond: the diverse biology of PPARgamma. *Annu Rev Biochem*. 2008;77:289-312.

32. Lefterova MI, Zhang Y, Steger DJ, et al. PPARgamma and C/EBP factors orchestrate adipocyte biology via adjacent binding on a genome-wide scale. *Genes Dev*. 2008;22:2941-2952.

33. Wu Z, Xie Y, Bucher NL, Farmer SR. Conditional ectopic expression of C/EBP beta in NIH-3T3 cells induces PPAR gamma and stimulates adipogenesis. *Genes Dev*. 1995;9:2350-2363.

34. Rosen ED, Sarraf P, Troy AE, et al. PPAR gamma is required for the differentiation of adipose tissue in vivo and in vitro. *Mol Cell*. 1999;4:611-617.

35. Frey E, Regenfelder F, Sussmann P, et al. Adipogenic and myogenic gene expression in rotator cuff muscle of the sheep after tendon tear. *J Orthop Res*. 2009;27:504-509.

36. Constantin D, Constantin-Teodosiu D, Layfield R, Tsintzas K, Bennett AJ, Greenhaff, PL. PPARdelta agonism induces a change in fuel metabolism and activation of an atrophy programme, but does not impair mitochondrial function in rat skeletal muscle. *J Physiol*. 2007;583:381-390.

37. Itoigawa Y, Kishmoto KN, Sano H, Kaneko K, Itoi E. Molecular mechanism of fatty degeneration in rotator cuff muscle with tendon rupture. *J Orthop Res*. 2011;29:861-866.

38. Meyer DC, Hoppeler H, von Rechenberg B, Gerber C. A pathomechanical concept explains muscle loss and fatty muscular changes following surgical tendon release. *J Orthop Res*. 2004;22:1004-1007.

39. Gerber C, Meyer DC, Frey E, et al. Neer Award 2007: reversion of structural muscle changes caused by chronic rotator cuff tears using continuous musculotendinous traction. An experimental study in sheep. *J Shoulder Elbow Surg*. 2009;18:163-171.

40. Liu X, Manzano G, Kim HT, Feeley BT. A rat model of massive rotator cuff tears. *J Orthop Res*. 2011;29(4):588-595.

41. Yan X, Chen YG. Smad7: not only a regulator, but also a cross-talk mediator of TGF-beta signalling. *Biochem J.* 2011;434:1-10.

42. Yan X, Liu Z, Chen Y. Regulation of TGF-beta signaling by Smad7. *Acta biochimica et biophysica Sinica.* 2009;41:263-272.

43. Sheppard D. Transforming growth factor beta: a central modulator of pulmonary and airway inflammation and fibrosis. *Proceedings of the American Thoracic Society.* 2006;3:413-417.

44. Li Y, Fu FH, Huard J. Cutting-edge muscle recovery: using antifibrosis agents to improve healing. *Physician and Sportsmedicine.* 2005;33:44-50.

45. Chan YS, Li Y, Foster W, Fu FH, Huard J. The use of suramin, an antifibrotic agent, to improve muscle recovery after strain injury. *Am J Sports Med.* 2005;33:43-51.

46. Foster W, Li Y, Usas A, Somogyi G, Huard J. Gamma interferon as an antifibrosis agent in skeletal muscle. *J Ortho Res.* 2003;21:798-804.

47. Chan YS, Li Y, Foster W, et al. Antifibrotic effects of suramin in injured skeletal muscle after laceration. *J Applied Physiol.* 2003;95:771-780.

48. Fukushima K, Badlani N, Usas A, Riano F, Fu F, Huard J. The use of an antifibrosis agent to improve muscle recovery after laceration. *Am J Sports Med.* 2001;29:394-402.

49. Cencetti F, Bernacchioni C, Nincheri P, Donati C, Bruni P. Transforming growth factor-beta1 induces transdifferentiation of myoblasts into myofibroblasts via up-regulation of sphingosine kinase-1/S1P3 axis. *Molecular Biology of the Cell.* 2010;21:1111-1124.

50. Sartori R, Milan G, Patron M, et al. Smad2 and 3 transcription factors control muscle mass in adulthood. *Am J Physiol Cell Physiol.* 2009;296:C1248-C1257.

51. Liu X, Manzano G, Kim HT, Feeley BT. A rat model of massive rotator cuff tears. *J Ortho Res.* 2011;29:588-595.

52. Gerber C, Meyer DC, Schneeberger AG, Hoppeler H, von Rechenberg B. Effect of tendon release and delayed repair on the structure of the muscles of the rotator cuff: an experimental study in sheep. *J Bone Joint Surg Am.* 2004;86-A:1973-1982.

53. Fabis J, Danilewicz M, Omuleck A. Rabbit supraspinatus tendon deatchment: effects of size and time after tenotomy on morphometric changes in the muscle. *Acta Orthop Scand.* 2001;72:282-286.

54. Matthews TJ, Hand GC, Rees JL, Athanasou NA, Carr AJ. Pathology of the torn rotator cuff tendon. Reduction in potential for repair as tear size increases. *J Bone Joint Surg Br.* 2006;88:489-495.

55. Nho SJ, Yadav H, Shindle MK, Macgillivray JD. Rotator cuff degeneration: etiology and pathogenesis. *Am J Sports Med.* 2008;36:987-993.

56. Yamamoto A, Takagishi K, Osawa T, et al. Prevalence and risk factors of a rotator cuff tear in the general population. *J Shoulder Elbow Surg.* 2010;19(1):116-120.

57. Yamaguchi K, Ditsios K, Middleton WD, Hildebolt CF, Galatz LM, Teefey SA. The demographic and morphological features of rotator cuff disease. A comparison of asymptomatic and symptomatic shoulders. *J Bone Joint Surg Am.* 2006;88:1699-1704.

58. Cofield RH, Parvizi J, Hoffmeyer PJ, Lanzer WL, Ilstrup DM, Rowland CM. Surgical repair of chronic rotator cuff tears. A prospective long-term study. *J Bone Joint Surg Am.* 2001;83-A:71-77.

59. Gladstone JN, Bishop JY, Lo IK, Flatow EL. Fatty infiltration and atrophy of the rotator cuff do not improve after rotator cuff repair and correlate with poor functional outcome. *Am J Sports Med.* 2007;35:719-728.

60. Shen PH, Lien SB, Shen HC, Lee CH, Wu SS, Lin LC. Long-term functional outcomes after repair of rotator cuff tears correlated with atrophy of the supraspinatus muscles on magnetic resonance images. *J Shoulder Elbow Surg.* 2008;17:1S-7S.

61. Warner JP, Krushell RJ, Masquelet A, Gerber C. Anatomy and relationships of the suprascapular nerve: anatomical constraints to mobilization of the supraspinatus and infraspinatus muscles in the management of massive rotator-cuff tears. *J Bone Joint Surg Am.* 1992;74:36-45.

62. Gladstone JN, Bishop JY, Lo IK, Flatow EL. Fatty infiltration and atrophy of the rotator cuff do not improve after rotator cuff repair and correlate with poor functional outcome. *Am J Sports Med.* 2007;35:719-728.

63. Burkhart SS, Danaceau SM, Pearce CE Jr. Arthroscopic rotator cuff repair: analysis of results by tear size and by repair technique-margin convergence versus direct tendon-to-bone repair. *Arthroscopy.* 2001;17:905-912.

64. Burkhart SS. Arthroscopic treatment of massive rotator cuff tears. *Clin Ortho Rel Res.* 2001:107-118.

65. Albritton MJ, Graham RD, Richards RS 2nd, Basamania CJ. An anatomic study of the effects on the suprascapular nerve due to retraction of the supraspinatus muscle after a rotator cuff tear. *J Shoulder Elbow Surg.* 2003;12:497-500.

66. Costouros JG, Porramatikul M, Lie DT, Warner JJ. Reversal of suprascapular neuropathy following arthroscopic repair of massive supraspinatus and infraspinatus rotator cuff tears. *Arthroscopy.* 2007;23:1152-1161.

67. Boykin RE, Friedman DJ, Zimmer ZR, Oaklander AL, Higgins LD, Warner JJ. Suprascapular neuropathy in a shoulder referral practice. *J Shoulder Elbow Surg.* 2011;20(6):983-988.

68. Dreyer HC, Glynn EL, Lujan HL, Fry CS, DiCarlo SE, Rasmussen BB. Chronic paraplegia-induced muscle atrophy downregulates the mTOR/S6K1 signaling pathway. *J Applied Physiol.* 2008;104:27-33.

69. Agata N, Sasai N, Inoue-Miyazu M, et al. Repetitive stretch suppresses denervation-induced atrophy of soleus muscle in rats. *Muscle Nerve.* 2009;39:456-462.

CHAPTER 5

HISTORY AND PHYSICAL EXAMINATION OF THE ROTATOR CUFF

Lee Jae Morse, MD and Christina Allen, MD

Obtaining a good history from a patient with shoulder complaints cannot be overemphasized. A good history begins with the sometimes forgotten chief complaint. The chief complaint, age of the patient, chronicity, hand dominance, mechanism of injury (if a specific event occurred), exacerbating and alleviating factors, occupation, activities, prior surgeries, pertinent past medical history (such as diabetes or thyroid problems), and prior injuries are essential components of the history. From the history, a differential diagnosis can be formulated that will direct the physical examination. There are numerous tests that evaluate different aspects of the shoulder, and it would be too time consuming and ultimately too confusing to use a shotgun approach. The worst case scenario would be obtaining a poor history and physical examination and relying solely on imaging for surgical decision making. This could lead to a surgery targeting an incidental pathology or artifact that is not the cause of the patient's symptoms. This is certainly a plausible scenario as 28% of asymptomatic patients 60 to 70 years of age have full-thickness rotator cuff tears while 65% of patients over 70 years of age have full-thickness tears. This applies to elite athletes as well. Miniaci and colleagues[1] found labral pathology in 79% of 14 asymptomatic professional baseball pitchers imaged with magnetic resonance imaging (MRI).

Patients with rotator cuff tears will most often complain of anterolateral shoulder pain, increased pain with overhead activities, night pain, loss of active shoulder motion, and generalized weakness. Younger patients may recall a specific incident associated with the onset of their shoulder symptoms, whereas older patients may relate a more insidious onset of shoulder pain and weakness due to rotator cuff pathology.

PHYSICAL EXAMINATION

Inspection and Palpation

It is imperative that both of the patient's shoulders and scapulae are fully exposed. Inspect for any deformities, such as prior clavicle fractures, acromioclavicular (AC) joint injuries, or scapular

Ma CB, Feeley BT, eds.
Basic Principles and Operative Management
of the Rotator Cuff (pp 61-76)
© 2012 SLACK Incorporated

winging. The examiner should look for shoulder asymmetry, muscle wasting, and whether the scapulae move appropriately with shoulder motion. Examine the neck for tenderness to palpation, assess range of motion, and ask about any radicular symptoms, as cervical stenosis may present as isolated shoulder pain. Palpate the clavicle starting at the sternoclavicular joint and move toward the AC joint, checking for deformity and tenderness. Palpate the bicipital groove to examine for biceps tenderness. Patients with rotator cuff tears will often have tenderness over the supraspinatus insertion (Codman point).[2] This is found by extending and internally rotating the shoulder and then palpating through the deltoid just distal to the anterolateral border of the acromion.

Range of Motion

Check active range of motion and then passive range of motion in both upper extremities. Checking the contralateral extremity is essential because some patients may compensate extremely well with partial or small full-thickness rotator cuff tears and deficits are subtle. Ensure that abduction is evaluated in the scapular plane with the arms adducted approximately 30 degrees versus raising the arms straight up from their sides. Normal range of abduction and forward elevation is 160 to 180 degrees. External rotation should be checked with the elbows flexed to 90 degrees and tucked in at the sides and also at 90 degrees of abduction in the coronal plane. External rotation with the elbows at the sides is normally 45 to 60 degrees, while 90 degrees of external rotation is normally achieved with the shoulder abducted to 90 degrees. Internal rotation can be checked by having the patient reach behind his or her back one extremity at a time and recording the most cephalad vertebrae reached by a hitch-hiking thumb. Patients with rotator cuff pathology will often have reduced abduction in the scapular plane, external rotation, and internal rotation, depending on the severity of the tear and which rotator cuff muscles are injured. The hallmark of rotator cuff injuries will be limited active range of motion with full passive range of motion.

IMPINGEMENT TESTS

Impingement tests are provocative maneuvers aimed at recreating rotator cuff impingement by forcing the greater tuberosity against the undersurface of the anterior acromion. Common tests for subacromial impingement are the Neer impingement sign, Hawkins-Kennedy impingement test, Jobe supraspinatus test (empty can test), Yocum test, and internal rotation resistance strength test.

Neer Impingement Sign

Neer first described this impingement sign in 1972[3] and further in 1983 when describing the 3 stages of impingement in rotator cuff disease (Figure 5-1).[4] The exam is performed with the patient seated or standing with the examiner standing at the patient's side. One hand is placed on the scapula to prevent scapular rotation while the other hand passively raises the patient's upper extremity, causing the greater tuberosity of the humerus to impinge on the anterior third of the acromion. A positive sign is pain with forward flexion usually in the range of 70 to 120 degrees. The exam can be augmented by a subacromial injection with a local anesthetic and repeating the maneuver. It is theorized that pain relief after injection is more specific for rotator cuff pathology than a positive Neer impingement sign alone. While a positive test is suggestive of rotator cuff disease, pain may also occur with many other shoulder pathologies. MacDonald and colleagues[5] showed the Neer impingement sign to be positive in 46% of patients with superior labrum anterior to posterior lesions, 25% of patients with Bankart lesions, and 69% of patients with AC joint arthritis. Park and colleagues[6] examined multiple tests to determine the accuracy of diagnosing rotator cuff disease and found that, in partial rotator cuff tears, Neer's sign had a sensitivity, specificity, and accuracy of 75%, 48%, and 51%, respectively. With full-thickness tears, the sensitivity, specificity, and accuracy was 59%, 47%, and 52%, respectively.

Figure 5-1. Neer impingement test. The patient is seated or standing with the examiner standing at the patient's side. One hand is placed on the scapula to prevent scapular rotation, while the other hand passively raises the patient's upper extremity. A positive sign is pain with forward flexion usually in the range of 70 to 120 degrees.

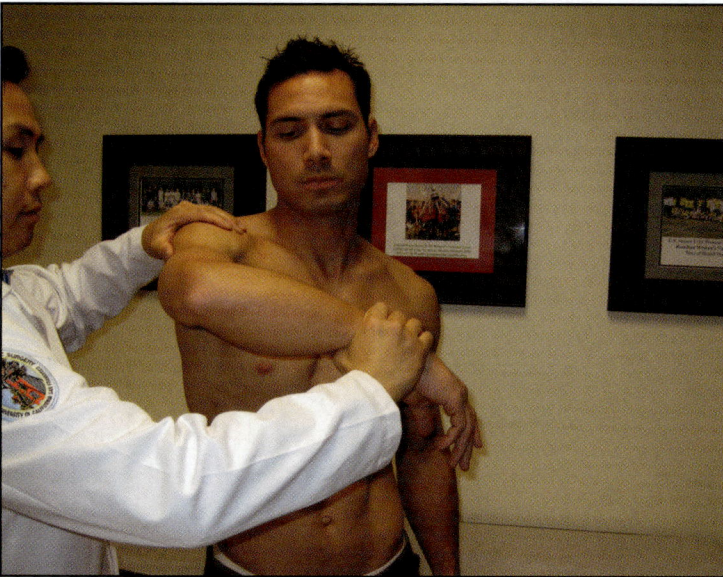

Figure 5-2. Hawkins-Kennedy impingement test. The patient is standing or sitting. The examiner forward flexes the shoulder to 90 degrees, flexes the elbow to 90 degrees, and internally rotates the shoulder by applying a downward force to the forearm. The opposite hand is used to stabilize the acromion. A positive test reproduces pain when the shoulder is internally rotated.

Hawkins-Kennedy Impingement Test

The Hawkins-Kennedy impingement test[7] was described in 1980 as an additional test for impingement of the supraspinatus (Figure 5-2). The test is performed with the patient standing or sitting. The examiner forward flexes the shoulder to 90 degrees, flexes the elbow to 90 degrees, and internally rotates the shoulder by applying a downward force to the forearm. The opposite hand is used to stabilize the acromion. Internal rotation of a forwardly flexed shoulder brings the greater tuberosity of the humerus into the coracoacromial (CA) arch directly impinging on the CA ligament. With progressive abduction, the greater tuberosity will impinge on the undersurface of the lateral acromion and the AC joint. Patients with impingement will have immediate pain when an internal rotation force is applied to the shoulder. MacDonald and colleagues[5] found this test to have a sensitivity of 88% and 92% for rotator cuff pathology and subacromial bursitis, respectively. Specificity was similar to the Neer test at 43% and 44% for rotator cuff pathology and subacromial bursitis, respectively.

Figure 5-3. Jobe supraspinatus test (empty can test). With the patient standing, the shoulders are abducted to 90 degrees, adducted horizontally 30 degrees, and fully internally rotated until the thumbs are pointing down toward the floor. Pain or weakness with resisted downward force is considered to be a positive test.

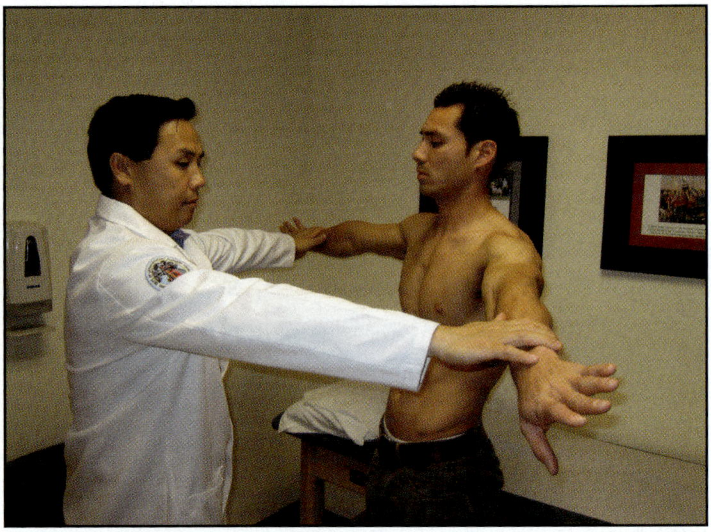

Jobe Supraspinatus Test (Empty Can Test)

Jobe and Jobe[8] described this provocative impingement test in 1983 with the goal of impinging an inflamed supraspinatus tendon against the CA arch (Figure 5-3). With the patient standing, the shoulders are abducted to 90 degrees, adducted horizontally 30 degrees, and fully internally rotated until the thumbs are pointing down toward the floor. Pain or weakness with resisted downward force is considered to be a positive test. Itoi and colleagues[9] found weakness to be a more accurate predictor of full-thickness supraspinatus tears. They performed the empty can test in 143 shoulders in 136 consecutive patients, and the results were recorded as pain, weakness, or both. The 143 shoulders were subsequently evaluated by MRI, and 35 shoulders were diagnosed with full-thickness supraspinatus tears. They found that weakness was 70% accurate in diagnosing a full-thickness supraspinatus tear, whereas pain was only 50% accurate.

Yocum Test

This test was described by Yocum[10] in 1983 for the diagnosis of subacromial impingement of the supraspinatus. The starting position is very similar to the bear-hug test with the injured arm adducted and the elbow flexed so the hand is over the contralateral shoulder (Figure 5-4). The patient is then asked to raise the elbow while keeping the shoulder still. A positive test is pain with elevation of the elbow. Silva and colleagues[11] found Yocum's test to have the highest sensitivity (79%) and accuracy (65.5%) in diagnosing MRI-positive subacromial impingement in comparison to the Neer impingement sign, Hawkins-Kennedy impingement test, Jobe supraspinatus test, Gerber lift-off test, and Patte maneuver.

Internal Rotation Resistance Strength Test

In an attempt to differentiate intra-articular impingement from subacromial outlet impingement, Zaslav[12] described the internal rotation resistance stress test (Figure 5-5). Intra-articular (internal) impingement is classically seen in overhead athletes. The posterior rotator cuff impinges on the posterior superior labrum in the late cocking phase of throwing, causing pain in the region of the infraspinatus insertion. The test is performed by having the patient abduct the shoulder to 90 degrees, flex the elbow 90 degrees, and externally rotate to 80 degrees. The patient is asked to further externally rotate against resistance and then internally rotate against resistance. The test is positive for internal impingement if the patient has good strength with external rotation but apparent weakness

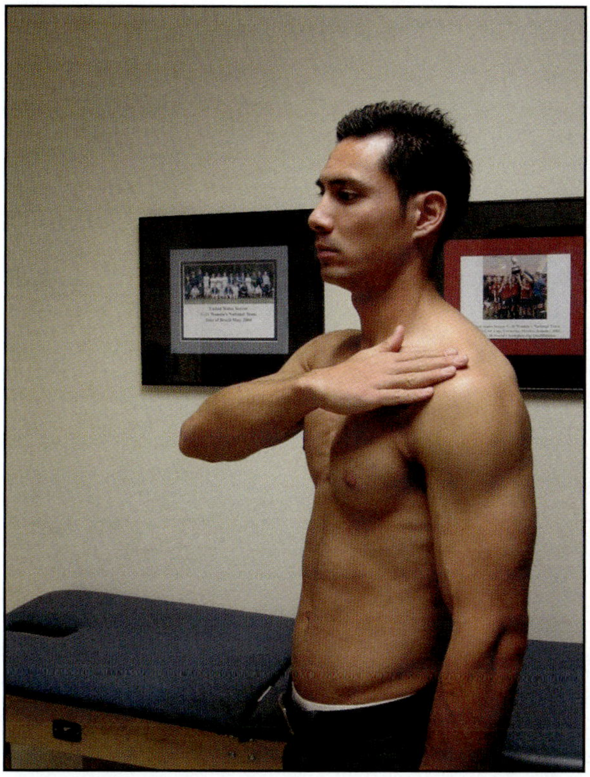

Figure 5-4. Yocum test. The starting position is very similar to the bear-hug test with the injured arm adducted and the elbow flexed so the hand is over the contralateral shoulder. The patient is then asked to raise the elbow while keeping the shoulder still. A positive test is pain with elevation of the elbow.

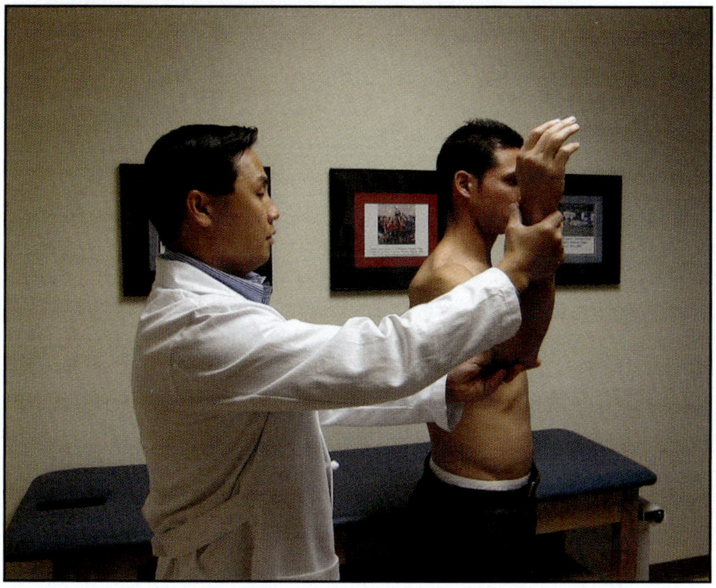

Figure 5-5. Internal rotation resistance strength test. The test is performed by having the patient abduct the shoulder to 90 degrees, flex the elbow 90 degrees, and externally rotate to 80 degrees. The patient is asked to further externally rotate against resistance and then internally rotate against resistance. The test is positive for internal impingement if the patient has good strength with external rotation but apparent weakness with internal rotation. Weakness with external rotation but not internal rotation indicates classic outlet impingement.

with internal rotation. Weakness with external rotation but not internal rotation indicates classic outlet impingement. A prospective study of 115 consecutive patients with arthroscopically confirmed pathology showed that the internal rotation resistance strength test had a positive and negative predictive value of 88% and 96%, respectively, and an accuracy of 94.5%.[12]

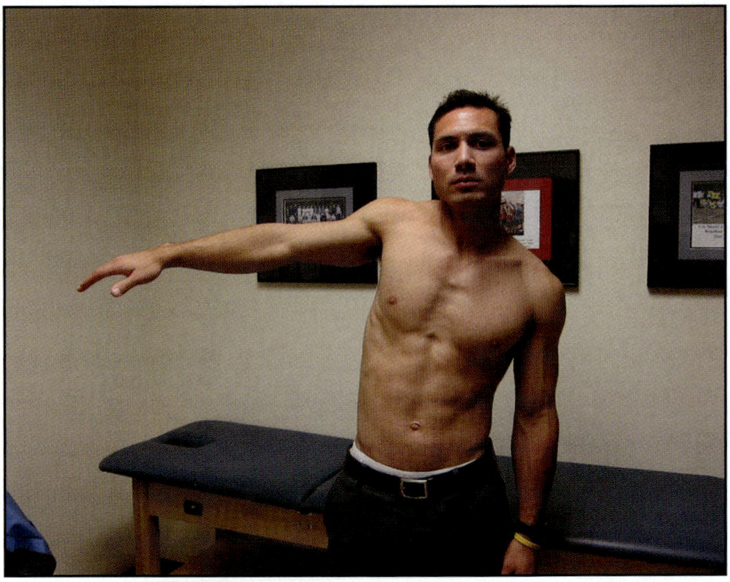

Figure 5-6. Drop-arm sign. The examiner abducts the injured arm to 90 degrees then releases the arm. The patient is instructed to maintain abduction then slowly lower the arm to the side. The test is positive if the arm drops suddenly or the patient has severe pain as he or she slowly lowers the arm.

ROTATOR CUFF STRENGTH TESTING

Evaluation of the Supraspinatus

The supraspinatus is the primary rotator cuff muscle that functions to abduct the shoulder in the scapular plane. The middle deltoid is also a primary shoulder abductor with secondary involvement of the anterior and posterior deltoid as well as the serratus anterior by its action on the scapula. Supraspinatus strength can be assessed as described by Jobe and Moynes[13] by having the patient abduct both shoulders 90 degrees, adduct each arm 30 degrees so they are in the scapular plane, then either internally rotate the arm or place it in a neutral position. The examiner then pushes down on each wrist to resist abduction.

Drop-Arm Sign

Codman[14] described the drop-arm sign, which is elicited by having the examiner abduct the injured arm to 90 degrees then release the arm (Figure 5-6). The patient is instructed to maintain abduction, then slowly lower the arm to the side. The test is positive if the arm drops suddenly or if the patient has severe pain as he or she slowly lowers the arm.

Full Can Test

The test is performed with the patient standing; the shoulders are abducted to 90 degrees, adducted horizontally 30 degrees, and externally rotated until the thumbs are pointing up toward the ceiling. Weakness with resisted downward force is considered a positive test (Figure 5-7). Kelly and colleagues[15] performed an electromyographic (EMG) study to assess different positions used for strength testing of the rotator cuff musculature. It was found that isolated supraspinatus strength was best evaluated with 90 degrees of elevation in the scapular plane and 45 degrees of external rotation with thumbs pointing up. They also found similar EMG results with the empty can test, but the full can test was less pain provocative. In a comparison of the empty can test versus the full can test for diagnosis of rotator cuff pathology, Itoi and colleagues[9] found that the full can test was slightly more accurate when weakness was used as a positive test, although it was not statistically significant (75% versus 70% for full can test and empty can test, respectively [$p=0.0707$]).

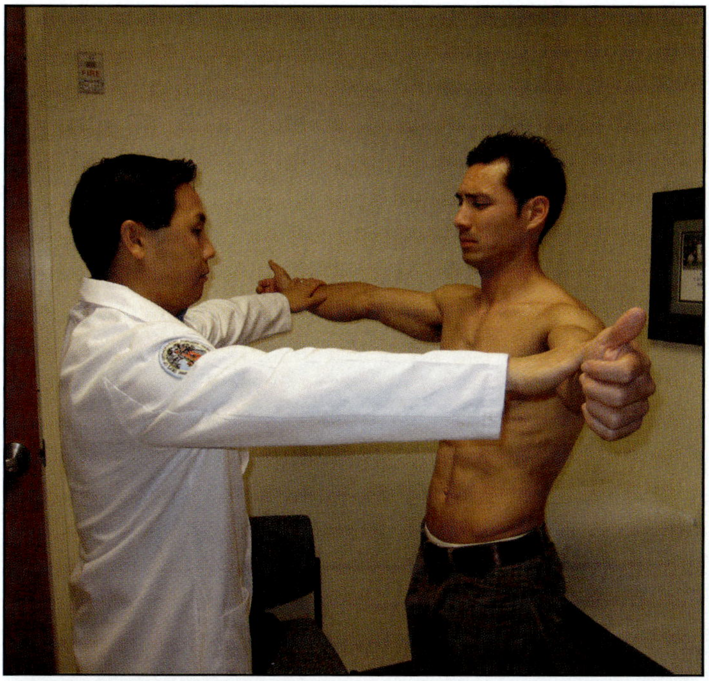

Figure 5-7. Full can test. With the patient standing, the shoulders are abducted to 90 degrees, adducted horizontally 30 degrees, and externally rotated until the thumbs are pointing up toward the ceiling. Pain or weakness or both with resisted downward force is considered a positive test.

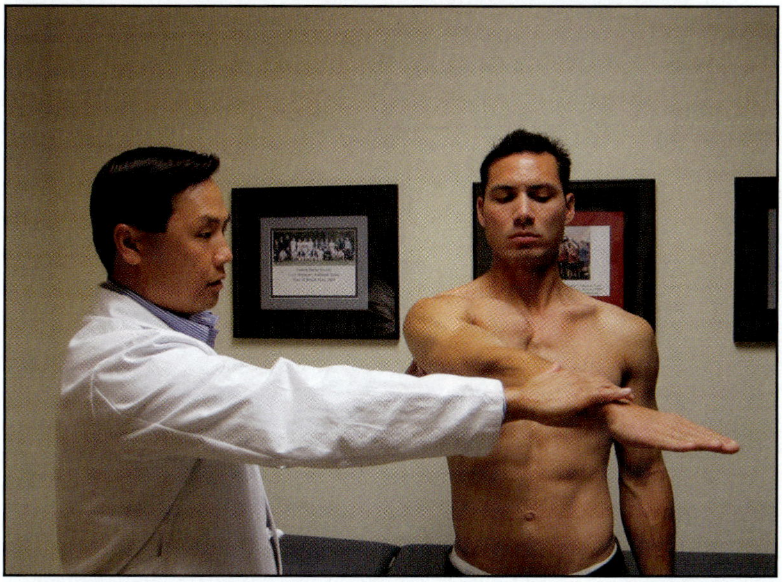

Figure 5-8. Whipple test. With the patient standing, the arm is forward flexed to 90 degrees and adducted until it is in front of the opposite shoulder with the palm down. The patient resists a downward force. The test is positive if there is weakness in comparison to the contralateral shoulder or if pain is present in the anterior shoulder.

Whipple Test

This test was developed to detect partial rotator cuff tears, specifically tears of the anterior supraspinatus (Figure 5-8).[16] While it was designed to assess partial supraspinatus tears, it will also be positive in full-thickness tears. The test is performed with the patient standing and the arm forward flexed to 90 degrees and adducted until it is in front of the opposite shoulder with the palm down. The patient is told to resist a downward force. The test is positive if there is weakness in comparison to the contralateral shoulder or if pain is present in the anterior shoulder.

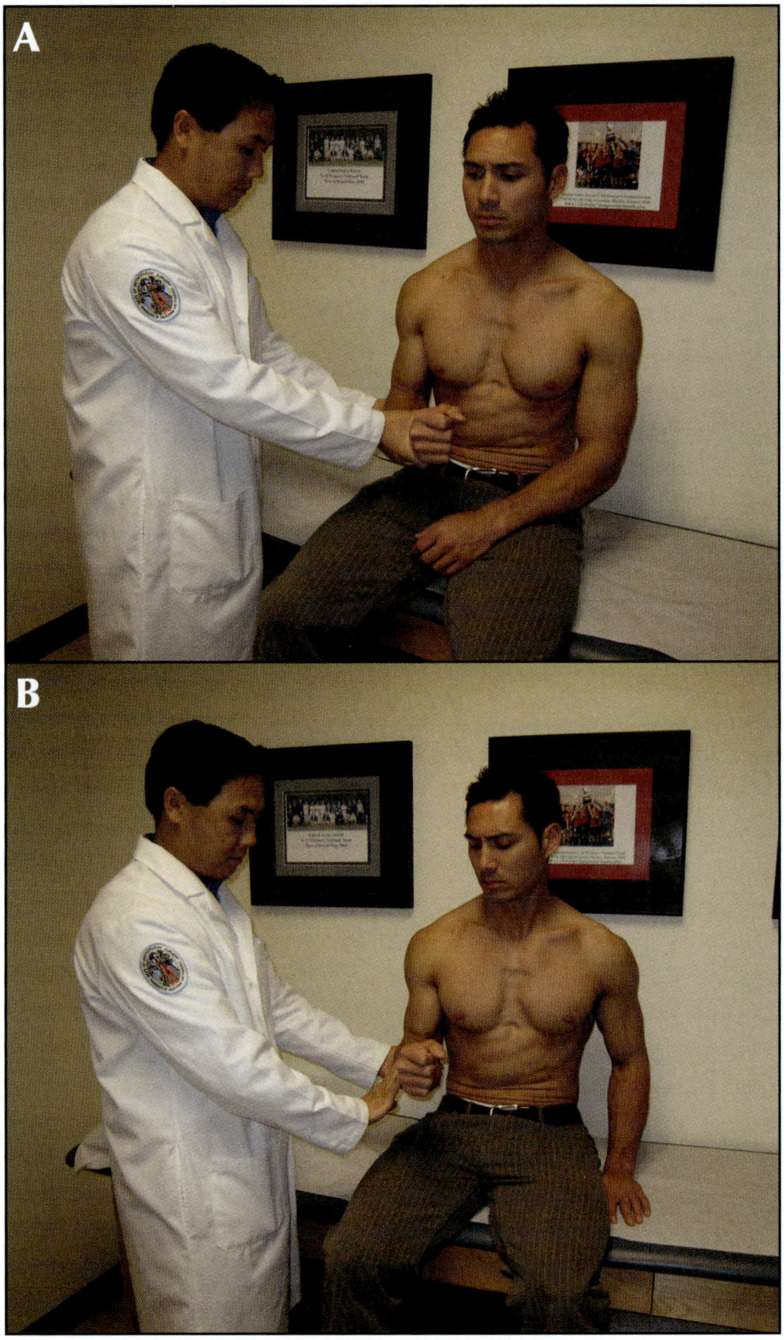

Figure 5-9. Evaluation of isolated infraspinatus strength. (A) The patient's elbow is tucked at the side and the shoulder is internally rotated 45 degrees. (B) The examiner places one hand on the elbow to stabilize it to the patient's side, and the other hand is used to resist external rotation.

Evaluation of the Infraspinatus and Teres Minor

The infraspinatus and teres minor are the primary external rotators of the shoulder with secondary contribution from the posterior deltoid. An EMG study by Kelly and colleagues[15] found that the optimal position for testing isolated infraspinatus strength was with the elbow tucked in at the side and with 45 degrees of humeral internal rotation (Figure 5-9). The examiner places one hand on the elbow to stabilize it to the patient's side, and the other hand is used to resist external rotation (Figure 5-9B). Starting in neutral or external rotation should be avoided as the deltoid is recruited,

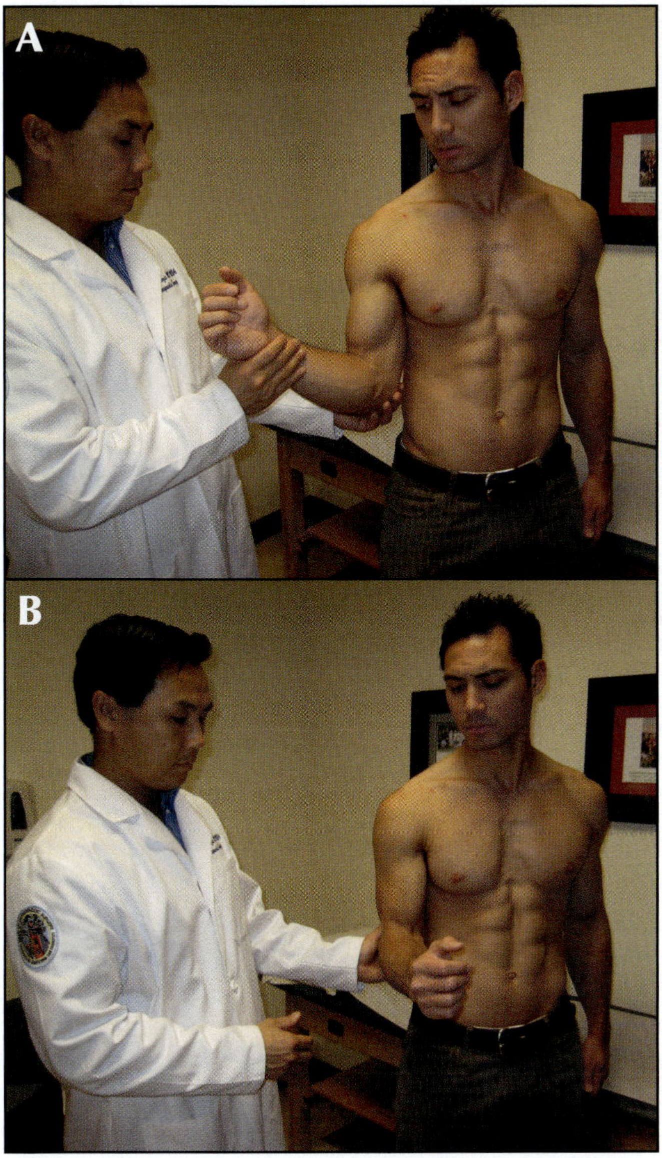

Figure 5-10. External rotation lag sign. (A) The test is performed with the patient seated or standing with the examiner standing behind the patient. The elbow is passively flexed to 90 degrees, the shoulder is elevated 20 degrees in the scapular plane, and the arm is maximally externally rotated and then decreased by 5 degrees to account for normal elastic recoil. (B) The examiner then releases the wrist while stabilizing the elbow. The test is positive if the patient is unable to maintain maximal active external rotation, as is demonstrated here.

which can mask any weakness of the infraspinatus. Additionally, a patient with a frozen shoulder will have limited external rotation, and thus it is crucial that his or her external rotation strength be tested from a starting position of 45 degrees of internal rotation.

External Rotation Lag Sign

To assess the integrity of the supraspinatus and infraspinatus tendons, the external rotation lag sign was described (Figure 5-10).[17] The test is performed with the patient seated or standing with the examiner standing behind the patient. The elbow is passively flexed to 90 degrees, the shoulder is elevated 20 degrees in the scapular plane, and the arm is maximally externally rotated and then decreased by 5 degrees to account for normal elastic recoil (Figure 5-10A). The examiner then releases the wrist while stabilizing the elbow. The test is positive if the patient is unable to maintain maximal active external rotation (Figure 5-10B). The amount of lag should be recorded to the nearest 5 degrees and compared to the contralateral side. It should also be noted whether the patient has

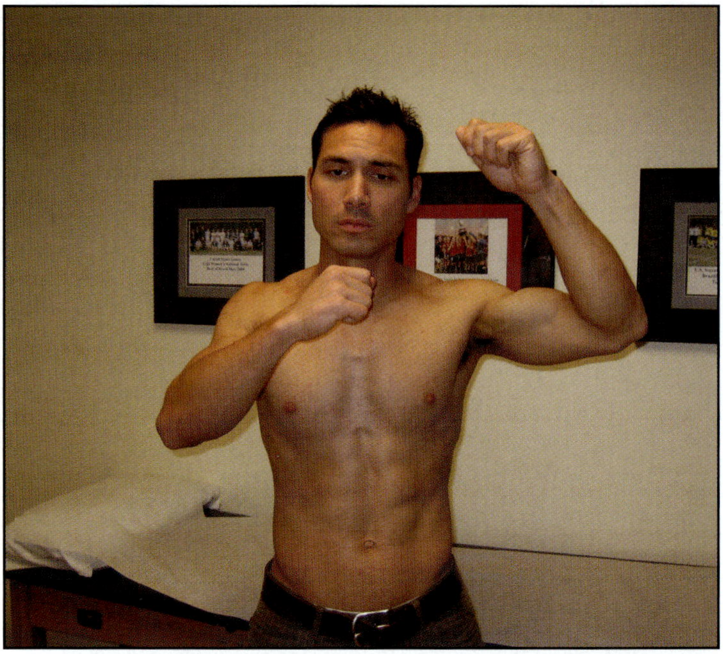

Figure 5-11. The hornblower's sign. With the patient standing, the test is performed with the shoulder abducted to 90 degrees and the elbow flexed to 90 degrees. The examiner places the arm in maximal external rotation. A patient with a torn infraspinatus and teres minor will be unable to maintain the external rotation, and the arm will drop to neutral at the level of the mouth. In this figure, the right shoulder is positive while the left shoulder is normal.

restricted passive external rotation because of contracture, which may give a false positive or negative result. Hertel and colleagues[17] found the external rotation lag sign to have a positive predictive value of 100%, but only a 56% negative predictive value.

Drop Sign

The drop sign is used to isolate the infraspinatus in external rotation. The test is performed with the patient seated or standing. With the examiner standing behind the patient, the injured arm is elevated 90 degrees in the scapular plane, the elbow is flexed to 90 degrees, and the arm is maximally externally rotated. Otis and colleagues[18] used an in vitro cadaver model to show that the infraspinatus is the primary rotator cuff muscle used to maintain external rotation in this position. Once in this position, the examiner releases the wrist while supporting the elbow. The test is positive if the patient is unable to maintain external rotation and the arm "sags" or drops.

The Hornblower's Sign

The hornblower's sign was first reported in the obstetrics literature in describing a child's difficulty in raising the hand to the mouth because of deficient external rotation caused by a brachial plexus birth palsy.[19] In one test used to elicit the hornblower's sign, the patient's shoulder is abducted to 90 degrees and the elbow is flexed to 90 degrees. The examiner then places the patient's arm in maximal external rotation. A patient with a torn infraspinatus and teres minor will be unable to maintain the external rotation, and the arm will drop to neutral at the level of the mouth (Figure 5-11). Walch and colleagues[20] determined the hornblower's sign to have 100% sensitivity and 93% specificity in detecting irreparable degeneration of the teres minor.

Walch and colleagues[20] and McCluskey[21] described another way to evaluate the external rotators and demonstrate the hornblower's sign. The patient is asked to bring both hands to his or her mouth. Patients with a tear of the infraspinatus and teres minor will abduct and internally rotate the affected shoulder to get their hands to their mouths because they have deficient external rotation (Figure 5-12).

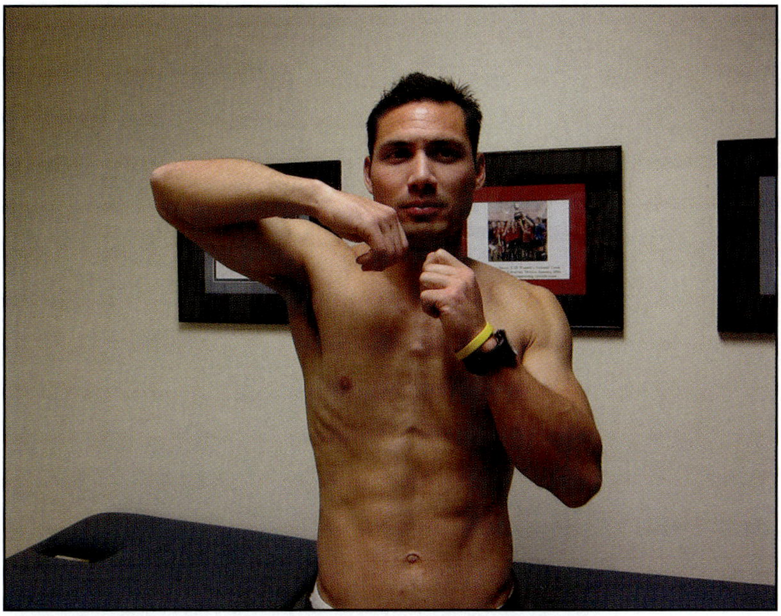

Figure 5-12. The patient is asked to bring both hands to his or her mouth. Patients with a large tear of the infraspinatus and teres minor will abduct and internally rotate the affected shoulder to get their hands to their mouths because they have deficient external rotation. In this figure, the right shoulder is positive while the left shoulder is normal.

Evaluation of the Subscapularis

The subscapularis is the primary muscle of the rotator cuff responsible for internal rotation of the shoulder. The pectoralis major, latissimus dorsi, and teres major also contribute to internal rotation. Internal rotation strength as a whole can be assessed by having patients tuck their elbows into their sides, flex the elbows to 90 degrees, and externally rotate their arms to 40 degrees with the forearms in neutral. The examiner then applies an outward force, pulling the patient's hands apart to evaluate resisted internal rotation. Isolated strength of the subscapularis can be evaluated with the lift-off test, which is described below. Kelly and colleagues[15] verified with EMG that resisted internal rotation with the lift-off maneuver provides optimal manual testing of the subscapularis.

Lift-Off Test and Internal Rotation Lag Sign

Gerber and Krushnell[22] evaluated a cohort of 16 patients with isolated subscapularis tears and found that they all had weakness with internal rotation, which is the foundation of the lift-off test (Figure 5-13). The test is performed by placing the dorsum of the ipsilateral hand against the patient's low back and having him or her push off to lift the hand off the back. A positive test is when the patient is unable to lift the dorsum of the hand off his or her back. Gerber and Krushnell described a positive test as a "pathologic lift-off test."[22]

Hertel and colleagues[17] subsequently described the internal rotation lift-off sign as a modification of the lift-off test. This is performed by having the examiner passively place the injured extremity in maximal internal rotation with the dorsum of the patient's hand off the middle lumbar region of the back. A patient with an intact subscapularis is able to hold maximal internal rotation after the examiner releases his or her hand. A positive sign is the patient's inability to maintain maximal internal rotation and the hand falls onto his or her back. In an evaluation of 100 consecutive painful shoulders composed of normal rotator cuffs and rotator cuffs with tears of varying muscles, Hertel and colleagues[17] found that the internal rotation lag sign was more sensitive and more accurate than the lift-off test with equal specificity ($p < 0.05$). The internal rotation lag sign had a positive predictive value of 97% and a negative predictive value of 96%, whereas the lift-off test had a 100% and 69% positive and negative predictive value, respectively.

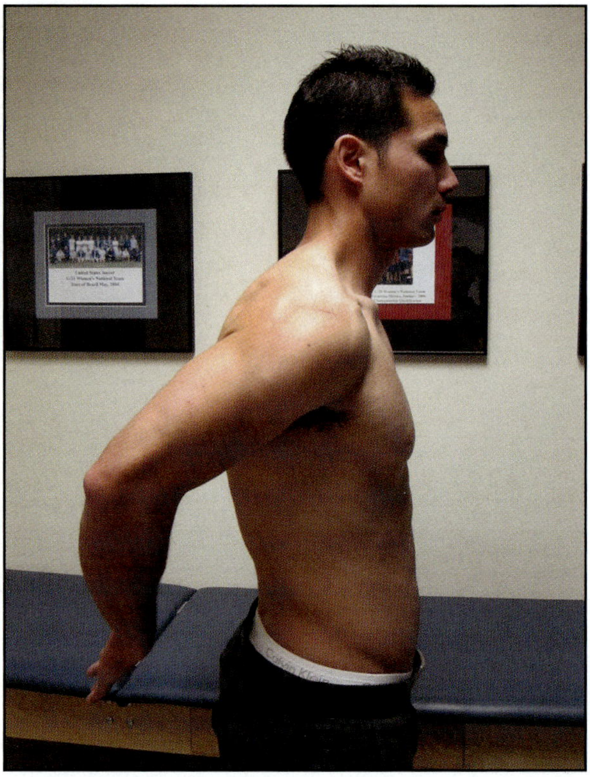

Figure 5-13. Lift-off test. The test is performed by placing the dorsum of the ipsilateral hand against the patient's low back and having him or her push off to lift the hand off the back. A positive test is when a patient is unable to lift the dorsum of the hand off his or her back.

Belly-Press Test

Gerber and colleagues[23] subsequently developed the belly-press test to evaluate for subscapularis tears in patients who were unable to perform the lift-off test because of impaired passive internal rotation (Figure 5-14A). The patient is instructed to place the palm of his or her ipsilateral hand against his or her belly, keeping the arm internally rotated. If the subscapularis is intact, the elbow will remain in front of the abdomen. A patient with a torn subscapularis will have weakness with internal rotation and will extend the shoulder in order to maintain internal rotation, thus causing the elbow to fall behind the plane of the trunk (Figure 5-14B). In Gerber's series of patients with isolated subscapularis tears, all 8 patients tested had a positive belly-press test.[23]

Napoleon Test

The Napoleon test is similar to the belly-press test, which was originally reported in 1999 by Schwamborn and Imhoff[24] and subsequently modified by Burkhart and Tehrany.[25] It was designed to distinguish the grade of subscapularis tendon tear. The palm of the hand is placed on the belly, and the patient is asked to push on his or her belly, keeping his or her wrist straight. This test was given its' name because the hand position is the same as that of Napoleon Bonaparte, who held his hand against his belly for all portraits. A negative test is when the patient is able to push against the belly while keeping the wrist straight. An intermediate result corresponds to a partial tear and is determined by the wrist flexing from 30 to 60 degrees to press against the belly. A positive test requires that the wrist be flexed to 90 degrees to achieve the belly-press, and this would be seen with a full tear of the subscapularis tendon.

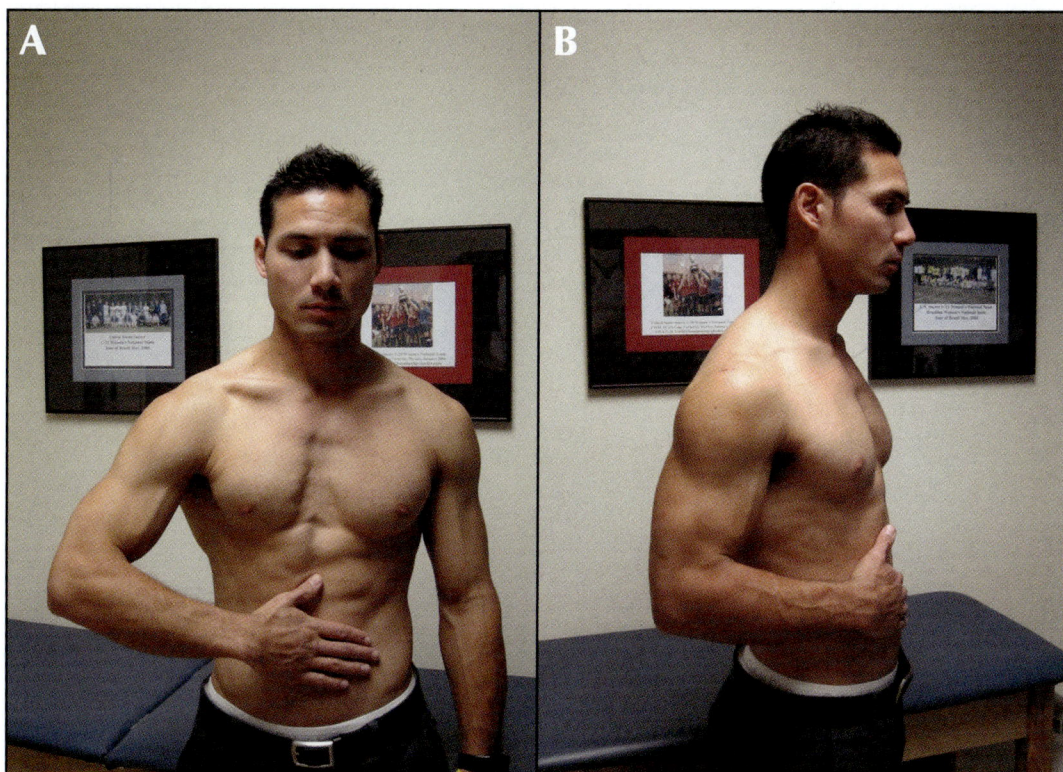

Figure 5-14. Belly-press test. (A) The patient is instructed to place the palm of his or her ipsilateral hand against his or her belly, keeping the arm internally rotated. If the subscapularis is intact, the elbow will remain in front of the abdomen. (B) A patient with a torn subscapularis will have weakness with internal rotation and will extend the shoulder in order to maintain internal rotation, thus causing the elbow to fall behind the plane of the trunk.

Bear-Hug Test

In 2006, Barth and colleagues[26] devised the bear-hug test to improve the diagnostic accuracy of evaluating subscapularis tears (Figure 5-15). The test is performed by having the patient place his or her ipsilateral hand on the contralateral shoulder with the fingers extended so that the palm is touching the shoulder. The examiner then holds the patient's wrist and lifts up, applying an external rotation force. The patient is instructed to maintain the palm on his or her shoulder (exerting resisted internal rotation). The test is considered positive if the patient is unable to hold his or her palm to the shoulder or if the patient's strength is less than 80% of the uninjured shoulder (Figure 5-15B). In a consecutive series of 68 patients with rotator cuff tears, 29.4% of which had subscapularis tears, Barth and colleagues[26] found the bear-hug test to be more sensitive (60%) than other tests of subscapularis function (lift-off, 25%; belly-press, 40%; and Napoleon test, 17.6%) and was particularly accurate in detecting tears of the upper portion of the subscapularis tendon. Specificities of all tests were high (lift-off test, 100%; Napoleon test, 97.9%; belly-press test, 97.9%; and bear-hug test, 91.7%). They determined that these tests were most useful in predicting the size of the subscapularis tear. A positive bear-hug and belly-press test used in combination is indicative of a subscapularis tear of at least 30%, whereas a Napoleon test detected tears greater than 50%. The lift-off test did not tend to be positive until at least 75% of the subscapularis tendon was torn.

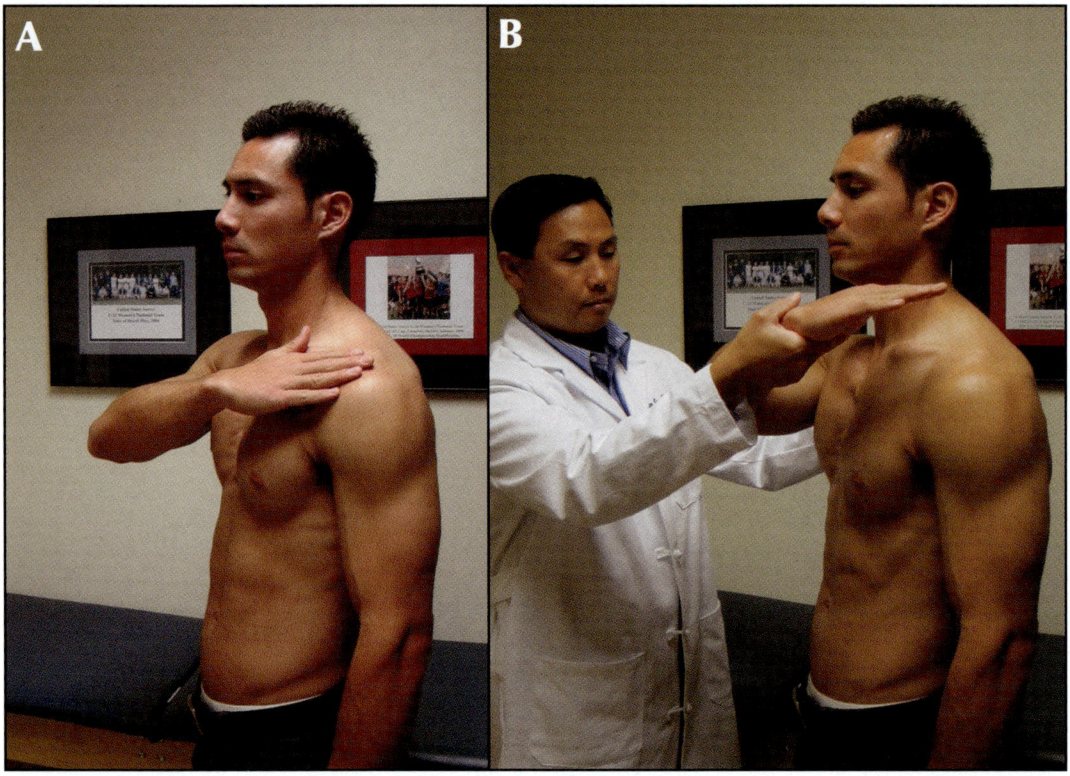

Figure 5-15. Bear-hug test. (A) The test is performed by having the patient place his or her ipsilateral hand on the contralateral shoulder with the fingers extended. The examiner then holds the patient's wrist and lifts up, applying an external rotation force. The patient is instructed to maintain his or her palm on his or her shoulder (exerting resisted internal rotation). (B) Demonstration of a positive test where the patient is unable to hold his or her palm to the shoulder because of deficiency of the subscapularis to maintain internal rotation. This test is also considered positive if the patient's strength is less than 80% of the uninjured shoulder.

CONCLUSION

It is imperative that a thorough yet concise history and physical examination be performed on every patient with a shoulder complaint before imaging is reviewed. Patients with rotator cuff injuries will often complain of pain with overhead activities, weakness, and night pain. The history is used to narrow the differential diagnosis so that a focused physical exam can be performed. There are several tests described for evaluation of the rotator cuff. While not exhaustive, this chapter provides a comprehensive list of tests organized by strength of individual rotator cuff muscles and provocative impingement maneuvers. It still remains unclear which test is the most accurate in diagnosing impingement or tears of individual rotator cuff muscles. Kelly and colleagues[15] used EMG to determine the optimal position for strength testing of the supraspinatus (see Figure 5-7), infraspinatus (see Figure 5-9), and subscapularis (see Figure 5-13). Another EMG study by Chao and colleagues[27] compared the bear-hug test at 0, 45, and 90 degrees of shoulder flexion with the belly-press and lift-off test. They found that the bear-hug test performed at 45 degrees of shoulder flexion and the belly-press test provided the greatest peak EMG activity in the upper subscapularis, while the bear-hug test positioned at 90 degrees of shoulder flexion had the highest EMG activity in the lower subscapularis. It is likely that tests used in combination more accurately assess the condition of the rotator cuff. Park and colleagues[6] looked at 8 tests for rotator cuff impingement: the Neer impingement sign, Hawkins-Kennedy impingement sign, painful arc sign, supraspinatus muscle strength test, Speed test, cross-body adduction test, drop-arm sign, and infraspinatus muscle strength test. They found that the Hawkins-Kennedy impingement sign, painful arc sign, and infraspinatus strength test in combination had the highest post-test probability for any degree of impingement (95%), whereas a combination of the drop-arm sign, infraspinatus strength test, and painful arc sign best diagnosed full-thickness rotator cuff tears (91%).

There are a number of tests to evaluate for impingement and strength of each of the rotator cuff muscles. It is likely that a combination of tests is more accurate in localizing the lesion. This chapter provides a comprehensive list of tests and some literature supporting their accuracy in identifying rotator cuff pathology. For the clinician, it is important to be familiar with each test but to develop a routine exam based on the individual patient in order to build experience that can discern the subtleties of each test and what truly is positive and negative.

ACKNOWLEDGMENTS

The authors would like to thank Joe Smith, MS, ATC and Derek Hirai, MS, ATC for their contribution to the figures.

REFERENCES

1. Miniaci A, Mascia AT, Salonen DC, Becker EJ. Magnetic resonance imaging of the shoulder in asymptomatic professional baseball pitchers. *Am J Sports Med.* 2002;30:66-73.
2. Codman EA, Akerson IB. The pathology associated with rupture of the supraspinatus tendon. *Ann Surg.* 1931;93:348-359.
3. Neer CS 2nd. Anterior acromioplasty for the chronic impingement syndrome in the shoulder: a preliminary report. *J Bone Joint Surg Am.* 1972;54:41-50.
4. Neer CS 2nd. Impingement lesions. *Clin Orthop Relat Res.* 1983;(173):70-77.
5. MacDonald PB, Clark P, Sutherland K. An analysis of the diagnostic accuracy of the Hawkins and Neer subacromial impingement signs. *J Shoulder Elbow Surg.* 2000;9:299-301.
6. Park HB, Yokota A, Gill HS, El Rassi G, McFarland EG. Diagnostic accuracy of clinical tests for the different degrees of subacromial impingement syndrome. *J Bone Joint Surg Am.* 2005;87:1446-1455.
7. Hawkins RJ, Kennedy JC. Impingement syndrome in athletes. *Am J Sports Med.* 1980;8:151-158.
8. Jobe FW, Jobe CM. Painful athletic injuries of the shoulder. *Clin Orthop Relat Res.* 1983;(173):117-124.
9. Itoi E, Kido T, Sano A, Urayama M, Sato K. Which is more useful, the "full can test" or the "empty can test," in detecting the torn supraspinatus tendon? *Am J Sports Med.* 1999;27:65-68.
10. Yocum LA. Assessing the shoulder. History, physical examination, differential diagnosis, and special tests used. *Clin Sports Med.* 1983;2:281-289.
11. Silva L, Andreu JL, Munoz P, et al. Accuracy of physical examination in subacromial impingement syndrome. *Rheumatology (Oxford).* 2008;47:679-683.
12. Zaslav KR. Internal rotation resistance strength test: a new diagnostic test to differentiate intra-articular pathology from outlet (Neer) impingement syndrome in the shoulder. *J Shoulder Elbow Surg.* 2001;10:23-27.
13. Jobe FW, Moynes DR. Delineation of diagnostic criteria and a rehabilitation program for rotator cuff injuries. *Am J Sports Med.* 1982;10:336-339.
14. Codman EA. *The Shoulder: Rupture of the Supraspinatus Tendon and Other Lesions in or About the Subacromial Bursa.* Boston, MA: T. Todd company; 1934.
15. Kelly BT, Kadrmas WR, Speer KP. The manual muscle examination for rotator cuff strength. An electromyographic investigation. *Am J Sports Med.* 1996;24:581-588.
16. Savoie FH 3rd, Field LD, Atchinson S. Anterior superior instability with rotator cuff tearing: SLAC lesion. *Orthop Clin North Am.* 2001;32:457-461, ix.
17. Hertel R, Ballmer FT, Lombert SM, Gerber C. Lag signs in the diagnosis of rotator cuff rupture. *J Shoulder Elbow Surg.* 1996;5:307-313.
18. Otis JC, Jiang CC, Wickiewicz TL, Peterson MG, Warren RF, Santner TJ. Changes in the moment arms of the rotator cuff and deltoid muscles with abduction and rotation. *J Bone Joint Surg Am.* 1994;76:667-676.
19. Arthuis M. [Obstetrical paralysis of the brachial plexus. I. diagnosis. B. Regression period. a. Clinical course during the regression period]. *Rev Chir Orthop Reparatrice Appar Mot.* 1972;58:Suppl 1:129-131.

20. Walch G, Boulahia A, Calderone S, Robinson AH. The 'dropping' and 'hornblower's' signs in evaluation of rotator-cuff tears. *J Bone Joint Surg Br.* 1998;80:624-628.

21. McCluskey GM. Classification and diagnosis of glenohumeral instability in athletes. *Sports Med Arthrosc Rev.* 2000;8:158-169.

22. Gerber C, Krushell RJ. Isolated rupture of the tendon of the subscapularis muscle. Clinical features in 16 cases. *J Bone Joint Surg Br.* 1991;73:389-394.

23. Gerber C, Hersche O, Farron A. Isolated rupture of the subscapularis tendon. *J Bone Joint Surg Am.* 1996;78:1015-1023.

24. Schwamborn T, Imhoff AB. [Diagnosis and classification of rotator cuff]. In: Imhoff AB, Konig U, eds. *Schulterinstabilitat-Rotatorenmanschette Darmstadt.* Heidelberg, Germany: Steinkopff Verlag; 1999:193-195.

25. Burkhart SS, Tehrany AM. Arthroscopic subscapularis tendon repair: technique and preliminary results. *Arthroscopy.* 2002;18:454-463.

26. Barth JR, Burkhart SS, De Beer JF. The bear-hug test: a new and sensitive test for diagnosing a subscapularis tear. *Arthroscopy.* 2006;22:1076-1084.

27. Chao S, Thomas S, Yucha D, Kelly JD, Driban J, Swanik K. An electromyographic assessment of the "bear hug": an examination for the evaluation of the subscapularis muscle. *Arthroscopy.* 2008;24:1265-1270.

CHAPTER 6

IMAGING OF THE ROTATOR CUFF

Lorenzo Nardo, MD and Thomas M. Link, MD

Shoulder pain is common with a 1-year prevalence reported up to 47% in the general population,[1,2] and it adversely affects daily living and work, causing substantial morbidity. Pain is the most common symptom related to shoulder problems, and it leads to a reduction in shoulder strength and functional impairment.[3] Rotator cuff disease related to subacromial impingement syndrome is one of the most frequently diagnosed clinical shoulder disorders.[4,5] Besides subacromial impingement, shoulder pain may be related to a wide range of pathologies, spanning from subacromial-subdeltoid bursitis and tendinopathy (sometimes associated with calcifications) to partial- and full-thickness rotator cuff tears.

Radiologic techniques are reliable in making the distinction between normal anatomy and abnormalities in the rotator cuff; they are indispensable in the therapeutic decision making, surgical planning, and postsurgical prognosis.[6] While standard radiographs give indirect evidence of mostly advanced rotator cuff disease, magnetic resonance imaging (MRI) allows direct visualization of the rotator cuff muscles and tendons. With advances in cross-sectional imaging over the past few years, better visualization of not only the muscle and tendons but also labrum and ligaments has been achieved. MRI allows direct assessment of rotator cuff tears, muscle atrophy, and denervation.[7] It will also demonstrate changes in the surrounding joint structures, which will affect the rotator cuff. However, MRI also has limitations, such as the visualization of calcific tendinitis; for this reason, a complete assessment of the rotator cuff will require both radiographs and MRI.[8]

Also, radiological and clinical findings must always be correlated to fully understand the underlying pathology. In the following chapter, we will review the different imaging techniques, the main important shoulder impingement syndromes and their sequelae, the various types and causes of rotator cuff injuries, and the radiological findings after shoulder surgery.

Ma CB, Feeley BT, eds.
*Basic Principles and Operative Management
of the Rotator Cuff (pp 77-102)*
© 2012 SLACK Incorporated

Figure 6-1. AP radiograph of the right shoulder demonstrating a high-riding humeral head, subacromial stenosis (double arrow), and degenerative changes at the acromion with increased sclerosis. In addition, there is an osteophyte at the acromion (arrow). These findings are indirect signs of a complete rotator cuff tear.

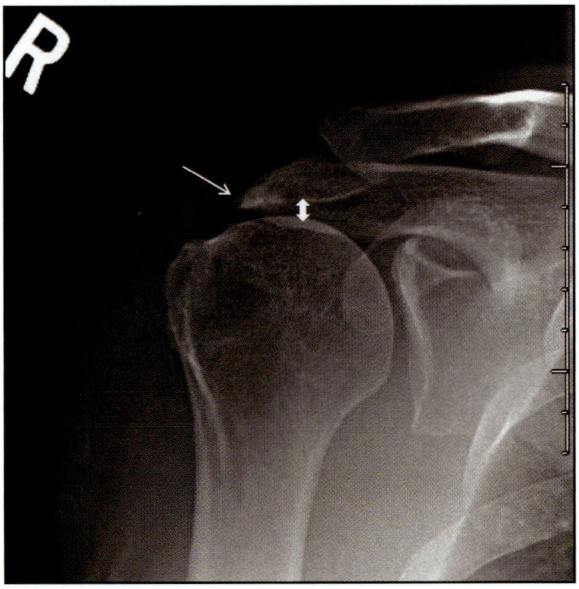

Techniques for Imaging of the Rotator Cuff

Different techniques are used to image the shoulder. In the following paragraph, standard techniques are described pertaining in particular to assessing abnormalities of the rotator cuff. These include standard radiographs, computed tomography (CT), MRI, and MR arthrography (MRA).

Conventional Radiographs

Conventional radiographs are usually the first step in the imaging examination performed on an individual suffering from shoulder pathology. Although numerous variations exist for several views to evaluate shoulder pathology, the basic examination of the shoulder consists of a standard anteroposterior (AP) view and a "true" AP view, 40-degree posterior oblique radiographs, called Grashey views.[9] Since the glenohumeral joint is tilted anteriorly about 40 degrees, on a standard AP view, the glenoid rim minimally overlaps the humeral head. This view can be obtained with the arm in the neutral position, internal and external rotation. With the arm internally rotated, the greater tuberosity is projected over the humerus head, and the lesser tuberosity may be superimposed over the glenohumeral joint. In this position, it is possible to assess calcification of subscapularis and infraspinatus muscles adjacent to the lesser tuberosity and on the lateral aspect of the humerus, respectively. With the arm externally rotated, supraspinatus calcifications are better demonstrated. Figure 6-1 shows an externally rotated view of the right shoulder with a high-riding humeral head and subacromial space narrowing consistent with advanced degenerative rotator cuff disease. The Grashey view of the scapula provides a tangent view of the glenohumeral joint, which is 35 to 45 degrees oblique to traditional shoulder AP radiography. This projection is very useful to assess glenohumeral joint space narrowing and inferior/superior humeral head migration.[10]

An axillary lateral view is performed for evaluating glenohumeral subluxation and may also detect fractures of the anterior glenoid rim (Bankart fracture; Figure 6-2). This projection is obtained with the patient supine, the arm abducted 90 degrees, and the x-ray beam aimed inferior to superior with 15 to 30 degrees of medial angulation. Variations have been developed to demonstrate different details, such as the West Point view and Stryker Notch view.[10] The West Point view is obtained by placing the patient prone with the arm abducted to 90 degrees and the elbow and forearm hanging over the edge of the table. The x-ray beam is directed 25 degrees in an anterior to superior direction

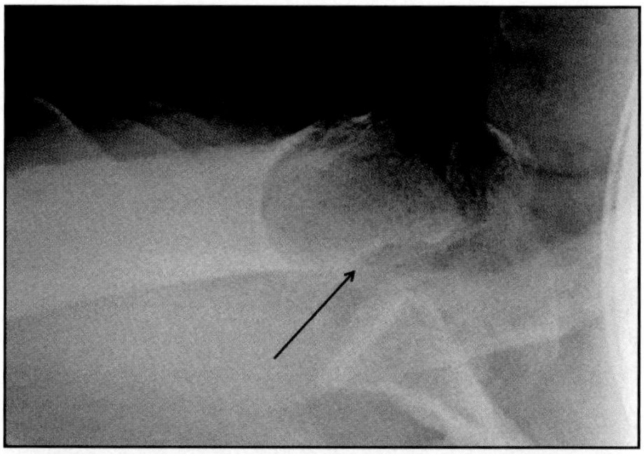

Figure 6-2. Axillary view of the shoulder demonstrating anterior dislocation of the right humeral head with a large Hill-Sachs deformity of the posterior humeral head (arrow).

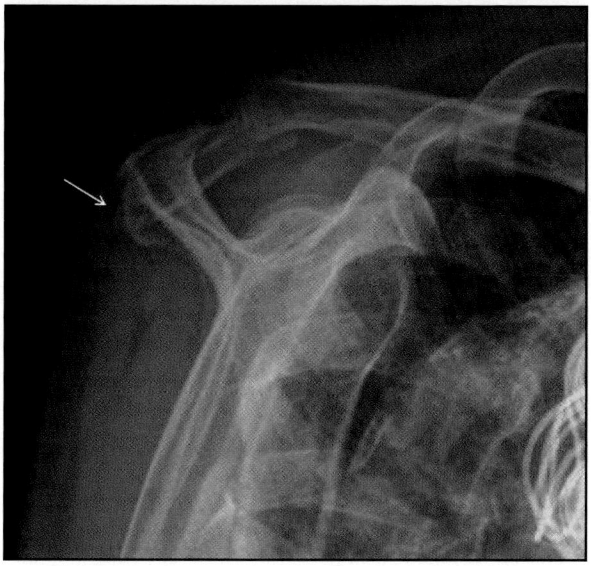

Figure 6-3. Scapular Y view demonstrating acromial fracture (arrow).

and 25 degrees medially tilted. This position improves visualization of the anteroinferior glenoid rim. West Point axillary views will demonstrate small osseous Bankart lesions of the anteroinferior glenoid rim and Bennett lesions.[11] The Stryker Notch view is obtained with the patient in the supine or upright position. The hand is placed on top of the head with the elbow flexed. The x-ray beam is tilted 10 degrees cephalic.[10] It depicts the posterolateral aspect of the humeral head and thus helps in the diagnosis of Hill-Sachs lesions; glenohumeral subluxation is difficult to evaluate with this projection.

The scapular Y view can be very helpful in different shoulder abnormalities, such as anterior or posterior humeral head subluxation or dislocation, fractures of the coracoid process, scapula, acromion process, and proximal humeral shaft (Figure 6-3); furthermore, it is useful to evaluate the type of the acromion. In the setting of acute trauma, this projection is preferable to the lateral axillary view because it is obtained without moving the arm of the patient; the patient is upright or prone, 40 degrees posteriorly rotated, and the beam is directed longitudinally down the axis of the scapular spine. The humeral head should be centered over the glenoid fossa.[12] The Y shape is formed by the projection of the acromion, scapular body, and coracoid.

A number of different projections have been used that are dedicated for different pathologies. For example, Neer and Rockwood views (AP with 30 degrees of caudal angulation of the x-ray beam) can evaluate the subacromial space for signs of impingement[9]; a superoinferior projection can well

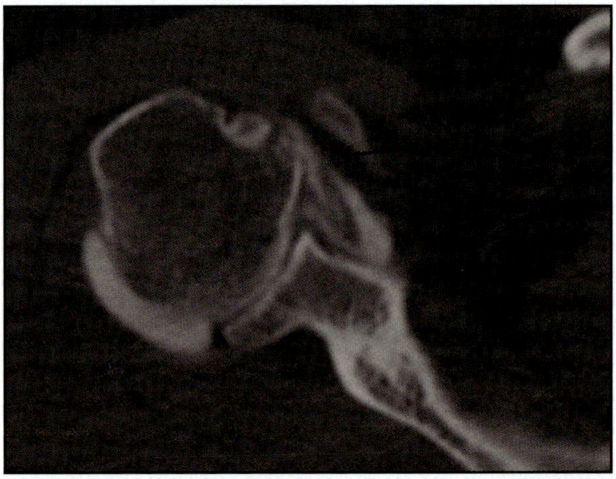

Figure 6-4. Axial CTA of the right shoulder. Contrast within the subscapularis tendon is seen (arrow) and is consistent with a full-thickness tear of the subscapularis near the lesser tuberosity attachment.

visualize the bicipital groove. Despite all of these different projections, usually only basic projections are obtained initially, and either MRI or CT scans are requested to assess additional pathologies/symptoms not demonstrated with standard radiographs.

Computed Tomography and Computed Tomography Arthrography

Although MRI and MRA represent the first choice in the diagnosis of most of the shoulder abnormalities, CT and CT arthrography (CTA) may be used successfully for some specific applications given CT's short time of acquisition and excellent contrast between bone (cortex), soft tissues (such as hyaline cartilage), and the iodinated contrast material (Figure 6-4).[12,13] Furthermore, specific indications of CT and CTA are absolute or relative contraindications to MRI or MRA, such as ferromagnetic implanted medical devices, claustrophobic or obese patients, and metal hardware.[8,13-15]

Standard and specific radiographic views are usually obtained before CTA in order to assess calcifications (calcific tendinitis or calcium pyrophosphate dihydrate), loose bodies, acromial shape (Y-view), and pathology of the bone contour deformities such as Hill-Sachs (Stryker Notch view) and Bankart lesion (West Point view).[10,16-20] CTA is performed when radiographs are not sufficient to solve the diagnostic request. Joint injection is performed by either an anterior or a posterior approach. The contrast media is injected into the glenohumeral joint space under fluoroscopic guidance and under sterile conditions. Double or mono-contrast techniques are described in the literature. Using double-contrast techniques, both iodinated contrast and room air are injected into the joint.[20] Double-contrast techniques are currently less frequently used in most institutions.[8] Mono-contrast techniques consist of injecting only iodinated contrast, which may be diluted with saline or local anesthetic; the injection is terminated when there is a palpable sense of an increase of pressure while injecting or if one reaches 12 to 14 mL of total injected volume to avoid capsular rupture. The CT should be performed as soon as possible after the joint injection to avoid resorption of contrast media, loss of capsular distension, and cartilage contrast imbibition.

CT exam is performed with the affected arm usually placed by the side of the body, in slightly external rotation. The contralateral arm is raised above the head to minimize radiation exposure.[8] After obtaining a scout view, the scanning is performed parallel to the humeral shaft from the superior margin of the acromioclavicular (AC) joint through proximal humeral diaphysis. The acquisition time with a multidetector CT (MDCT) is very short, and, thus, the examination can be performed in apnea. MDCT scanners with submillimeter section acquisition (0.6 mm), almost isotropic data acquisition, and excellent spatial resolution are very helpful in the diagnosis of most of the shoulder pathologies.[21] Multiplanar reformations are obtained in the coronal oblique and sagittal oblique planes; the coronal oblique plane is reformatted parallel to the long axis of the

TABLE 6-1. STANDARD SHOULDER MAGNETIC RESONANCE PROTOCOL						
SEQUENCE #	1	2	3	4	5	6
SEQUENCE TYPE	FSE T2 fat saturation	FSE PD	FSE T2 fat saturation	FSE T1	FSE T2 fat saturation	FSE PD
PLANE	Axial	Axial	Coronal oblique	Coronal oblique	Sagittal oblique	Sagittal oblique
FIELD OF VIEW (CM)	12	12	12	12	12	12
SLICE THICKNESS (MM)	4	4	4	4	4	4
REPETITION TIME IN MS	3500	2500	3500	500	3500	2500
ECHO TIME IN MS	55	30	55	8	55	30

FSE = fast spin echo; PD = proton density-weighted

supraspinatus muscle and the sagittal oblique perpendicular to the latter.[22] In case of specific concerns such as internal posterosuperior impingement (PSI), a lesion of posterior glenoid, evaluation of the deep fibers of the suprascapular muscle, an acquisition with the shoulder in the abduction external rotation (ABER) position, may be helpful.[23,24]

Magnetic Resonance Imaging/Arthrography

Shoulder MRI should be performed with a dedicated surface coil to provide the best possible visualization of shoulder anatomic structures. The shoulder is scanned with the patient placed supine with the arm at the patient's side in a neutral position or slight external rotation for a standard examination; the rotation of the arm influences the position of the anatomic structures on the MR images and is therefore very critical for image interpretation.[25,26] Imaging is obtained using a 13- to 16-mm field of view, with 3- to 4-mm thick slices and 1-mm interslice space in 3 planes: coronal oblique, axial, and sagittal oblique.[27] The coronal oblique images are acquired in a plane perpendicular to the glenoid cavity or parallel to the supraspinatus tendon, including all the volume between infraspinatus and subscapularis muscles. The axial images are obtained from the top of the acromion to the inferior margin of the glenohumeral joint using a coronal scout image as a localizer. The oblique sagittal images extend from the lateral aspect of the greater tuberosity through the scapular body and are acquired with cuts perpendicular to the supraspinatus tendon. A typical shoulder MR protocol consists of the following sequences (Table 6-1): axial proton density-weighted and fat-saturated T2-weighted fast spin echo (FSE) sequences, oblique coronal T1-weighted and fat-saturated T2-weighted FSE sequences, and sagittal oblique proton density-weighted and fat-saturated T2-weighted FSE sequences.

Shoulder MRA is performed after intra-articular injection of diluted gadolinium-based contrast agents (eg, Magnevist); the typical MR protocol is described in detail in Table 6-2. Initially, local anesthesia is performed using 5 cc of lidocaine (1%) and 0.5 cc of sodium bicarbonate (8.4%). Subsequently, the correct needle position is confirmed with 2 to 4 mL of a mixture of 10 cc of iodinated contrast agent and 10 cc of bacteriostatic saline. Once contrast agent is demonstrated in the joint, a mixture of 10 cc of bacteriostatic saline, 10 cc of ropivacaine (local anesthetic Naropin), and 0.1 cc of Magnevist are injected. The ropivacaine is used because it is less toxic to the chondrocytes than other local anesthetics. In the literature, different approaches are described: anterior, posterior, and, recently, the rotator interval approach.[28,29] The majority of the radiologists are trained in fluoroscopy-guided procedures using an anterior injection. Thus, this approach is the most commonly used: coracoid process and anterior humeral head are localized, and the needle is inserted

TABLE 6-2. SHOULDER MAGNETIC RESONANCE ARTHROGRAPHY PROTOCOL

SEQUENCE #	1	2	3	4	5	6	7 (ABER position)
SEQUENCE TYPE	FSE T1 fat saturation	FSE T1 fat saturation	FSE T1 fat saturation	FSE T2 fat saturation	FSE T2 fat saturation	FSE T1	FSE T1 fat saturation
PLANE	Axial	Axial	Coronal oblique	Coronal oblique	Sagittal oblique	Sagittal oblique	Sagittal oblique
FIELD OF VIEW (CM)	12	12	12	12	12	12	12
SLICE THICKNESS (MM)	4	4	4	4	4	4	4
REPETITION TIME IN MS	600	3000	600	3000	3000	600	600
ECHO TIME IN MS	8	50	8	50	50	8	8

FSE = fast spin echo

under fluoroscopy guidance inferiorly to the coracoid toward the glenohumeral joint space.[30] The posterior approach[31] has been advocated in order to avoid potential damage to the stabilizing structures of the shoulder (disadvantages of an anterior approach), including labrocapsular complex and inferior glenohumeral ligament, especially when joint anterior instability is suspected.[32,33] Also, if there is concern for subscapularis abnormalities, the posterior approach may be useful. The rotator cuff interval approach[33] is the most recent; this approach can avoid damage to the anterosuperior labrum, anteroinferior labrum, subscapularis muscle and tendon, and inferior glenohumeral ligament. The injection site is the rotator interval, between the supraspinatus and the subscapularis tendons. In order to avoid traumatic lesion of the biceps, the biceps muscle should be lateralized by externally rotating the shoulder.

PATHOLOGY OF THE ROTATOR CUFF

Shoulder Impingement

Shoulder impingement syndromes are usually classified into extrinsic (also known as external) and intrinsic impingements, which refer to extra- and intra-articular impingements of the rotator cuff tendons, respectively.[34] The impingement may result from abnormalities of the anatomical structures, including muscles, tendons, bones, and bursae. The radiological and MR findings associated with impingement may consist of tendinosis or tears of the tendons, degenerative cysts, sclerosis, osseous hypertrophy of the greater tuberosity and/or humeral head, bursitis, and narrowing of acromion-humeral associated with superior humeral migration.[11,35-41]

Extrinsic Impingement

Extrinsic impingement may be either primary or secondary. Primary external impingement results from subacromial and subcoracoid compression, while secondary extrinsic impingement results from glenohumeral instability.[40]

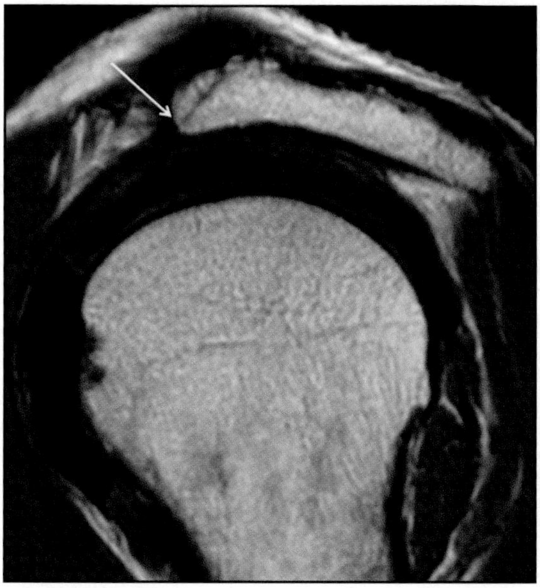

Figure 6-5. Proton density-weighted sagittal MRI of the right shoulder demonstrating type II morphology of the acromion, which is curved (arrow) but has no hook.

Subacromial Impingement

The supraspinatus tendon, the long head of the biceps, and the subacromial-subdeltoid bursa are contained in the coracoacromial (CA) arch, which is the structure surrounding the supraspinatus outlet. The CA arch consists of coracoid and CA ligament anteriorly, the acromion superiorly, and the humeral head posteriorly.[42] All conditions that decrease the space within the CA arch can potentially result in clinical impingement. The subacromial impingement syndrome is a condition characterized by acute or chronic pain induced by internal rotation and elevation of the shoulder or by external rotation and abduction of the shoulder.[7,41] The most important causes of subacromial impingement include the following:

- Morphology of the undersurface of the acromion: According to the Bigliani-Gagey classification, the acromial shape is classified based either on the appearance of the undersurface on scapular Y view radiographs or on sagittal oblique MRI. Four types are differentiated: type I, flat (12%); type II, curved (50%; Figure 6-5); and type III, hooked (29%); type IV (3%) with a convex inferior surface. Type III has been associated with subacromial impingement.[43] Enthesophytes are usually localized at the site of the CA ligament insertion on the acromion. They are significantly more common with type III acromion, and this combination is particularly associated with subacromial impingement syndrome and rotator cuff tears.[43]
- AC relation to the humeral head: Anterior or lateral down-sloping of the acromion and a low-lying acromion have been associated with subacromial impingement.[44]
- AC joint degenerative changes with osteophytes and thickening of the capsule.
- Os acromiale (Figure 6-6): Best evaluated on axial images; normally, it is fused in patients older than 25 years, but in up to 15% of the population, it is unfused and is frequently a bilateral condition. Different types of os acromiale have been differentiated; based on their position, they can be classified as mesoacromion, meta-acromion, basiacromion, and preacromion.[45-49]
- Thickening of the CA ligament: The CA ligament usually consists of 2 distinct ligamentous bands: the anterolateral band and the posteromedial band. Spurs usually grow in the antero-lateral band due to load-bearing mechanisms.[42] The thickness of the CA ligament varies from 2 to 5.6 mm.[50]
- Post-traumatic deformity of the acromion.
- Muscular hypertrophy causing subacromial stenosis.

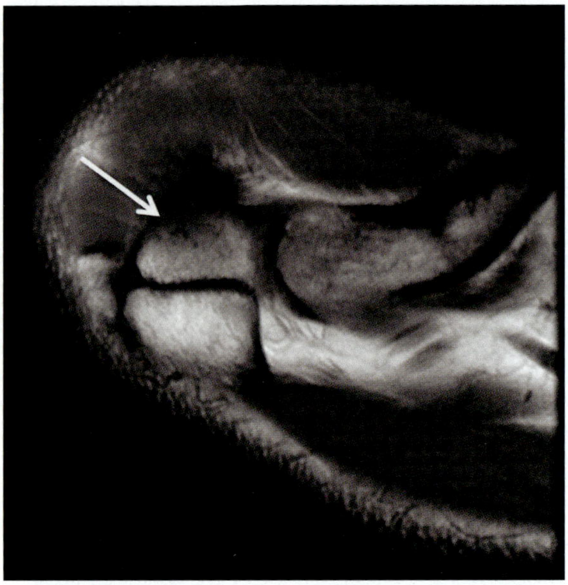

Figure 6-6. Os acromiale. Proton density-weighted axial image of the right shoulder in a 40-year-old patient. At the level of the AC joint, a separate os acromiale (arrow) is demonstrated. This condition may lead to subacromial impingement.

Subcoracoid Impingement

The coracohumeral (CH) interval is bounded by the coracoid process anteriorly and the humeral head posteriorly. The term *subcoracoid impingement syndrome* refers to entrapment of subscapularis tendon and muscle in the CH interval.[51] On the axial MRI images, the CH distance can be assessed as the narrowest distance between the apex of the coracoid and the humeral head/lesser tuberosity. Normally, the CH interval is about 10 mm; the suggested cut-off to consider subcoracoid stenosis is 6 mm.[52-54] Any conditions that may reduce the CH distance fewer than 6 mm may lead to subcoracoid impingement. The causes of subcoracoid impingement have been categorized as traumatic, idiopathic (developmental enlargement or downward sloping of the coracoid), and iatrogenic.[38] MR findings associated with subcoracoid impingement include tendinosis/tear of the subscapularis tendon, abnormalities of the long head of biceps, subcoracoid bursitis, and cortical irregularities of the lesser tuberosity.[34]

Secondary Extrinsic Impingement

Extrinsic impingement can be distinguished from primary impingement in that there are no abnormalities in the CA arch architecture; secondary extrinsic impingement results from glenohumeral instability. The instability related to the glenohumeral joint may increase the strain of the rotator cuff muscles and tendon, causing cuff fatigue. The direct consequence of this instability is the superior migration of the humeral head, which narrows the AC arch.[55-57] MRA can be helpful for the assessment of secondary extrinsic impingement evaluating capsular laxity and ruling out the presence of anatomical factors responsible for primary extrinsic impingement.

Internal Impingement

The term *internal impingement* refers to the entrapment of the supraspinatus and/or infraspinatus muscle fibers and the glenoid labrum due to abnormal contact between the greater tuberosity and the glenoid. With regard to the portion of the involved glenoid, it is classified into anterior and posterior internal impingement.[41] PSI of the shoulder is a pathologic condition characterized by excessive or repetitive contact of the posterosuperior aspect of the glenoid against the greater tuberosity of the humeral head when the arm is in the ABER position.[39,41] This leads to entrapment of the posterior fibers of the supraspinatus tendon, anterior fibers of the infraspinatus tendon, and the posterosuperior labrum. The majority of patients who suffer from this kind of impingement are overhead athletes, such as swimmers, volleyball players, tennis players, baseball players, and racquet sport athletes. Three radiographic findings that have been described in association with PSI include (1) Bennett lesion, exostosis of the posteroinferior glenoid rim due to repetitive traction of the posterior capsule; (2) sclerotic and cystic changes of the greater tuberosity sometimes associated with geodes of the posterior humeral head; and (3) bony remodeling or rounding of the posterior glenoid rim.[41] On MRI images, there is a triad of direct signs of PSI: (1) marrow edema and/or subcortical cystic changes within the posterolateral aspect of the humeral head; (2) tendinosis and/or articular surface tears of the infraspinatus and posterior supraspinatus tendon; and (3) abnormal signal or a frank tear of the posterosuperior labrum.[34] Other MRI findings may include anterior capsule laxity and instability as well as posterior capsule thickening.[9] Adding an ABER sequence to the standard MRI shoulder protocol makes it possible to clearly demonstrate the basic mechanism of the PSI: abnormal contact between the glenoid and greater tuberosity.[58] Most of the described findings (on both MRI and radiographs) may also be seen in the asymptomatic shoulder; thus, radiologic findings must always be evaluated in light of the history and clinical findings.[41]

Anterosuperior impingement (ASI) of the shoulder is a pathologic condition characterized by the entrapment of the undersurface of the reflective pulley system and the articular surface of the subscapularis tendon against the anterosuperior glenoid rim, when the arm is elevated, adducted, and internally rotated.[34] The reflective pulley system consists of the CH ligament, superior glenohumeral ligament, anterior aspect of supraspinatus tendon, and superior aspect of subscapularis tendon.[59] The main important function of the pulley system is to protect the long head of the biceps against anterior shearing stress and keep it within the bicipital groove, stabilizing the glenohumeral joint during movements of the shoulder. An injury of the reflective pulley system can result from acute or chronic repetitive trauma, especially repetitive and forceful anterior elevation, horizontal adduction, and internal rotation (common movements in the overhead athletes). A torn reflective pulley in turn may lead to instability of the long head of the biceps in its intra-articular course, resulting in anterior translation and superior migration of the humeral head. An injured pulley, especially when associated with a partial articular-side subscapularis and supraspinatus tendon, may result in ASI.

The physiologic contact between the rotator cuff and the superior labrum becomes abnormal in the presence of pulley lesions and a partial subscapularis tear located on the articular side.[34] Clinically, ASI is characterized by chronic anterior shoulder pain that is unresponsive to subacromial anesthetic infiltration and usually affects overhead athletes, such as swimmers and tennis players.[38]

MRI or MRA can demonstrate findings associated with ASI; conventional MR axial sequences demonstrate long head of the biceps subluxation and the subscapularis tendon tears. Sagittal sequences delineate the superior subscapularis tears, deep surface anterior supraspinatus tears, and the tear of the pulley ligaments. Arthro-MRI can diagnose a pulley lesion by detecting irregularity of the superior margin of the subscapularis tendon, extra-articular contrast medium collection, and long head of the biceps tendon subluxation.[40,44] According to Bennett's classification, lesions of the biceps pulley can be classified into 5 grades[37]:

- Grade I: Tears of superior fibers of the subscapularis
- Grade II: Tear of the CH ligament-superior glenohumeral ligament complex
- Grade III: Tears of both subscapularis fibers and the CH ligament-superior glenohumeral ligament complex
- Grade IV: Lesions of the CH ligament and the most anterior fibers of the supraspinatus
- Grade V: Combination of tears of all the structures of the pulley

Grade I and II lesions are associated with medial subluxation within the groove; grade III lesions are associated with dislocation of the long head of the biceps into the joint; grade IV lesions are associated with dislocation of the long head of the biceps anterior to the subscapularis muscle and CH ligament; and grade V lesions are associated with dislocation from the groove either anteriorly or into the joint.[60]

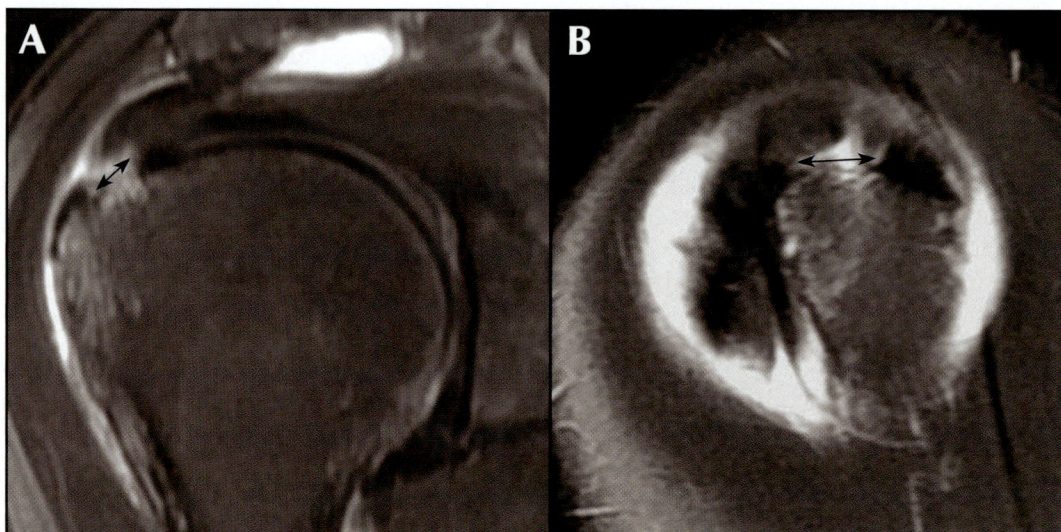

Figure 6-7. Small full-thickness tears of the supraspinatus muscle (arrows) in (A) oblique coronal and (B) sagittal fluid-sensitive fat-saturated FSE sequences of the right shoulder.

Sequelae and Radiologic Findings of Impingement

Ultrasound, CT, and MRI provide information that is helpful to the orthopedic surgeon in managing patients with rotator cuff tears. These imaging modalities can assess intrinsic tear characteristics, such as dimensions, thickness, shape, status of the remaining tendon, and tear relationship with the surrounding structures; muscle atrophy; size of muscle cross-sectional area; and fatty degeneration. Furthermore, they can provide information concerning rotator cuff impingement.[44]

Classification of Rotator Cuff Tears

Rotator cuff tears can be classified according to their depth and geometry. Both depth and geometry of the tear are important for the surgical plan. As to the depth, tears can be classified into full-thickness and partial-thickness tears. Full-thickness tears extend from the undersurface to the bursal surface of the tendon, and partial-thickness tears can occur on either the articular surface or the bursal surface of the rotator cuff or only within the substance of the rotator cuff without surfacing.[7]

Full-thickness tears, which need surgery, can be classified into 4 types[61,62]: type I, crescent-shape; type II, longitudinal (U-shape or L-shape); type III, massive contractive; and type IV, cuff tear arthropathy. MRI is helpful to classify each tear according to its AP and lateromedial length in the sagittal and coronal plane, respectively (Figure 6-7). Measuring either on T2-weighted sequences or T1-weighted MRA studies allows an accurate evaluation. The medial-to-lateral length of type I tears is less than the anterior-to-posterior width (short and wide). Type II tears are U-shaped and L-shaped; the medial-to-lateral length of these tears is greater than the anterior-to-posterior width (long and narrow, Figure 6-8). Type III tears are massive contracted tears, which are long and wide (Figure 6-9). Type IV are massive tears associated with significant glenohumeral osteoarthritis and loss of the subacromial space (Figure 6-10). This classification associates the type of tear with surgical treatment[61,63,64]: end-to-bone repair for type I tears, margin convergence for type II, and interval slides or partial repair for type III. Type IV tears are considered to be irreparable and may require arthroplasty.

Figure 6-8. Fluid-sensitive fat-suppressed (A) coronal oblique and (B) sagittal oblique images illustrating a Type II, longitudinal, full-thickness tear with the medial-to-lateral length greater than the anterior-to-posterior width (the double arrow indicates the extent of the tear).

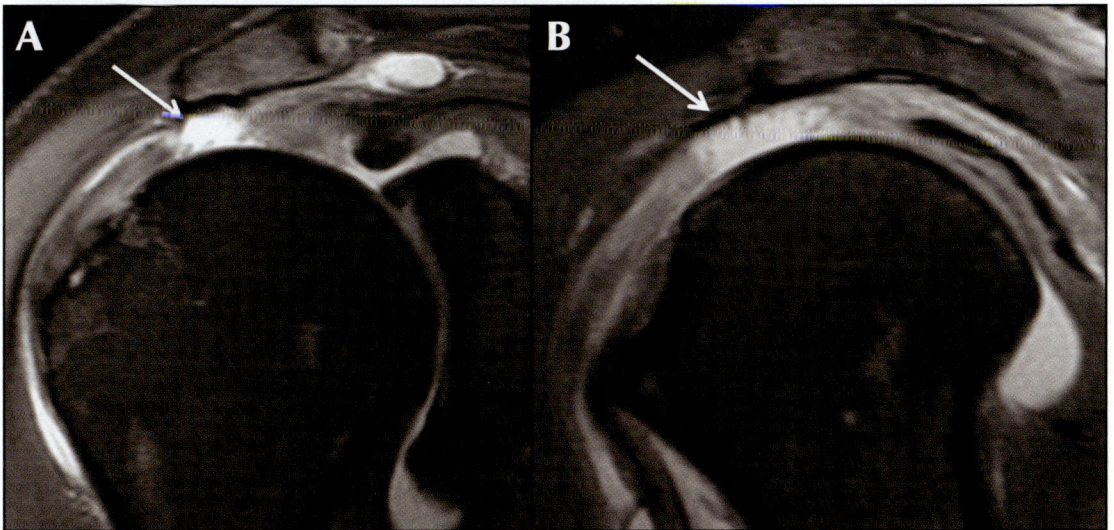

Figure 6-9. Fluid-sensitive fat-suppressed (A) coronal oblique and (B) sagittal oblique images showing a Type III, massive contracted tear measuring 35.2 x 21 mm (the arrows indicate the site of the tear).

Partial-Thickness Tears

In these tears, a partial-thickness T2 signal abnormality as bright as fluid is found, which extends across a portion of the tendon but not through its entire thickness.[65] Different types of partial tears may occur according to the surface of the tendon involved: undersurface/articular surface, intra-substance/intratendinous, and bursal surface.[40,66] The more the depth of a partial-thickness tear increases, the more the strain increases in the remaining tendon and in the other rotator cuff tendons.[67] As stated in Ellman's classification, partial-thickness tears can be scored according to their depth, as either grade 1 (<3 mm), grade 2 (3 to 6 mm), or grade 3 (>6 mm).[68] Because the normal rotator cuff is 10- to 12-mm thick, grade 1 tears involve up to 25% of the cuff thickness, grade 2 tears up to 50%, and grade 3 tears more than 50% of the cuff thickness (Figures 6-11 and 6-12).

Figure 6-10. Fluid-sensitive fat-suppressed coronal oblique image with Type IV cuff tear arthropathy: massive rotator cuff tears associated with significant glenohumeral osteoarthritis, superior migration of the humeral head (double arrow) with loss of the entire subacromial space (short arrow). Sclerotic changes are seen at the greater tuberosity (long arrow).

Figure 6-11. High-grade partial tear of the supraspinatus muscle. T2-weighted fat-suppressed oblique coronal image of a shoulder MRA. There is a high-grade partial-thickness tear of the supraspinatus tendon at the critical zone and footprint. High-signal fluid (long arrow) fills the defect. There are prominent subchondral cystic changes at and adjacent to the supraspinatus tendon insertion (short arrow).

Figure 6-12. Partial-thickness tear of the infraspinatus muscle. T2-weighted fat-suppressed oblique coronal image of a shoulder MRA. High-grade articular surface partial tear involving the footprint of the infraspinatus muscle. High-signal fluid (long arrow) fills the defect.

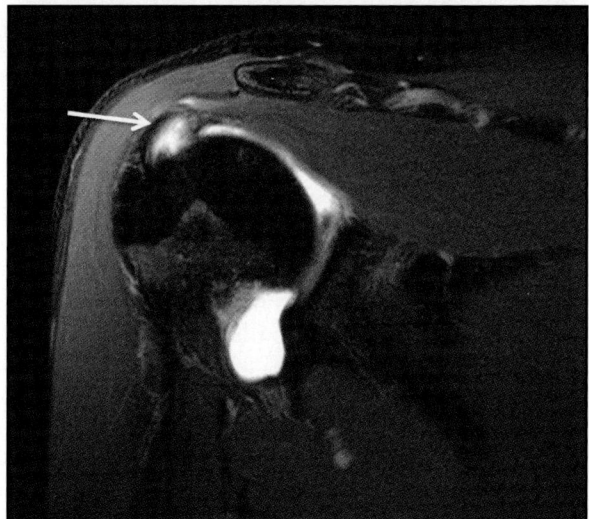

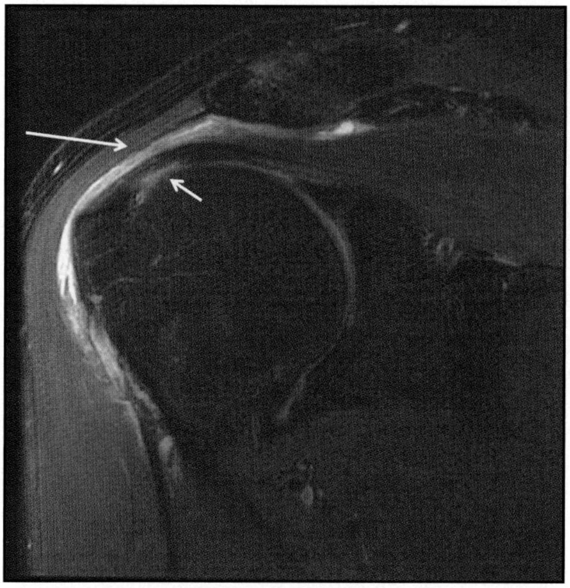

Figure 6-13. Subacromial-subdeltoid bursitis. T2-weighted fat-suppressed oblique sagittal image of the shoulder in a 29-year-old swimmer suffering from subacromial-subdeltoid bursitis. A fluid collection is demonstrated in the subacromial-subdeltoid bursa, containing synovial debris (long arrow). In addition, a low-grade partial tear of the supraspinatus is demonstrated (short arrow).

Articular surface tears are the most common type of partial-thickness tear and can be easily diagnosed on MRI when joint effusion is present as a focal area of tendon discontinuity filled with T2 bright signal. Fat-suppressed sequences improve the evaluation of the fluid-filled tendon gaps. Granulation tissue or scarring may seal off the gap, making the identification of tears difficult, especially when joint effusion is very mild or absent.[40] MRA has been shown to improve the evaluation of partial-thickness undersurface tears: a cuff tear is diagnosed when intra-articular contrast fills the gap in the substance of the tendon. Also, using specialized positioning, such as ABER position (abduction and external rotation), may improve the conspicuity of these tears.[64] A rim-rent tear, also called a partial articular supraspinatus tendon avulsion lesion, is an articular surface partial-thickness tear of anterior fibers of the rotator cuff at its insertion on the greater tuberosity. It usually occurs in young athletic patients with shoulder pain, and these lesions can easily be missed on MRI.[69]

Bursal surface partial tears are characterized by a focal extra-articular fluid-filled gap in the bursal surface of the tendon. They are generally hidden on T1-weighted MRA images as the intra-articular contrast cannot fill the gap. The presence of subacromial-subdeltoid bursal fluid (Figure 6-13) makes the MRI diagnosis easier if a T2-weighted sequence is acquired; thus, the MRA protocol must include at least one T2-weighted sequence.

Intrasubstance tears are characterized by a T2 fluid signal within the tendon that does not extend to the bursal or to the articular surface; these lesions do not communicate with the joint space and, thus, cannot be reached by contrast media. Furthermore, they are occult to macroscopic inspection during surgery.[44]

Full-Thickness Tear

A tear is classified as full thickness when there is complete discontinuity of the tendon fibers extending from the articular surface of the rotator cuff to the subacromial-subdeltoid bursa. In 10% of full-thickness tears, there is low signal intensity on T2-weighted images due to chronic scarring.[40] In this case, retraction of the myotendinous junction is a helpful sign of full-thickness tear. MRA signs of full-thickness tear are the communication between the glenohumeral joint and the subacromial-subdeltoid bursa highlighted by contrast media.[40] DeOrio and Cofield's classification is the most frequently used by orthopedic surgeons. This classification, based on the greatest diameter of the tear, grades them as either small (<1 cm), medium (1 to 3 cm), large

(3 to 5 cm), or massive (>5 cm). The dimensions of a rotator cuff tear have important implications for the surgical treatment choice, postoperative prognosis, and tear recurrence.[70] As to surgical planning, primary repair is often not possible when both the length and the width of the tear exceed 4 cm on preoperative MR; it is helpful for the surgeon to know both the mediolateral (for deciding the surgical approach, open surgery versus arthroscopy) and the AP dimensions (it adds information regarding the status of the other rotator cuff muscles). As to postoperative prognosis, recovery of strength after large and massive rotator cuff tears is much slower and less consistent than with smaller tears. As to the risk of tear recurrence, the larger the tear, the greater the likelihood of recurrence.[44]

Very important findings, such as fatty degeneration, muscle atrophy, tendon retraction, fluid in the subacromial-subdeltoid bursa (see Figure 6-13), sentinel cysts, and superior humeral head migration, are secondary signs of tears with implications for the surgical management of the tear; thus, they deserve a separate discussion.[71,72]

Fatty Degeneration

In the literature, the relationship between fatty infiltration of the rotator cuff muscles and tears of the corresponding tendons has been well studied. Fatty degeneration of rotator cuff muscles may occur as a result of chronic tears or denervation and glenohumeral osteoarthritis. The natural history of fatty infiltration has been described as an irreversible and often progressive process; for this reason, it is important to treat the patient with rotator cuff tears before this process develops. For the assessment of fatty infiltration, CT and MRI-based classifications have been established by Goutallier and colleagues[73] and by Fuchs and colleagues,[74] respectively. Goutallier's classification is a standard 5-grade scoring system for muscle fatty infiltration of the rotator cuff: normal muscle (grade 0), some fatty streaks within muscle (grade 1), fatty degeneration of less than 50% but still more muscle than fat (grade 2), fatty degeneration of 50% (grade 3), and fatty degeneration of more than 50% (grade 4). The 5 grades in Goutallier's system were reduced by Fuchs and colleagues to 3 stages by grouping: Goutallier's grades 0 and 1 are classified as normal muscle, grade 2 as moderately pathologic muscle, and grades 3 and 4 as advanced degeneration. The fatty tissue is better seen on T1-weighted images as strands of high signal within the muscle fibers. High grade of fatty degeneration is associated with a high rate of repair failure and more limitations in the achievable outcome in the postoperative period, even though some studies have demonstrated that repairing the rotator cuff in patients with a high grade of fatty degeneration can still provide significant functional improvement.[75]

Muscle Atrophy

Atrophy of the rotator cuff muscles is seen as decreased muscle bulk (Figure 6-14). Measuring muscle cross-sectional area may provide important information because this measurement correlates with muscle strength. Loss of normal bulk of the supraspinatus muscle is characterized by a reduced muscle filling of the suprascapular fossa with more surrounding fat. The evaluation of the supraspinatus muscle makes use of the scapular ratio and the tangent sign. The scapular ratio is calculated on sagittal oblique images and stands for the ratio of the cross-sectional area of the supraspinatus muscle to the area of the supraspinatus fossa. In supraspinatus muscle atrophy, this ratio is less than 50%.[76] The tangent sign is assessed on a T1-weighted sagittal oblique image: the normal supraspinatus muscle belly crosses a line drawn between the superior aspect of the scapular spine and the superior margin of the coracoids process. If the muscle belly does not cross this line, supraspinatus atrophy is diagnosed.[77,78]

Tendon Retraction

The extent of a tendon tear and its retraction is important information for the surgical planning (Figure 6-15).[44] The most accurate description of the extent of a tear should be achieved in all reports because it may change the surgical plan and the outcome prognosis; for instance, a tear of the supraspinatus has a worse prognosis if it also extends anteriorly into the rotator interval

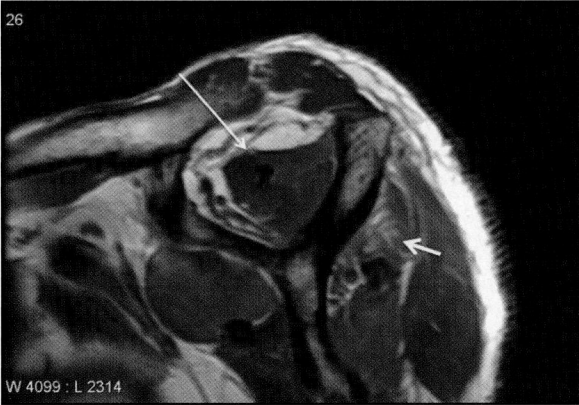

Figure 6-14. Muscle atrophy of the supraspinatus and infraspinatus muscles. T1-weighted sagittal oblique image of the shoulder. The supraspinatus (long arrow) and the infraspinatus (short arrow) muscles are atrophied and demonstrate fatty infiltration, which creates a speckled appearance compared to the normal subscapularis muscle. These findings are caused by compression of the supraspinatus nerve (SSN) at the suprascapular notch due to a paralabral cyst.

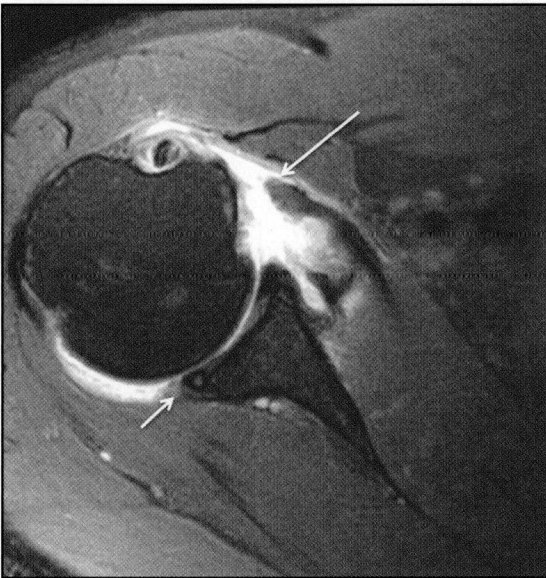

Figure 6-15. Full-thickness tear of the subscapularis muscle with tendon retraction. T2-weighted fat-suppressed axial image of a shoulder MRA. The subscapularis tendon demonstrates severe tendinosis and full-thickness tear with retraction of the tendon (long arrow). T2 prolongation within the posterior labrum represents intrasubstance degeneration (short arrow).

and subscapularis tendon fibers and posteriorly to the infraspinatus muscle fibers than an isolated supraspinatus tear.[79] The involvement of the subscapularis muscle may require a different surgical approach, such as a deltopectoral approach.[79-81] Regarding tear retraction, a torn tendon should be adjacent to the attachment site to avoid any tension within the surgical fixation.[63] The more the tendon is dislocated, the stronger the tension of the repair is; a tendon tear is considered to be irreparable if it is retracted to the medial aspect of the glenoid fossa.[44]

Fluid in Subacromial-Subdeltoid Bursa

A full-thickness tear of the rotator cuff tendon allows communication between the joint space and the subacromial-subdeltoid bursa. The fluid may further extend into the AC joint, especially in case of chronic full-thickness cuff tear and after subacromial decompression. On MRA, this is described as a *geyser sign*.[82]

Sentinel Cysts

These are intramuscular fluid collections that result from the communication between joint fluid and the muscle tissue. These cysts are easily identified on T2-weighted sequences as round areas of high signal; the detection of these findings suggests the presence of associated rotator cuff pathology.[83]

Figure 6-16. Calcific tendinitis (radiograph). AP projection of the left shoulder: large amorphous soft tissue density is seen in the subacromial space and represents hydroxyapatite deposition disease (arrow).

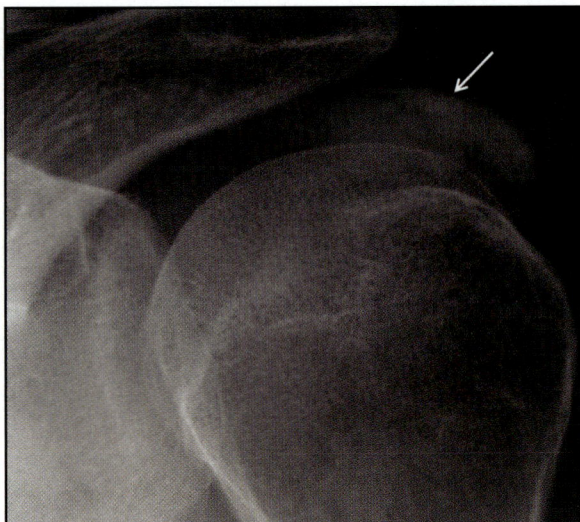

Superior Humeral Head Migration

This finding is usually associated with a full-thickness tear and retraction of the tendon; it can be determined on an outlet view or on sagittal MR sequences if the acromiohumeral distance measures less than 5 mm. The size of the rotator cuff tear and the degree of fatty degeneration of the infraspinatus and supraspinatus muscle are the most important factors determining the supraspinatus outlet.[84] Mild superior subluxation of the humeral head may be caused also by capsular tightening or scarring as a consequence of chronic instability, for instance.[85]

TENDINOPATHY/TENDINOSIS

Tendinosis represents a degenerative process of the tendon due to multiple etiologic factors including aging, overuse, trauma, underlying conditions that weaken the tendon, and impingement. Tendinosis does not involve active cellular infiltration to indicate inflammation; hence, the term *tendinitis* is not appropriate.[40] Tendinosis is diagnosed on MRI, and it is characterized by increased intrasubstance signal on short echo time sequence that is lower than that of the fluid. The involved tendon may be normal or thicker and swollen but intact. Sometimes, the differential diagnosis between partial tear and tendinosis can be challenging on MRI; even in normal tendons, tendinosis may be suggested due to the presence of magic angle phenomenon and partial volume averaging with the adjacent tissue.[78]

Calcific Tendinitis

Calcific tendinitis is a painful rotator cuff disease due to the deposition of calcium hydroxyapatite (Figures 6-16 and 6-17). The most common site is the supraspinatus tendon (82% of all the shoulder calcific deposits), where the calcific deposits usually are located 1.5 to 2 cm from the greater tuberosity.[86] The calcifications may grow and work their way into the glenohumeral joint or into the subacromial bursa (calcific bursitis). On radiographs, the calcifications are easily seen in the AP projection with the shoulder externally rotated or in an outlet view in the subacromial space. On MRI, the calcifications have low signal intensity on all sequences, similar to the normal tendon; therefore, they are sometimes difficult to visualize. Irregular morphology and thickening or thinning of the tendon may be associated with calcific tendinitis.[87]

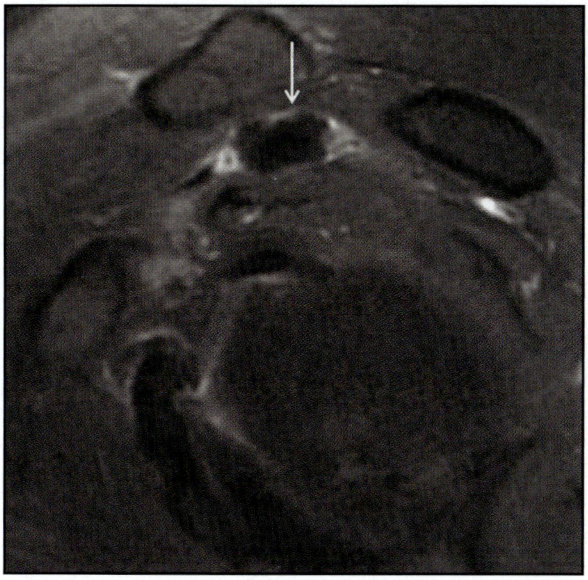

Figure 6-17. Calcific tendinitis MRI. T2-weighted fat-suppressed oblique sagittal image of the left shoulder; a round low signal area adjacent to the superior aspect of the supraspinatus muscle is demonstrated (arrow). The finding is consistent with hydroxyapatite deposition disease.

POSTSURGICAL SHOULDER

The radiological interpretation of images of the postoperative shoulder may present many challenges. Findings that indicate pathology in presurgical patients are interpreted differently in a shoulder after surgery.[19] Different techniques such as MRI, MRA, CT, and CTA can be used for the evaluation of the patients who have undergone surgery for shoulder impingement or rotator cuff tears.[19,88] The choice of which technique should be used is based on the personal experience of the radiologist evaluating the advantages and disadvantages of each technique from case to case.

Conventional radiographs should be regarded as the first imaging step to perform after shoulder surgery. The protocol of views to obtain after shoulder surgery should include a true AP (Grashey view) or AP in intra- and extra-rotation and an outlet view. Axillary views can best demonstrate an insufficient resection of the posterior portion of the acromion.[89] Furthermore, conventional radiographs can assess how metal artifacts may impair the quality of MRI or CT studies and thus help in the choice of the diagnostic management. The quality of MR images obtained after surgery can be minimally impaired to not interpretable due to the presence of metallic hardware and metallic shavings.[90,91] In general, the kind of metal and its dimensions are the most important factor for determining the severity of the artifacts: titanium hardware and metal anchors create little artifacts, whereas cobalt chrome and prostheses are responsible for severe artifacts. In the presence of metallic hardware, in order to reduce artifacts, it is advised to avoid standard (spectral selective) fat-suppression and gradient echo sequences; short T1 inversion recovery and low echo time sequences are preferred. Also, the strength of the magnetic field has importance in the production of artifact with higher strength fields producing more severe artifacts.

The use of MDCT in the postoperative shoulder is helpful for assessing bony abnormalities and the depiction of complications related to metallic implants that are not well visualized by radiography, such as loosening, particle disease, and displaced device. Furthermore, specific indications for CTA are all the absolute and relative contraindications for MRA (implanted medical devices, claustrophobic or obese patients).[89]

Radiological Findings After Subacromial Decompression

Postoperative persistence of symptoms can result from suboptimal surgical decompression with residual subacromial stenosis or spur[42] or from another, so far undiagnosed, pathology that mimics symptoms of subacromial impingement.[85] Following acromioplasty, a comparison between pre- and postoperative radiographs shows a flattened undersurface of the acromion and loss of the anterior aspect of the acromion.[92] Outlet views can detect the eventual presence of remaining spurs. When the Mumford procedure is performed, the AC distance is increased to 1 to 2 cm and should not be misdiagnosed as an AC joint separation.[19,89]

On MRI, the resection of the anterior part of the acromion and the flattering of its undersurface are usually associated with bone marrow edema or signal loss within the acromial bone marrow. Bone marrow edema pattern has been attributed to postoperative change and should not be misinterpreted as a sign of osteomyelitis.[21] Low-signal artifacts from metallic burr due to acromioplasty are frequently seen due to surgical shavings. In place of the subacromion/subdeltoid bursa, granulation tissue with different signal intensity depending on time from surgery can be demonstrated on MRI.[93] Fluid in the subacromial-subdeltoid bursa is a normal finding and may persist for years as long as it does not increase on the follow-up or is present in a large amount.[94] Subacromial fluid may communicate with fluid within the AC joint, resulting in the so-called geyser sign.[82,95] This common finding may result from the iatrogenic injury of the acromial undersurface. When metal artifacts in MR images are too severe, an MDCT may be useful, especially if high voltage (up to 145 kVp) and high exposure (up to 300 mAs) are used. Furthermore, if bony structures need to be better evaluated, CT may help to evaluate the shape of the acromion and of heterotopic ossifications.[96-98]

Radiological Findings After Rotator Cuff Repair

Following rotator cuff surgery, a combination of AP radiographs and outlet views are usually obtained to assess the correct position of hardware and the distance from acromion to humeral head, which is normally about 1 cm.[19] So far, the exact role of CTA in the shoulder after surgery has not been determined. CTA is able to detect undersurface partial- and full-thickness tear; also, the evaluation of soft tissue shows useful information, such as the degree of fatty infiltration and muscle atrophy.[99,100]

The normal appearance of rotator cuff tendon postsurgery is much different from the preoperative appearance (Figure 6-18). In the majority of rotator cuff repairs, the signal of the tendon is not low in all the sequences as it is in the normal preoperative tendon, but it is increased on T2 sequences; this may be related to the presence of fluid within sutures, granulation tissue, scar formations, metallic abrasion artifacts, chemical shift artifact from sutures, and quality of the tendon itself.[19]

A small amount of fluid within the subacromial-subdeltoid bursa and bone characterized by bone marrow edema in correspondence to the greater tuberosity should be considered as normal and may persist over time. Full-thickness retears can result from different causes, such as suture-failure or anchor pull-out and can be diagnosed by the presence of fluid signal intensity extending from the undersurface throughout the entire thickness of the repaired tendon.

It has to be considered that not all the repairs are water tight, and the presence of the leakage of joint fluid or contrast into the subacromial bursa can be a normal finding rather than a sign of tear.[21] A clinically relevant parameter in the assessment of a full-thickness tear is the size, described as the maximum diameter of the defect; it has been demonstrated that tears larger than 1 cm are more related to symptoms than smaller-sized tears.[94]

The diagnosis of a partial-thickness tear is not very reliable on MRI. After a normal rotator cuff repair, the expected findings include intermediate/low signal within the tendon, indicating scar and fibrosis and irregular morphology characterized by irregular surface and thickening or thinning of the tendon. For this reason, clinical information regarding symptoms and comparison with preoperative MRI are recommended.

The evaluation of muscle quality is important to predict the clinical outcome of the rotator cuff repair. Fatty infiltration can be assessed using a semi-quantitative classification, such as Goutallier's classification. A Goutallier score lower than or equal to 2 (fatty infiltration less than muscle tissue) predicts a good clinical outcome. If a score higher than 2 (fatty infiltration equal to or more than muscle) is found, a second surgical treatment may be contraindicated.[72]

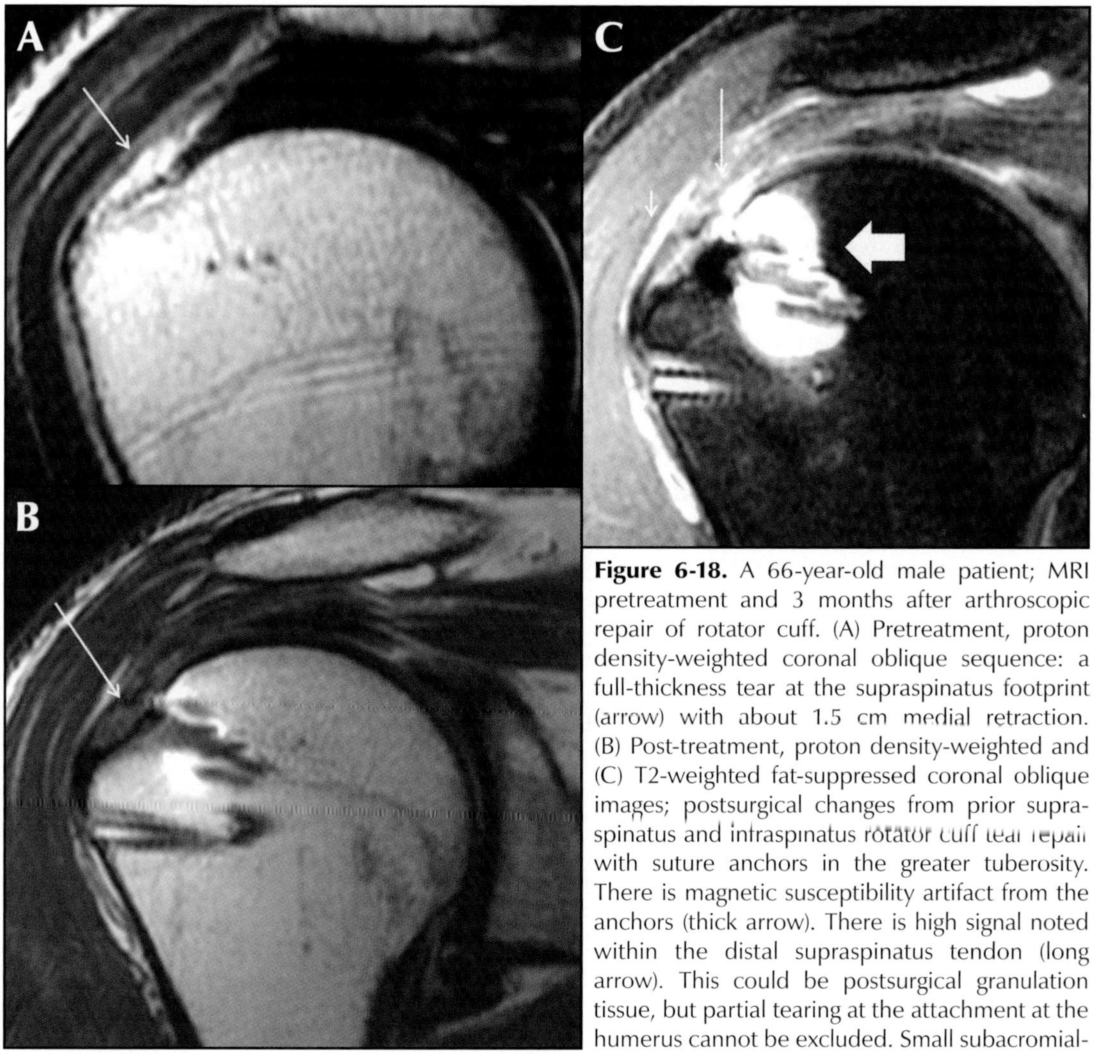

Figure 6-18. A 66-year-old male patient; MRI pretreatment and 3 months after arthroscopic repair of rotator cuff. (A) Pretreatment, proton density-weighted coronal oblique sequence: a full-thickness tear at the supraspinatus footprint (arrow) with about 1.5 cm medial retraction. (B) Post-treatment, proton density-weighted and (C) T2-weighted fat-suppressed coronal oblique images; postsurgical changes from prior supraspinatus and infraspinatus rotator cuff tear repair with suture anchors in the greater tuberosity. There is magnetic susceptibility artifact from the anchors (thick arrow). There is high signal noted within the distal supraspinatus tendon (long arrow). This could be postsurgical granulation tissue, but partial tearing at the attachment at the humerus cannot be excluded. Small subacromial-subdeltoid effusion is seen (short arrow).

Complications After Rotator Cuff Repair

Common complications of rotator cuff repair may be fixation failures, deltoid detachment, nerve injury, and infection.[92] Misplaced or detached staples, tracks, or screws can result in cartilage injury by sticking out of the bone into the joint, leading to degenerative changes or functioning as a loose body within the joint.[19] Radiographs can evaluate the misplacement and migration of metallic devices (not all of the devices are radio-opaque), loosening, and osteolysis. In case of loosening or osteolysis, further exams may be required. For example, loosening can be seen on CT images as an area of lucency, larger than 2 mm, around the devices; osteolysis around biodegradable material can be demonstrated as an area of low signal on T1-weighted images and high signal on T2-weighted images and contrast-enhanced MRI.[21]

The prevalence of detachment of the deltoid muscle from its insertion on the acromion, after rotator cuff surgery, is 8%.[101] This complication can result from either incorrect reattachment during surgery or excessive tension on the suture in the postsurgical period. MRI is important to evaluate the size of the detachment, which is seen as a retraction of the deltoid with fluid filling the defect; if the detachment is greater than 3 cm, patients need to undergo revision surgery.

A detached deltoid may lead to a loss of strength in the shoulder movements, and when the condition is chronic, the muscle belly becomes atrophic and fatty; this can be demonstrated as high T1 signal within the muscle belly.[89]

Iatrogenic nerve injury can result from direct laceration or suture entrapment or after surgery for intraoperative tissue retraction.[102] The affected nerves during rotator cuff repair are the axillary and the suprascapular nerves (SSNs). Injury of the axillary nerve may result in denervation of deltoid and/or teres minor depending on the site of the injury; injury of the SSN may lead either to denervation of supraspinatus and infraspinatus or only of the infraspinatus muscle when the injury site is the suprascapular notch or the spinoglenoid notch, respectively.[103] MRI can indirectly diagnose denervation. According to the stage of the denervation, the muscle presents different findings: in the early stages, the edema within the muscle is seen as increased signal on short T1 inversion recovery or fat-suppressed T2-weighted images; in the following stages, the muscle bulk can decrease and be infiltrated by fatty tissue seen on T1-weighted imaging without fat suppression as streaks of increased signal.

Hematoma formation, septic arthritis, periarticular soft tissue infection, and osteomyelitis represent rare complications of shoulder surgery.[92] The imaging has a primary role of the diagnosis of these complications. On radiographs, findings like joint space narrowing, erosions, osteopenia, and soft tissue swelling should raise the suspicion of infection in the presence of the appropriate clinical picture. MRI can show findings consistent with soft tissue infection, abscess formation, and osteomyelitis; the needle aspiration in turn can provide the final diagnosis and the isolation of the pathogenic agent.[21]

Neurogenic Rotator Cuff Pathologies

Nerve Impingement

Shoulder neuropathies are diagnosed on the basis of clinical history, physical examination, electrophysiologic studies, and MRI. MRI can investigate the lesion responsible for the nerve injury and determine the extent of muscle damage. Initially, the principal finding of denervation consists of muscle edema seen as high signal on fluid-sensitive images; in the latter phases, findings consist of muscular atrophy and fatty infiltration. Electromyography (EMG) is the gold standard in the diagnosis of muscle denervation, but MRI can detect findings of denervation after 48 hours, while EMG can detect them only after 15 to 20 days.[103] The most common injured nerves at the shoulder region are the suprascapular and axillary nerves.

The most common site of entrapment for the axillary nerve is the quadrilateral space.[104] The cause of nerve injury can be traumatic or atraumatic. Traumatic causes include acute glenohumeral dislocation, fracture of the scapula or proximal humerus, and surgical or arthroscopic procedure. Atraumatic causes include mass lesions such as hematoma, tumors, posteroinferior labral cysts (between 6 and 9 o'clock), bony callus, and hypertrophy of the muscles bounding the quadrilateral space or fibrous bands. Also, large osteophytes in severe osteoarthritis of the glenohumeral joint may cause compression or traction of the nerve. Radiographs can usually exclude fractures or severe degenerative changes. On MRI, both direct and indirect signs of axillary nerve dysfunction can be seen. Direct signs consist of the detection of a mass in the quadrilateral space. Indirect signs consist of abnormalities in the teres minor and/or deltoid muscles; MRI shows classical changes related to muscle denervation: edema in early phases, detected as high-signal intensity on T2-weighted sequences, and atrophy and fatty degeneration in the later stages seen as a decreasing muscle bulk and high signal on T1-weighted sequences within the muscle.

The more common sites of SSN entrapment are the suprascapular notch and the spinoglenoid notch. The SSN courses through the suprascapular notch with motor fibers for both infraspinatus and supraspinatus muscles and through the spinoglenoid notch with motor fiber for only the infraspinatus muscle. The infraspinatus muscle alone or both the infraspinatus and supraspinatus

Figure 6-19. Paralabral cyst and full-thickness supraspinatus tear with retraction. T2-weighted fat-suppressed coronal oblique image of the shoulder. An ovoid fluid collection consistent with paralabral cyst (white arrow) is noted extending into the suprascapular notch (black arrow). It contains synovial debris having the appearance of "rice" bodies and results in compression of the SSN. In addition, there is large joint effusion and full-thickness supraspinatus tear with retraction.

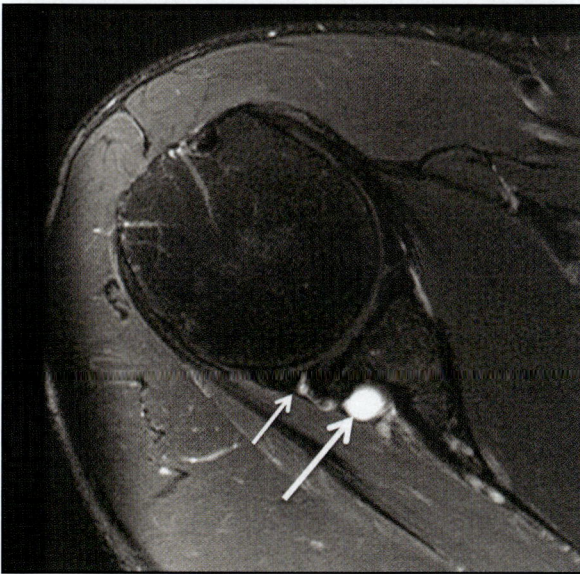

Figure 6-20. Paralabral cyst in the spinoglenoid notch. T2-weighted fat-suppressed axial image of the shoulder. A round fluid collection is detected at the spinoglenoid notch (large arrow), which originates from a labral tear (small arrow). It causes SSN entrapment.

muscles may be involved depending on the site of SSN entrapment. Traumatic causes usually include scapular fracture or iatrogenic surgical injury. Atraumatic causes include mass lesions such as ganglion cysts, usually associated with superior labral tear (Figures 6-19 and 6-20), enlarged varicosities (Figure 6-21A), and tumors. In these cases, MRI is useful to demonstrate the mass in the notch and the fatty atrophy of the affected muscle (Figure 6-21B).

PARSONAGE-TURNER SYNDROME

Parsonage-Turner syndrome, also referred to as *acute brachial neuritis*, results from a viral inflammation of the brachial plexus. Clinically, it is characterized by severe pain in the shoulder girdle. The pain disappears usually in 1 to 3 weeks and is followed by muscular weakness. The MR finding most typical of this syndrome is that of diffuse T2 high signal involving one or more muscles innervated by the brachial plexus; this finding is consistent with interstitial muscle edema associated with denervation.[105] Fatty replacement and decreased bulk of the affected muscles may be seen on T1-weighted MR in later stages.

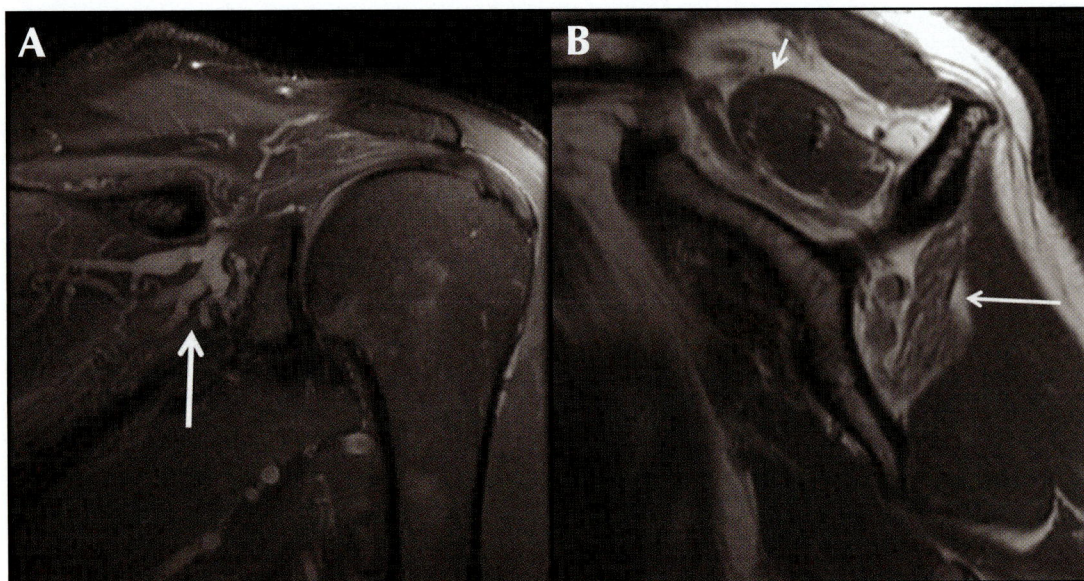

Figure 6-21. Prominent vessels leading to nerve compression in the spinoglenoid and suprascapular notches. (A) T1-weighted coronal oblique image of the shoulder. Prominent vessels noted within the suprascapular and spinoglenoid notches (arrow). (B) These findings result in SSN entrapment with atrophy of the supraspinatus (short arrow) and infraspinatus muscles (long arrow) as demonstrated in this proton density-weighted sagittal oblique image.

Conclusion

Radiologic techniques are very important in the assessment of rotator cuff pathology both pre-operatively[44,51,71,73,106-108] and postoperatively.[78,88-90,94,97,109-113] In the preoperative phase, these techniques can assess all the conditions that may predispose to impingement,[42,52,102,114-116] characterize underlying pathologies that may lead to rotator cuff tears,[35,37,40,117] and evaluate the pertinent pathologic anatomy related to tendon and muscle such as size of tear, muscle and tendon retraction, and muscle atrophy, thus helping orthopedic surgeons in diagnostic decision making.[44,70,73,78] In the postoperative phase, radiologic techniques can help in assessing possible complications, such as fixation failures, retears, nerve injury, and infection.[19,36,40,85,89,94,106,113,118,119]

References

1. Miranda H, Viikari-Juntura E, Heistaro S, Heliovaara M, Riihimaki H. A population study on differences in the determinants of a specific shoulder disorder versus nonspecific shoulder pain without clinical findings. *Am J Epidemiol*. 2005;161(9):847-855.
2. Luime JJ, Koes BW, Hendriksen IJ, et al. Prevalence and incidence of shoulder pain in the general population: a systematic review. *Scand J Rheumatol*. 2004;33(2):73-81.
3. Lewis JS. Rotator cuff tendinopathy. *Br J Sports Med*. 2009;43(4):236-241.
4. Roquelaure Y, Ha C, Rouillon C, et al. Risk factors for upper-extremity musculoskeletal disorders in the working population. *Arthritis Rheum*. 2009;61(10):1425-1434.
5. Lewis JS. Rotator cuff tendinopathy/subacromial impingement syndrome: is it time for a new method of assessment? *Br J Sports Med*. 2009;43(4):259-264.
6. Ekeberg OM, Bautz-Holter E, Juel NG, Engebretsen K, Kvalheim S, Brox JI. Clinical, socio-demographic and radiological predictors of short-term outcome in rotator cuff disease. *BMC Musculoskelet Disord*. 2010;11:239. PMCID: 2978136.

7. Opsha O, Malik A, Baltazar R, et al. MRI of the rotator cuff and internal derangement. *Eur J Radiol.* 2008;68(1):36-56.

8. Lecouvet FE, Simoni P, Koutaissoff S, Vande Berg BC, Malghem J, Dubuc JE. Multidetector spiral CT arthrography of the shoulder. Clinical applications and limits, with MR arthrography and arthroscopic correlations. *Eur J Radiol.* 2008;68(1):120-136.

9. Goud A, Segal D, Hedayati P, Pan JJ, Weissman BN. Radiographic evaluation of the shoulder. *Eur J Radiol.* 2008;68(1):2-15.

10. Sanders TG, Jersey SL. Conventional radiography of the shoulder. *Semin Roentgenol.* 2005;40(3):207-222.

11. Drakos MC, Rudzki JR, Allen AA, Potter HG, Altchek DW. Internal impingement of the shoulder in the overhead athlete. *J Bone Joint Surg Am.* 2009;91(11):2719-2728.

12. Sanders TG, Zlatkin M, Montgomery J. Imaging of glenohumeral instability. *Semin Roentgenol.* 2010;45(3):160-179.

13. Rydberg J, Buckwalter KA, Caldemeyer KS, et al. Multisection CT: scanning techniques and clinical applications. *Radiographics.* 2000;20(6):1787-1806.

14. De Filippo M, Bertellini A, Sverzellati N, et al. Multidetector computed tomography arthrography of the shoulder: diagnostic accuracy and indications. *Acta Radiol.* 2008;49(5):540-549.

15. Farron A, Theumann N. [Indications to complementary radiological exams for pathologies of the shoulder]. *Rev Med Suisse.* 2006;2(92):2913-2917.

16. Babacan M, Kesmezacar H, Ogut T, Cansu E, Erginer R. [Radiologic evaluation of shoulder instability: conventional radiography, computed tomography and magnetic resonance imaging]. *Acta Orthop Traumatol Turc.* 2005;39 (Suppl 1):24-33.

17. Edwards TB, Boulahia A, Walch G. Radiographic analysis of bone defects in chronic anterior shoulder instability. *Arthroscopy.* 2003;19(7):732-739.

18. Natsis K, Totlis T, Tsikaras P, Appell HJ, Skandalakis P, Koebke J. Proposal for classification of the suprascapular notch: a study on 423 dried scapulas. *Clin Anat.* 2007;20(2):135-139.

19. Woertler K. Multimodality imaging of the postoperative shoulder. *Eur Radiol.* 2007;17(12):3038-3055.

20. Yang SO, Cho KJ, Kim MJ, Ro IW. Assessment of anterior shoulder instability by CT arthrography. *J Korean Med Sci.* 1987;2(3):167-171.

21. Lecouvet FE, Dorzee B, Dubuc JE, Vande Berg BC, Jamart J, Malghem J. Cartilage lesions of the glenohumeral joint: diagnostic effectiveness of multidetector spiral CT arthrography and comparison with arthroscopy. *Eur Radiol.* 2007;17(7):1763-1771.

22. Cochet H, Couderc S, Pele E, Amoretti N, Moreau-Durieux MH, Hauger O. Rotator cuff tears: should abduction and external rotation (ABER) positioning be performed before image acquisition? A CT arthrography study. *Eur Radiol.* 2010;20(5):1234-1241.

23. Mulligan ME. CT-guided shoulder arthrography at the rotator cuff interval. *AJR Am J Roentgenol.* 2008;191(2):W58-W61.

24. Buckwalter KA. CT arthrography. *Clin Sports Med.* 2006;25(4):899-915.

25. Davis SJ, Teresi LM, Bradley WG, Ressler JA, Eto RT. Effect of arm rotation on MR imaging of the rotator cuff. *Radiology.* 1991;181(1):265-268.

26. Kwak SM, Brown RR, Trudell D, Resnick D. Glenohumeral joint: comparison of shoulder positions at MR arthrography. *Radiology.* 1998;208(2):375-380.

27. Lee SU, Lang P. MR and MR arthrography to identify degenerative and posttraumatic diseases in the shoulder joint. *Eur J Radiol.* 2000;35(2):126-135.

28. Chung CB, Corrente L, Resnick D. MR arthrography of the shoulder. *Magn Reson Imaging Clin N Am.* 2004;12(1):25-38, v, vi.

29. Chung CB, Dwek JR, Feng S, Resnick D. MR arthrography of the glenohumeral joint: a tailored approach. *AJR Am J Roentgenol.* 2001;177(1):217-219.

30. Sahin G, Demirtas M. An overview of MR arthrography with emphasis on the current technique and applicational hints and tips. *Eur J Radiol.* 2006;58(3):416-430.

31. Catalano OA, Manfredi R, Vanzulli A, et al. MR arthrography of the glenohumeral joint: modified posterior approach without imaging guidance. *Radiology.* 2007;242(2):550-554.

32. Chung CB, Dwek JR, Cho GJ, Lektrakul N, Trudell D, Resnick D. Rotator cuff interval: evaluation with MR imaging and MR arthrography of the shoulder in 32 cadavers. *J Comput Assist Tomogr.* 2000;24(5):738-743.

33. Porat S, Leupold JA, Burnett KR, Nottage WM. Reliability of non-imaging-guided glenohumeral joint injection through rotator interval approach in patients undergoing diagnostic MR arthrography. *AJR Am J Roentgenol.* 2008;191(3):W96-W99.

34. Mulyadi E, Harish S, O'Neill J, Rebello R. MRI of impingement syndromes of the shoulder. *Clin Radiol.* 2009;64(3):307-318.

35. Castagna A, Garofalo R, Cesari E, Marcopoulos N, Borroni M, Conti M. Anterior and posterior internal impingement: an evidence-based review. *Br J Sports Med.* 2010;44(5):382-388.

36. Ellman H, Kay SP. Arthroscopic subacromial decompression for chronic impingement. Two- to five-year results. *J Bone Joint Surg Br.* 1991;73(3):395-398.

37. Garofalo R, Karlsson J, Nordenson U, Cesari E, Conti M, Castagna A. Anterior-superior internal impingement of the shoulder: an evidence-based review. *Knee Surg Sports Traumatol Arthrosc*. 2010;18(12):1688-1693.

38. Gerber C, Sebesta A. Impingement of the deep surface of the subscapularis tendon and the reflection pulley on the anterosuperior glenoid rim: a preliminary report. *J Shoulder Elbow Surg*. 2000;9(6):483-490.

39. Grainger AJ. Internal impingement syndromes of the shoulder. *Semin Musculoskelet Radiol*. 2008;12(2):127-135.

40. Habermeyer P, Magosch P, Pritsch M, Scheibel MT, Lichtenberg S. Anterosuperior impingement of the shoulder as a result of pulley lesions: a prospective arthroscopic study. *J Shoulder Elbow Surg*. 2004;13(1):5-12.

41. Heyworth BE, Williams RJ 3rd. Internal impingement of the shoulder. *Am J Sports Med*. 2009;37(5):1024-1037.

42. Fealy S, April EW, Khazzam M, Armengol-Barallat J, Bigliani LU. The coracoacromial ligament: morphology and study of acromial enthesopathy. *J Shoulder Elbow Surg*. 2005;14(5):542-548.

43. Natsis K, Tsikaras P, Totlis T, et al. Correlation between the four types of acromion and the existence of enthesophytes: a study on 423 dried scapulas and review of the literature. *Clin Anat*. 2007;20(3):267-272.

44. Morag Y, Jacobson JA, Miller B, De Maeseneer M, Girish G, Jamadar D. MR imaging of rotator cuff injury: what the clinician needs to know. *Radiographics*. 2006;26(4):1045-1065.

45. Abboud JA, Silverberg D, Pepe M, et al. Surgical treatment of os acromiale with and without associated rotator cuff tears. *J Shoulder Elbow Surg*. 2006;15(3):265-270.

46. Carlson DW, Kim DH. Os acromiale. *Am J Orthop (Belle Mead NJ)*. 2002;31(8):458.

47. Case DT, Burnett SE, Nielsen T. Os acromiale: population differences and their etiological significance. *Homo*. 2006;57(1):1-18.

48. Demetracopoulos CA, Kapadia NS, Herickhoff PK, Cosgarea AJ, McFarland EG. Surgical stabilization of os acromiale in a fast-pitch softball pitcher. *Am J Sports Med*. 2006;34(11):1855-1859.

49. Edelson JG, Zuckerman J, Hershkovitz I. Os acromiale: anatomy and surgical implications. *J Bone Joint Surg Br*. 1993;75(4):551-555.

50. Bencardino JT, Garcia AI, Palmer WE. Magnetic resonance imaging of the shoulder: rotator cuff. *Top Magn Reson Imaging*. 2003;14(1):51-67.

51. Giaroli EL, Major NM, Lemley DE, Lee J. Coracohumeral interval imaging in subcoracoid impingement syndrome on MRI. *AJR Am J Roentgenol*. 2006;186(1):242-246.

52. Ferreira Neto AA, Almeida AM, Maiorino R, Zoppi Filho A, Benegas E. An anatomical study of the subcoracoid space. *Clinics (Sao Paulo)*. 2006;61(5):467-472.

53. Gerber C, Terrier F, Zehnder R, Ganz R. The subcoracoid space. An anatomic study. *Clin Orthop Relat Res*. 1987;215:132-138.

54. Lo IK, Burkhart SS. The etiology and assessment of subscapularis tendon tears: a case for subcoracoid impingement, the roller-wringer effect, and TUFF lesions of the subscapularis. *Arthroscopy*. 2003;19(10):1142-1150.

55. Allegrucci M, Whitney SL, Irrgang JJ. Clinical implications of secondary impingement of the shoulder in freestyle swimmers. *J Orthop Sports Phys Ther*. 1994;20(6):307-318.

56. Belling Sorensen AK, Jorgensen U. Secondary impingement in the shoulder. An improved terminology in impingement. *Scand J Med Sci Sports*. 2000;10(5):266-278.

57. Hovis WD, Dean MT, Mallon WJ, Hawkins RJ. Posterior instability of the shoulder with secondary impingement in elite golfers. *Am J Sports Med*. 2002;30(6):886-890.

58. Giaroli EL, Major NM, Higgins LD. MRI of internal impingement of the shoulder. *AJR Am J Roentgenol*. 2005;185(4):925-929.

59. Krief OP. MRI of the rotator interval capsule. *AJR Am J Roentgenol*. 2005;184(5):1490-1494.

60. Petchprapa CN, Beltran LS, Jazrawi LM, Kwon YW, Babb JS, Recht MP. The rotator interval: a review of anatomy, function, and normal and abnormal MRI appearance. *AJR Am J Roentgenol*. 2010;195(3):567-576.

61. Davidson J, Burkhart SS. The geometric classification of rotator cuff tears: a system linking tear pattern to treatment and prognosis. *Arthroscopy*. 2010;26(3):417-424.

62. Davidson JF, Burkhart SS, Richards DP, Campbell SE. Use of preoperative magnetic resonance imaging to predict rotator cuff tear pattern and method of repair. *Arthroscopy*. 2005;21(12):1428.

63. Davidson PA, Rivenburgh DW. Rotator cuff repair tension as a determinant of functional outcome. *J Shoulder Elbow Surg*. 2000;9(6):502-506.

64. Kandemir U, Allaire RB, Debski RE, Lee TQ, McMahon PJ. Quantification of rotator cuff tear geometry: the repair ratio as a guide for surgical repair in crescent and U-shaped tears. *Arch Orthop Trauma Surg*. 2010;130(3):369-373. PMCID: 2814036.

65. Kassarjian A, Bencardino JT, Palmer WE. MR imaging of the rotator cuff. *Radiol Clin North Am*. 2006;44(4):503-523, vii, viii.

66. Finnan RP, Crosby LA. Partial-thickness rotator cuff tears. *J Shoulder Elbow Surg*. 2010;19(4):609-616.

67. Yang S, Park HS, Flores S, et al. Biomechanical analysis of bursal-sided partial thickness rotator cuff tears. *J Shoulder Elbow Surg*. 2009;18(3):379-385.

68. Lee SY, Lee JK. Horizontal component of partial-thickness tears of rotator cuff: imaging characteristics and comparison of ABER view with oblique coronal view at MR arthrography initial results. *Radiology*. 2002;224(2):470-476.

69. Vinson EN, Helms CA, Higgins LD. Rim-rent tear of the rotator cuff: a common and easily overlooked partial tear. *AJR Am J Roentgenol*. 2007;189(4):943-946.

70. Thomazeau H, Boukobza E, Morcet N, Chaperon J, Langlais F. Prediction of rotator cuff repair results by magnetic resonance imaging. *Clin Orthop Relat Res.* 1997;344:275-283.

71. Oh JH, Kim SH, Choi JA, Kim Y, Oh CH. Reliability of the grading system for fatty degeneration of rotator cuff muscles. *Clin Orthop Relat Res.* 2010;468(6):1558-1564. PMCID: 2865616.

72. Pfirrmann CW, Schmid MR, Zanetti M, Jost B, Gerber C, Hodler J. Assessment of fat content in supraspinatus muscle with proton MR spectroscopy in asymptomatic volunteers and patients with supraspinatus tendon lesions. *Radiology.* 2004;232(3):709-715.

73. Goutallier D, Postel JM, Bernageau J, Lavau L, Voisin MC. Fatty muscle degeneration in cuff ruptures. Pre- and postoperative evaluation by CT scan. *Clin Orthop Relat Res.* 1994;304:78-83.

74. Fuchs B, Weishaupt D, Zanetti M, Hodler J, Gerber C. Fatty degeneration of the muscles of the rotator cuff: assessment by computed tomography versus magnetic resonance imaging. *J Shoulder Elbow Surg.* 1999;8(6):599-605.

75. Jost B, Pfirrmann CW, Gerber C, Switzerland Z. Clinical outcome after structural failure of rotator cuff repairs. *J Bone Joint Surg Am.* 2000;82(3):304-314.

76. Thomazeau H, Rolland Y, Lucas C, Duval JM, Langlais F. Atrophy of the supraspinatus belly. Assessment by MRI in 55 patients with rotator cuff pathology. *Acta Orthop Scand.* 1996;67(3):264-268.

77. Zanetti M, Gerber C, Hodler J. Quantitative assessment of the muscles of the rotator cuff with magnetic resonance imaging. *Invest Radiol.* 1998;33(3):163-170.

78. Schaefer O, Winterer J, Lohrmann C, Laubenberger J, Reichelt A, Langer M. Magnetic resonance imaging for supraspinatus muscle atrophy after cuff repair. *Clin Orthop Relat Res.* 2002;403:93-99.

79. Ide J, Tokiyoshi A, Hirose J, Mizuta H. Arthroscopic repair of traumatic combined rotator cuff tears involving the subscapularis tendon. *J Bone Joint Surg Am.* 2007;89(11):2378-2388.

80. Kasten P, Loew M, Rickert M. Repair of large supraspinatus rotator-cuff defects by infraspinatus and subscapularis tendon transfers in a cadaver model. *Int Orthop.* 2007;31(1):11-15. PMCID: 2267529.

81. Patten RM. Tears of the anterior portion of the rotator cuff (the subscapularis tendon): MR imaging findings. *AJR Am J Roentgenol.* 1994;162(2):351-354.

82. Craig EV. The geyser sign and torn rotator cuff: clinical significance and pathomechanics. *Clin Orthop Relat Res.* 1984;191:213-215.

83. Yamaguchi K, Tetro AM, Blam O, Evanoff BA, Teefey SA, Middleton WD. Natural history of asymptomatic rotator cuff tears: a longitudinal analysis of asymptomatic tears detected sonographically. *J Shoulder Elbow Surg.* 2001;10(3):199-203.

84. Saupe N, Pfirrmann CW, Schmid MR, Jost B, Werner CM, Zanetti M. Association between rotator cuff abnormalities and reduced acromiohumeral distance. *AJR Am J Roentgenol.* 2006;187(2):376-382.

85. Mohana-Borges AV, Chung CB, Resnick D. MR imaging and MR arthrography of the postoperative shoulder: spectrum of normal and abnormal findings. *Radiographics.* 2004;24(1):69-85.

86. Cho NS, Lee BG, Rhee YG. Radiologic course of the calcific deposits in calcific tendinitis of the shoulder: does the initial radiologic aspect affect the final results? *J Shoulder Elbow Surg.* 2010;19(2):267-272.

87. Zubler C, Mengiardi B, Schmid MR, Hodler J, Jost B, Pfirrmann CW. MR arthrography in calcific tendinitis of the shoulder: diagnostic performance and pitfalls. *Eur Radiol.* 2007;17(6):1603-1610.

88. Owen RS, Iannotti JP, Kneeland JB, Dalinka MK, Deren JA, Oleaga L. Shoulder after surgery: MR imaging with surgical validation. *Radiology.* 1993;186(2):443-447.

89. McMenamin D, Koulouris G, Morrison WB. Imaging of the shoulder after surgery. *Eur J Radiol.* 2008;68(1):106-119.

90. Zanetti M, Hodler J. MR imaging of the shoulder after surgery. *Radiol Clin North Am.* 2006;44(4):537-551, viii.

91. Peh WC, Chan JH. Artifacts in musculoskeletal magnetic resonance imaging: identification and correction. *Skeletal Radiol.* 2001;30(4):179-191.

92. Zlatkin MB. MRI of the postoperative shoulder. *Skeletal Radiol.* 2002;31(2):63-80.

93. Longobardi RS, Rafii M, Minkoff J. MR imaging of the postoperative shoulder. *Magn Reson Imaging Clin N Am.* 1997;5(4):841-859.

94. Zanetti M, Jost B, Hodler J, Gerber C. MR imaging after rotator cuff repair: full-thickness defects and bursitis-like subacromial abnormalities in asymptomatic subjects. *Skeletal Radiol.* 2000;29(6):314-319.

95. Holibka A, Holibkova A, Laichman S, Ruzickova K. Some peculiarities of the rotator cuff muscles. *Biomed Pap Med Fac Univ Palacky Olomouc Czech Repub.* 2003;147(2):233-237.

96. Gazielly DF, Gleyze P, Montagnon C, Bruyere G, Prallet B. [Functional and anatomical results after surgical treatment of ruptures of the rotator cuff. 1: Preoperative functional and anatomical evaluation of ruptures of the rotator cuff]. *Rev Chir Orthop Reparatrice Appar Mot.* 1995;81(1):8-16.

97. Gazielly DF, Gleyze P, Montagnon C, Bruyere G, Prallet B. [Functional and anatomical results after surgical treatment of ruptures of the rotator cuff. 2: postoperative functional and anatomical evaluation of ruptures of the rotator cuff]. *Rev Chir Orthop Reparatrice Appar Mot.* 1995;81(1):17-26.

98. Gazielly DF, Gleyze P, Montagnon C. Functional and anatomical results after rotator cuff repair. *Clin Orthop Relat Res.* 1994;304:43-53.

99. Reilly P, Amis AA, Wallace AL, Emery RJ. Mechanical factors in the initiation and propagation of tears of the rotator cuff. Quantification of strains of the supraspinatus tendon in vitro. *J Bone Joint Surg Br.* 2003;85(4):594-599.

100. Reilly P, Amis AA, Wallace AL, Emery RJ. Supraspinatus tears: propagation and strain alteration. *J Shoulder Elbow Surg.* 2003;12(2):134-138.

101. Gumina S, Di Giorgio G, Perugia D, Postacchini F. Deltoid detachment consequent to open surgical repair of massive rotator cuff tears. *Int Orthop.* 2008;32(1):81-84. PMCID: 2219931.

102. Ogata S, Uhthoff HK. Acromial enthesopathy and rotator cuff tear. A radiologic and histologic postmortem investigation of the coracoacromial arch. *Clin Orthop Relat Res.* 1990;254:39-48.

103. Linda DD, Harish S, Stewart BG, Finlay K, Parasu N, Rebello RP. Multimodality imaging of peripheral neuropathies of the upper limb and brachial plexus. *Radiographics.* 2010;30(5):1373-1400.

104. Blum A, Lecocq S, Louis M, Wassel J, Moisei A, Teixeira P. The nerves around the shoulder. *Eur J Radiol.* 2011 May 4. [Epub ahead of print].

105. Gaskin CM, Helms CA. Parsonage-Turner syndrome: MR imaging findings and clinical information of 27 patients. *Radiology.* 2006;240(2):501-507.

106. Cole BJ, McCarty LP 3rd, Kang RW, Alford W, Lewis PB, Hayden JK. Arthroscopic rotator cuff repair: prospective functional outcome and repair integrity at minimum 2-year follow-up. *J Shoulder Elbow Surg.* 2007;16(5):579-585.

107. Goutallier D, Postel JM, Bernageau J, Lavau L, Voisin MC. Fatty infiltration of disrupted rotator cuff muscles. *Rev Rhum Engl Ed.* 1995;62(6):415-422.

108. Helms CA. The impact of MR imaging in sports medicine. *Radiology.* 2002;224(3):631-635.

109. Go PM, Dunselman GA. Anatomic and functional results of surgical repair after total perineal rupture at delivery. *Surg Gynecol Obstet.* 1988;166(2):121-124.

110. Wright RW, Heller MA, Quick DC, Buss DD. Arthroscopic decompression for impingement syndrome secondary to an unstable os acromiale. *Arthroscopy.* 2000;16(6):595-599.

111. DeFranco MJ, Bershadsky B, Ciccone J, Yum JK, Iannotti JP. Functional outcome of arthroscopic rotator cuff repairs: a correlation of anatomic and clinical results. *J Shoulder Elbow Surg.* 2007;16(6):759-765.

112. Zanetti M, Hodler J. MR imaging of the shoulder after surgery. *Magn Reson Imaging Clin N Am.* 2004;12(1):169-183, viii.

113. Magee TH, Gaenslen ES, Seitz R, Hinson GA, Wetzel LH. MR imaging of the shoulder after surgery. *AJR Am J Roentgenol.* 1997;168(4):925-928.

114. Paraskevas G, Raikos A, Lazos L, Economou Z, Natsis K. Co-existence of os acromiale with suprascapular osseous bridge: a case report and review of the literature. *Folia Morphol (Warsz).* 2009;68(2):109-112.

115. Gonzales JB, Pearson SE, Beach WR. Fusion of unstable os acromiale. *J Shoulder Elbow Surg.* 2001;10(2):197-198.

116. Granieri GF, Bacarini L. A little-known cause of painful shoulder: os acromiale. *Eur Radiol.* 1998;8(1):130-133.

117. Struhl S. Anterior internal impingement: an arthroscopic observation. *Arthroscopy.* 2002;18(1):2-7.

118. Holibka R, Kalina R, Pach M, Ruzickova K. Arthroscopic treatment of ruptures of the rotator cuff. *Biomed Pap Med Fac Univ Palacky Olomouc Czech Repub.* 2005;149(2):277-280.

119. Peckett WR, Gunther SB, Harper GD, Hughes JS, Sonnabend DH. Internal fixation of symptomatic os acromiale: a series of twenty-six cases. *J Shoulder Elbow Surg.* 2004;13(4):381-385.

CHAPTER 7

ULTRASOUND OF THE ROTATOR CUFF

Anthony Luke, MD, MPH and Alison R. I. Spouge, MD, FRCPC

Musculoskeletal ultrasound continues to be a growing field, especially with advances in technology. Sound waves are generated from an ultrasound transducer, reflected back by underlying structures, and received by the ultrasound transducer using piezoelectric crystals in the ultrasound probe with frequency determinants around 5 to 12 MHz (range: 4 to 17 MHz). The ultrasound image is created from reflected sound waves. Attenuation occurs when sound energy is rapidly lost as it passes through tissue. Attenuation can involve reflection, absorption, and scattering. Higher frequencies are attenuated more quickly; thus, higher frequency transducers have less imaging depth but higher resolution capabilities. Understanding how sound waves behave and create the image can help the clinician understand more about the details of the underlying structures. Tendons consist of multiple parallel collagen bundles that cause maximal reflection of the ultrasound waves when the ultrasound beam is oriented perpendicular to the tendon, resulting in a distinctive echogenic fibrillar appearance. If the sound waves are not oriented perpendicular to the tendon, the bright reflective echo is lost and replaced with an area of decreased echogenicity, creating the impression of tendinosis or a tear. This phenomenon is termed *anisotropy* and is a common artifact encountered in shoulder ultrasound due to the curved geometry of the tendons (Figure 7-1).[1] Other artifacts can suggest the shape, density, or consistency of tissues (ie, refractile shadowing, acoustic enhancement, etc). Color or power Doppler is useful for assessing neovascularity in tendons related to inflammation or repair. In color Doppler, signals related to the mean frequency shift/velocity and direction of flow are displayed (conventionally set so that blue denotes flow away from the transducer and red toward the transducer). Power Doppler displays the total power of the Doppler shift, without regard for direction or velocity of flow, and is very sensitive to flow. The best mode (color versus power Doppler) for detection of flow is controversial; however, it is generally unique to an individual ultrasound unit.[2]

Ultrasound is highly accurate for evaluating the rotator cuff and is used as a first-line investigation in many Canadian and European centers. Advantages of ultrasound over other imaging modalities include a lack of ionizing radiation, ability to perform dynamic evaluation of joints and soft

Ma CB, Feeley BT, eds.
Basic Principles and Operative Management
of the Rotator Cuff (pp 103-120)
© 2012 SLACK Incorporated

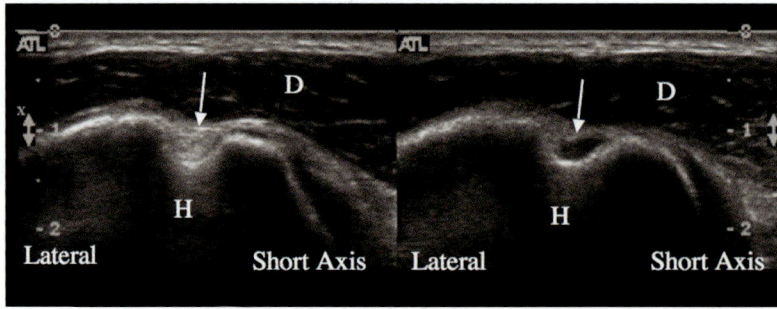

Figure 7-1. Anisotropy. Short-axis view of the biceps (arrows). On the left, the sound waves generated by the transducer are oriented at 90 degrees to the normal tendon, resulting in an echogenic appearance. When the sound waves insonate the tendon off 90 degrees (right), the tendon appears hypoechoic due to anisotropic artefact. The overlying deltoid (D) and proximal humerus (H) are visible.

TABLE 7-1. STANDARD CONVENTIONS FOR RECORDING AND VIEWING IMAGES

- Left side of screen = Posterior, superior
- Right side of screen = Anterior, inferior
- Orthogonal views relative to the structure of interest should be evaluated
- Findings are typically labeled and described in the short and long axis of the structure of interest

tissue structures, and immediate point of care service for the patient. Common concerns for adopting use of ultrasound are variable accuracy related to operator experience, need for special training, cost of ultrasound equipment, and relatively long examination times required to perform the test.

Musculoskeletal ultrasound is performed mostly using linear probes, though curvilinear and small footprint probes can be used. The positioning of the probe in relation to the structure of focus is important because reflectivity is greatest when the desired surface is at 90 degrees to ultrasound beam to avoid anisotropy. The image quality can be adjusted by the operator using basic controls, such as the following:

- Gain and time gain compensation, which changes the signal amplification (amplitude) for better visualization
- Depth of the field of view
- Frequency of the probe
- Depth of focus (focal zone; Table 7-1)

ULTRASOUND TECHNIQUE FOR EXAMINATION OF THE SHOULDER

The patient is typically seated on a rotating stool in front of the ultrasound machine with the operator in front or behind. The depth of the ultrasound beam needs to be focused to accommodate for differences in soft-tissue bulk among the patients, usually between 3 and 5 cm. Technically, the operator should take care to push lightly on the probe and not too hard to prevent distortion of the shape of the underlying structures. One finger can be placed on the patient's skin to support the operator's hand holding the probe. A standard examination of the shoulder includes systematic evaluation of the biceps tendon, the rotator cuff (supraspinatus, infraspinatus, teres minor, and subscapularis), acromioclavicular (AC) joint, and posterior glenohumeral joint as well as dynamic assessment of impingement.[3]

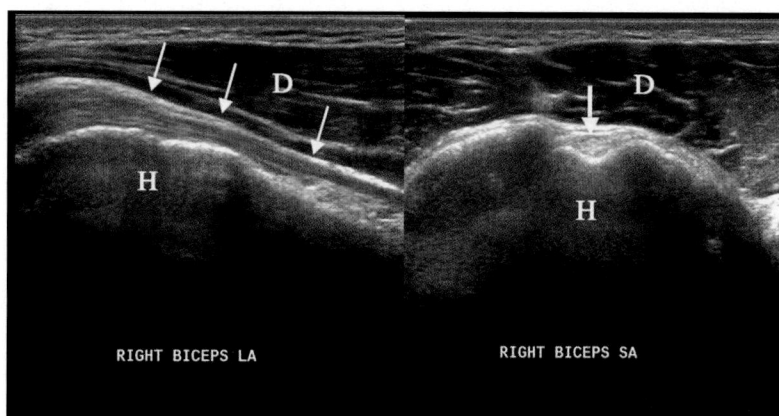

Figure 7-2. Biceps tendon long and short axis. (Left) Long- and (Right) short-axis views of the biceps tendon (arrows) situated within the bicipital groove (H, humerus; D, deltoid).

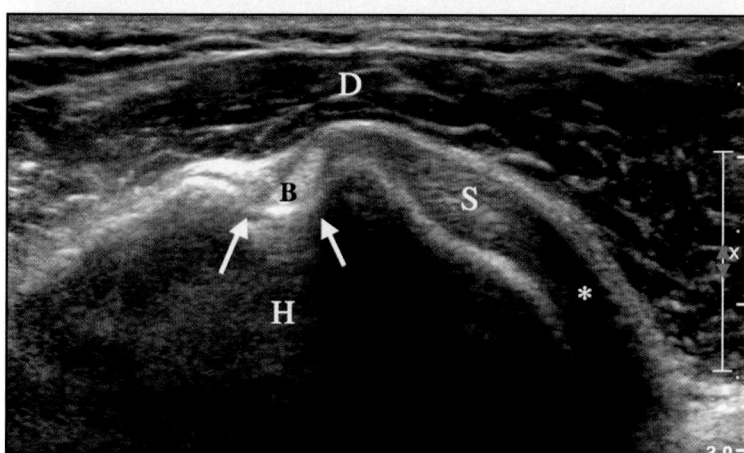

Figure 7-3. Subscapularis long axis and biceps short axis. Transverse image at the level of the proximal humerus (H) with the arm positioned in neutral displaying the relationship between the distal subscapularis (S) and biceps (B) tendons. The medial aspect of the subscapularis tendon is hypoechoic (*) due to anisotropy from the curved anatomy relative to the angle of insonation. The bicipital groove (arrows) is manifested by a concave contour of the bone.

Images of the biceps tendon are obtained in short and long axes, with the hand positioned on the thigh with the palm turned up (Figure 7-2). The heel/toe maneuver is performed for optimal visualization of the long axis of the tendon, whereby the distal end of the transducer is pushed in to compress the soft tissues alternating with compression of the proximal end of the transducer, rocking back and forth to continuously realign the ultrasound beam perpendicular to the tendon. This technique is used to reduce anisotropic artifact in other tendons that have curvilinear anatomy.

The subscapularis tendon is evaluated with the palm up and the elbow flexed 90 degrees and held close to the patient's side. It can be seen in its long and short axes with the transducer oriented parallel and perpendicular to the tendon insertion, respectively (Figures 7-3 and 7-4). The subscapularis is a multipennate tendon with several tendon slips (versus a single tendon) converging within the muscle to form a single tendon unit in the distal third. The appearance can produce an inhomogeneous appearance sonographically. Dynamic imaging of the subscapularis and biceps tendons can be observed by the patient actively rotating the shoulder from internal to external rotation.

The supraspinatus tendon is examined primarily in the modified Crass (or Middleton) position with the patient's arm placed posteriorly, placing the palm down on the superior aspect of the iliac wing with the elbow tucked in, flexed 90 degrees, and directed posteriorly ("hand on the back pocket"). The transducer is placed anterior to the AC joint and oriented 45 degrees to demonstrate the longitudinal course of the tendon (Figure 7-5A) and then rotated 90 degrees to demonstrate the transverse plane of the tendon (Figure 7-5B). The heel/toe maneuver is used to avoid anisotropic hypoechoic tendon artifacts.

Figure 7-4. Subscapularis long axis. Long-axis view with the arm externally rotated shows the full length of the subscapularis tendon (arrows). Areas of anisotropy are present both proximally and distally (*). This artifact can be eliminated by reorienting the transducer with the heel/toe maneuver. The biceps (B) has been rotated laterally and is no longer optimally demonstrated (H, humerus; D, deltoid).

Figure 7-5. (A) Supraspinatus tendon long axis. Long-axis sonogram of a normal supraspinatus tendon (arrows) showing the typical fibrillar hyperechoic appearance. The deltoid muscle (D) covers the supraspinatus muscle and the humeral head (H) lies deep to it. (B) Supraspinatus tendon short axis. Short-axis sonogram of a normal supraspinatus tendon (arrows). An adjustable color Doppler sample box outlined in white has been placed over the tendon, which shows no neovascularity either within the tendon substance or other adjacent tissues (H, humerus; D, deltoid).

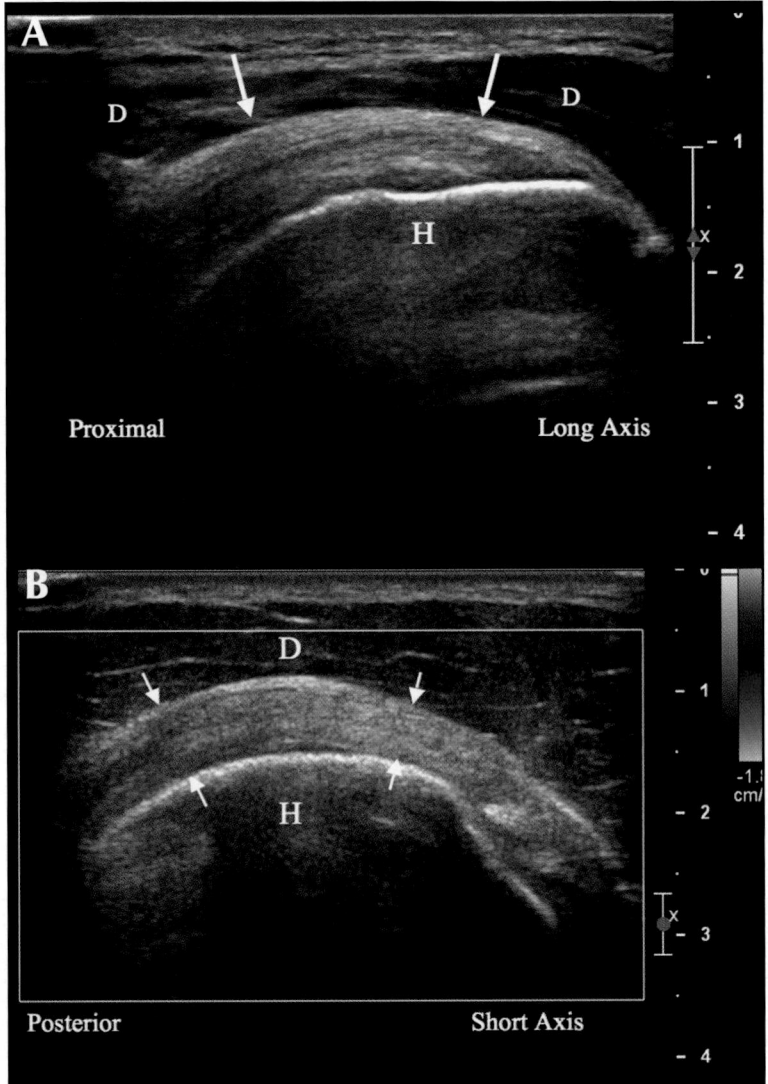

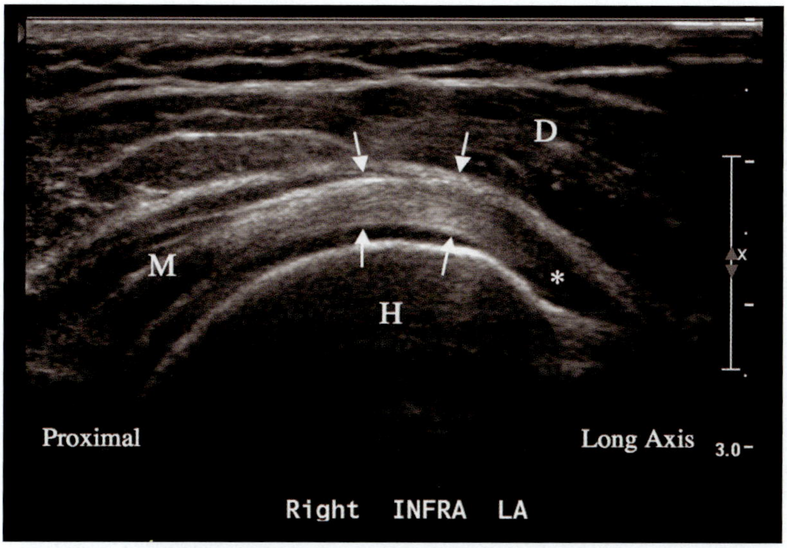

Figure 7-6. Infraspinatus tendon long axis. Long-axis view of a normal infraspinatus tendon. The tendon is manifest as a hyperechoic fibrillar structure (arrows) overlying the humeral head (H), deep to the deltoid muscle (M). The infraspinatus myotendinous junction is evident medially (D). A focal area of hypoechogenicity (*) is present corresponding to anisotropy where the tendon curves to its insertion.

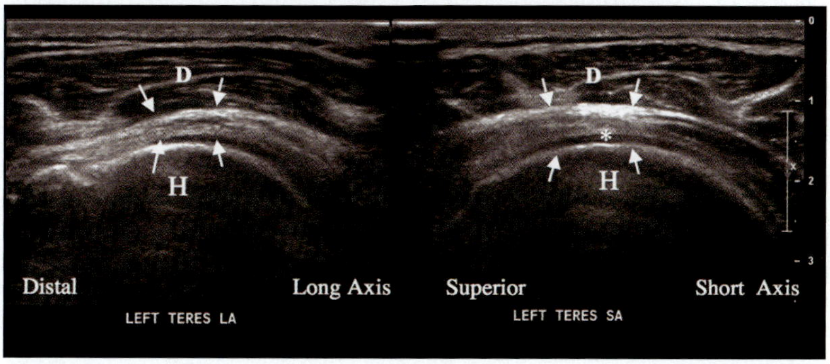

Figure 7-7. Teres minor long and short axis. (Left) Long- and (right) short-axis views of the normal teres minor tendon (arrows) overlying the humeral head (H) and deep to the deltoid (D), demonstrating the typical fibrillar echogenic appearance of normal tendons. The articular cartilage of the humeral head (*) is often apparent with current generation ultrasound equipment.

The infraspinatus tendon is viewed longitudinally with the hand on the anterior aspect of the opposite shoulder and the transducer positioned just inferior and parallel to the spine of the scapula. The infraspinatus muscle may then be followed laterally as it crosses the posterior glenohumeral joint where it becomes tendinous (Figure 7-6). More inferiorly, the teres minor can be seen just below the infraspinatus (Figure 7-7). Short-axis views of both tendons are obtained by rotating the ultrasound transducer 90 degrees from the long-axis position.

Rotator Cuff Interval and Insertion

The rotator cuff interval is the space between the anterior margin of the supraspinatus and superior border of the subscapularis tendon and can be seen in an anteriorly positioned short-axis view of the supraspinatus (Figure 7-8). It serves as an important landmark that defines the anterior margin of the supraspinatus tendon. The rotator interval contains the biceps tendon with the coracohumeral (CH) ligament, forming the roof of the interval. Together, the CH ligament with the superior glenohumeral ligament (inferior to biceps) form the rotator cuff pulley. Burkhart described the rotator crescent as the thin, crescent-shaped sheet of rotator cuff composing the distal portions of the supraspinatus and infraspinatus insertions. He termed the rotator cable as a structure of thick bundles of

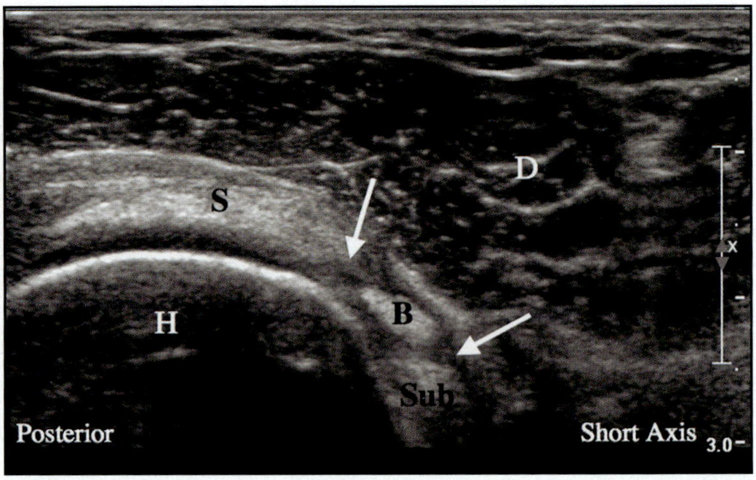

Figure 7-8. Rotator interval. Short-axis view showing the rotator cuff interval (arrows) as a space between the anterior margin of the supraspinatus (S) and superior border of the subscapularis (Sub) tendons. The long head of biceps runs through the interval, seen as an oval hyperechoic structure (B) (H, humerus; D, deltoid).

fibers that run perpendicular to the fibers of the distal supraspinatus tendon, potentially functioning to augment and reinforce the distal tendon.[4] The rotator cable fibers arch anteriorly to posteriorly to attach onto the humerus and are an extension of the CH ligament. The rotator cuff cable may be identified on ultrasound and has been described in cadaveric shoulders as an articular-sided fibrillar hyperechoic structure running perpendicular to the supraspinatus tendon fibers, most prominent along its undersurface (average thickness and width, 1.2 and 4.5 mm, respectively). Ultrasound of asymptomatic shoulders depicted the rotator cable in 3 (11%) shoulders located 1.1 to 1.5 cm medial to the greater tuberosity.[5] Younger patients may have more involvement of the cable (usually anterior edge of the rotator cuff tear), especially with tear extension either anteriorly or posteriorly, involving the subscapularis and/or the biceps pulley leading to subluxation of the biceps medially.

The AC joint is assessed in the long axis with the arms positioned by the patient's side, and stability is assessed dynamically during adduction of the ipsilateral arm by positioning the hand against the contralateral shoulder.

The posterior labrum and glenohumeral joint are visualized in the transverse plane after evaluation of the infraspinatus and teres minor. The posterior labrum is seen as a triangular echogenic structure (Figure 7-9). Usually, only a small amount of fluid is present in the posterior glenohumeral joint. The spinoglenoid notch containing the suprascapular nerve and artery can then be assessed by moving the transducer slightly superior and medial in the transverse plane from the posterior joint.

The dynamic assessment of subacromial (anterosuperior) impingement[6] can be recorded by placing the transducer in the coronal plane with its medial margin at the lateral margin of the acromion, aligned to the long axis of the supraspinatus tendon. The coracoacromial (CA) ligament can be visualized by identifying the coracoid in transverse plane then rotating the lateral aspect of the probe. During dynamic assessment, the patient abducts the arm while in internal rotation similar to Hawkins and Neer impingement tests of the shoulder on physical examination.[7] Normally, the tendon glides freely underneath the acromion and CA ligament during this maneuver. Impingement of the supraspinatus tendon against the CA ligament or undersurface of the acromion manifests as indentation of superior aspect of the tendon and/or bursa or milk-back of fluid into the lateral aspect of the bursa (Figure 7-10).

MAGNETIC RESONANCE IMAGING VERSUS ULTRASOUND

Studies demonstrate that ultrasound in the hands of an experienced examiner yields similar diagnostic capabilities for rotator cuff tears as magnetic resonance imaging (MRI).[8] In a study of

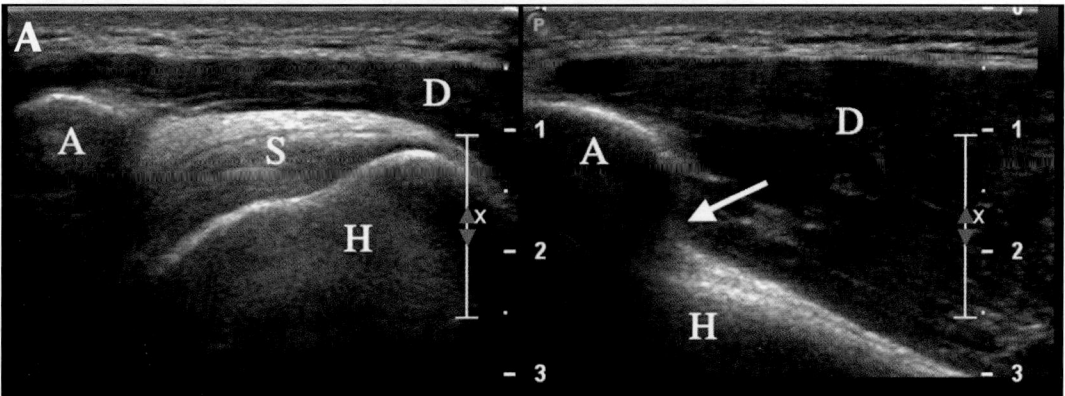

Figure 7-9. Posterior joint and labrum. Image at the level of the posterior glenohumeral joint shows the reflective echoes of the cortical bone of the posterior margin of the glenoid process (G) and adjacent posterior humeral head (H). The posterior labrum (L) is identified as a smooth triangular hyperechoic structure adjacent to the glenoid. The deltoid (D) and infraspinatus (IS) muscles are evident superficial to the joint. No effusion or other periarticular fluid collection is evident.

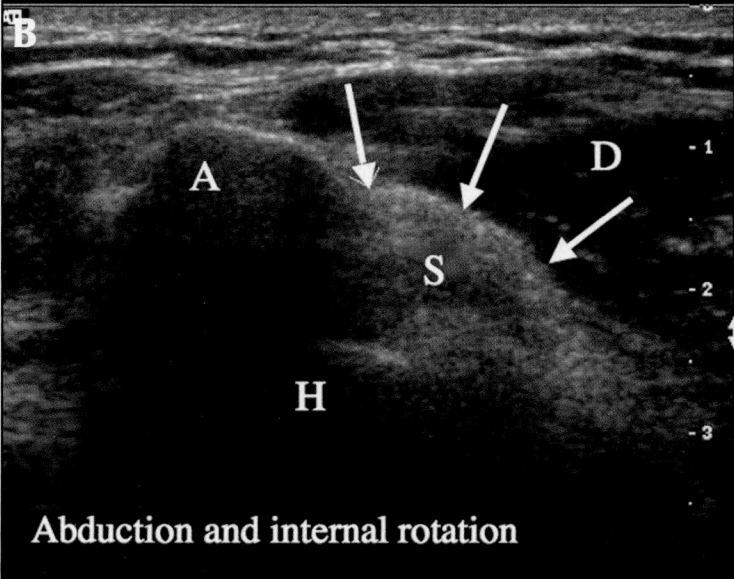

Figure 7-10. Impingement. (A) Normal appearance of the supraspinatus (S) during forward abduction and internal rotation as part of the standard dynamic assessment for impingement. The subacromial soft tissues glide freely underneath the acromion (A), without mechanical compression of either the bursa or tendon or extrusion of bursal fluid (arrow). (B) Impingement manifested by protrusion and bunching of the supraspinatus tendon (S) between the acromion (A) and humerus (H) with the upper extremity positioned in abduction and internal rotation (D, deltoid).

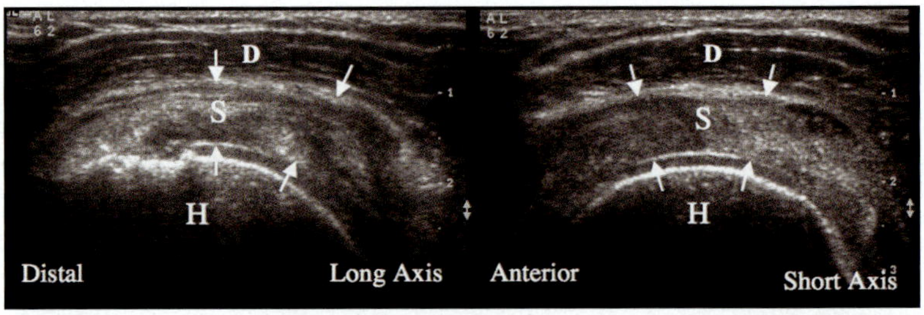

Figure 7-11. Rotator cuff tendinosis. (Left) Long- and (right) short-axis sonograms of the supraspinatus tendon (S, arrows) showing mild thickening and prominent heterogeneous hypoechogenicity (H, humerus; D, deltoid).

88 patients who underwent surgery, the accuracy in the detection of full-thickness tears was 98% and 100% for ultrasound and MRI, respectively. Similarly, for partial-thickness tears, ultrasound performed equivalent to MRI imaging. The accuracy for detecting partial-thickness tears was 87% for ultrasonography and 90% for MRI.[9] Ultrasound had a sensitivity of 95.6%, a specificity of 70%, an accuracy of 91%, and a positive predictive accuracy of 93.6% compared to MRI, which had measures of 97.7% sensitivity, 63.6% specificity, 91% accuracy, and 91.7% positive predictive accuracy, respectively.[10] Another study suggested that the overall accuracy for both imaging tests was 87%.[11] Ultrasound may be less reliable in distinguishing between full- versus partial-thickness tears with some false-negatives for moderate-size tears that were incorrectly assessed as partial-thickness and false-positives overdiagnosed as small full-thickness tears when they were only partially torn and had 2 intact cuffs. Estimation of tear size was more accurate for large and massive tears at 96.5% than for moderate (88.8%) and small tears (91.6%).[12] Many of the published reports on the accuracy of ultrasound diagnosis of partial-thickness tears were based on sonography prior to 2000. Given the ongoing advances in ultrasound technology, these studies likely underestimate the accuracy of sonographic diagnosis of partial-thickness tears currently achieved in experienced hands. A meta-analysis of 65 papers comparing MR arthrography (MRA), noncontrast MRI, and ultrasound reported sensitivities of 95.4, 92.1, and 92.3 for detection of full-thickness tears, respectively, and sensitivities of 85.9, 63.6, and 66.7 for partial-thickness rotator cuff tears.[13] The authors found specificities that were similar for MRI and ultrasound, though slightly higher for MRA. In summary, MRI and ultrasound results for detecting rotator cuff tears are comparable.

PATHOLOGIC FINDINGS ON ULTRASOUND

Rotator Cuff Tendinosis

The term *tendinosis* is preferred over tendinitis as no inflammatory cells are identified pathologically. Patients with tendinosis are usually 40 years old or younger. Older patients typically demonstrate degenerative changes to the rotator cuff and may have asymptomatic tears:
- Ill-defined hypoechoic region (Figure 7-11)
- Focal enlargement of tendon (no volume loss)
- Calcification (calcific tendinosis)
- Neovascularity on color or power Doppler (Figure 7-12)

Rotator Cuff Tears (Table 7-2)

Partial Rotator Cuff Tear

Partial rotator cuff tears can be difficult to detect at times. They can occur on both the bursal surface (superior) of the tendon and the articular side (inferior) of the tendon. Tears can be asymptomatic and are classified often by the depth of the tear. The depth of the tear can be helpful to surgeons for surgical planning. Tears less than 50% are often simply débrided, while tears involving greater than 50% of the tendon may warrant surgical repair.

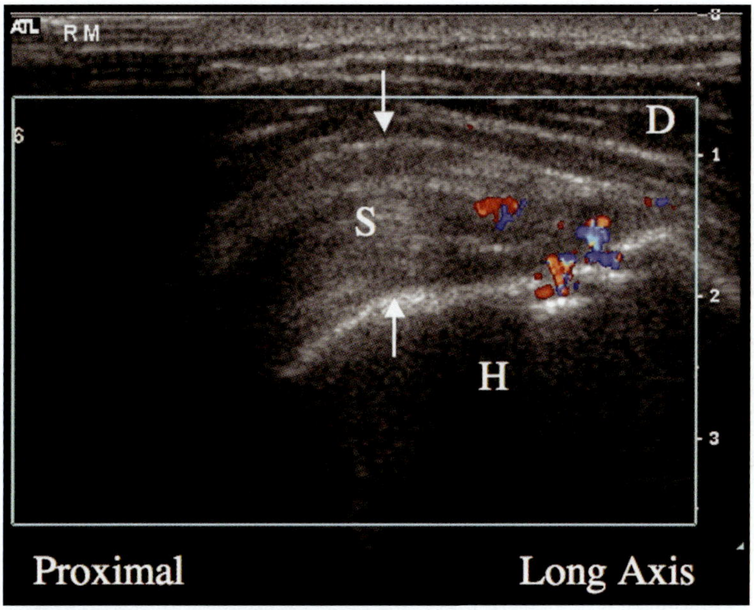

Figure 7-12. Rotator cuff tendinosis (color Doppler). Long-axis sonogram of the supraspinatus tendon (S, arrows) with color Doppler interrogation (green box), showing prominent focal blood flow at the tendon insertion as a manifestation of neovascularity related to inflammation and/or reparative change. The background supraspinatus tendon adjacent to the blood flow shows heterogeneous decreased echogenicity (H, humerus; D, deltoid).

TABLE 7-2. PEARLS FOR ULTRASOUND OF THE ROTATOR CUFF

Rotator cuff tears can have a diverse appearance consisting of both primary and secondary sonographic abnormalities. On ultrasound, the following characteristics of a rotator cuff tear should be described:

- Which tendon is involved (extension into adjacent tendon)?
- Where in the long axis of the tendon (proximal, mid, or distal)?
- Partial (articular or bursal side) versus full-thickness?
- The size of the tear (measured in millimeters)?
- Tear morphology?
- Retraction?

Primary/Direct Findings

- Well-defined hypoechoic defect involving the articular or bursal surfaces or intrasubstance portion of the tendon (Figure 7-13).
- Occasionally or mixed hyper- and hypoechoic or purely hyperechoic.
- An intrasubstance tear is confined to the center of the tendon without extension through either the articular or bursal surface.

Secondary/Indirect Findings (Table 7-3)

- Flattening of the bursal surface with focal tendon thinning. The deltoid may dip into the tear as a result of herniation of subdeltoid fat plane (Figure 7-14).
- Cartilage interface or naked cartilage sign: Visualization of the linear reflective echo produced by the underlying articular cartilage. This phenomenon occurs as the loss of rotator cuff tendon allows more sound to be transmitted to and reflected off the articular cartilage and becomes more pronounced with larger tendon defects. This sign is less specific using current-generation high-frequency transducers, as the articular cartilage of the humerus can often be demonstrated in the presence of an intact cuff (Figure 7-15).

Figure 7-13. Bursal side partial-thickness tear. (Left) Long- and (right) short-axis images of the supraspinatus tendon (S) show an irregular bursal surface tear (arrows) distally involving slightly more than 50% of the thickness of the tendon (H, humerus; D, deltoid).

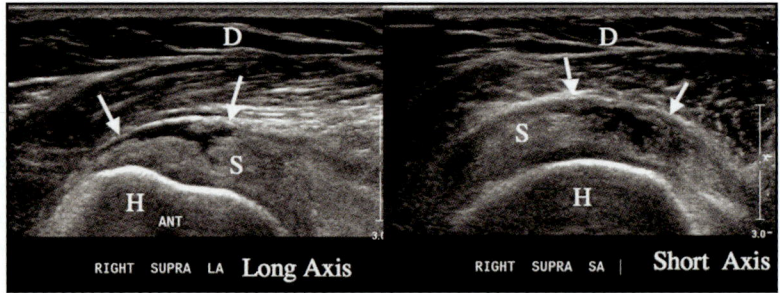

TABLE 7-3. CLASSIFICATION OF PARTIAL-THICKNESS TEARS

- Grade 1: <3 mm deep
- Grade 2: 3 to 6 mm deep (50% cuff thickness)
- Grade 3: 6 mm deep (>50% involved)

Figure 7-14. Articular and bursal partial-thickness tear. Short-axis sonogram showing an anechoic defect (short arrows) on the articular side of the tendon and focal thinning on the bursal side where the subacromial-subdeltoid bursal fat and deltoid muscle (long arrow) have herniated into the focally attenuated tendon. The tear involves slightly more than 50% of the thickness of the tendon (H, humerus; D, deltoid).

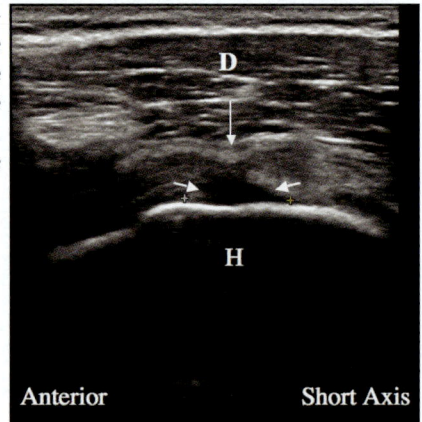

Figure 7-15. Articular surface tear. Short-axis sonogram shows a well-defined anechoic defect (arrows) in the articular surface of the supraspinatus tendon involving less than 50% of the tendon thickness. The "cartilage interface" sign is apparent deep to the tear (H, humerus; D, deltoid).

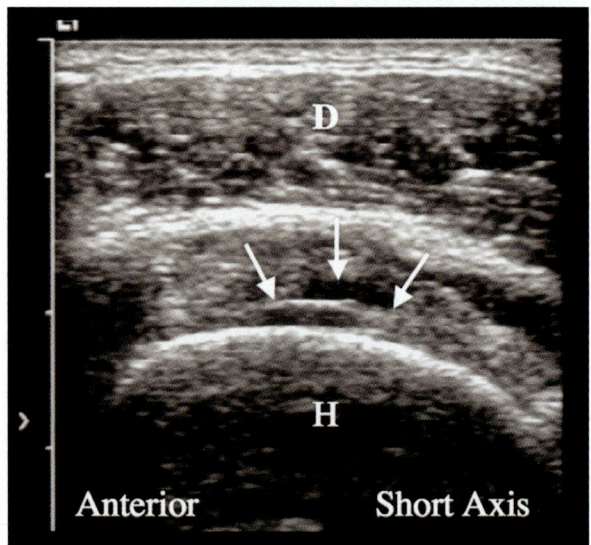

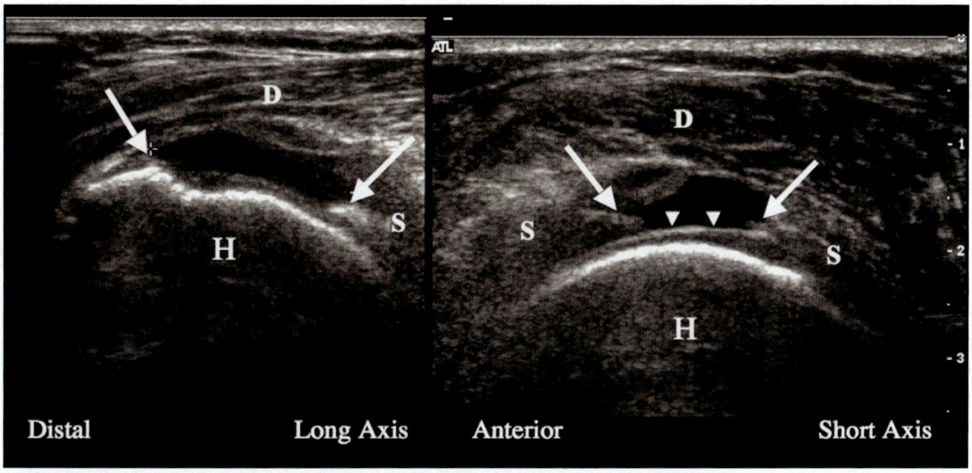

Figure 7-16. Full-thickness supraspinatus tear. (Left) Long- and (right) short-axis sonograms of the supraspinatus tendon (S) show a full-thickness tear manifested by a moderated-sized fluid filled defect tear in the mid-distal tendon (arrows) with a prominent cartilage interface evident (arrowheads) (H, humerus; D, deltoid).

TABLE 7-4. TIPS FOR IDENTIFYING FULL-THICKNESS ROTATOR CUFF TEARS

- Absence of structures (ie, rotator cuff layer)
- Demonstrate the tear in 2 planes
- Correct anisotropy: Tilt the probe to eliminate anisotropy and avoid misdiagnosis of a tear
- Sonopalpation: Compression with the probe may reveal fluid, bubbles, and movement of subdeltoid fat plane

---

Full-Thickness Rotator Cuff Tear

Full-thickness tears show findings similar to partial-thickness tears but are typically more pronounced (Figure 7-16). A complete tear may be difficult to identify if there is echogenic granulation tissue in-situ. Patient-related factors, including obesity and restricted motion, also compromise the ability to detect complete tears. Several signs of full-thickness rotator cuff tears have been described on ultrasound (Table 7-4).[14]

Primary Signs
- Well-defined focal full-thickness hypoechoic defect (less commonly hyperechoic).
- Nonvisualization of the tendon. Deltoid muscle lies directly on the humeral head (loss of muscle layers; Figure 7-17).
- Retraction of the tendon.

Secondary Signs of Rotator Cuff Tear[14]
- Volume loss with herniation of the deltoid muscle into the defect.
- Cartilage interface sign (similar to partial-thickness tear).
Additional less specific findings:
- Excessive fluid in the subacromial/subdeltoid bursa (Figure 7-18).
- Biceps tendon fluid.
- Joint effusion (specificity 95%): Joint effusion is present in 60% of tears and is present in 10% of normal.

Figure 7-17. Full-thickness tear of the supraspinatus tendon. (Left) Long- and (right) short-axis sonogram in the region of the distal supraspinatus tendon show complete absence of the tendon (arrows). The deltoid muscle (D) and peribursal fat (arrowheads) have filled the space normally occupied by the tendon (H, humerus).

Figure 7-18. Subacromial-subdeltoid bursa. (A) Long-axis sonogram of the supraspinatus tendon (S) showing a linear echogenic structure superficial to it (arrows) representing a normal subacromial-subdeltoid bursal fat stripe. (B) Long-axis image sonogram (left) of the region of the distal supraspinatus tendon in another patient, showing absence of the tendon due to a large full-thickness tear with a small amount of fluid within the adjacent bursa (arrows). An extended field of view sonogram in the same patient (right) positioned over the anterolateral aspect of the proximal arm shows a large amount of fluid has accumulated in the bursa distally (arrows) (H, humerus; D, deltoid).

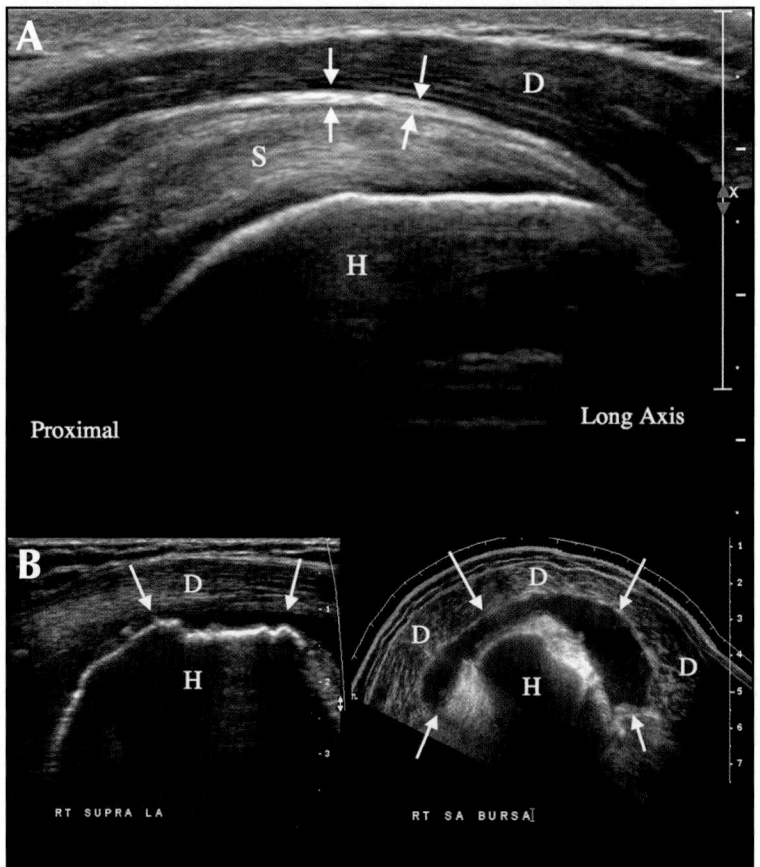

- Inhomogeneity of the tendon substance.
- Synovial thickening or fibrosis of the subacromial-subdeltoid bursa.
- Greater tuberosity cortical irregularity (Figure 7-19)[14]: Bones spurs, cortical pitting, hyperostosis poor, positive predictive value 80%, normal 40%.
- Calcification flecks.
- Enthesopathy.

Figure 7-19. Cortical irregularity of the humerus. Long-axis image showing irregularity of the cortical surface of the humeral head (arrows) due to entheseal resorptive change. This finding is regarded as an indirect sign of rotator cuff tendinopathy and/or tear. The distal supraspinatus tendon (S) shows heterogeneous echogenicity, consistent with tendinosis (H, humerus; D, deltoid).

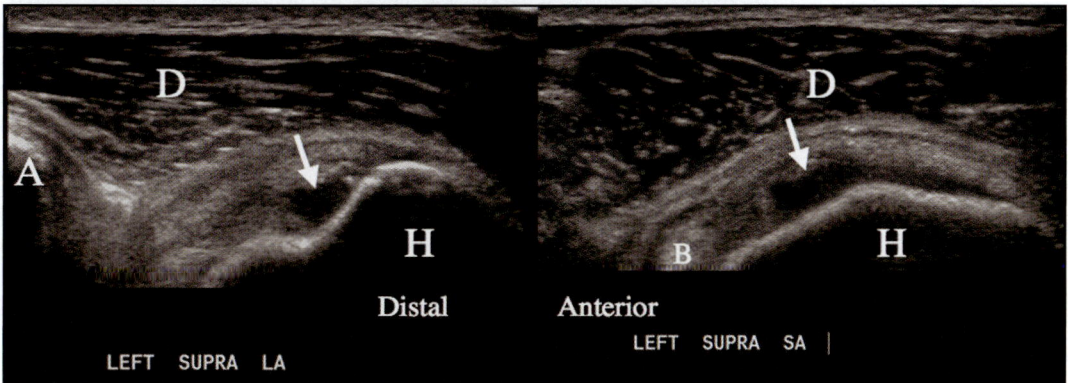

Figure 7-20. Rim rent tear. (Left) Long- and (right) short-axis view of the anterodistal supraspinatus tendon show a focal area of decreased echogenicity (arrows) involving the articular surface. The short-axis view shows the biceps (B) within the rotator interval confirming the anterior location of the tear (A, acromion; H, humerus; D, deltoid).

Supraspinatus Tear

Free edge tears can occur in younger patients and are often located near the rotator cuff interval and the biceps tendon, seen best on long-axis view of the supraspinatus similar to an axial view on MRI. A rim-rent tear occurs when a partial-thickness articular surface tear develops on the footprint at the insertion on the greater tuberosity (Figure 7-20).[15]

Subscapularis Tear

Subscapularis tears are associated with CH or anterior superior impingement. Injuries may occur anteriorly and superiorly (near the cable) as an extended tear.

Infraspinatus and Teres Minor Tears

Injury to the infraspinatus tendon usually results as an extension of a supraspinatus tendon tear (Figure 7-21), when there are signs suggesting posterosuperior impingement. These occur more commonly in elderly patients and in throwing athletes where posterosuperior labral tears can occur in conjunction with the tendon injury. Labral pathology is typically difficult to see on ultrasound, though paralabral cysts can be visualized (Figure 7-22). Tears of the teres minor tendon are rare.

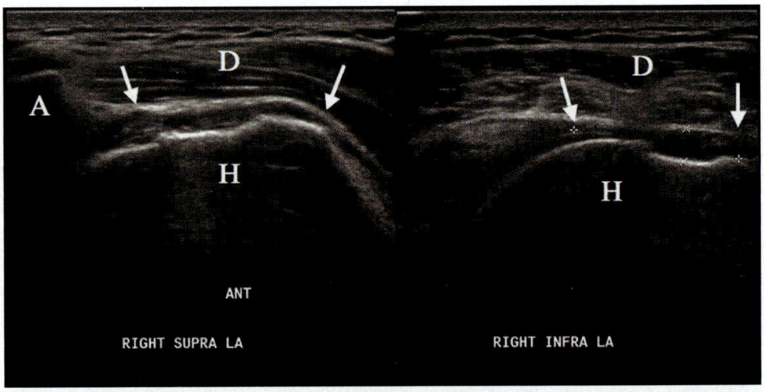

Figure 7-21. Infraspinatus tear as extension of supraspinatus tear. Long-axis views of supraspinatus (left) and infraspinatus (right) show full-thickness tears (arrows) that were in continuity at real time (A, acromion; H, humerus; D, deltoid).

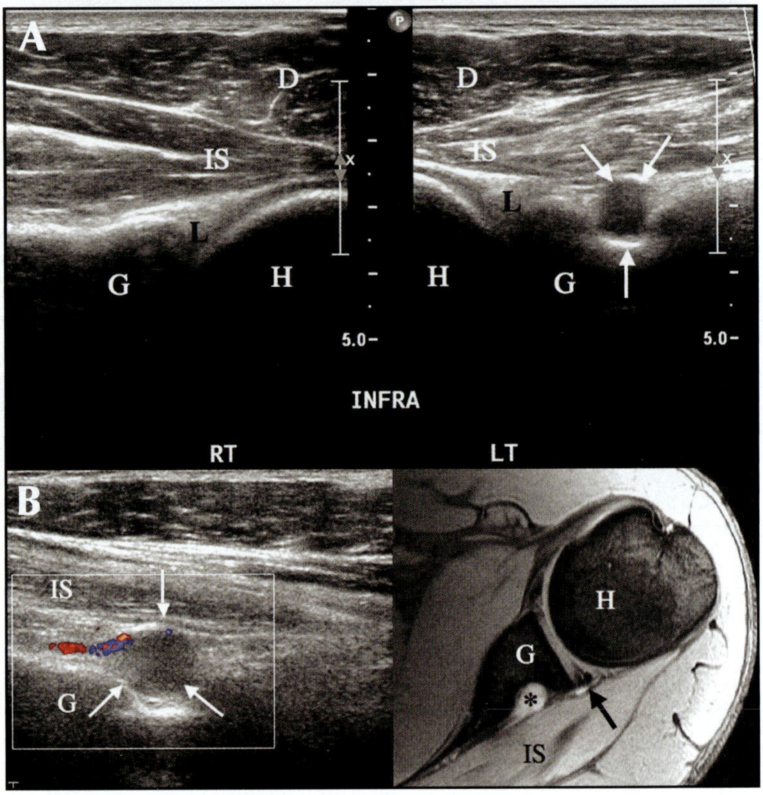

Figure 7-22. Spinoglenoid notch. (A) Normal spinoglenoid notch (left) and spinoglenoid notch cyst (arrows, right) seen posterior to the glenoid (G) and deep to the infraspinatus muscle (IS). The infraspinatus muscle on the side of the cyst shows mild increased echogenicity, suggesting the presence of early fatty infiltration. The glenoid labrum (L) is visible bilaterally. (B) Spinoglenoid notch cyst on ultrasound and MR. Sonogram (left) of the spinoglenoid region with a color Doppler box (white rectangle) placed over the cyst (white arrows) shows no internal flow, eliminating the possibility of a suprascapular varix. Transverse MR gradient echo image of the same region confirms the cyst (*) and a small tear in the posterior labrum with an adjacent linear extension of the cyst arising from the tear (arrows) (H, humeral head; D, deltoid; G, glenoid).

Atrophy and Fatty Infiltration

Ultrasound can be used to grade atrophy in the rotator cuff.[16] A simple side-to-side comparison of muscle bulk with the unaffected side may demonstrate muscle atrophy (Figure 7-23). The cross-sectional surface area of the supraspinatus muscle belly can be assessed as proposed by Strobel and colleagues[17] using a sagittal plane at the scapular notch with the spine of scapula on one side and the clavicle on the other similar to a "Y" view on MRI. This can be divided by the area of the supraspinatus fossa. A ratio greater than 0.6 is consistent with supraspinatus atrophy. Fatty infiltration can be evaluated by comparing the echogenicity of the supraspinatus muscle with that of the trapezius

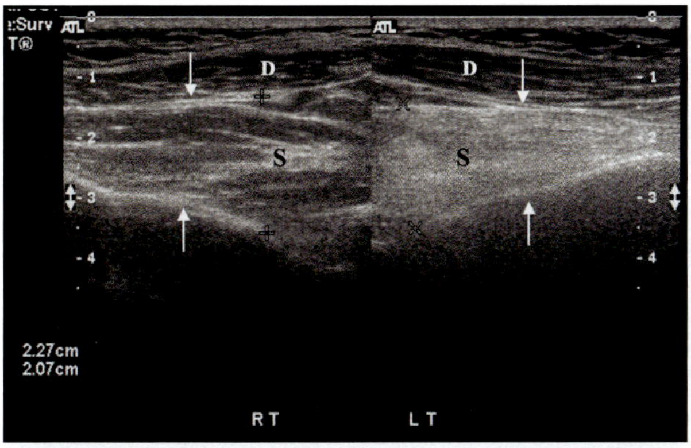

Figure 7-23. Supraspinatus muscle atrophy. Split-screen coronal side-to-side images of a normal (left) and atrophic (right) supraspinatus (S) muscle. On the normal side, the pennate pattern is preserved. On the atrophic side, diffuse hyperechogenicity is evident with loss of the pennate pattern and reduction in muscle bulk, corresponding to Goutallier grade 4 atrophy.

muscle and its pennate pattern. Interobserver agreement was moderate for supraspinatus (kappa = 0.55) and substantial for infraspinatus (kappa = 0.71) muscles compared to MRI.[18] Fatty atrophy and effacement of the fascicular pattern has been studied by Goutallier using computed tomography (CT), who suggested the percentage of atrophy in the cuff based on fascicular patterns.[19] Khoury and colleagues indicate that it can be difficult to distinguish from the surrounding fat in the supraspinatus fossa with similar echogenicity and proposed the following findings on ultrasound for the Goutallier grading system: In the absence of fatty infiltration (Goutallier grade 0), echogenicity is normal and the pennate pattern is preserved. With mild fatty infiltration (Goutallier grades 1 and 2), there is mild hyperechogenicity and an effaced pennate pattern. With moderate to severe fatty infiltration (Goutallier grades 3 and 4), there is marked hyperechogenicity and an absent pennate pattern (see Figure 7-23).[16]

Ultrasound Procedures

The widespread availability of ultrasound equipment and lack of ionizing radiation are features that favor the use of sonography over traditional fluoroscopic or CT-guided shoulder-related procedures. Use of real-time ultrasound guidance enabling direct visualization of needle placement for procedures is technically challenging. Localizing the needle can be difficult if the transducer is not perfectly aligned with the ultrasound waves as perpendicular as possible to the needle in the long axis. The learning curve for developing this skill is relatively long.

GLENOHUMERAL JOINT INJECTION

Indications for glenohumeral joint injection include osteoarthritis and adhesive capsulitis. The patient is positioned prone oblique with the affected shoulder in internal rotation. A posterior approach is used with real-time ultrasound guidance, aiming the tip of the needle between the articular surface of the humeral head and the posterior labrum.[20] The normal capacity of the shoulder joint is around 10 to 15 cc. Patients with frozen shoulders often have much smaller volumes due to capsular scarring, while those patients with instability often have increased volumes.[21]

SUBACROMIAL INJECTION

Only 30% to 80% of blind injections of steroid and local anesthetic reach the subacromial-subdeltoid bursa. Ultrasound enables direct visualization and accurate guidance of needle placement for bursal injections. However, a recent publication reported that ultrasound-guided subacromial injection of steroid provided no significant improvement in shoulder pain compared to administration of a systemic gluteal injection of steroid.[22]

CHAPTER 8

NATURAL HISTORY OF ROTATOR CUFF TEARS

Warren R. Dunn, MD, MPH and Brian T. Feeley, MD

Rotator cuff tears are unique in that they are one of the few tendon tears in the body that we as physicians allow to be treated in a nonoperative fashion as a primary mode of treatment. Despite this, there are relatively few data as to the natural history of rotator cuff tears. As surgeons, we often are well equipped to teach patients about how a surgical procedure is done and what the expected postoperative course and outcomes will be. However, we are often unable to inform the patient about what would happen in the setting of nonoperative management for particular disease processes. Due to the recent efforts of many researchers, there is now a better understanding of the natural history of asymptomatic, symptomatic, and massive rotator cuff tears when treated nonoperatively. The focus of this chapter is to review the natural history of rotator cuff tears when treated nonoperatively. Outcomes from surgical procedures for rotator cuff tears are the focus of other chapters.

INCIDENCE AND PREVALENCE OF ROTATOR CUFF TEARS

The prevalence of rotator cuff disease is reported to be quite high, particularly as we increase in age. Reilly and colleagues performed a review of cadaveric and radiologic imaging studies to determine the incidence of partial- and full-thickness rotator cuff tears.[1] In 2553 shoulders of patients with an average age of 70.1 years, there was a 12% incidence of partial-thickness tears and an 18% incidence of full-thickness tears. The overall incidence of rotator cuff tears when assessed by ultrasound was 41% and 49% when assessed by magnetic resonance imaging (MRI). Although there are many limitations to this retrospective review, it does highlight the high incidence of rotator cuff tears in the general population. MRI of asymptomatic volunteers demonstrated partial or complete tears of the rotator cuff in 4% of patients younger than 40 years of age and in 54% of those older than 60 years of age with 28% having full-thickness tears.[2] Similar findings of asymptomatic subjects using ultrasound detected a prevalence of rotator cuff tears in 40% of subjects older than 50 years of age; when subjects were stratified by age, a graded response was seen:

Ma CB, Feeley BT, eds.
Basic Principles and Operative Management
of the Rotator Cuff (pp 121-126)
© 2012 SLACK Incorporated

13% in quinquagenarians (50 year olds), 20% in sexagenarians (60 year olds), 31% in septuagenarians (70 year olds), and 51% in octogenarians (80 year olds).[3] Yamaguchi and colleagues performed a study evaluating 588 patients with ultrasound. Of these, 212 had an intact rotator cuff bilaterally, 199 had a unilateral rotator cuff tear (either partial or full thickness), and 177 had a bilateral tear (either partial or full thickness).[4] The authors found that the prevalence of rotator cuff disease correlated considerably with age. The average age was 48 years for patients with no rotator cuff tear, 58 years for those with a unilateral tear, and 68 years for those with a bilateral tear. They also showed that there is a 56.3% chance of a rotator cuff tear in the contralateral, asymptomatic shoulder if a patient presents with a painful full-thickness tear in one shoulder. Studies of cadaveric shoulders demonstrate similar findings of increasing prevalence of full-thickness tears with increasing age.[1] This evidence suggests that rotator cuff disease is found in a large number of asymptomatic individuals. It is believed that there are 57 million people older than age 60 in the United States; applying a conservative estimate that 10% of subjects in the United States older than age 60 have full-thickness rotator cuff tears, this amounts to 5.7 million individuals in the United States with rotator cuff tears. To put this in perspective, this is greater than the population of most states. Although the actual number of rotator cuff repairs that are performed per annum in the United States is not known, it is likely an order of magnitude less than the number of tears. Thus, the number of rotator cuff tears in the general population is quite high, and the number of patients with asymptomatic and minimally symptomatic shoulder pain from rotator cuff tears suggests that many people can compensate quite well with a cuff tear.

ASYMPTOMATIC ROTATOR CUFF TEARS

An asymptomatic rotator cuff tear is defined as the presence of a rotator cuff tear found by diagnostic (usually radiologic) evaluation in a patient who does not complain of shoulder dysfunction. As a shoulder surgeon, one of the most common questions asked is whether a tear that is asymptomatic will progress to a problematic tear causing pain and dysfunction. Fortunately, many recent studies have addressed this question. Moosmayer and colleagues evaluated 420 asymptomatic volunteers from 50 to 79 years of age.[5] Full-thickness cuff tears were detected in 32 subjects (7.6%). The prevalence increased with age: 50 to 59 years, 2.1%; 60 to 69 years, 5.7%; and 70 to 79 years, 15%. The mean size of the tear was less than 3 cm, and the tear was limited to the supraspinatus tendon in most cases (78%). Flexion strength was significantly less when compared between those patients with and without tears. A similar radiographic study found that a full-thickness supraspinatus tear occurred in 6% of all asymptomatic patients aged 18 to 85 years with an average age of 67 years for those with a tear.[6] Strength in these patients was lower than in those patients without a cuff tear.

Yamaguchi and colleagues reported on the natural history of asymptomatic rotator cuff tears.[7] Patients treated for unilateral symptomatic rotator cuff tears underwent ultrasound on the contralateral asymptomatic side, and nearly 40% of the patients had a tear on the asymptomatic shoulder. These authors followed patients with asymptomatic rotator cuff tears with ultrasound examinations and showed that 51% became symptomatic, on average, 2.8 years following their initial ultrasound. They were able to get follow-up ultrasound studies on about half the cohort (23 of 45 subjects), which showed progression of the tear in 9 of the 23 subjects (39%). Two of the 9 were in asymptomatic shoulders, and 7 were in subjects who had developed symptoms. In their cohort, symptomatic tears were significantly larger than in those patients with asymptomatic tears. Mall and colleagues prospectively evaluated 195 patients with asymptomatic rotator cuff tears as identified with ultrasound.[8] There were 44 patients (22%) who developed symptoms during the study period (1 year). These patients were compared to 55 patients who remained asymptomatic. In patients who became symptomatic, there was a significant difference in cuff tear width, but no difference in tear length or cuff tear area at the time of enrollment. This suggests that the absolute size of an asymptomatic tear may be an important predictor of future pain development. Importantly, the presence of pain was an important predictor of an increase in rotator cuff tear size, and those who remained pain-free likely did not have an increase in tear size. Not surprisingly, shoulder function decreased as asymptomatic tears became symptomatic.

Kim and colleagues evaluated the shoulder strength in asymptomatic individuals with rotator cuff tears and compared them to those without a torn rotator cuff.[9] Two hundred thirty-seven health volunteers with no history of shoulder pain were screened with ultrasound. Forty-one (17%) patients were found to have a rotator cuff tear in at least one side. Tears were more common in older patients than younger patients, and large full-thickness tears were found primarily in elderly patients. The prevalence of rotator cuff tears was 0% for the subjects between 40 and 49 years old; 10% for those between 50 and 59 years old; 20% for those between 60 and 69 years old; and 40.7% for those 70 years old or older. A loss of abduction strength was associated with a large or massive asymptomatic tear. However, not all of the shoulders with an asymptomatic rotator cuff tear were found to be weaker than those shoulders with an intact rotator cuff. In the presence of a large or massive full-thickness tear in a shoulder, abduction strength was significantly decreased compared with the contralateral shoulder with an intact cuff, a partial-thickness tear, or a small or medium full-thickness tear.

Taken together, the available literature suggests that asymptomatic tears are common, especially in the elderly patient population. These tears can be associated with weakness that is not appreciated by the patient. Approximately 20% to 30% of patients can expect to progress to a symptomatic tear over the following year, and this progression may suggest an increase in tear size.

PARTIAL-THICKNESS ROTATOR CUFF TEARS

Perhaps the most challenging problem faced by shoulder surgeons is the patient with a painful shoulder and an MRI report of a partial-thickness rotator cuff tear and tendinosis. Partial-thickness rotator cuff tears are common, especially in the supraspinatus tendon. Lohr and Uhthoff noted a 32% incidence of partial-thickness tears in a study of 306 cadaveric shoulders.[10] Similarly, Fukuda et al reported an incidence of 13% partial-thickness and 7% full-thickness rotator cuff tears in a cadaveric study.[11] Articular-sided tears appear to be more common, with Payne and colleagues noting that articular-sided tears comprise 91% of all partial-thickness tears.[12]

The natural history of these tears is difficult to determine because relatively few studies exist and there is no long-term follow-up using a standardized treatment protocol. Further, there is no distinction in the studies that do exist between articular, intrasubstance, and bursal-sided tears. Studies suggest that partial-thickness tears do not typically heal on their own. In a small series, Yamanaka and Matsumoto evaluated 40 partial-thickness tears with arthrography over a 2-year period and found that 80% of them had enlarged or progressed to a full-thickness tear.[13] Twenty percent of the tears had healed completely or had reduced in size. Predictors of worsening symptoms and tear progression included older age, larger tear size, and the absence of a history of trauma. Similarly, Weber found that partial-thickness tears that had been débrided during a first arthroscopy had no evidence of healing at a second arthroscopy.[14,15] In a recent MRI study, Maman et al evaluated a series of patients with symptomatic partial- and full-thickness tears.[16] In the partial-thickness group, only 8% progressed over the time of the study. Importantly, none of the partial-thickness tears developed muscle atrophy or fatty infiltration during the study.

Despite the improvements in rotator cuff imaging, there remains a paucity of data on the natural history of symptomatic partial-thickness rotator cuff tears. It appears that these tears are common and many do not heal on their own. In patients with a documented partial-thickness symptomatic tear, it is likely that symptom progression represents an increase in tear size with a possible progression to a full-thickness rotator cuff tear.

FULL-THICKNESS ROTATOR CUFF TEARS

Based on the data provided by Yamaguchi and others, the reported prevalence of full-thickness rotator cuff tears is dependent on age, but occurs in up to 50% to 80% of the population.[4,17,18] When counseling a patient as to whether to have surgery for his or her rotator cuff tear, it is important for the patient to understand the natural progression of the full-thickness tear. Reports in the literature are conflicting, with some studies showing that most tears progress in size and symptoms, while other studies do show acceptable outcomes with nonoperative treatment with no increase in symptoms.[19,20] It remains difficult to predict which patients will progress with an increase in tear size or symptoms.

Multiple recent studies have evaluated factors that are associated with tear progression in full-thickness tears. Maman and colleagues evaluated 59 shoulders in 54 patients with an average age of 59 years. In the subgroup of patients with symptomatic full-thickness rotator cuff tears, 24% of patients increased more than 5 mm, 27% increased from 2 to 5 mm, and 36% had not changed.[16] Twelve percent decreased in size. None of the larger (more than one tendon) rotator cuff tears decreased in size. The study found that being older (older than 60 years of age), having full-thickness tears, and the presence of fatty infiltration increased the risk of progression. The authors concluded that use of MRI was a safe and effective technique to evaluate patients nonoperatively for tear progression. In a younger patient population, nonoperative treatment of symptomatic rotator cuff tears is more controversial. Safran and colleagues followed a cohort of younger (younger than 60 years old) patients with symptomatic rotator cuff tears for a mean of 29 months.[21] The authors found that there was nearly a 50% chance that the tear would progress over the study period. Increase in tear size correlated with an increase in pain reported by the patients. The authors concluded that younger patients with symptomatic rotator cuff tears treated nonoperatively should be routinely monitored for increases in tear size. Because larger tears predictably result in higher retear rates, it is important to counsel younger patients who wish to treat their rotator cuff tears nonoperatively. In multiple studies, the presence of increased pain is an indicator of tear progression and should be taken seriously by the patient and the treating shoulder surgeon.

Rotator cuff tears lead to degeneration of the cuff muscles with the degree of muscular degeneration and fatty infiltration increasing with the size of the tear. This is demonstrated in elderly populations with massive tears—rotator cuff muscles often demonstrate marked muscle atrophy and fatty infiltration seen by both computed tomography and MRI and on visual inspection at the time of surgical intervention. Goutallier and colleagues proposed grading fatty infiltration based on the ratio of fat to muscle.[22] This grading system is important as the level of fatty infiltration significantly increases with tear severity.[23] This system also correlates the decrease in muscle function seen following massive tears with the levels of fatty infiltration at time of repair. Patients graded with pathologic levels of fatty infiltration clinically exhibit limited range of active external rotation compared to those graded 2 or less.[24] The quantity of fatty infiltration is not only important due to its effects on decreased muscle function, but also because there is a degree of fatty infiltration that can be irreversible, even following repair.[25]

The natural history of muscle atrophy and fatty infiltration in the rotator cuff has been well studied in the past few years. In a series of retrospective reviews, Melis and colleagues performed a review of 1688 patients with rotator cuff tears to determine the natural history of fatty infiltration and atrophy.[23,26,27] Fatty infiltration was related to increased patient age, larger tears, and delay between onset and diagnosis. Perhaps most importantly, the authors found that fatty infiltration occurred an average of 4 years after the onset of symptoms. Thus, patients should be counseled that a delay of 4 years may increase the risk of poorer outcomes due to the amount of fatty infiltration within the rotator cuff. Muscle atrophy was also influenced by the degree of fatty infiltration, number of tendons involved, time after diagnosis, and age of the patient. A recent study by Cheung and colleagues described the prevalence and relationship of fatty infiltration with the significance of muscle tears.[28]

The authors reported that the prevalence of fatty infiltration in the infraspinatus and supraspinatus muscles increases with worsening tear of the respective muscles; however, the prevalence of higher grade fatty infiltration is much higher in the infraspinatus muscle. More interestingly, the findings of worsening fatty infiltration in the untorn infraspinatus muscle is related to the worsening degree of supraspinatus tendon. This finding pointed out the interrelationship between the infraspinatus and supraspinatus muscle and the complexity of the pathway of muscle deterioration.

Many patients with chronic massive rotator cuff tears are treated with nonoperative modalities due to medical comorbidities and the high rates of retear and complications associated with surgical treatment options. Zingg and colleagues evaluated the natural history of 19 patients with massive cuff tears treated nonoperatively for an average of 4 years.[29] The mean relative constant score was 83%, and the score for pain averaged 11.5 points on a 0- to 15-point scale in which 15 points represented no pain. The active range of motion did not change over the time of the study. Forward flexion and abduction averaged 136 degrees; external rotation, 39 degrees; and internal rotation, 66 degrees. Glenohumeral osteoarthritis progressed, and the acromiohumeral distance decreased. The authors also found that the size of the tear increased and the grade of fatty infiltration increased as well. Patients with a 3-tendon tear showed more progression of osteoarthritis than those with a 2-tendon tear. Fifty percent of the rotator cuff tears that were graded as reparable at the time of the diagnosis became irreparable at the time of final follow-up. Thus, although the disease process likely progresses in patients with massive rotator cuff tears, the symptoms may remain tolerable with acceptable function. However, patients should be counseled that their tear may become irreparable over a period of time.

At this point in time, management of full-thickness symptomatic rotator cuff tears is controversial. Patients should be aware that these usually do not heal on their own, and many will progress over time. Patients should also know that the muscle will undergo changes over time, and these changes may make the outcome of repair less successful. However, many patients with a massive rotator cuff tear and progression will continue to do well.

CONCLUSION

Much of our knowledge about the natural history of full-thickness cuff tears comes indirectly from a limited number of studies. The lack of understanding regarding the natural history of cuff disease and the puzzling clinical entity of asymptomatic cuff tears begs a number of questions regarding the treatment of rotator cuff disease. Future studies will have to answer the following questions:

- What factors predict successful nonoperative treatment (converting a symptomatic, full-thickness tear to an asymptomatic state)?
- If this is successful, which individuals will experience progression of the tear with time, potentially making later surgical repair more difficult or even impossible?
- Is there an ideal interval during the natural history or along the continuum of disease to repair a full-thickness rotator cuff tear?

Determining the answers to these questions will help us understand the natural history of rotator cuff tears better and improve the clinical and functional outcomes of this large cohort of patients.

REFERENCES

1. Reilly P, Macleod I, Macfarlane R, Windley J, Emery RJ. Dead men and radiologists don't lie: a review of cadaveric and radiological studies of rotator cuff tear prevalence. *Ann R Coll Surg Engl.* 2006;88(2):116-121.
2. Sher JS, Uribe JW, Posada A, Murphy BJ, Zlatkin MB. Abnormal findings on magnetic resonance images of asymptomatic shoulders. *J Bone Joint Surg Am.* 1995;77(1):10-15.
3. Tempelhof S, Rupp S, Seil R. Age-related prevalence of rotator cuff tears in asymptomatic shoulders. *J Shoulder Elbow Surg.* 1999;8(4):296-299.

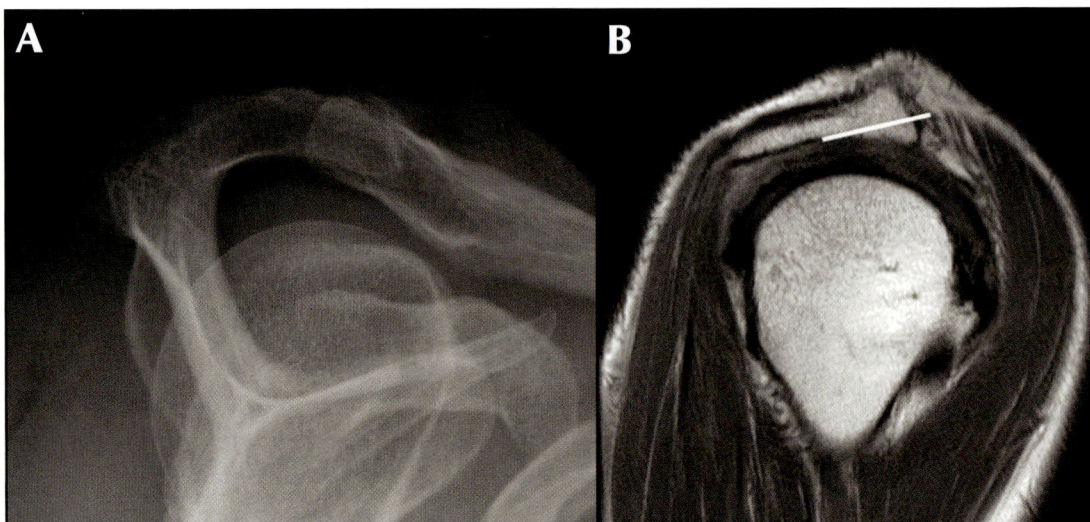

Figure 9-1. (A) A radiographic view of a type III or hooked acromion. A hooked acromion is thought to contribute to subacromial impingement. (B) A magnetic resonance image of sagittal T1 evaluation of the anterior acromion. The normal flat projection of the acromion is seen with the white line. The patient has a type III acromion.

DIAGNOSIS AND MANAGEMENT

History

Because the subacromial space is maximally narrowed during shoulder abduction and flexion, most patients suffering from impingement often complain of symptoms when performing overhead activities, such as combing hair, placing dishes into cupboards, and any other actions that place the arm between 70 and 100 degrees of elevation. Pain is generally localized to the anterolateral shoulder from the acromioclavicular (AC) joint to the lateral deltoid insertion. Night pain is another common presenting symptom, presumably because the humeral head is either directly compressed or positioned in abduction.

Impingement syndrome usually occurs in middle-aged individuals or in younger athletes, such as swimmers, or laborers who perform repetitive overhead activities. While the onset of symptoms is often insidious, some attribute a vigorous workout or activity as the inciting event. Weakness associated with a traumatic episode, such as a fall onto an outstretched arm, may herald an acute rotator cuff tear or a proximal humerus fracture and should prompt more aggressive imaging. Radicular pain, numbness, tingling, and neck pain should be specifically sought to eliminate a cervical etiology of symptoms.

A thorough review of any interventions, such as injections, medications, surgeries, and therapy, will help guide future treatments and avoid redundancies in care. The location of the injection (subacromial, AC, or glenohumeral) and its efficacy provide invaluable information on the source of pain and limit diagnoses to an anatomic region. Knowledge of the patient's previous procedures not only helps determine the diagnosis but may aid in prognosticating the success of future interventions.

Finally, the overall medical and social history must be determined to optimize treatment. Key historical highlights include presence of chronic or metastatic diseases, diabetes mellitus, tobacco use, hand dominance, occupation, and overall functional requirements.

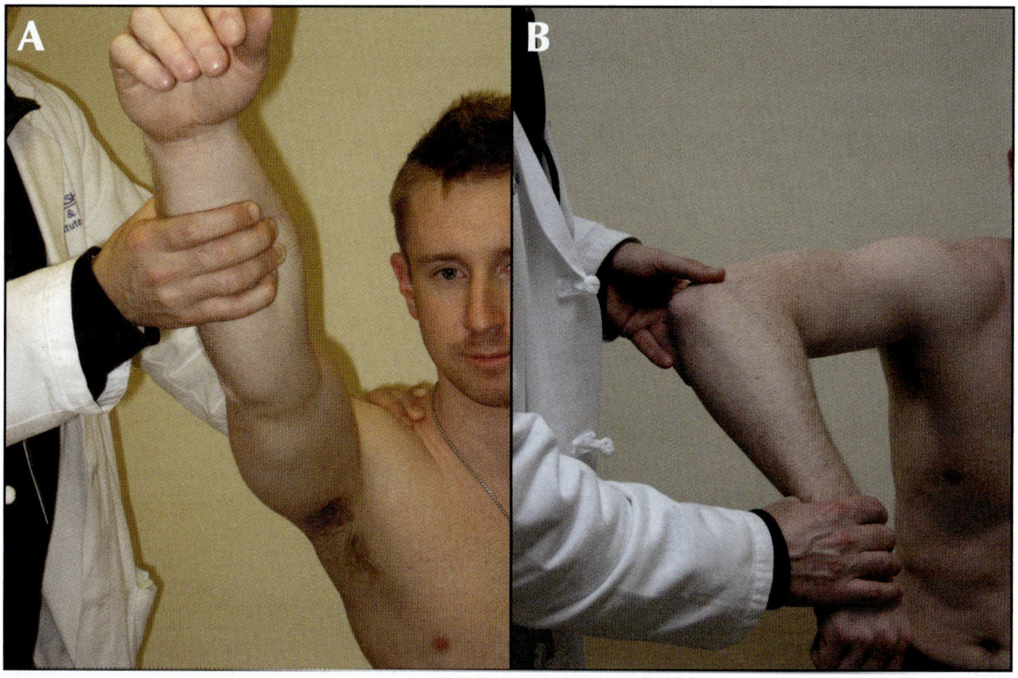

Figure 9-2. (A) Neer impingement sign. Passive forward elevation of the shoulder with the scapula manually stabilized elicits pain. (B) Hawkins impingement test. With the arm abducted 90 degrees in the plane of the scapula, the elbow flexed, and the scapula stabilized, internal rotation of the arm produces pain. *(continued)*

Physical Examination

Although much attention has been focused in the literature on the accuracy of specific maneuvers to diagnose various ailments, the physical examination should include the basics of any musculoskeletal evaluation: observation, palpation, range of motion, motor strength, sensation, and pulses. Patients suffering from subacromial impingement do not demonstrate a characteristic appearance but are generally reluctant to raise their arm overhead. Though often painful above 75 degrees of elevation, passive abduction and forward elevation are symmetric to the contralateral limb. Patients can have tenderness at the supraspinatus tendon insertion into the greater tuberosity or bicipital groove adjacent to the anterior acromion. If a tight posterior capsule is contributing to the pathologic state, internal rotation at 90 degrees of abduction will be limited compared to the contralateral limb.

Provocative tests, such as those described by Neer (Figure 9-2A), Hawkins (Figure 9-2B), and Yocum (Figure 9-2C), elicit symptoms by decreasing the available subacromial space. Published reports of the effectiveness of these tests in predicting pathology is highly variable (Table 9-1). Likewise, the Jobe test (Figure 9-2D) is classically used to predict rotator cuff tears but can be positive in some cases of impingement syndrome with a rotator cuff tear.

With the high variability in reported sensitivity and specificity with common physical exam tests, the Neer injection test remains the gold standard for diagnosing subacromial impingement.[10] The test is considered positive if pain is significantly reduced and provocative tests are painless moments after the injection of 10 mL of xylocaine anesthetic within the subacromial space.[11,12]

Imaging Findings

Radiographs are relatively inexpensive, form the framework for interpretation of other studies, and are useful to exclude many common shoulder ailments, such as fractures and/or dislocations,

Figure 9-2 (continued). (C) Yocum maneuver. With the hand on the contralateral shoulder, pain is experienced if the flexed elbow is directed superiorly without moving the shoulder. (D) Jobe test. With the arm abducted 90 degrees in the plane of the scapula and maximally internally rotated and with the elbow extended, pain occurs with resistance to a downward-directed force.

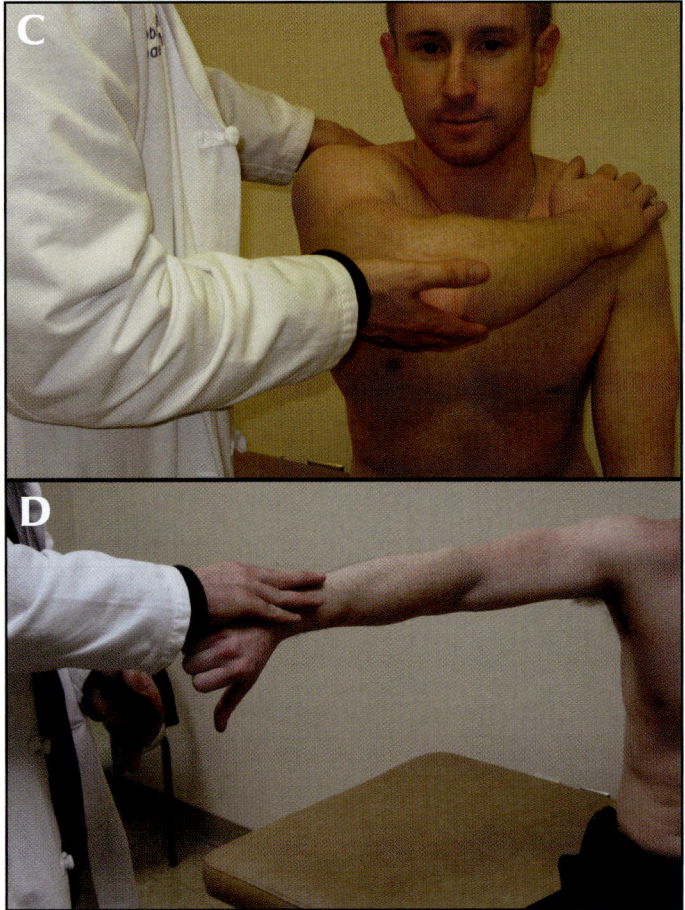

TABLE 9-1. SENSITIVITY AND SPECIFICITY OF COMMON TESTS OF IMPINGEMENT SYNDROME

TEST	TECHNIQUE	SENSITIVITY	SPECIFICITY
Neer	Pain with forced forward elevation	39 to 89	0 to 98
Hawkins	Pain with internal rotation at 90 degrees abduction	72 to 95	25 to 78
Yocum	Pain with elbow elevation and arm adducted	78 to 79	40
Jobe	Pain and/or weakness with forced abduction	52 to 74	30 to 53

Table created with data compiled from Hegedus et al,[18] Tennent et al,[19] Silva et al,[20] Leroux et al,[21] Calis et al,[22] MacDonald et al,[23] and Kelly et al.[24]

degenerative joint disease of both the glenohumeral and AC joints, and tumors. A standard impingement series consists of anteroposterior, axillary lateral, and supraspinatus outlet views, which help define the morphology of the anterior acromion.[13] Three distinct acromial morphologies have been described (Table 9-2)[14] and are often thought to contribute to subacromial impingement; however, the correlation between morphology type and rotator cuff pathology remains controversial.[15,16] Other radiographic findings that may be suggestive of subacromial impingement and/or rotator cuff pathology include os acromiale, acromial and/or greater tuberosity sclerosis, AC joint narrowing, and/or osteophytes.[17]

TABLE 9-2. ACROMIAL MORPHOLOGY

TYPE	APPEARANCE	% OF POPULATION
I	Flat	17%
II	Curved	43%
III	Hooked	40%

Table created with data compiled from Kelly SM, Brittle N, Allen GM. The value of physical tests for subacromial impingement syndrome: a study of diagnostic accuracy. *Clin Rehabil.* 2010;24(2):149-158.

TABLE 9-3. STAGES OF THE SUBACROMIAL IMPINGEMENT SYNDROME

STAGE	AGE GROUP	PATHOLOGY
Edema/hemorrhage	<25 years	Inflamed bursa
Fibrosis/tendinosis	25 to 40 years	Bursal fibrosis and rotator cuff tendinosis
Bone spurs/tears	>40 years	Rotator cuff tendon tear

Table created with data compiled from Neer CS 2nd. Impingement lesions. *Clin Orthop Relat Res.* 1983;173:70-77.

Magnetic resonance imaging (MRI) and ultrasonography are useful adjuncts to detect the presence of rotator cuff pathology. Bursal-sided tendinitis and/or partial-thickness tears that are detected using MRI may be suggestive of subacromial impingement. A disadvantage of MRI remains a high false-positive rate in older patients: up to 54% of asymptomatic patients over age 60 will demonstrate signal abnormality within the supraspinatus tendon consistent with a tear.[26] Unlike MRI, ultrasonography allows for dynamic assessment and may provide direct visualization of the impinging structures. However, ultrasonography is limited by the availability and skill of able radiologists trained to interpret these studies. Both studies should be correlated with history and physical examination. A failure to do so may subject patients to unnecessary and overly aggressive treatment because studies have demonstrated that rotator cuff abnormalities are detected in up to 35% of MRI[26] and 23% of ultrasonography[27] exams performed in asymptomatic shoulders.

Recently, single photon emission computerized tomography (SPECT) has been advocated to confirm the diagnosis and evaluate the prognosis after surgical intervention.[28] With this technique, increased uptake within the greater tuberosity preoperatively correlated with improved outcome postoperatively.[28] Further investigation is needed to determine if SPECT has clinical utility in the diagnosis of impingement.

NONOPERATIVE MANAGEMENT AND OUTCOMES

The subacromial impingement syndrome typically proceeds to rotator cuff tears in a series of stages (Table 9-3).[11] Staging of disease helps to formulate a plan to guide diagnostics and treatment. Because pathology is generally limited to inflammation of bursa in earlier stages, less aggressive diagnostic imaging and treatment strategies are chosen because most generally respond to conservative therapy, including rest, activity modification, nonsteroidal anti-inflammatory medications, and physical therapy. Conversely, more advanced stages may require interventions, such as injections and surgical procedures, to rectify more long-standing disease.

Most treatment protocols begin with physical therapy and a regimen to decrease inflammation, using either oral or injected medications. Physical therapy progresses from control of pain and restoration of motion to specific muscle strengthening to eventually sport- and work-specific activities.

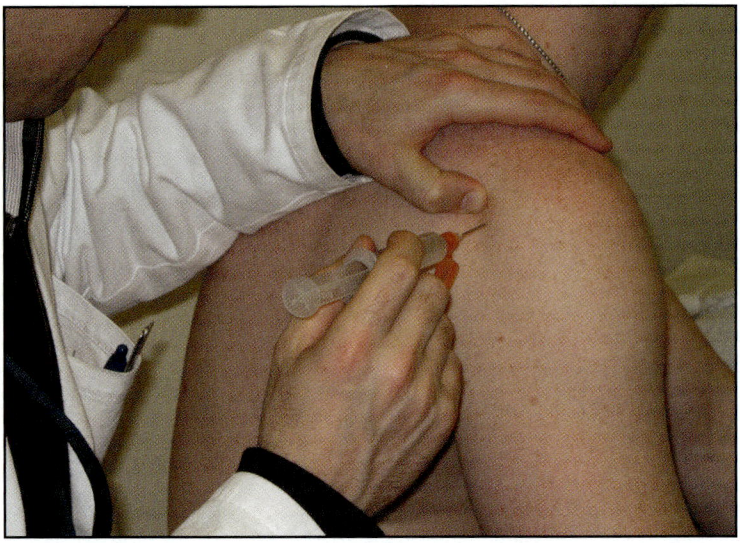

Figure 9-3. Subacromial steroid injection. The posterolateral border of the acromion is palpated. Using a sterile technique, a needle is inserted inferior and parallel to the acromion and directed anteriorly.

Often, a nonsteroidal anti-inflammatory medication or an injection into the subacromial space (Figure 9-3) is administered to alleviate pain to maximize therapy efforts. Presence of a rotator cuff tear greater than 1 cm, pretreatment symptoms lasting more than 1 year, and functional impairment portend a worse prognosis for successful nonoperative management.[29]

Several meta-analyses have confirmed the efficacy of physical therapy, especially when an exercise program is combined with joint mobilization.[30,31] In one cohort of patients originally scheduled for operative treatment of subacromial impingement, physical therapy reduced the need for operative intervention in more than 25%.[32] Evidence suggests that home exercise programs are as effective as therapist-led sessions.[30,33] Conversely, modalities such as ultrasound, extracorporeal shock wave therapy, and laser have minimal effectiveness in the treatment of subacromial impingement.[30,34-38]

The role of subacromial steroid injections remains controversial in treating those with subacromial impingement. While most report significant short-term relief following subacromial steroid injections,[39,40] studies addressing the long-term effectiveness of this treatment modality have produced conflicting results.[31,41] Combined with exercise, subacromial steroid injections offer significant improvements in pain and disability at 1- and 6-week intervals when compared to exercise alone; however, these differences fade at 12- and 24-week follow-up periods.[42]

SURGICAL MANAGEMENT

Indications for Surgery

Surgical intervention for isolated subacromial impingement should be reserved for anyone suspected of suffering from subacromial impingement and who has failed conservative methods for at least 6 months and has persistent functional impairment despite physical therapy and/or subacromial steroid injections.

Surgical procedures usually include débridement of the subacromial and/or subdeltoid bursae, release of the CA ligament, and/or flattening of the anterior acromion to decompress the subacromial space.

Positioning

While the subacromial space can be easily inspected with the patient placed into the lateral decubitus position, our preferred technique involves the beach chair position. Advantages of the beach chair position include anatomic positioning, ease in conversion to an open procedure, and mobility of the operative arm.[43]

Prior to configuring the operative bed into the beach chair position, several measures are taken to ensure the patient will be safely positioned once the head of the bed is raised. With the patient supine and centered from side to side on the operative table, he or she is brought cephalad such that his or her iliac crests are cephalad to most cephalad break in the operative table. If the patient's pelvis is equal to or caudad to this break, he or she will slouch or slide down the bed. The head is secured by head straps into the helmet and, depending upon the stability of the cervical spine, the neck may be further stabilized with a cervical collar. Sequential compressive devices are wrapped around and a pillow is placed behind each ankle and calf.

The bed is slowly configured into the beach chair position by raising the head of the bed, dropping the foot of the bed, and manipulating the bed into the Trendelenburg position to prevent the patient from sliding down the bed. The anesthesiologist should be informed prior to any positional change to maintain control of the airway and cervical spine and to monitor changes in blood pressure. Rapid drops in blood pressure can lead to decreased cerebral perfusion and cerebral ischemic injury.[44,45] To more closely monitor cerebral perfusion, cerebral oximetry has been suggested.[46,47]

Once prepped and draped, the extremity can be manipulated by an arm holder. Current models are pneumatic or hydraulic. The pneumatic devices are less expensive and are somewhat easier to manipulate, while hydraulic types offer more precise placement of the extremity. To work within the subacromial space, the arm is positioned in neutral rotation with inferior traction placed onto the arm to provide maximal space between the undersurface of the acromion and humeral head.

Surgical Technique

Acromioplasty is rarely an isolated procedure. Most often, the procedure is associated with another procedure, such as rotator cuff repair, biceps tenotomy/tenodesis, and/or distal clavicle excision. Therefore, in addition to performing an acromioplasty, careful attention should be directed at recognizing pathology and providing the appropriate treatment.

Once the adequate positioning has been obtained, a posterior portal is created. The typical location of the posterior portal is 1 cm medial and 2 cm inferior to the posterolateral corner of the acromion. After the glenohumeral joint has been visualized and all intra-articular pathology addressed, the arthroscope is directed into the subacromial space. The trocar is placed just inferior to the undersurface of the acromion and is directed from the posterior portal to the anterolateral corner of the acromion. The trocar is gently swept medially. Passage of the arthroscope in this sequence increases the likelihood that the arthroscope is above the subacromial bursal tissue. A lateral portal is created 2 cm distal to the acromion's lateral border and is centered between the anterior and posterior borders of the acromion. A suction shaver device, such as a full radius resector, and radiofrequency ablation device are used to débride any inflamed bursal tissue.

The bursectomy proceeds in a step-wise fashion. First, the soft tissue adherent to the undersurface of the acromion is removed using a radiofrequency ablation device. Removal of this tissue assists in defining the anatomical relationships within the subacromial space. Second, the bursal tissue is débrided from the lateral subdeltoid region so that the undersurface of the acromion and the rotator cuff tendon are visualized as separate entities. Bursal tissue can be differentiated from the underlying rotator cuff tendon by the following: bursal tissue extends to the deltoid, and bursal tissue is readily consumed by the suction-shaver device with the blade directed 90 degrees away from the underlying tissue and using a sweeping motion. Once the bursal tissue is removed from the lateral subdeltoid region, the arthroscope is switched to the lateral portal. Débridement of the bursal tissue from the anterior and posterior subdeltoid and medial subacromial regions can be readily performed from this view. These regions are extremely vascularized and often result in brisk hemorrhaging. Therefore, an electrocautery ablation device should be readily available when débriding bursal tissue from these areas. To avoid thermal injury from the electrocautery device, the surgeon should ensure that there is adequate fluid flow, the electrocautery device is set at the lowest energy to produce the desired effect, and the heating probe is continuously moved (Figure 9-4A).[47]

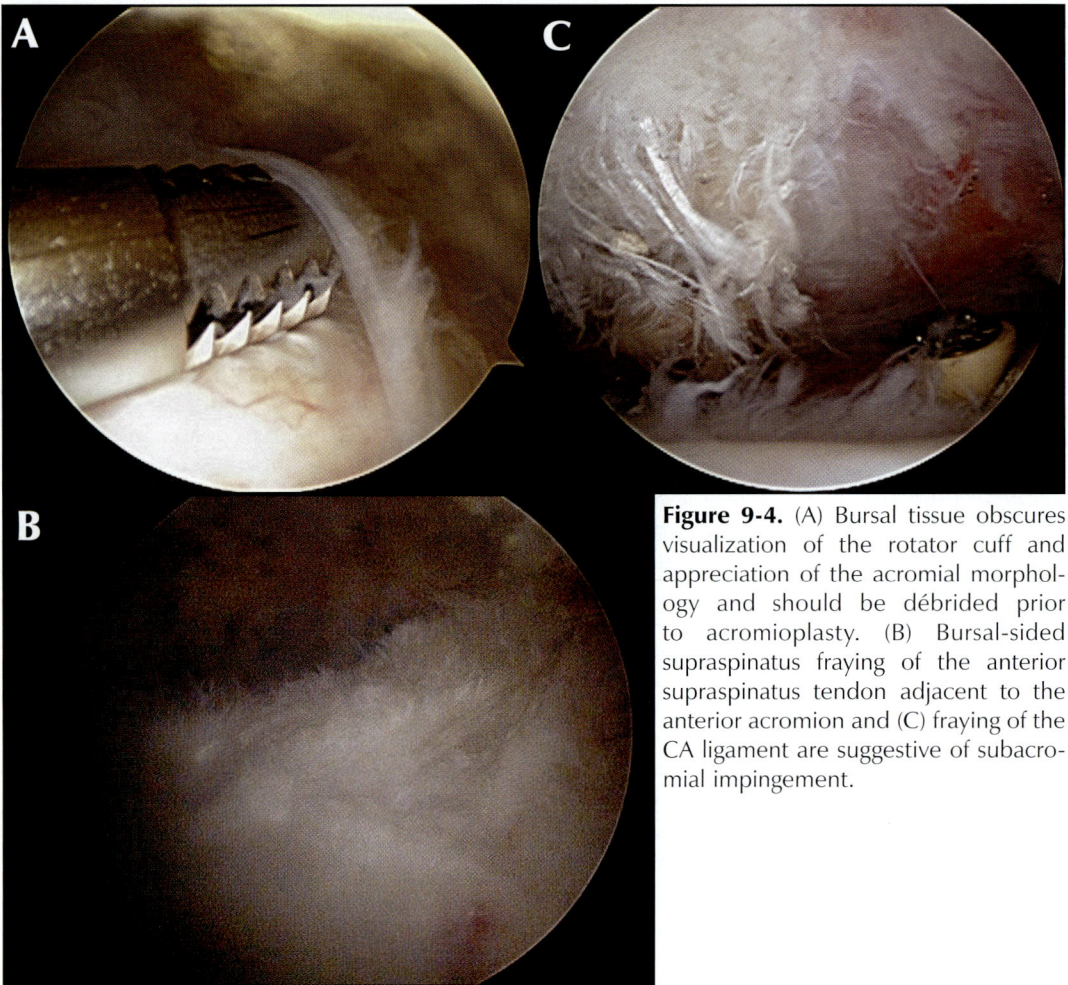

Figure 9-4. (A) Bursal tissue obscures visualization of the rotator cuff and appreciation of the acromial morphology and should be débrided prior to acromioplasty. (B) Bursal-sided supraspinatus fraying of the anterior supraspinatus tendon adjacent to the anterior acromion and (C) fraying of the CA ligament are suggestive of subacromial impingement.

Following the bursectomy, key anatomic structures are inspected, searching for signs of pathologic impingement. With the arthroscope in the lateral portal, supraspinatus and infraspinatus tendons are visualized. The arm can be externally rotated to improve visualization of the supraspinatus tendon's leading edge, which is the most common site of tendon injury. A partial-thickness tear or fraying of the bursal side of the supraspinatus tendon adjacent to the anterior edge of the acromion offers objective evidence of subacromial impingement (Figure 9-4B). Further confirmation of subacromial impingement is fraying of the CA ligament, which is most easily viewed with the arthroscope in the posterior portal (Figure 9-4C).

While the anterior acromion, especially a type II or III variant, is generally assumed to be the primary source of subacromial impingement, the coracohumeral ligament and distal clavicle are other potential contributors to subacromial impingement. The morphology of the acromion is most readily appreciated viewing from the lateral portal. Often, a straight object, such as a probe or Wissinger rod, is helpful to provide orientation. If a distal clavicular osteophyte is thought to be a contributor to impingement, the undersurface of the distal clavicle should be débrided to define the morphology of the distal clavicle. The distal clavicle should only be exposed if thought to contribute to the impingement, as coplaning of the distal clavicle has been associated with increasing laxity within the AC joint.[48]

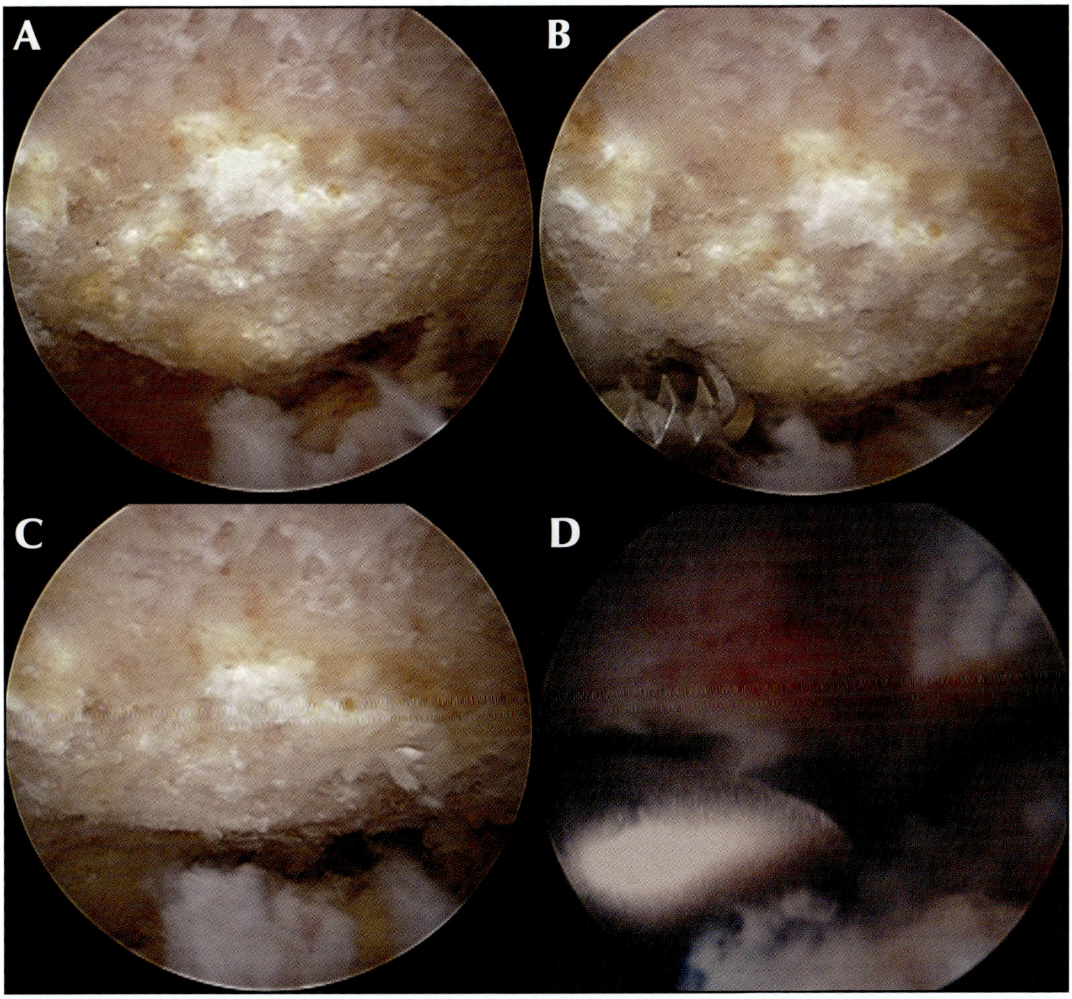

Figure 9-5. (A) With the arthroscope in the posterior viewing portal, the CA ligament is detached to fully expose the anterior acromion. (B) Anterior acromioplasty proceeds from lateral to medial using an arthroscopic bur. (C) Anterior acromion resection is completed once the normal contour of the acromion is restored and approximately 4 mm of insertional tissue exposed. (D) With the arthroscope in the lateral portal, final resection is performed to ensure a flattened undersurface of the acromion.

Once the decision to perform an acromioplasty has been made, the CA ligament is detached from its acromial insertion. Release of the CA ligament decreases subacromial pressure by 72%.[4] The CA ligament is released from lateral to medial using an electrocautery device and viewing from the posterior portal. Though resection of the CA ligament has been associated with anterolateral escape of the humeral head, evidence suggests that the CA ligament regrows within 3 years.[49,50]

The anterior edge of the acromion should be defined prior to acromioplasty. The anterior insertional fibers of the deltoid are clearly visualized from the posterior portal (Figure 9-5A). An arthroscopic bur is passed through the lateral portal and, from lateral to medial, progressively removes the anterior lip of the acromion (Figure 9-5B). Resection proceeds until approximately 4 mm of "white" insertional tissue is appreciated (Figure 9-5C). The arthroscope is switched into the lateral portal, and acromial morphology is appreciated. Because the majority of the resection involved the anterior acromion, the middle section of the acromion can be prominent. Using a cutting block technique,[51] the bur is passed from the posterior portal and is used to contour the undersurface of the acromion to a flattened surface (Figure 9-5D). The adequacy of the acromioplasty is confirmed by alternating between the posterior and lateral viewing portals. A satisfactory acromioplasty is confirmed by placing a Wissinger rod through the posterior portal and comparing its straightness to the recontoured acromion. The two should be parallel.

If a distal clavicular osteophyte is a suspected contributor to impingement of the supraspinatus, the undersurface of distal clavicular is defined using an electrocautery ablation device. The distal clavicular osteophyte can be easily resected using a motorized arthroscopic bur.

Postoperative Management and Rehabilitation

In the early postoperative period, patients are instructed to wear a sling as tolerated and to begin a series of simple exercises, including table slides, wall climbs, and Codman exercises. At the 2-week postoperative visit, sutures are removed, and range of motion is examined. If range of motion has failed to reach 90 degrees of abduction and forward elevation and 60 degrees of external rotation, a course of supervised physical therapy is initiated. Nonetheless, no clear benefit with regard to functional limitations and duration of disability exists between a supervised exercise program and a self-directed protocol.[52]

Potential Complications

The majority of complications after acromioplasty stem from overaggressive resection of the acromion. While arthroscopic acromioplasty has gained wide acceptance due to assumed preservation of the anterior deltoid attachment, multiple studies have confirmed that resection of the anterior acromion may compromise the deltoid origin.[53] Cadaveric studies have demonstrated that a 4.0-mm acromioplasty releases 41% to 56% of the deltoid insertional fibers, while resections of 5.5 mm and greater result in detachments of 69% to 77% of the tendinous insertion.[53,54] However, other studies have suggested that the anterior deltoid fibers, which are frequently detached during arthroscopic acromioplasty, may not be as clinically important as the superior and anterosuperior deltoid fibers, which are usually preserved during arthroscopic acromioplasty.[55] Although the functional consequence of partial deltoid release has not been clearly determined, complete deltoid origin disruption has been associated with poor function.[56]

The deltoid origin is not the only structure affected by acromioplasty: the mechanical properties of the acromion, clavicle, and AC joint are altered by acromioplasty. Overenthusiastic acromioplasty can weaken the acromion and lead to fracture, which can be problematic to treat due to excessive deltoid muscle forces coupled with poor bone stock. Release of the inferior AC joint capsule during anterior acromioplasty has been correlated with AC joint instability.[48,57,58] This biomechanical alteration may result in distal clavicle osteolysis or "vanishing distal clavicle."[59]

Release of the CA ligament causes a significant increase in anterosuperior humeral head migration, which is amplified by acromioplasty.[60] Some studies suggest that this effect can be mitigated to a variable degree with muscle strengthening simulations and/or regrowth of the CA ligament, which takes at least 3 years to return to normal strength.[61] Nonetheless, anterosuperior migration is a significant concern following acromioplasty, especially when performed in those with a massive rotator cuff tear.

While most of the complications following acromioplasty are the result of overzealous resection of the acromion and associated structures, inadequate decompression can lead to recurrent impingement symptoms. The persistence of symptoms is usually attributed to the formation of thick, fibrous adhesions and/or inadequate or uneven resection.[62] Less frequently, severe heterotopic ossification and spur reformation can cause recurrent impingement symptoms.[63,64]

TABLE 9-4. OUTCOMES FOLLOWING ARTHROSCOPIC ACROMIOPLASTY

AUTHOR	YEAR	TOTAL PTS	MEAN F/U	CONCLUSIONS
Henkus et al[9]	2009	30	31 mo	18.5-point increase in constant score 3.0 decrease in visual analogue scale for pain
Ketola et al[8]	2009	70	24 mo	3.9 decrease in visual analogue scale for pain 65% pain-free
Odenbring et al[65]	2008	31	13 yrs	77% excellent or good outcomes 13-point increase in UCLA
Lim et al[66]	2007	42	15 mo	83% excellent or good outcomes
Stephens et al[67]	1998	82	8 yrs	81% excellent to good outcomes 15% required additional procedure for pain
Roye et al[68]	1995	88	41 mo	93% satisfied

TABLE 9-5. OUTCOMES FOLLOWING OPEN ACROMIOPLASTY

AUTHOR	YEAR	TOTAL PTS.	MEAN F/U	CONCLUSIONS
Chin et al[69]	2007	32	25 yrs	88% satisfied
Hyvonen et al[70]	1998	93	9 yrs	72% excellent and good outcomes
Skoff[71]	1995	25	24 mo	80% very satisfied; none dissatisfied

Outcomes

Many studies have published the efficacy of anterior acromioplasty for the treatment of subacromial impingement. Collectively, objective and subjective success rates approach 82% and 90%, respectively,[72] with satisfaction maintained at up to 25 years following the procedure.[69] There is no definite relationship between amount of resection and clinical outcome.[66] Despite the high rates of sustained patient satisfaction, the role of acromioplasty in halting the progression of rotator cuff disease remains controversial.[69,70,73-75]

While the current trend has shifted from open to arthroscopic acromioplasty, multiple studies have demonstrated no statistically significant differences in ultimate clinical outcomes and complication rates between the 2 techniques.[72,76-78] Selected results for arthroscopic and open acromioplasty are outlined in Tables 9-4 and 9-5. Arthroscopic acromioplasty does appear to hasten recovery. Those undergoing arthroscopic acromioplasty have a decreased length of hospital stay and time to return to work and a more accelerated postoperative rehabilitation.[72,77,79] Therefore, due to prolonged recovery and the potential morbidity associated with deltoid detachment during open acromioplasty and improved visualization of adjacent structures using arthroscopy, open acromioplasty is generally reserved for revision cases of persistent and/or recurrent impingement.

Recently, several prospective, randomized studies have questioned the role of acromioplasty in the treatment of subacromial impingement.[8,9] A study by Henkus and colleagues found no difference in pain and functional outcome between arthroscopic acromioplasty with bursectomy versus bursectomy alone.[9] Ketola and colleagues reported that arthroscopic acromioplasty conferred no clinically important advantages in subjective outcome and cost at 2 years compared to a structured physical therapy program.[8] In fact, the type of acromion and severity of symptoms appear to have a greater influence on ultimate outcome following treatment than does the presence of an acromioplasty.[9]

Pearls and Pitfalls

- Common physical examination tests are highly variable and are generally more sensitive than specific.
- The Neer injection test is the gold standard for diagnosing subacromial impingement.
- At the 2-year follow-up, physical therapy produces equivalent outcomes to acromioplasty. Therefore, an extensive course of nonoperative treatment, including exercise and/or subacromial injection, should be attempted prior to acromioplasty.
- Arthroscopic and open acromioplasty produce equivalent outcomes.
- Due to improved visualization of surrounding structures and perceived lower risk of deltoid injury, an arthroscopic acromioplasty is preferred over an open acromioplasty.
- Overaggressive acromioplasty can result in acromial fracture or detachment of the anterior fibers of the deltoid.

References

1.   Neer CS 2nd. Anterior acromioplasty for the chronic impingement syndrome in the shoulder: a preliminary report. *J Bone Joint Surg Am.* 1972;54(1):41-50.
2.   Nordt WE 3rd, Garretson RB 3rd, Plotkin E. The measurement of subacromial contact pressure in patients with impingement syndrome. *Arthroscopy.* 1999;15(2):121-125.
3.   Payne LZ, Deng XH, Craig EV, Torzilli PA, Warren RF. The combined dynamic and static contributions to subacromial impingement. A biomechanical analysis. *Am J Sports Med.* 1997;25(6):801-808.
4.   Denard PJ, Bahney TJ, Kirby SB, Orfaly RM. Contact pressure and glenohumeral translation following subacromial decompression: how much is enough? *Orthopedics.* 2010;33(11):805.
5.   Altchek DW, Carson EW. Arthroscopic acromioplasty. Current status. *Orthop Clin North Am.* 1997;28(2):157-168.
6.   Vitale MA, Arons RR, Hurwitz S, Ahmad CS, Levine WN. The rising incidence of acromioplasty. *J Bone Joint Surg Am.* 2010;92(9):1842-1850.
7.   Yu E, Cil A, Harmsen WS, Schleck C, Sperling JW, Cofield RH. Arthroscopy and the dramatic increase in frequency of anterior acromioplasty from 1980 to 2005: an epidemiologic study. *Arthroscopy.* 2010;26(9 Suppl):S142-S147.
8.   Ketola S, Lehtinen J, Arnala I, et al. Does arthroscopic acromioplasty provide any additional value in the treatment of shoulder impingement syndrome? A two-year randomised controlled trial. *J Bone Joint Surg Br.* 2009;91(10):1326-1334.
9.   Henkus HE, de Witte PB, Nelissen RG, Brand R, van Arkel ER. Bursectomy compared with acromioplasty in the management of subacromial impingement syndrome: a prospective randomised study. *J Bone Joint Surg Br.* 2009;91(4):504-510.
10.   Cohen RB, Williams GR Jr. Impingement syndrome and rotator cuff disease as repetitive motion disorders. *Clin Orthop Relat Res.* 1998;351:95-101.
11.   Neer CS 2nd. Impingement lesions. *Clin Orthop Relat Res.* 1983;173:70-77.
12.   Gartsman GM. Arthroscopic management of rotator cuff disease. *J Am Acad Orthop Surg.* 1998;6(4):259-266.
13.   Kitay GS, Iannotti JP, Williams GR, Haygood T, Kneeland BJ, Berlin J. Roentgenographic assessment of acromial morphologic condition in rotator cuff impingement syndrome. *J Shoulder Elbow Surg.* 1995;4(6):441-448.
14.   Bigliani DS, April EW. The morphology of the acromion and its relationship to rotator cuff tears. *Orthop Trans.* 1986;10:228.
15.   Hyvonen P, Paivansalo M, Lehtiniemi H, Leppilahti J, Jalovaara P. Supraspinatus outlet view in the diagnosis of stages II and III impingement syndrome. *Acta Radiol.* 2001;42(5):441-446.
16.   Lee SB, Itoi E, O'Driscoll SW, An KN. Contact geometry at the undersurface of the acromion with and without a rotator cuff tear. *Arthroscopy.* 2001;17(4):365-372.
17.   Tytherleigh-Strong G, Hirahara A, Miniaci A. Rotator cuff disease. *Curr Opin Rheumatol.* 2001;13(2):135-145.
18.   Hegedus EJ, Goode A, Campbell S, et al. Physical examination tests of the shoulder: a systematic review with meta-analysis of individual tests. *Br J Sports Med.* 2008;42(2):80-92; discussion 92.
19.   Tennent TD, Beach WR, Meyers JF. A review of the special tests associated with shoulder examination. Part I: the rotator cuff tests. *Am J Sports Med.* 2003;31(1):154-160.
20.   Silva L, Andreu JL, Munoz P, et al. Accuracy of physical examination in subacromial impingement syndrome. *Rheumatology (Oxford).* 2008;47(5):679-683.
21.   Leroux JL, Thomas E, Bonnel F, Blotman F. Diagnostic value of clinical tests for shoulder impingement syndrome. *Rev Rhum Engl Ed.* 1995;62(6):423-428.
22.   Calis M, Akgun K, Birtane M, Karacan I, Calis H, Tuzun F. Diagnostic values of clinical diagnostic tests in subacromial impingement syndrome. *Ann Rheum Dis.* 2000;59(1):44-47.

23. MacDonald PB, Clark P, Sutherland K. An analysis of the diagnostic accuracy of the Hawkins and Neer subacromial impingement signs. *J Shoulder Elbow Surg.* 2000;9(4):299-301.

24. Kelly SM, Brittle N, Allen GM. The value of physical tests for subacromial impingement syndrome: a study of diagnostic accuracy. *Clin Rehabil.* 2010;24(2):149-158.

25. Bigliani LU, Levine WN. Subacromial impingement syndrome. *J Bone Joint Surg Am.* 1997;79(12):1854-1868.

26. Sher JS, Uribe JW, Posada A, Murphy BJ, Zlatkin MB. Abnormal findings on magnetic resonance images of asymptomatic shoulders. *J Bone Joint Surg Am.* 1995;77(1):10-15.

27. Tempelhof S, Rupp S, Seil R. Age-related prevalence of rotator cuff tears in asymptomatic shoulders. *J Shoulder Elbow Surg.* 1999;8(4):296-299.

28. Park JY, Park SG, Keum JS, Oh JH, Park JS. The diagnosis and prognosis of impingement syndrome in the shoulder using quantitative SPECT assessment: a prospective study of 73 patients and 24 volunteers. *Clin Orthop Surg.* 2009;1(4):194-200.

29. Bartolozzi A, Andreychik D, Ahmad S. Determinants of outcome in the treatment of rotator cuff disease. *Clin Orthop Relat Res.* 1994;308:90-97.

30. Kromer TO, Tautenhahn UG, de Bie RA, Staal JB, Bastiaenen CH. Effects of physiotherapy in patients with shoulder impingement syndrome: a systematic review of the literature. *J Rehabil Med.* 2009;41(11):870-880.

31. Faber E, Kuiper JI, Burdorf A, Miedema HS, Verhaar JA. Treatment of impingement syndrome: a systematic review of the effects on functional limitations and return to work. *J Occup Rehabil.* 2006;16(1):7-25.

32. Dickens VA, Bhamra MS. Role of physiotherapy in the treatment of subacromial impingement syndrome: a prospective study. *Physiotherapy.* 2005;91(3):159-164.

33. Walther M, Werner A, Stahlschmidt T, Woelfel R, Gohlke F. The subacromial impingement syndrome of the shoulder treated by conventional physiotherapy, self-training, and a shoulder brace: results of a prospective, randomized study. *J Shoulder Elbow Surg.* 2004;13(4):417-423.

34. Nykanen M. Pulsed ultrasound treatment of the painful shoulder a randomized, double-blind, placebo-controlled study. *Scand J Rehabil Med.* 1995;27(2):105-108.

35. Schmitt J, Tosch A, Hunerkopf M, Haake M. [Extracorporeal shockwave therapy (ESWT) as therapeutic option in supraspinatus tendon syndrome? One year results of a placebo controlled study]. *Orthopade.* 2002;31(7):652-657.

36. Speed CA, Richards C, Nichols D, et al. Extracorporeal shock-wave therapy for tendonitis of the rotator cuff. A double-blind, randomised, controlled trial. *J Bone Joint Surg Br.* 2002;84(4):509-512.

37. Downing DS, Weinstein A. Ultrasound therapy of subacromial bursitis. A double blind trial. *Phys Ther.* 1986;66(2):194-199.

38. Vecchio PC, Hazleman BL, King RH. A double-blind trial comparing subacromial methylprednisolone and lignocaine in acute rotator cuff tendinitis. *Br J Rheumatol.* 1993;32(8):743-745.

39. Karthikeyan S, Kwong HT, Upadhyay PK, Parsons N, Drew SJ, Griffin D. A double-blind randomised controlled study comparing subacromial injection of tenoxicam or methylprednisolone in patients with subacromial impingement. *J Bone Joint Surg Br.* 2010;92(1):77-82.

40. Blair B, Rokito AS, Cuomo F, Jarolem K, Zuckerman JD. Efficacy of injections of corticosteroids for subacromial impingement syndrome. *J Bone Joint Surg Am.* 1996;78(11):1685-1689.

41. Alvarez-Nemegyei J, Canoso JJ. Evidence-based soft tissue rheumatology. Part I: subacromial impingement syndrome. *J Clin Rheumatol.* 2003;9(3):193-199.

42. Crawshaw DP, Helliwell PS, Hensor EM, Hay EM, Aldous SJ, Conaghan PG. Exercise therapy after corticosteroid injection for moderate to severe shoulder pain: large pragmatic randomised trial. *BMJ.* 2010;340:c3037.

43. Peruto CM, Ciccotti MG, Cohen SB. Shoulder arthroscopy positioning: lateral decubitus versus beach chair. *Arthroscopy.* 2009;25(8):891-896.

44. Pohl A, Cullen DJ. Cerebral ischemia during shoulder surgery in the upright position: a case series. *J Clin Anesth.* 2005;17(6):463-469.

45. Dippmann C, Winge S, Nielsen HB. Severe cerebral desaturation during shoulder arthroscopy in the beach-chair position. *Arthroscopy.* 2010;26(9 Suppl):S148-S150.

46. Fischer GW, Torrillo TM, Weiner MM, Rosenblatt MA. The use of cerebral oximetry as a monitor of the adequacy of cerebral perfusion in a patient undergoing shoulder surgery in the beach chair position. *Pain Pract.* 2009;9(4):304-307.

47. Gryler EC, Greis PE, Burks RT, West J. Axillary nerve temperatures during radiofrequency capsulorrhaphy of the shoulder. *Arthroscopy.* 2001;17(6):567-572.

48. Edwards SG. Acromioclavicular stability: a biomechanical comparison of acromioplasty to acromioplasty with coplaning of the distal clavicle. *Arthroscopy.* 2003;19(10):1079-1084.

49. Hansen U, Levy O, Even T, Copeland SA. Mechanical properties of regenerated coracoacromial ligament after subacromial decompression. *J Shoulder Elbow Surg.* 2004;13(1):51-56.

50. Levy O, Copeland SA. Regeneration of the coracoacromial ligament after acromioplasty and arthroscopic subacromial decompression. *J Shoulder Elbow Surg.* 2001;10(4):317-320.

51. Sampson TG, Nisbet JK, Glick JM. Precision acromioplasty in arthroscopic subacromial decompression of the shoulder. *Arthroscopy.* 1991;7(3):301-307.

52. Andersen NH, Johannsen HV, Sneppen O. Self-training versus physiotherapist-supervised rehabilitation of the shoulder in patients treated with arthroscopic subacromial decompression: a clinical randomized study. *J Shoulder Elbow Surg.* 1999;8(2):99-101.

53. Torpey BM, Ikeda K, Weng M, van der Heeden D, Chao EY, McFarland EG. The deltoid muscle origin. Histologic characteristics and effects of subacromial decompression. *Am J Sports Med.* 1998;26(3):379-383.

54. Green A, Griggs S, Labrador D. Anterior acromial anatomy: relevance to arthroscopic acromioplasty. *Arthroscopy.* 2004;20(10):1050-1054.

55. Kumar VP, Satku K, Liu J, Shen Y. The anatomy of the anterior origin of the deltoid. *J Bone Joint Surg Br.* 1997;79(4):680-683.

56. Sher JS, Iannotti JP, Warner JJ, Groff Y, Williams GR. Surgical treatment of postoperative deltoid origin disruption. *Clin Orthop Relat Res.* 1997;343:93-98.

57. Deshmukh AV, Perlmutter GS, Zilberfarb JL, Wilson DR. Effect of subacromial decompression on laxity of the acromioclavicular joint: biomechanical testing in a cadaveric model. *J Shoulder Elbow Surg.* 2004;13(3):338-343.

58. Kuster MS, Hales PF, Davis SJ. The effects of arthroscopic acromioplasty on the acromioclavicular joint. *J Shoulder Elbow Surg.* 1998;7(2):140-143.

59. Pouliart N, Casteleyn PP. Vanishing distal clavicle after arthroscopic acromioplasty. *Arthroscopy.* 2000;16(8):855-857.

60. Su WR, Budoff JE, Luo ZP. The effect of coracoacromial ligament excision and acromioplasty on superior and anterosuperior glenohumeral stability. *Arthroscopy.* 2009;25(1):13-18.

61. Hunt JL, Moore RJ, Krishnan J. The fate of the coracoacromial ligament in arthroscopic acromioplasty: an anatomical study. *J Shoulder Elbow Surg.* 2000;9(6):491-494.

62. Connor PM, Yamaguchi K, Pollock RG, Flatow EL, Bigliani LU. Comparison of arthroscopic and open revision decompression for failed anterior acromioplasty. *Orthopedics.* 2000;23(6):549-554.

63. Boynton MD, Enders TJ. Severe heterotopic ossification after arthroscopic acromioplasty: a case report. *J Shoulder Elbow Surg.* 1999;8(5):495-497.

64. Anderson K, Bowen MK. Spur reformation after arthroscopic acromioplasty. *Arthroscopy.* 1999;15(7):788-791.

65. Odenbring S, Wagner P, Atroshi I. Long-term outcomes of arthroscopic acromioplasty for chronic shoulder impingement syndrome: a prospective cohort study with a minimum of 12 years' follow-up. *Arthroscopy.* 2008;24(10):1092-1098.

66. Lim KK, Chang HC, Tan JL, Chan BK. Arthroscopic subacromial decompression for stage-II impingement. *J Orthop Surg (Hong Kong).* 2007;15(2):197-200.

67. Stephens SR, Warren RF, Payne LZ, Wickiewicz TL, Altchek DW. Arthroscopic acromioplasty: a 6- to 10-year follow-up. *Arthroscopy.* 1998;14(4):382-388.

68. Roye RP, Grana WA, Yates CK. Arthroscopic subacromial decompression: two- to seven-year follow-up. *Arthroscopy.* 1995;11(3):301-306.

69. Chin PY, Sperling JW, Cofield RH, Stuart MJ, Crownhart BS. Anterior acromioplasty for the shoulder impingement syndrome: long-term outcome. *J Shoulder Elbow Surg.* 2007;16(6):697-700.

70. Hyvonen P, Lohi S, Jalovaara P. Open acromioplasty does not prevent the progression of an impingement syndrome to a tear. Nine-year follow-up of 96 cases. *J Bone Joint Surg Br.* 1998;80(5):813-816.

71. Skoff HD. Conservative open acromioplasty. *J Bone Joint Surg Br.* 1995;77(6):933-936.

72. Checroun AJ, Dennis MG, Zuckerman JD. Open versus arthroscopic decompression for subacromial impingement. A comprehensive review of the literature from the last 25 years. *Bull Hosp Jt Dis.* 1998;57(3):145-151.

73. Kartus J, Kartus C, Rostgard-Christensen L, Sernert N, Read J, Perko M. Long-term clinical and ultrasound evaluation after arthroscopic acromioplasty in patients with partial rotator cuff tears. *Arthroscopy.* 2006;22(1):44-49.

74. Liem D, Alci S, Dedy N, Steinbeck J, Marquardt B, Mollenhoff G. Clinical and structural results of partial supraspinatus tears treated by subacromial decompression without repair. *Knee Surg Sports Traumatol Arthrosc.* 2008;16(10):967-972.

75. Cordasco FA, Backer M, Craig EV, Klein D, Warren RF. The partial-thickness rotator cuff tear: is acromioplasty without repair sufficient? *Am J Sports Med.* 2002;30(2):257-260.

76. Spangehl MJ, Hawkins RH, McCormack RG, Loomer RL. Arthroscopic versus open acromioplasty: a prospective, randomized, blinded study. *J Shoulder Elbow Surg.* 2002;11(2):101-107.

77. Davis AD, Kakar S, Moros C, Kaye EK, Schepsis AA, Voloshin I. Arthroscopic versus open acromioplasty: a meta-analysis. *Am J Sports Med.* 2010;38(3):613-618.

78. Barfield LC, Kuhn JE. Arthroscopic versus open acromioplasty: a systematic review. *Clin Orthop Relat Res.* 2007;455:64-71.

79. Kinnard P, Van Hoef K, Major D, Lirette R. Comparison between open and arthroscopic acromioplasties: evaluation of absenteeism. *Can J Surg.* 1996;39(1):21-23.

Please see video on the accompanying Web site at http://www.slackbooks.com/rotatorcuffvideos

CHAPTER 10

PARTIAL-THICKNESS TEARS OF THE ROTATOR CUFF

Richard K. N. Ryu, MD and William H. Dunbar V, MD

The accurate diagnosis and treatment of the partial-thickness rotator cuff tear has improved as diagnostic and treatment options have become more sophisticated. During the past decade, we have benefited from a more thorough understanding of the anatomy, pathoanatomy, natural history, and treatment strategies for partial rotator cuff tears. As noted with full-thickness tears, which are well documented to be asymptomatic in a percentage of the population, not all partial-thickness rotator cuff tears require treatment. A rigorous understanding of the histopathology, clinical evaluation, diagnostic imaging choices, and treatment algorithm of the partial-thickness tear is prudent if one is to appropriately manage this challenging clinical entity.

INCIDENCE OF PARTIAL-THICKNESS CUFF TEARS

Since the classic study by Codman[1] in 1934 in which he observed rotator cuff tears in one-third of cadaveric specimens, several studies have more accurately depicted the incidence of partial-thickness rotator cuff tears. The incidence of partial rotator cuff tears has been strongly correlated with advancing age. Lohr and Uhthoff[2] reported that approximately 90 of 306 shoulders studied post mortem demonstrated a partial-thickness cuff tear. Sher and colleagues[3] imaged 2 groups: those aged 19 to 39 years and those older than 60 years of age. As anticipated, the incidence of rotator cuff pathology increased with age in these asymptomatic shoulders with a 4% incidence of partial-thickness tears in the younger age group and a 26% incidence in the asymptomatic over-60-years age group. In 1987, Fukuda et al[4] reported a 13% incidence of partial-thickness rotator cuff tears, subdivided into articular-sided (27%), bursal-sided (18%), and intratendinous (55%) categories, all in older specimens. Although the supraspinatus is the most common tendon affected,[5] Sakurai and colleagues described partial tears of the subscapularis in 17 of 46 cadaveric specimens.[6]

Throughout the literature, the ratio of articular-sided to bursal-sided partial-thickness tears consistently approaches a ratio of greater than 2:1. Nakajima et al's histologic and biomechanical

Ma CB, Feeley BT, eds.
*Basic Principles and Operative Management
of the Rotator Cuff (pp 141-160)*
© 2012 SLACK Incorporated

study of the supraspinatus tendon established that the articular surface of the rotator cuff demonstrates half the strength in a test of stress to failure compared to the bursal surface.[7] This was further supported by Mazzocca and colleagues, who noted increasing articular-sided strain within the remaining tendon in tears greater than 25% with no significant difference noted on the bursal side.[8,9] This again lends credence to the argument that many tears initiate on the articular side and propagate to the bursal surface.[10-12] Noteworthy were the additional findings of Mazzocca and colleagues who determined that repair of articular-sided partial-thickness cuff tears of greater than 25% returned the strain patterns to a near-normal state.

Although several studies have delineated a significant incidence of post-mortem partial cuff tears, the relevance of cadaveric correlation with actual clinical symptomatology is lacking. Much like the full-thickness rotator cuff tear, many patients with a partial tear may be asymptomatic.

Natural History of Partial-Thickness Cuff Tears

The current conventional belief is that the natural history of partial-thickness tears is one of progressive tearing. Several studies[13-15] have demonstrated that subacromial decompression does not prevent progressive tearing of the partial cuff tear and that clinical efforts that fail to address the partial tear itself lead to inferior outcomes when compared to attempts to repair the partial tear. Kartus et al[13] in 2006 reported on a 35% (9 of 26 patients) incidence of progressive full-thickness tearing following subacromial decompression for a partial-thickness tear. Yamanaka and Matsumoto[16] in 1994 established through the use of arthrographic techniques that the spontaneous healing rate of partial-thickness cuff tears was approximately 10% (4 of 40 patients) while 25% progressed to a full-thickness tear and more than 50% were noted to be larger in size with follow-up studies. Conversely, Lo reported on 46 patients with partial-thickness rotator cuff tears who averaged 54 years of age and were followed for 4 years on average (Unpublished data, 2010). Using magnetic resonance arthrography (MRA), 24% of the partial tears progressed in size, 65% were noted to demonstrate no change in dimensions, while 11% showed healing. He concluded that, contrary to previous reports, 76% of partial-thickness tears either stayed the same or improved in tear size over a 4-year follow-up. He did note, however, that those partial-thickness tears less than 50% were much less likely to progress in size (14%) as compared to tears exceeding 50% of the thickness (55%).

Pathogenesis

The etiology of rotator cuff disease is often multifactorial with the final common denominator being fiber failure. Two broad categories, intrinsic and extrinsic, have historically served as the basis for why partial tears occur.

The argument for the extrinsic pathogenesis of rotator cuff disease was originally proposed by Neer[17,18] and provided a counterargument to Codman's theory that senescent changes in the rotator cuff were the primary cause for rotator cuff disease. Neer elegantly detailed a mechanical, anatomic explanation of rotator cuff pathogenesis and outlined the causes of subacromial impingement in a seminal description of the morphologic variations in acromial anatomy. Commonly referred to as primary extrinsic impingement, Neer's explanation has been augmented to include not only pathologic acromial morphology, but also acromial slope, hypertrophy of the coracoacromial (CA) ligament, traumatic tuberosity deformity, os acromiale, and even enthesopathy at the acromioclavicular (AC) joint.[19-24]

When considering the intrinsic causes of partial-thickness cuff tears, the well-described age-related changes in the composition of the rotator cuff, including diminished vascularity, loss of collagen, dystrophic calcification, and decreased cellularity, all contribute to a degraded tissue quality and concomitant stunted healing potential. Degenerative tearing occurs with little chance of intrinsic healing and reinforces the concept of the age-related incidence of partial-thickness tears.

In many instances, a combination of this intrinsic degeneration with the concomitant diminution of normal-functioning "force couples" serves to propagate the compromised rotator cuff to a more diseased status. This phenomenon can lead to confusion when trying to ascertain etiology. With intrinsic cuff degeneration and the subsequent loss of humeral head containment, superior migration of the humeral head can lead to secondary impingement in which the cuff "moves to the arch." A secondary traction spur can form in the CA ligament, and bursal-sided rotator cuff damage can ensue. When this occurs, the distinction between primary extrinsic impingement as described by Neer[17,18] and predicated on some form of outlet stenosis and a secondary bursal-sided partial cuff tear based on intrinsic cuff dysfunction can be blurred, and a definitive etiology can be difficult to ascertain as both the intra-articular and subacromial spaces reveal cuff pathology.

Shoulder instability and scapular dyskinesis are 2 common entities in which secondary cuff compromise can be encountered. Of importance is that the treatment be directed toward the underlying condition and not focused on opening the subacromial outlet, which often only serves to magnify underlying instability.[25]

Partial-thickness tears of the subscapularis tendon can be seen in 2 distinct patient populations. Younger patients demonstrate isolated, traumatic tears of the subscapularis tendon. Degenerative tears, seen in the older patient population, can result from anterosuperior rotator cuff disease where additional stress is placed on the subscapularis from concomitant rotator cuff dysfunction and remote tearing.[26] Impingement is another possible cause of subscapularis pathology. In subcoracoid impingement, the subscapularis is compromised as it passes beneath the coracoid process. Partial-thickness tears can take the form of articular-sided tears, such as the "TUFF" (traumatic undersurface fiber failure). These TUFF lesions are theorized to result from impingement under the coracoid process best described as a "roller wringer effect."[27] Tearing at the superior margin of the subscapularis tendon can be associated with an impingement phenomenon or may simply represent tensile failure from repetitive microtrauma. Subscapularis pathology can often lead to concomitant biceps pain and instability within the bicipital groove.[28]

Internal impingement can also lead to secondary subacromial changes and describes a unique pathology generally discovered in the overhand throwing athlete.[28-30] Rather than a tensile failure related to cuff degeneration, this entity is seen in much younger patients with multiple theories as to the dynamics of this injury. Morgan and colleagues[31,32] described a pathologic cascade in which a tight posterior capsule resulting in a glenohumeral internal rotation deficit shifts the humeral head into a posterosuperior position, allowing for not only hyperexternal rotation of the rotator cuff resulting in an articular-sided partial tear at the supraspinatus-infraspinatus junction, but also a "peel back" of the posterosuperior labrum. Others[33-37] have proposed physical contact between the posterosuperior glenoid and labrum with the articular surface of the rotator cuff, leading to cuff failure. This can be on a physiologic to pathologic basis in which contact is normal but the repetitive microtrauma eventually leads to fiber failure. The internal impingement lesion has also been hypothesized to result from anterior capsular insufficiency,[38,39] as well as from the various scapular dyskinesis patterns that can occur in the throwing athlete.[40]

CLASSIFICATION

While partial-thickness tears had been incompletely described in the literature, it was Ellman's classification system that first addressed the subject in a way that has proven most useful, both from a diagnostic and treatment standpoint.[41,42] His classification system is based on findings at 120 arthroscopic subacromial decompressions and is based on 2 primary criteria: location (articular sided, bursal sided, or intratendinous) and depth of the tear. Grade 1 partial tears were less than 3 mm, Grade 2 were 3 to 6 mm, and Grade 3 were greater than 6 mm (Table 10-1). Snyder and colleagues[43] also proposed an alternative classification system for partial-thickness tears of the rotator cuff, based on the location, articular- versus bursal-sided, and the severity of the tear (Table 10-2).

TABLE 10-1. ELLMAN CLASSIFICATION FOR PARTIAL-THICKNESS ROTATOR CUFF TEARS

CLASSIFICATION FOR PARTIAL TEARS: BASED ON DEPTH OF DEFECT*		
Articular Surface		
Bursal Surface		
Grade 1 <¼ thickness (~3 mm)	**Grade 2** <½ thickness (3 to 6 mm)	**Grade 3** >½ thickness (6+ mm)

*Indicates area of defect: Base of tear x maximum retraction = mm²

TABLE 10-2. SNYDER CLASSIFICATION FOR PARTIAL-THICKNESS ROTATOR CUFF TEARS

LOCATION OF TEAR		
A—articular	B—bursal	C—full thickness
Grade	0 Normal cuff	
	1 Inflamed synovium and superficial fraying <1 cm	
	2 Moderate tear with actual fiber disruption 1 to 2 cm	
	3 Disruption and fragmentation of tissues 2 to 3 cm	
	4 Complex partial-thickness rotator cuff tear (flap formation and retraction) >3 cm	

Reprinted from *Arthroscopy*, vol 7, iss 1, Snyder SJ, Pachelli AF, Del Pizzo W, Friedman MJ, Ferkel RD, Pattee G, Partial thickness rotator cuff tears: results of arthroscopic treatment, pp 1-7, Copyright 1991, with permission from Elsevier.

Other classification systems have been proposed,[44,45] but Kuhn and colleagues have noted that there is little interobserver reliability.[46] Ellman's system appears to have endured as the most clinically useful grading system available. With improved knowledge of the anatomic footprint of the rotator cuff, more precise measurements of the depth of the tear have been attainable. The depth of the tear is estimated as the distance from the exposed footprint to the intact tendon. This can be estimated with an instrument of known dimensions, such as an arthroscopic probe or shaver. Several studies[1,47,48] have documented the average dimensions of the supraspinatus tendon footprint with the medial-to-lateral length approximating 12 mm. It is noteworthy that recently some have challenged the purported attachment sites and dimensions of the rotator cuff footprint.[49] Accurate grading of the tear depth becomes a critical step when attempting to decide whether a tear should or should not be repaired.

PATIENT PRESENTATION AND DIAGNOSIS

History

The common complaint that brings a patient to the office with a partial-thickness tear of the rotator cuff is pain. While these patients may complain of pain, other common concerns include stiffness, weakness, and occasionally a sense of instability. The shoulder pain experienced by these patients and their relevant clinical findings are by no means specific to partial-thickness tears. Patients often complain of significant night pain, insomnia, and pain with overhead activities, and they may have real or perceived weakness associated with vigorous activities. Such complaints can mimic those seen in other conditions including impingement, labral and biceps pathology, and even full-thickness rotator cuff tears.

Despite the nonspecific nature of a patient's presenting complaints, there is evidence in the literature that the history and examination of patients with partial-thickness tears may provide some insight into making the diagnosis. Fukuda compared pain levels prior to surgery in patients with subacromial bursitis and/or partial-thickness tears to patients with full-thickness tears.[5] He noted that more patients (73%) with subacromial bursitis and/or partial-thickness tears rated their pain at a higher level (visual analogue scale >5) when compared to patients with full-thickness tears (50%). He also reported that bursal-sided tears were considered more painful than those on the articular side. These findings may reflect a mechanical, anatomic impingement that is associated with a painful arc, but may also indicate that a rotator cuff in the process of tearing can generate more pain than that associated with a completed cuff tear. One study[50] noted that levels of substance P and immunoreactive nerve fibers were higher in those patients with partial-thickness tears when compared to those with full-thickness tears. This may again reflect an active process versus a more quiescent environment after a complete tear.

Clinical Examination

A thorough clinical examination of the patient is warranted given the difficulty of making an accurate diagnosis of a partial-thickness cuff tear. A detailed shoulder exam begins with a visual inspection of the shoulder girdle to evaluate for atrophy or asymmetry. A complete examination of active range of motion should then be performed and documented with comparison to the contralateral (normal) side. This should include abduction, forward flexion, as well as internal and external rotation at 0 and 90 degrees of abduction. Passive range of motion is then similarly evaluated. Normal scapulothoracic synchrony should be ascertained by viewing the patient from behind.

It is crucial to measure range of motion bilaterally in the overhead athlete. One should consider not only the limits of internal and external range of motion, but the total arc of motion as well. In the overhead athlete, the total arc of motion is often the same as the contralateral nondominant side with external rotation increased and a concomitant decrease in internal rotation as an adaptive change. If the overall arc of motion is decreased relative to the uninvolved side or if the difference in internal rotation exceeds 15 to 20 degrees, the possibility of a glenohumeral internal rotation deficit and its association with the internal impingement lesion must be considered.

Palpation of the shoulder adds to the clinical picture by geographically mapping areas of tenderness. Unfortunately, areas of tenderness do not always correspond to an anatomic lesion, as "radiating pain" often fails to pinpoint the underlying pathology. Palpation of the biceps tendon that elicits significant pain suggests biceps pathology but may also implicate the superior border of the subscapularis given the association of biceps instability and subscapularis tendon pathology. Codman's point can be evaluated with the shoulder extended and internally rotated with tenderness elicited at the supraspinatus insertion site. AC joint tenderness should be clearly documented and should serve as the basis for whether this joint requires concomitant treatment if the partial tear is treated operatively. Radiographic findings of AC degenerative change are common, and clinical tenderness must be present to warrant any invasive treatment.

Strength testing should then be carefully preformed to evaluate the integrity of the rotator cuff. Resisted abduction in the scapular plane focuses on the supraspinatus tendon. Both the empty[51] or full[52] can test have been shown to be similarly accurate in demonstrating rotator cuff pathology.[53] Despite a recent electromyogram study disputing the ability of either test to adequately isolate the supraspinatus, pain registered during this stress test leads one to suspect supraspinatus involvement. The infraspinatus is isolated during resisted external rotation with the elbow at the side. Pain or weakness may suggest a tear that involves or extends into the infraspinatus. The subscapularis can be evaluated with the belly-press test[52] (Napoleon test).[53] Subtle weakness patterns can indicate a partial tear.

The physical exam is then complemented with additional tests, such as the Hawkins test in which the shoulder is forward flexed to 90 degrees and internally rotated, attempting to elicit cuff pain. The Neer test in which an anesthetic is injected into the subacromial space can confirm rotator cuff involvement when preinjection pain is eliminated following the injection. A positive Jobe relocation test in which pain is eliminated with an anterior-to-posterior force while the arm is abducted and externally rotated can signal an internal impingement lesion and partial cuff tear in conjunction with anterior instability.

DIAGNOSTIC IMAGING

Shoulder radiographs offer a limited, first step in the evaluation of rotator cuff tears. A reduced acromiohumeral distance is suggestive of a chronic complete cuff tear. Calcific tendinitis may be offered as an alternative diagnosis. The presence of AC degenerative joint disease, subacromial spurring, an os acromiale, an abnormal acromial slope, or an abnormal acromial shape can be used to infer the presence of shoulder impingement. Magnetic resonance imaging (MRI) and MRA represent the mainstay of imaging partial-thickness rotator cuff tears. Conventional MRI findings of partial-thickness tears include focal defects on the T2-weighted images at the articular or bursal surfaces. Fat suppression and the use of a coronal oblique plane are also key elements in the imaging of rotator cuff tears (Figures 10-1 through 10-3).

A recent prospective study of 48 patients who had a preoperative MRI performed on a 3.0 tesla magnet followed by arthroscopy found a positive predictive value of 92% for partial-thickness tears and a positive predictive value of 100% for full-thickness tears.[54] The addition of contrast material has further elevated the sensitivity and specificity for MRI.[55] The advantages of MRA over standard MRI are the fluid distension of the glenohumeral joint, which highlights articular surface partial cuff lesions while also affording a thorough evaluation of the labrum, capsule, and glenohumeral ligaments.

Previous studies have established the utility of positioning the shoulder in the abduction-externally rotated position while imaging for undersurface tears of the rotator cuff.[56] It is critical to understand that, in the abduction-externally rotated position, contact between the glenoid and rotator cuff insertion sites is physiologic and may be mistakenly interpreted as evidence of superior glenoid and labral pathology in throwing athletes (Figure 10-4).[57]

Figure 10-1. (A) Arrow demonstrates a bursal-sided partial-thickness tear on coronal oblique T2 fat saturation. (B) Arrow demonstrates the same bursal-sided image on coronal oblique inversion recovery sequence.

Figure 10-2. Red arrow depicts an articular-sided partial-thickness tear on coronal oblique inversion recovery.

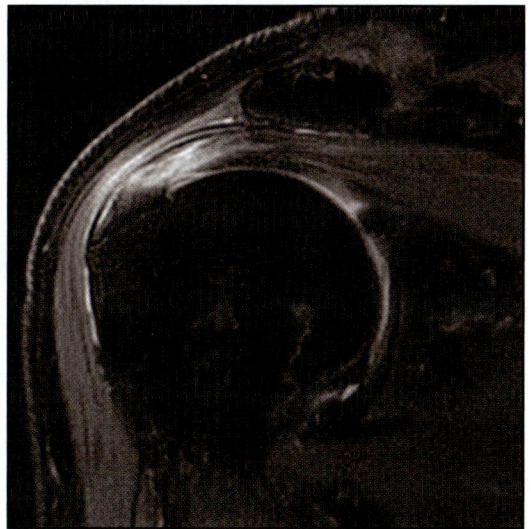

Figure 10-3. Intratendinous tear of the supraspinatus tendon.

Although the use of musculoskeletal ultrasonography has been widespread internationally, its use in North America has historically been limited with the availability of MRI. However, increasing cost consciousness, technologic advances in spatial resolution, and the appeal of an office setting exam have augmented the practice by radiologists and nonradiologists alike. The current disadvantages of ultrasound include extreme operator dependence and the inability to evaluate associated shoulder pathology.

With experienced operators, an accuracy rate of 94% has been reported in discriminating partial-thickness from full-thickness tears, using the finding of "focal heterogeneous hypoechogenicity."[58] The principal findings on ultrasound that suggest partial-thickness rotator cuff tearing are focal areas of decreased echogenicity. A normal convexity of the overlying tendon distinguishes it from a full-thickness tear.

Figure 10-4. The abduction-externally rotated position view of MRA demonstrating labral pathology (white arrow) and fraying of the undersurface of the supraspinatus tendon (red arrow).

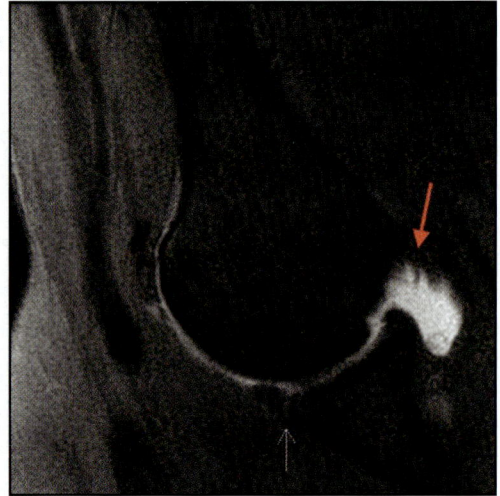

An increasing body of literature supports the equivalence of ultrasound and MRI. A 2009 meta-analysis of 65 studies using operative findings as the gold standard found no statistical difference in the ability of either MRI or ultrasound to identify partial-thickness cuff tears, citing a sensitivity and specificity of 67% and 94% for ultrasound and 64% and 92%, respectively, for MRI. MRA statistically outperformed both modalities ($p<0.001$) with a sensitivity of 86% and specificity of 96%.[55]

Nakagawa et al reported on a unique MR finding, which they termed the *greater tuberosity notch sign*. These humeral head "notches" were noted in throwing athletes with partial-thickness cuff tears and were initially misread as atypical Hill-Sachs lesions. The size of the notches corresponded closely with the actual size of the partial-thickness articular-sided tears.[59]

TREATMENT ALTERNATIVES

Nonoperative Treatment

Nonoperative management of partial-thickness rotator cuff tears should be attempted before any surgical intervention. A carefully supervised rehabilitation program must take into account the patient's expectations, quality of life concerns, ability to modify aggravating activities, and ability to participate in a rehabilitation program. If a nonoperative regimen is selected, a reasonable course of treatment should allow for improvement over a minimum 3- to 6-month period. As gains are made subjectively and clinically and the patient remains satisfied, rehabilitation may continue until the symptoms resolve or have resolved to a level satisfying the patient.

Conservative management consists of a program using nonsteroidal anti-inflammatory medication, strict avoidance of aggravating activities, and a well-supervised shoulder rehabilitation program. Physical therapy should focus on minimizing inflammation while restoring balance and function to both the front and back of the shoulder. Range-of-motion exercises followed by core and scapular strengthening allow the rotator cuff to be rehabilitated in a safe manner.

Although there is a paucity of evidence in the literature with regard to the use of corticosteroid injections for partial-thickness tears, the judicious use of corticosteroid injections can be very helpful in the management of pain associated with impingement symptoms and rotator cuff pathology. Additionally, the response to such injections combined with local anesthetics can often provide information that helps establish the diagnosis.

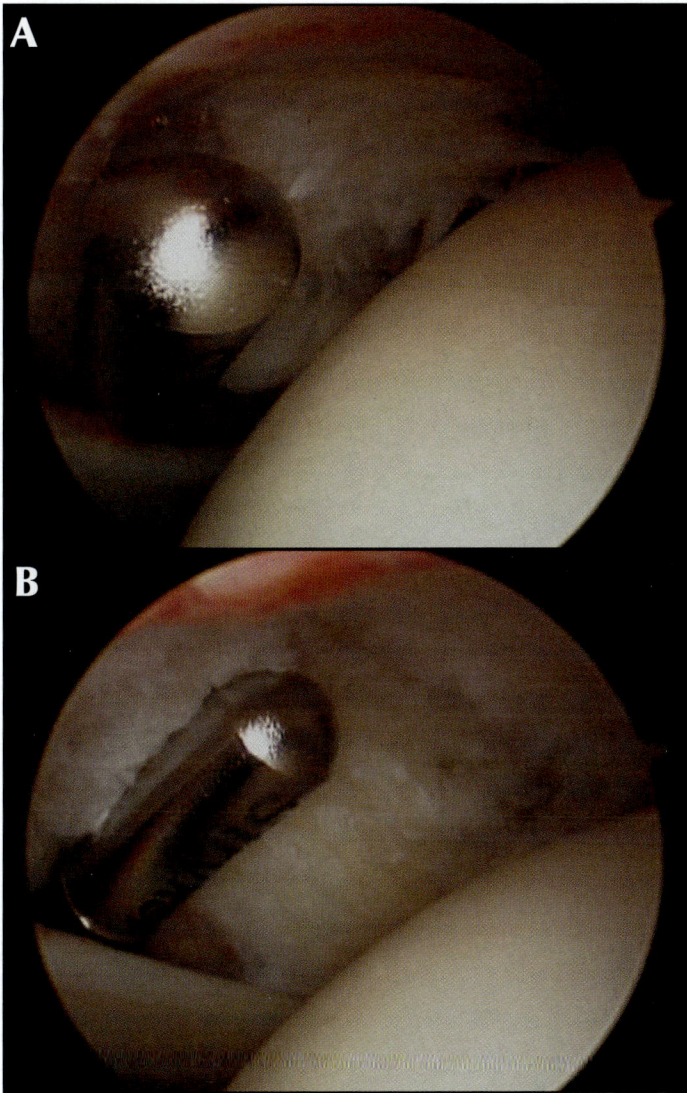

Figure 10-5. (A) Articular view of articular-sided partial rotator cuff tear prior to débridement. (B) Débridement of undersurface fraying of the rotator cuff partial tear.

SURGICAL TECHNIQUE: TRANSTENDON REPAIR OF ARTICULAR-SIDED PARTIAL-THICKNESS ROTATOR CUFF TEAR

The technique in which the partial tear is converted to a full-thickness lesion followed by a standard arthroscopic repair, double or single row, is described elsewhere in this textbook. The technique description that follows is pertinent to the transtendon approach.

Once a decision has been made that the remaining bursal attachment of the cuff is of sufficient quality and a high-grade partial tear (partial articular-sided tendon avulsion) has been identified on the articular margin (Figures 10-5 and 10-6), the arthroscope is introduced into the subacromial space. If there is evidence of the impingement phenomenon, namely bursal-sided cuff fraying or CA roughening, an acromioplasty is appropriate even if the changes are secondary in nature. If not, the bursal space is débrided in order to provide access to the suture tails, which will be tied in the subacromial space. Failure to prepare the subacromial space leads to potential suture compromise if a débridement is performed after the transtendon sutures have been placed.

Figure 10-6. Articular view of a partial articular-sided tendon avulsion tear showing exposure of the footprint of the supraspinatus tendon.

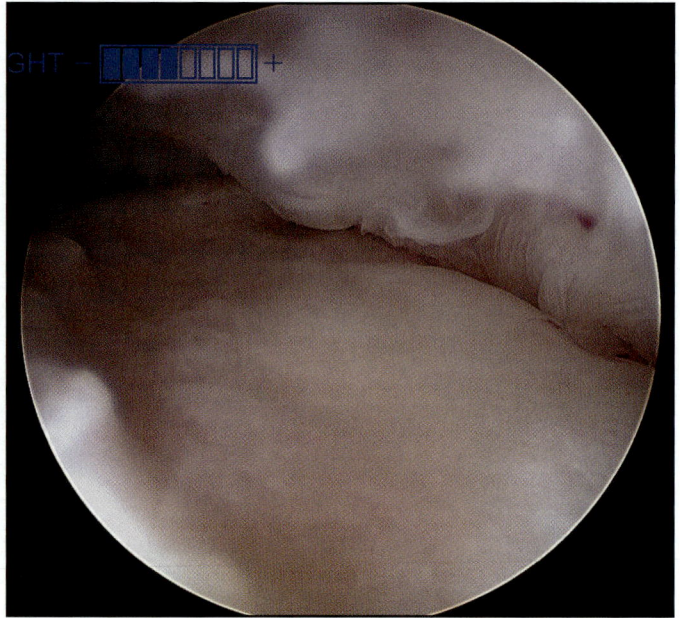

Figure 10-7. Suture anchor introduced transtendon on to the footprint of the supraspinatus.

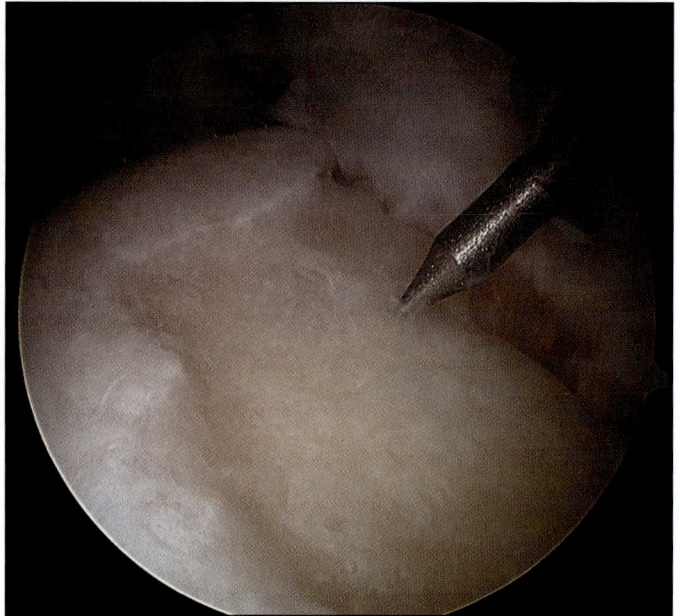

A grasper from the anterior portal can be used to reduce the partial tear and to determine its mobility. The footprint is prepared with a shaver, and the exposed margin is measured with an instrument of known dimensions. Once a partial tear of 5 to 6 mm or greater is established, a spinal needle is used to establish the angle of penetration for the suture anchor, which will penetrate the intact bursal portion of the cuff. This is followed by introduction of the cannula (Figure 10-7), which should be of the smallest diameter possible that is compatible with the correct anchor choice. The direction of insertion should be lateral to medial to avoid inadvertent penetration of the humeral head. Adduction of the shoulder can assist in the accurate and safe passage of the cannula followed by insertion of a double-loaded suture anchor.

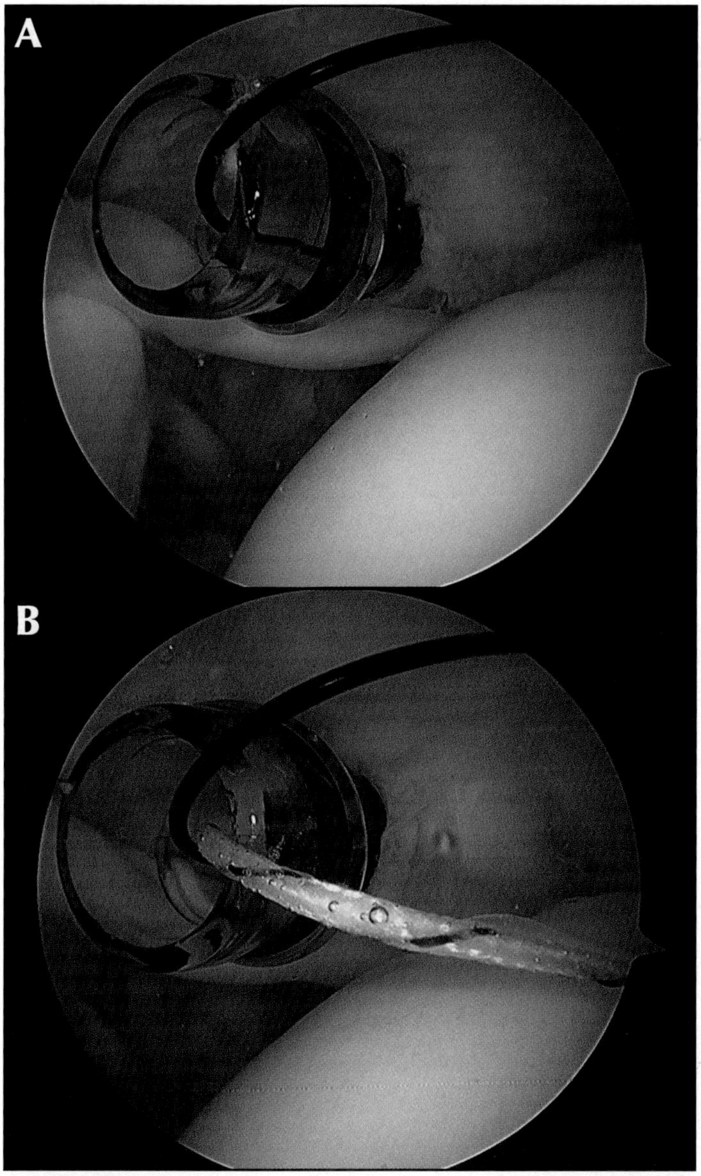

Figure 10-8. (A) Percutaneous monofilament suture shuttle passed and then (B) retrograded with suture from anchor (braided appearance) tied into the shuttle.

Two suture limbs are brought through the anterior cannula with their respective limbs remaining in the subacromial space. Using a spinal needle loaded with a monofilament suture ("poor man's suture shuttle"), the edge of the tear is pierced percutaneously, and the suture is retrieved through the anterior cannula. The passing suture is loaded with the appropriate suture match and then retrograded through the cuff edge into the subacromial space (Figure 10-8). This is performed until all of the sutures have been passed retrograde through the torn cuff (Figure 10-9). Cinching the sutures reduces the tear back to the footprint for an anatomic repair (Figure 10-10).

It is critically important to reduce the tear while passing the spinal needle during the repair in an effort to avoid a length mismatch between the bursal and articular surfaces of the tear. Such a mismatch can lead to significant stiffness and more perioperative discomfort. The sutures are then retrieved in the subacromial space and tied as pairs once a cannula is introduced into the subacromial space (Figure 10-11). The surgeon can then place the camera back into the glenohumeral joint and visualize the repair to confirm that an adequate reduction has been achieved.

Figure 10-9. Two limbs of the suture anchor passed through the edge of the articular-sided partial tear prior to tying the knots on the bursal side.

Figure 10-10. Appearance of the articular-sided partial tear after anatomic reduction to the footprint.

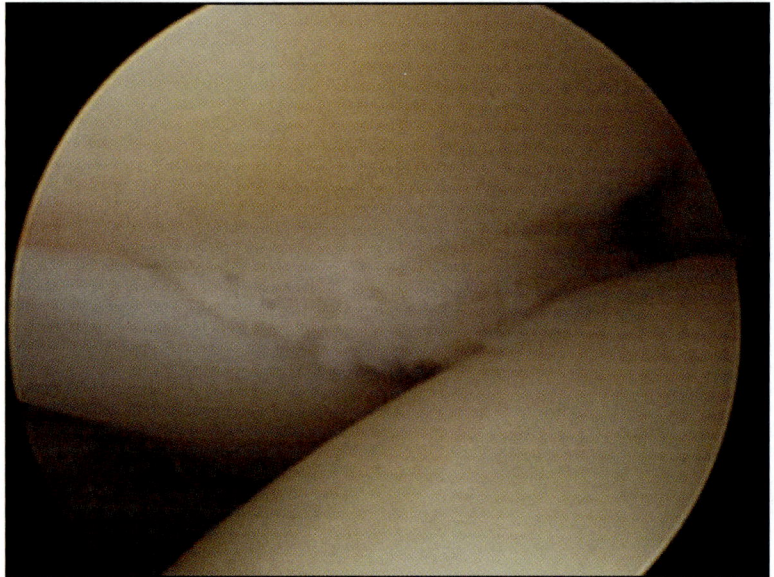

In the overhand athlete, repair of an articular-sided partial-thickness rotator cuff tear may be necessary, but great care should be taken in making this decision. There may be an adaptive role reflected in the exposed footprint, allowing greater rotation and velocity. These partial articular-sided tendon avulsion lesions, which can result from the internal impingement phenomenon described earlier in this chapter, can also have an intratendinous extension component (posterior articular-surface intratendinous) that may also need to be treated.[60] Larger intratendinous partial tears in this population may require a formal takedown, débridement, and repair, while those of smaller dimension can be addressed with side-to-side sutures placed percutaneously, much like the transtendon approach.

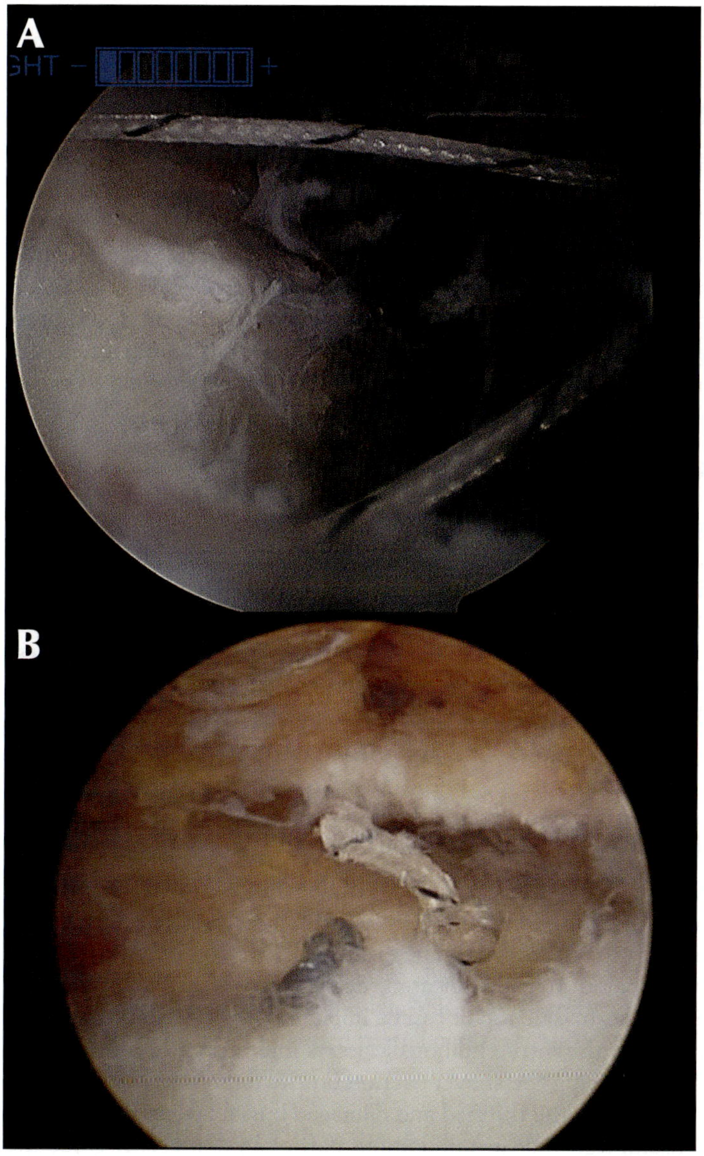

Figure 10-11. (A) Sutures captured in the subacromial space and tied. (B) Final appearance of transtendon repair of partial articular-sided tendon avulsion lesion while viewing from the subacromial space.

REHABILITATION

Following a transtendon repair, even though the bursal layer remains intact and some stress shielding may be present, the rehabilitation should not be accelerated. Tensile stress on the repair is present based on shoulder position, and the repair must be protected. A shoulder immobilizer is used for 5 to 6 weeks, and simple gravity exercises are initiated as soon as the patient is comfortable. Progressive active-assisted motion is started at 6 weeks, and resistance exercises are delayed for 10 to 12 weeks. Scapular setting exercises are initiated early in the protocol while a resumption of normal activities is permitted at 5 to 6 months postoperatively.

to tear completion with dual-row repair. However, caution must be exercised when attempting to determine if the remaining cuff is of sufficient quality, especially in the older patient. Ide and colleagues[71] in 2005 were one of the first to report on results with transtendon repair in a study of 17 patients with 3 years of follow-up. The average age was 42, and these authors reported good or excellent results in 16 of the 17. It is noteworthy that only 2 of 6 overhand athletes returned to the same proficiency level. More recently, Castagna and colleagues[72] reported on 54 patients who had undergone a transtendon repair with a patient satisfaction rate of 98%. As might be anticipated, those who were younger and experienced a traumatic, acute injury fared the best.

The option of completing the tear and performing a full-thickness repair is a valuable alternative, especially if the remaining tissue is of poor or suspect quality. Furthermore, this technique can allow for better mobilization, débridement, and improved fixation with a variety of constructs available that are not applicable to the transtendon technique. In addition to the Weber study,[68] which clearly delineated a better outcome with mini-open repair and decompression for the high-grade partial rotator cuff tear, other studies have shared similar outcomes. Deutsch[73] reported on 41 patients with high-grade partial tears treated prospectively with a complete and single-row simple repair technique. A nearly 100% satisfaction rate was achieved with strength testing revealing no deficits compared to the contralateral extremity. In 2009, Kamath and colleagues[74] evaluated tendon integrity and functional outcome after converting a high-grade partial tear to a complete tear followed by an arthroscopic repair. They reported that 88% of the patients demonstrated an intact cuff with ultrasound testing while the overall patient satisfaction rate was 93%. The 5 patients with a persistent cuff defect were noteworthy for an average age of nearly 63 years compared to the cuff-intact group, which averaged 52 years of age. It is also noteworthy that the conversion of a high-grade tear to a complete one followed by a formal repair of the cuff has met with little success in the overhead throwing population[75] and emphasizes that this unique population of patients must be managed conservatively whenever feasible.

CONCLUSION

Partial-thickness rotator cuff tears remain one of the most challenging treatment decisions for shoulder surgeons. Many patients will present with MRI findings of a partial-thickness cuff tear, but will not require surgical intervention and will do well with a nonoperative treatment program that includes activity modification, anti-inflammatories, and physical therapy. When surgical treatment is decided upon, choosing one technique over the other when faced with a high-grade partial-thickness rotator cuff tear can be a difficult clinical decision, and criteria such as age, quality of the remaining tendon, surgical expertise, as well as patient expectations all play a role in the decision making. The outcomes of partial-thickness rotator cuff repair are quite good, and patients should be encouraged to return to full activities after they complete the rehabilitation process.

REFERENCES

1. Codman EA. *The Shoulder: Rupture of the Supraspinatus Tendon and Other Lesions in or About the Sub-Acromial Bursa.* Boston, MA: Thomas Todd; 1934.
2. Lohr JF, Uhthoff HK. The pathogenesis of degenerative rotator cuff tears. *Orthop Trans.* 1987;11:715-725.
3. Sher JS, Uribe JW, Posada A, Murphy BJ, Zlatkin MB. Abnormal findings on magnetic resonance images of asymptomatic shoulders. *J Bone Joint Surg Am.* 1995;77:10-15.
4. Fukuda H, Mikasa M, Yamanaka K. Incomplete thickness rotator cuff tears diagnosed by subacromial bursography. *Clin Orthop Relat Res.* 1987:51-58.
5. Fukuda H. Partial-thickness rotator cuff tears: a modern view on Codman's classic. *J Shoulder Elbow Surg.* 2000;9:163-168.
6. Sakurai G, Osaki J, Tomita Y, et al. Incomplete tears of the subscapularis tendon associated with tears of the supraspinatus tendon: cadaveric and clinical studies. *J Shoulder Elbow Surg.* 1998;7:510-515.

7. Nakajima T, Rokuuma N, Hamada K, et al. Histologic and biomechanical characteristics of the supraspinatus tendon: a reference to rotator cuff tearing. *J Shoulder Elbow Surg.* 1994;3:79-87.

8. Mazzocca AD, Rincon LM, O'Connor RW, et al. Intra-articular partial-thickness rotator cuff tears: analysis of injured and repaired strain behavior. *Am J Sports Med.* 2008;36:110-116.

9. Sano H, Wakabayashi I, Itoi E. Stress distribution in the supraspinatus tendon with partial-thickness tears: an analysis using two-dimensional finite element model. *J Shoulder Elbow Surg.* 2006;15:100-105.

10. Bey MJ, Ramsey ML, Soslowsky LJ. Intratendinous strain fields of the supraspinatus tendon: effect of a surgically created articular-surface rotator cuff tear. *J Shoulder Elbow Surg.* 2002;11:562-569.

11. Reilly P, Amis AA, Wallace AL, Emery RJ. Supraspinatus tears: propagation and strain alteration. *J Shoulder Elbow Surg.* 2003;12:134-138.

12. Yang S, Park HS, Flores S, et al. Biomechanical analysis of bursal-sided partial-thickness rotator cuff tears. *J Shoulder Elbow Surg.* 2009;18:379-385.

13. Kartus J, Kartus C, Rostgard-Christensen L, Sernert N, Read J, Perko M. Long-term clinical and ultrasound evaluation after arthroscopic acromioplasty in patients with partial rotator cuff tears. *Arthroscopy.* 2006;22:44-49.

14. Weber SC. Arthroscopic débridement and acromioplasty versus mini-open repair in the treatment of significant partial-thickness rotator cuff tears. *Arthroscopy.* 1999;15:126-131.

15. Hyvönen P, Loji S, Jalovaara P. Open acromioplasty does not prevent the progression of an impingement syndrome to a tear: nine-year follow-up of 96 cases. *J Bone Joint Surg Br.* 1998;80:813-816.

16. Yamanaka K, Matsumoto T. The joint side tear of the rotator cuff: a follow-up study by arthrography. *Clin Orthop Relat Res.* 1994:68-73.

17. Neer CS II. Anterior acromioplasty for the chronic impingement syndrome in the shoulder: a preliminary report. *J Bone Joint Surg Am.* 1972;54:41-50.

18. Neer CS II. Impingement lesions. *Clin Orthop.* 1983;173:70-77.

19. Gohlke F, Barthel T, Gandorfer A. The influence of variations of the coracoacromial arch on the development of rotator cuff tears. *Acta Orthop Trauma Surg.* 1993;113:28-32.

20. Burns WC, Whipple TL. Anatomic relationships in the shoulder impingement syndrome. *Clin Orthop.* 1993;294:96-102.

21. Payne LZ, Deng XH, Craig EV, et al. The combined dynamic and static contributions to subacromial impingement: a biomechanical analysis. *Am J Sports Med.* 1997;25:801-808.

22. Rockwood CA, Lyons FR. Shoulder impingement syndrome: diagnosis, radiographic evaluation, and treatment with a modified Neer acromioplasty. *J Bone Joint Surg Am.* 1993;74:409-424.

23. Zuckerman JD, Klummer FJ, Cuomo F, et al. The influence of the coracoacromial arch anatomy on rotator cuff tears. *J Shoulder Elbow Surg.* 1992;1:4-14.

24. Ozaki J, Fujimoto S, Nakagawa Y, et al. Tears of the rotator cuff of the shoulder associated with pathological changes in the acromion: a study in cadaver. *J Bone Joint Surg Am.* 1988;70:1224-1230.

25. Lee TQ, Black AD, Tibone JE, McMahon PJ. Release of the coracoacromial ligament can lead to glenohumeral laxity: a biomechanical study. *J Shoulder Elbow Surg.* 2001;10(1):68-72.

26. Burkhart S, Ochoa E. Subscapularis tendon tears: diagnosis and treatment strategies. *Curr Ortho Pract.* 2008;19(5):542-547.

27. Lo IK, Burkhart SS. The etiology and assessment of subscapularis tendon tears: a case for subcoracoid impingement, the roller-wringer effect, and TUFF lesions of the subscapularis. *Arthroscopy.* 2003;19(1):1142-1150.

28. Drakos MC, Rudzki JR, Allen AA, Potter HG, Altchek DW. Internal impingement of the shoulder in the overhead athlete. *J Bone Joint Surg Am.* 2009;91(11):2719-2728.

29. Kirchhoff C, Imhoff AB. Posterosuperior and anterosuperior impingement of the shoulder in overhead athletes-evolving concepts. *Int Orthop.* 2010;34(7):1049-1058.

30. Greiwe RM, Ahmad CS. Management of the throwing shoulder: cuff, labrum and internal impingement. *Orthop Clin North Am.* 2010;41(3):309-323.

31. Burkhart SS, Morgan CD, Kibler WB. Shoulder injuries in overhead athletes. The "dead arm" revisited. *Clin Sports Med.* 2000;19(1):125-158.

32. Morgan CD, Burkhart SS, Palmeri M, Gillespie M. Type II SLAP lesions: three subtypes and their relationships to superior instability and rotator cuff tears. *Arthroscopy.* 1998;14(6):553-565.

33. Walch G, Liotard JP, Boileau P, Noël E. Postero-superior glenoid impingement. Another shoulder impingement. *Chir Orthop Reparatrice Appar Mot.* 1991;77(8):571-574.

34. Jobe CM. Posterior superior glenoid impingement: expanded spectrum. *Arthroscopy.* 1995;11:530-536.

35. Edelson G, Teitz C. Internal impingement in the shoulder. *J Shoulder Elbow Surg.* 2000;9:308-315.

36. Paley KJ, Jobe FW, Pink MM, Kvitne RS, ElAttrache NS. Arthroscopic findings in the overhand throwing athlete: evidence for posterior internal impingement of the rotator cuff. *Arthroscopy.* 2000;16:35-40.

37. Kim T, McFarland S. Internal impingement of the shoulder in flexion. *Clin Orthop Relat Res.* 2004;421:112-119.

38. Jazrawi LM, McCluskey GM, Andrews JR. Superior labral anterior and posterior lesions and internal impingement in the overhead athlete. *Instr Course Lect.* 2003;52:43-63.

39. Kvitne RS, Jobe FW, Jobe CM. Shoulder instability in the overhand or throwing athlete. *Clin Sports Med.* 1995;14(4):917-935.

40. Uhl TL, Kibler WB, Gecewich B, Tripp BL. Evaluation of clinical assessment methods for scapular dyskinesis. *Arthroscopy*. 2009;25(11):1240-1248.

41. Ellman H. Diagnosis and treatment of incomplete rotator cuff tears. *Clin Orthop Relat Res*. 1990;(254):64-74.

42. Ellman H, Gartsman GM. *Arthroscopic Shoulder Surgery and Related Procedures*. Philadelphia, PA: Lea & Febiger; 1993.

43. Snyder SJ, Pachelli AF, Del Pizzo W, et al. Partial thickness rotator cuff tears: results of arthroscopic treatment. *Arthroscopy*. 1991;7(1):1-7.

44. Conway JE. Arthroscopic repair of partial-thickness rotator cuff tears and SLAP lesions in professional baseball players. *Orthop Clin North Am*. 2001;32:443-456.

45. Habermeyer P, Kreiter C, Tang KL, et al. A new arthroscopic classification of articular-sided supraspinatus footprint lesions: a prospective comparison of Snyder's and Ellman's classification. *J Shoulder Elbow Surg*. 2008;17:909-913.

46. Kuhn JE, Dunn WR, Ma B, et al. Multicenter Orthopaedic Outcomes Network—Shoulder (MOOM Shoulder Group). Interobserver agreement in the classification of rotator cuff tears. *Am J Sports Med*. 2007;35:437-441.

47. Ruotolo C, Fow JE, Nottage WM. The supraspinatus footprint: an anatomic study of the supraspinatus insertion. *Arthroscopy*. 2004;20:246-249.

48. Dugas JR, Campbell DA, Warren RF, et al. Anatomy and dimensions of rotator cuff insertions. *J Shoulder Elbow Surg*. 2002;11:498-503.

49. Mochizuki T, Sugaya H, Uomizu M, et al. Humeral insertion of the supraspinatus and infraspinatus. New anatomical findings regarding the footprint of the rotator cuff. *J Bone Joint Surg Am*. 2008;90(5):962-969.

50. Gotoh M, Hamada K, Yamakawa H, et al. Increased substance P in the subacromial bursa and shoulder pain in rotator cuff diseases. *J Orthop Res*. 1998;16:618-621.

51. Itoi E, Kido T, Sano A, et al. Which is more useful, the "full can test" or the "empty can test," in detecting the torn supraspinatus tendon? *Am J Sports Medicine*. 1999;27:65-68.

52. Gerber C, Hersche O, Farron A. Isolated rupture of the subscapularis tendon. *J Bone Joint Surg Am*. 1996;78:1015-1023.

53. Schwamborn T, Imhoff AB. Diagnostik und klassifikation der rotatorenmanschettenlasionen. In: Imhoff AB, Konig U, eds, *Schulterinstabilitat-Rotatorenmanschette*. Darmstadt: Steinkopff Verlag; 1999:193-195.

54. Lambert A, Loffroy R, Guiu B, et al. Rotator cuff tears: value of 3.0T MRI. *J Radiol*. 2009;90(5 Pt 1):583-588.

55. de Jesus J, Parker L, Frangos A, et al. Accuracy of MRI, MR arthrography, and ultrasound in the diagnosis of rotator cuff tears: a meta-analysis. *Am J Roentgenol*. 2009;192(6):1701-1707.

56. Tirman PF, Bost FW, Steinbach LS, et al. MR arthrographic depiction of tears of the rotator cuff: benefit of abduction and external rotation of the arm. *Radiology*. 1994;192:851-856.

57. Gold G, Pappas G, Blemker S, et al. Abduction and external rotation in shoulder impingement: an open MR study on healthy volunteers—initial experience. *Radiology*. 2007;244:815-822.

58. Yen C, Chiou H, Chou Y, et al. Six surgery-correlated sonographic signs for rotator cuff tears: emphasis on partial-thickness tear. *Clin Imaging*. 2004;28(1):69-76.

59. Nakagawa S, Yoneda M, Hayashida K, et al. Greater tuberosity notch: an important indicator of articular-side partial rotator cuff tears in the shoulders of throwing athletes. *Am J Sports Med*. 2001;29(6):762-772.

60. Conway JE. The management of partial thickness rotator cuff tears in throwers. *Oper Tech Sports Med*. 2002;10:75-85.

61. Lo IK, Gonzalez M, Burkhart SS. The bubble sign: an arthroscopic indicator of an intratendinous rotator cuff tear. *Arthroscopy*. 2002;18:1029-1033.

62. Fukuda H, Hamada K, Nakajima T, Tomonaga A. Pathology and pathogenesis of the intratendinous tearing of the rotator cuff viewed from en bloc histologic sections. *Clin Orthop Relat Res*. 1994;(304):60-67.

63. Stetson WB, Ryu RKN, Bittar ES. Arthroscopic treatment of partial rotator cuff tears. *Oper Tech Sports Med*. 2004;12:135-148.

64. Ryu RK. Arthroscopic subacromial decompression: a clinical review. *Arthroscopy*. 1992;8(2):141-147.

65. Park JY, Yoo MJ, Kim MH. Comparison of surgical outcome between bursal and articular partial thickness rotator cuff tears. *Orthopedics*. 2003;26:387-390.

66. Reynolds SB, Dugas JR, Cain EL, McMichael CS, Andrews JR. Débridement of small partial-thickness rotator cuff tears in elite overhead throwers. *Clin Orthop Relat Res*. 2008;466(3):614-621.

67. Vitale MA, Arons RR, Hurwitz S, Ahmad CS, Levine WN. The rising incidence of acromioplasty. *J Bone Joint Surg Am*. 2010;92(9):1842-1850.

68. Weber SC. Arthroscopic débridement and acromioplasty versus mini-open repair in the treatment of significant partial thickness rotator cuff tears. *Arthroscopy*. 1999;15:126-131.

69. Liem D, Alci S, Dedy N, et al. Clinical and structural results of partial supraspinatus tears treated by subacromial decompression without repair. *Knee Surg Sports Traumatology Arthroscopy*. 2008;16(10):967-972.

70. Gonzalez-Lomas G, Kippe MA, Brown GD, et al. In situ transtendon repair outperforms tear completion and repair for partial articular-sided supraspinatus tendon tears. *J Shoulder Elbow Surg*. 2008;17(5):722-728.

71. Ide J, Maeda S, Takagi K. Arthroscopic transtendon repair of partial-thickness articular-side tears of the rotator cuff: anatomical and clinical study. *Am J Sports Med*. 2005;33(11):1672-1679.

72. Castagna A, Delle Rose G, Conti M, et al. Predictive factors of subtle residual shoulder symptoms after transtendinous arthroscopic cuff repair: a clinical study. *Am J Sports Med.* 2009;37(1):103-108.

73. Deutsch A. Arthroscopic repair of partial-thickness tears of the rotator cuff. *J Shoulder Elbow Surg.* 2007;16(2):193-201.

74. Kamath G, Galatz LM, Keener JD, Teefey S, Middleton W, Yamaguchi K. Tendon integrity and functional outcome after arthroscopic repair of high-grade partial-thickness supraspinatus tears. *J Bone Joint Surg Am.* 2009;91(5):1055-1062.

75. Mazoué, CG Andrews, JR. Repair of full-thickness rotator cuff tears in professional baseball players. *Am J Sports Med.* 2006;34:182-189.

Please see video on the accompanying Web site at
http://www.slackbooks.com/rotatorcuffvideos

CHAPTER 11

MANAGEMENT OF FULL-THICKNESS SUPRASPINATUS TEARS

Todd C. Moen, MD and William N. Levine, MD

Full-thickness tears of the supraspinatus tendon are a common problem in the shoulder, with an increasing prevalence with age. The clinical manifestations of supraspinatus tears are highly variable; some tears can be asymptomatic with little or no functional consequence for the patient, while others can be profoundly painful and debilitating. Therefore, multiple factors must be considered when evaluating a patient with a full-thickness supraspinatus tear. The patient's clinical history, physical examination, and imaging studies must all be considered when determining nonoperative or operative treatment. With appropriate indications and a well-executed plan, both nonoperative and operative management strategies can effectively relieve pain and restore optimal function to patients with full-thickness supraspinatus tears.

ANATOMY

Although the anatomy of the rotator cuff in general is discussed in a previous chapter, it is appropriate to review the relevant anatomy of the supraspinatus. The supraspinatus inserts onto the greater tuberosity footprint of the proximal humerus, specifically the superior facet and the superior half of the middle facet. Different studies have cited subtly differing dimensions for the footprint, but the approximate dimensions are 12 to 14 mm medial to lateral and 22 to 24 mm anterior to posterior.[1-6] These data are of critical importance and are the basis of anatomic repairs of supraspinatus tears.

HISTORY

The evaluation of any patient presenting with shoulder pain begins with a thorough history, physical examination, and appropriate imaging studies. Patients with symptomatic supraspinatus

Ma CB, Feeley BT, eds.
*Basic Principles and Operative Management
of the Rotator Cuff (pp 161-180)*
© 2012 SLACK Incorporated

tears typically complain of pain localized to the lateral aspect of the shoulder about the deltoid and subacromial space. The acuity of onset, duration, and severity of the pain can be highly variable. Certain activities, specifically overhead activities, may be cited as exacerbating factors. Patients may also complain of weakness, most pronounced with overhead activities, and/or varying losses in function in addition to pain.

When a supraspinatus tear is suspected, the surgeon must further obtain specific information that will aid in the therapeutic decision making for the patient. Tear acuity determination is critically important as an acute traumatic tear is often treated with early surgery more so than a chronic, degenerative tear. In the case of an isolated traumatic event, such as a fall or subluxation/dislocation event, the determination between acute and chronic is typically straightforward. However, when a patient has a more insidious onset of symptoms, with no specific inciting event, the age of the tear is more difficult to determine. Nevertheless, clues such as a dramatic increase in pain or an abrupt decompensation in function can help. Another critical component of a patient's history is age, as the incidence and size of rotator cuff tears increase with age.[7-11] Additionally, rotator cuff repair has been shown to be more effective when performed in younger patients. However, it is determining the patient's physiologic age, more so than true chronological age, that is critical.[12] A patient's physiologic age is hard to explicitly define; however, a patient's general health, occupation, and preferred activities can aid in delineating young versus old. For example, a 65-year-old with no medical problems who plays tennis 4 times per week should be considered younger than an inactive 50-year-old with type II diabetes mellitus, hypertension, and hypercholesterolemia. Physiologic age is an important aspect of a patient's history to obtain, as a more aggressive approach to the treatment of rotator cuff tears has been advocated in younger patients, as surgical repair may allow for earlier return to activities.[13,14]

PHYSICAL EXAMINATION

The physical examination of the shoulder should be tailored to the individual patient based on the patient's history. For the patient with a suspected rotator cuff tear, it is critical to inspect the shoulder girdle, palpate the bony and soft tissue prominences, measure the patient's active and passive range of motion, test the strength and integrity of the cuff, and evaluate for evidence of subacromial impingement. A thorough physical exam review has been described in Chapter 5, but relevant findings are repeated here.

All examinations of the shoulder should begin with inspection of the shoulder girdle. Muscular atrophy and asymmetry are typically suggestive of a chronic tear, while previous surgical scars are obviously indicative of prior operative intervention. Particular attention should be given to asymmetry in the supraspinatus and infraspinatus fossa as a marker for chronic cuff atrophy. The shoulder is then palpated for points of tenderness, paying particular attention to tenderness at the acromioclavicular (AC) joint, as this suggests symptomatic AC pathology. Next, upright active range of motion (forward elevation, external rotation with the elbow at the side, external rotation in 90 degrees of abduction, and internal rotation behind the back) is assessed. Both shoulders should be evaluated in all cases, even though an asymptomatic tear may be present. Inability to fully actively forward elevate and/or externally rotate the shoulder can be suggestive of a rotator cuff tear. If there are any deficits in range of motion, the patient's passive range of motion should then be re-examined with the patient lying supine. A difference between upright and supine range of motion can help discern between patient guarding due to pain and adhesive capsulitis. range of motion that is equally diminished when the patient is upright and supine is suggestive of adhesive capsulitis.

The most critical portion of the examination is determinating the patient's strength and cuff integrity. Examination of rotator cuff strength can be clouded by a patient's lack of effort due to shoulder pain; nevertheless, subtle differences in strength can usually be detected. Supraspinatus strength is tested by resisted forward elevation to 90 degrees in the plane of the scapula. The infraspinatus is tested by resisted external rotation with the patient's arm at the side, in neutral rotation, with the elbow flexed to 90 degrees. The subscapularis can be tested by resisted internal rotation with the patient's arm at his or her side, in neutral rotation, with the elbow flexed to 90 degrees. The subscapularis can also be tested by the lift-off test or belly-press test.[15,16] When weakness is demonstrated, an examiner can gain a better understanding of the extent of the tear based on lag signs.[17,18] A positive external or internal rotation lag sign indicates a tear of the infraspinatus or subscapularis, respectively. Typically, in a patient with an isolated supraspinatus tear, lag signs will be negative.

Finally, the patient should be examined for evidence of subacromial impingement. Neer described the impingement sign in 1972[19] as pain localized to the anterolateral subacromial region with forward elevation.[20] Hawkins described a test in which the shoulder is forward-flexed to 90 degrees with the elbow flexed and then internally rotated; pain with this maneuver is considered a positive test.[21] The Jobe test is a test in which the shoulder is forward elevated to 90 degrees in the plane of the scapula, internally rotated, and tested against resistance. Pain or weakness with this test is considered positive and suggestive of rotator cuff pathology and/or impingement.[22] The utility of these tests can be improved with the use of selective subacromial injections with local anesthetic and/or corticosteroid. Relief of pain and reversal of provocative maneuvers (Neer, Hawkins, and Jobe signs) in subacromial testing can help confirm and strengthen the certainty of the diagnosis of subacromial impingement.

IMAGING

With a history and physical examination suggestive of a supraspinatus cuff tear, the final components of the evaluation to confirm the diagnosis are imaging studies. The standard shoulder trauma series should be obtained including true anteroposterior (AP), scapular outlet, and axillary views. The anatomy of the subacromial space and acromial morphology has been associated with subacromial impingement and disorders of the rotator cuff. The AP and scapular outlet views should be scrutinized for acromial spurs, which may impinge on the rotator cuff. Additionally, the morphology of the acromion should be determined. Bigliani described the acromion as being of 3 types: type 1—flat, type 2—curved, and type 3—hooked; with types 2 and 3 being associated with subacromial impingement, predisposing a patient to rotator cuff pathology. The chronicity of rotator cuff tears has been shown to adversely affect bone quality at the rotator cuff footprint[23]; this osteopenia can adversely affect suture anchor fixation and should be noted prior to proceeding to the operating room for rotator cuff repair.

Although x-rays are indispensable in the evaluation of the shoulder, magnetic resonance imaging (MRI) is the imaging study of choice, given its ability to image subtle soft tissue and osseous abnormalities not seen on plain films.[24] When evaluating an MRI of the shoulder, it is best to approach the study systematically[25] and not rely on the radiologist's report; the surgeon has the unique perspective of being able to bring together the patient's history, physical exam, and imaging findings to make the most accurate diagnosis. Coronal T2 images are the most effective for evaluating supraspinatus pathology. Rotator cuff disease exists as a spectrum, ranging from tendinopathy to partial-thickness fraying and ending with a full-thickness tear.[26-28] A full-thickness tear of the supraspinatus appears as a complete discontinuity of the tendon to the footprint, extending from inferior to superior (Figure 11-1). This can be visualized on T1 images, but may be more readily apparent on T2 images, in which fluid is visualized in the gap between the tendon and footprint, extending into the subacromial space. The size of the tear can be estimated on coronal imaging based on the number of image cuts in which the tear appears; for example, assuming an MRI protocol of 5-mm cuts, a tear that appears in 3 consecutive images can be estimated to be 1.5 cm in size. Additionally, coronal images allow visualization of the degree of retraction of the tear. Sagittal images are valuable for the localization of the tear in the AP direction, as well as quantification of

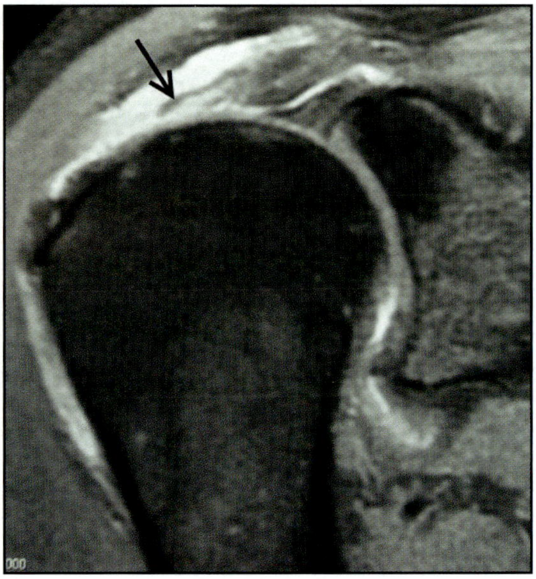

Figure 11-1. Fifty-three-year-old woman with rheumatic heart disease with a right shoulder full-thickness supraspinatus tear. T2 coronal MRI demonstrating full-thickness supraspinatus tear (arrow) with retraction to the mid-humeral level. (Courtesy of Columbia Center for Shoulder, Elbow and Sports Medicine.)

the size of the tear. Rotator cuff muscular atrophy and fatty infiltration should be determined on sagittal images. Goutallier et al reported a classification system describing fatty atrophy of the rotator cuff muscles.[29] This information is valuable as an increasing degree of fatty atrophy portends a poor prognosis regarding the ability of the rotator cuff repair to heal. Anterior supraspinatus tears can be associated with upper border subscapularis tears, which can easily be overlooked.[30] Finally, all MRI images should be evaluated for any associated shoulder pathology. For example, bone edema of the AC joint recognized on T2 images in a patient with a symptomatic AC joint should generate consideration to performing a distal clavicle excision.[31] Taken together, the information from all 3 imaging planes from an MRI of the shoulder can aid the surgeon in discerning the extent, location, size, amount of retraction, and degree of atrophy associated with a tear of the supraspinatus, as well as any associated pathology; this information is critical in determining the appropriate management of the tear, as well as the surgical management of any associated pathology.

TEAR CLASSIFICATION

Rotator cuff tears are classified as partial- and full-thickness tears and are further classified by tear size and degree of retraction. Most of this information is gained preoperatively with MRI. Tear size is measured in the AP direction (best seen on sagittal MRI evaluation), and tears are divided into small (less than 1 cm), medium (1 to 3 cm), large (3 to 5 cm), and massive (more than 5 cm) tears. By definition, a large and massive rotator cuff tear consists of a 2-tendon tear. Despite this classification system, most surgeons use the term *massive tear* to convey a tear with significant medial retraction, muscle atrophy, and fatty infiltration. Medial retraction is identified and characterized by coronal MRI. The degree of retraction is important as it helps the surgeon determine if a repair is possible. However, using techniques such as interval slides and margin convergence, many "irreparable" tears are actually repairable.

Further classification of rotator cuff tears is based primarily on the work of Burkhart. Tears are classified into crescent, U-shaped, L-shaped, and massive retracted tears. Crescent-shaped tears are small tears that have no retraction or minimal retraction of the tendon from the footprint (Figure 11-2). These tears are often adequately fixed with a single anchor or small transosseous-equivalent technique. These are the easiest to fix and the most common tear encountered by most orthopedic surgeons. Because these tears are small and not retracted, the outcomes of these repairs are usually very good.

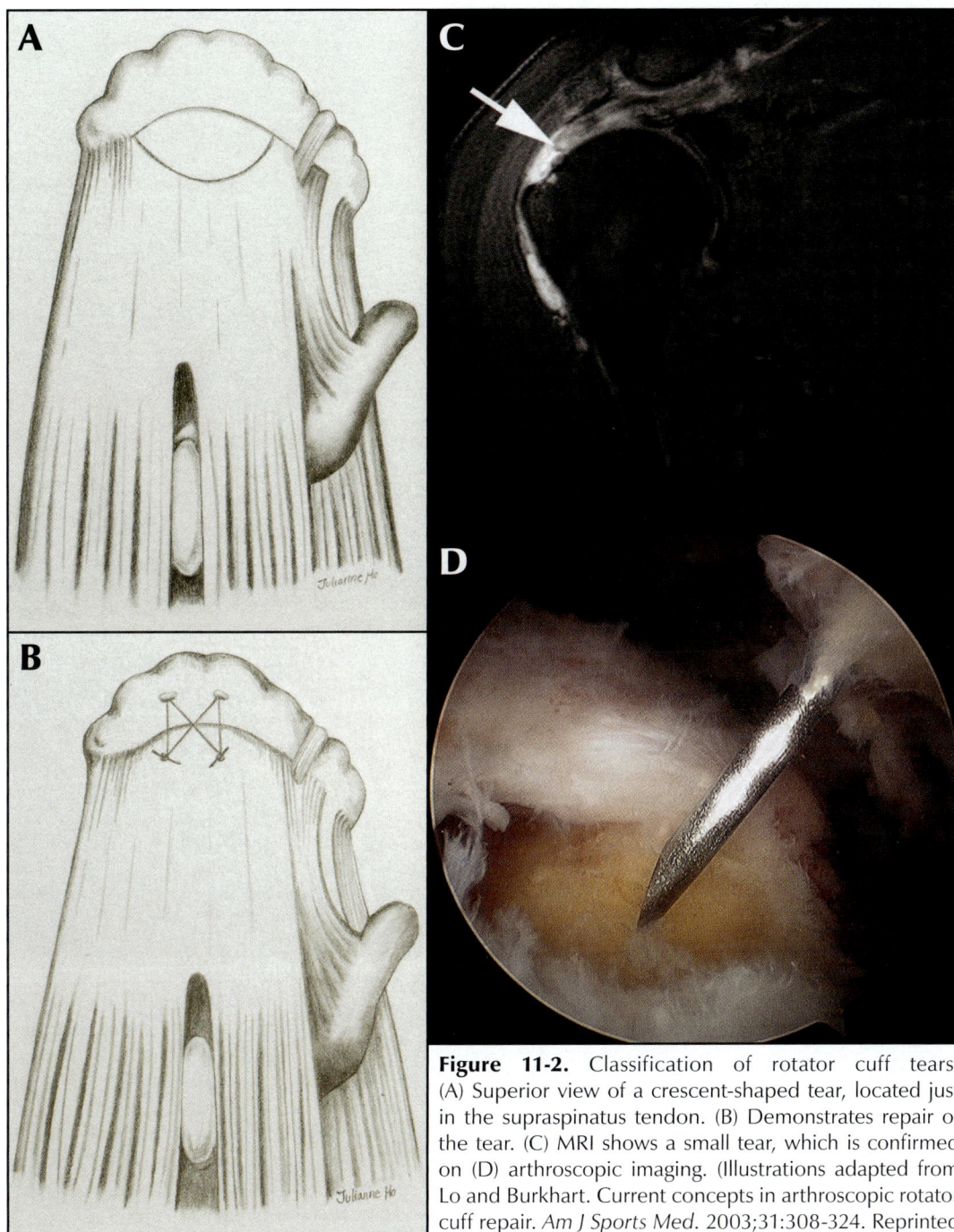

Figure 11-2. Classification of rotator cuff tears. (A) Superior view of a crescent-shaped tear, located just in the supraspinatus tendon. (B) Demonstrates repair of the tear. (C) MRI shows a small tear, which is confirmed on (D) arthroscopic imaging. (Illustrations adapted from Lo and Burkhart. Current concepts in arthroscopic rotator cuff repair. *Am J Sports Med.* 2003;31:308-324. Reprinted with permission of Julianne Ho.)

U-shaped tears are usually larger tears that encompass 2 tendons (Figure 11-3), but can sometimes be very narrow isolated supraspinatus tears. These tears typically demonstrate considerable retraction on the sagittal MRI through the supraspinatus, but often the leading edge of the supraspinatus remains attached. Identification of this tear pattern is critical because attempting to medially mobilize and repair the apex of the tear to the greater tuberosity can result in overwhelming tensile stresses in the middle of the repaired rotator cuff tendon, which can lead to failure of the repair.

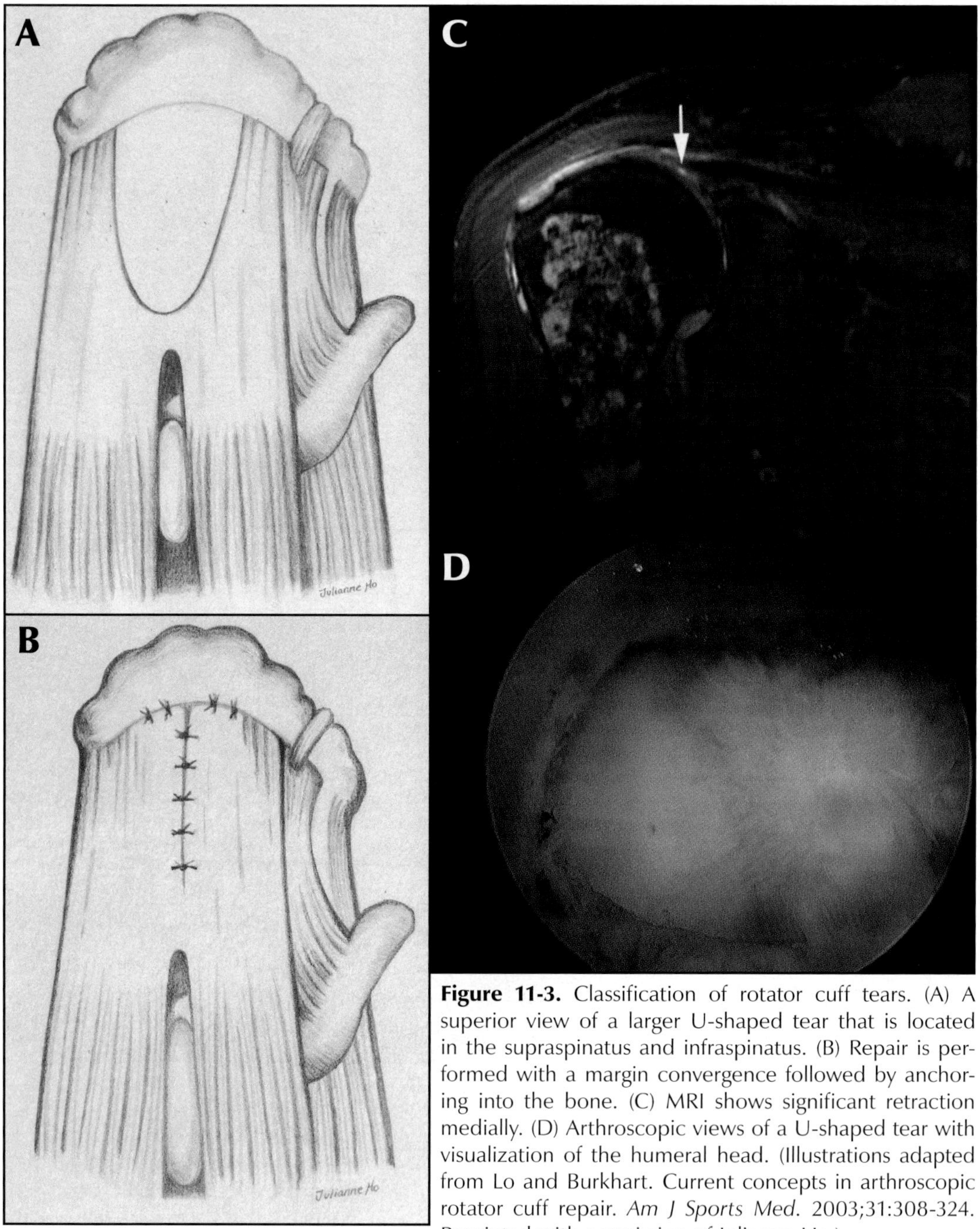

Figure 11-3. Classification of rotator cuff tears. (A) A superior view of a larger U-shaped tear that is located in the supraspinatus and infraspinatus. (B) Repair is performed with a margin convergence followed by anchoring into the bone. (C) MRI shows significant retraction medially. (D) Arthroscopic views of a U-shaped tear with visualization of the humeral head. (Illustrations adapted from Lo and Burkhart. Current concepts in arthroscopic rotator cuff repair. *Am J Sports Med.* 2003;31:308-324. Reprinted with permission of Julianne Ho.)

The preferred technique to repair these tears is to perform a side-to-side repair, or margin convergence, first, and then secure the tendon to bone with anchors into the greater tuberosity. The technique of margin convergence allows the repair of "irreparable" tears and decreases the strain at the repair site. Arthroscopic repair of these tears is usually performed easier than if the repair was performed open.

The L-shaped tears are similar to U-shaped tears. However, one of the leaves (usually the posterior leaf) is more mobile than the other leaf and can be easily brought to the greater tuberosity (Figure 11-4). For L-shaped tears, side-to-side suturing is first performed along the longitudinal

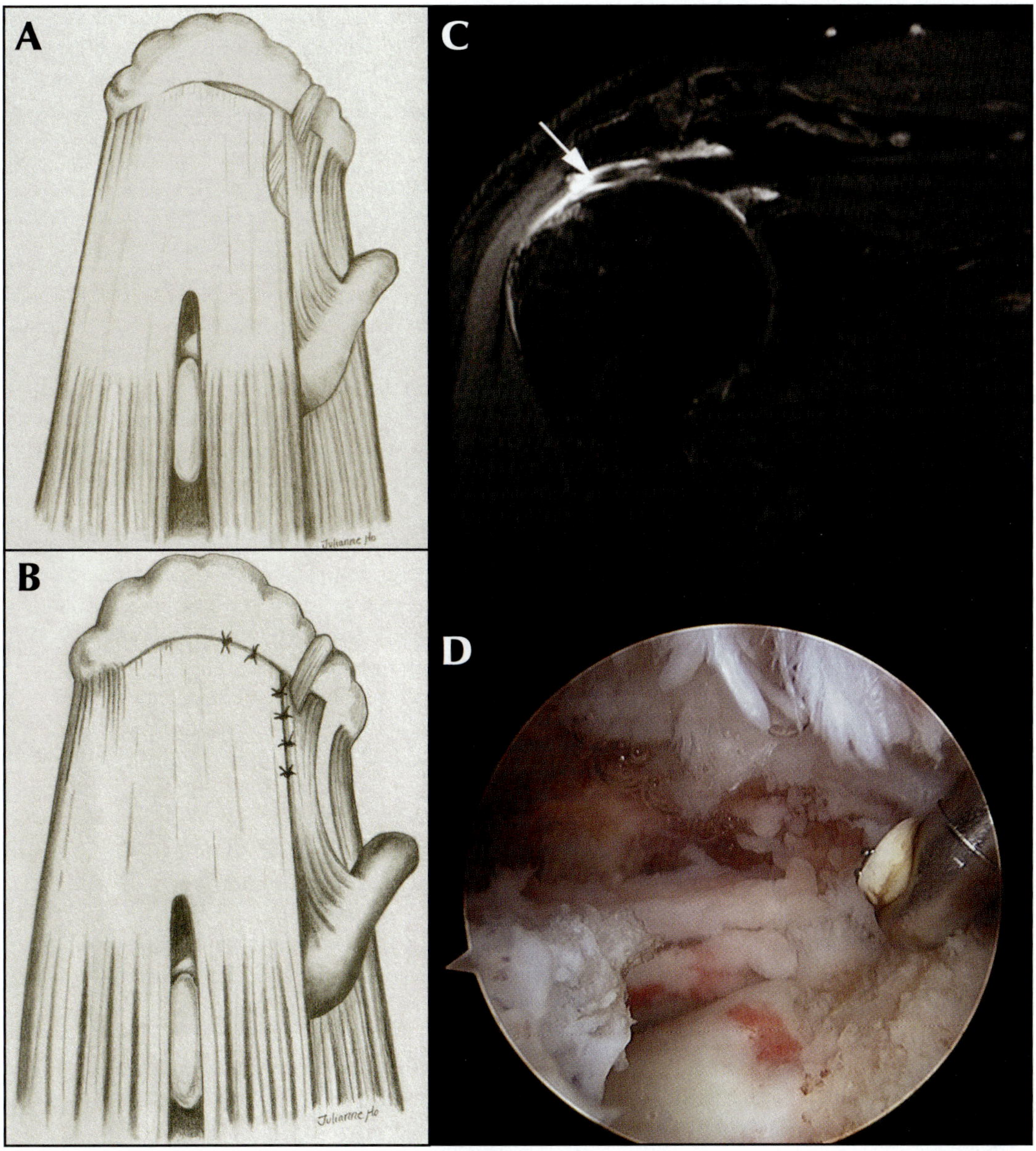

Figure 11-4. Classification of rotator cuff tears. (A) A superior view of an anterior-based L-shaped tear. (B) These are repaired based on the mobility of the leafs of the rotator cuff tendon. (C) MRI of an L-shaped tear shows anterior retraction of the supraspinatus. (D) Arthroscopic imaging demonstrates a tear of the anterior supraspinatus with medial retraction of the anterior border. Repair is performed with margin convergence and an anchor. (Illustrations adapted from Lo and Burkhart. Current concepts in arthroscopic rotator cuff repair. *Am J Sports Med.* 2003;31:308-324. Reprinted with permission of Julianne Ho.)

split similar to those performed for U-shaped tears. These sutures often are in the rotator interval to secure the leading edge of the supraspinatus back to its anatomic location. The anchor is then placed in the leading corner, and the repair is secured down to bone.

Massive retracted tears are those tears that consist of 2-tendon tears that have significant medial retraction. Although these tears are uncommon, it is important to recognize these tears preoperatively in order to determine if a repair is feasible and prepare the patient accordingly for a possible open procedure. It is particularly important in these patients to determine the degree of muscle atrophy and fatty infiltration, as this may help determine the predicted outcome in these cases should a repair be attempted. If repair is to be attempted, advanced techniques such as those described in Chapter 20, such as anterior and posterior interval slides, are used. In some cases, it may be preferable to perform a reverse shoulder arthroplasty if the muscle quality precludes an acceptable outcome.

SURGICAL INDICATIONS

After a diagnosis of a full-thickness rotator cuff tear has been made based on history, physical examination, and imaging, the surgeon must decide how to manage this tear. The specific indications for nonoperative and operative treatment of rotator cuff tears is a source of controversy among orthopedic surgeons, due largely to the imprecisely characterized natural history of rotator cuff tears, their propagation, and their effect on symptoms and function in patients. Nevertheless, studies on the natural history of rotator cuff tears and clinical results following nonoperative and operative treatment have delineated broad principles of how to approach the management of rotator cuff tears.[12,32]

Whether rotator cuff tears arise as a result of an extrinsic or intrinsic degenerative process remains highly controversial; however, it is clear that degeneration of the rotator cuff is an expected phenomenon of normal aging.[10,11,33,34] A rotator cuff tear does not necessarily cause pain and/or weakness, and the specific factors that relate to a rotator cuff becoming symptomatic remain poorly defined. However, asymptomatic rotator cuff tears are likely to produce symptoms in due time.[11] Additionally, rotator cuff tears tend to progress in size with aging.[7,9-11,35] As a rotator cuff tear increases in size, the cuff musculature progressively atrophies and becomes infiltrated with fat.[29,36] The amount of atrophy is inversely related to the cuff's ability to heal after operative repair.[29,36] If left untreated for a long period of time, a rotator cuff tear may evolve from an isolated damaged tendon to florid joint degeneration and cuff tear arthropathy.[37]

The indications for surgery are most straightforward in the case of an acute injury. A rotator cuff tear caused by a fall or glenohumeral dislocation is best treated with prompt repair. When a tear is more chronic and degenerative in nature, the indications are based on the patient's symptoms. For patients who have symptomatic rotator cuff tears that fail nonoperative management (4 to 6 months of physical therapy, nonsteroidal anti-inflammatory drugs, activity modification, cortisone injections), surgical intervention is often warranted.

Clinical series have shown that the younger the patient's age, the more successful the outcomes of repair of the rotator cuff, thus encouraging operative repair of rotator cuff tears in young patients.[38-41] Regardless, a patient's expectations should be assessed, and the patient should be counseled on the potential outcomes given his or her specific situation.

SURGICAL TECHNIQUE

The optimal technique for rotator cuff repair remains controversial. Although open rotator cuff was historically considered the "gold standard," excellent pain relief and functional improvements have been reported to support open, mini-open, and arthroscopic rotator cuff repairs. Our preference, however, is to repair full-thickness supraspinatus tears arthroscopically. The current state-of-the-art techniques of arthroscopic repair allow the surgeon to reliably and reproducibly identify tear configuration, build biomechanically durable repair constructs to allow for tendon-to-bone healing, and address concomitant shoulder pathology while avoiding potential morbidity of open repair (deltoid dehiscence).

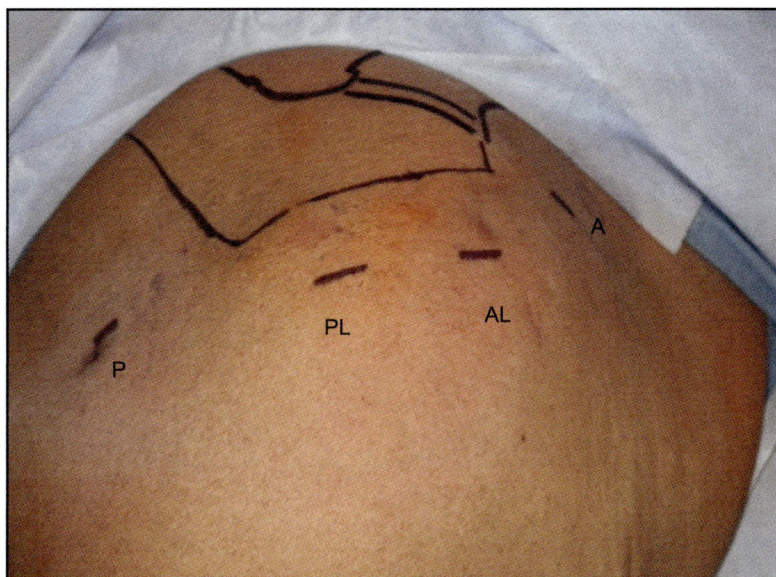

Figure 11-5. Same patient from Figure 11-1. Right shoulder in the beach chair position (AL, anterolateral subacromial portal; PL, posterolateral subacromial portal; A, anterior portal; P, posterior portal). (Courtesy of Columbia Center for Shoulder, Elbow and Sports Medicine.)

Set-Up and Portal Placement

We prefer regional anesthesia with an interscalene block for most patients. The patient is positioned in a modified beach chair position using a specifically designed operating table. Beginning at the medial clavicle and base of the cervical spine, the patient's entire upper extremity is prepped and draped free to allow access to the entire shoulder. A commercially available arm positioner (Spider Limb Positioner, Tenet Medical Engineering, Calgary, Canada) is used to facilitate intraoperative positioning of the shoulder.

The relevant osseous anatomy and planned portals are outlined with a marking pen (Figure 11-5). Standard posterior, lateral, and anterior portals are used. However, small modifications in portal placement can facilitate the performance of the operation dependent on the preoperative and intraoperative findings. The standard posterior portal is typically placed 2 cm inferior and 1 cm medial to the posterolateral border of the acromion. A standard anterior portal can be made under direct visualization with a spinal needle to localize using an outside-in technique. If it is anticipated that a distal clavicle excision is to be performed, the anterior portal is moved more proximal to afford easier access to the AC joint.

A lateral working portal is made for work in the subacromial space. The lateral working portal should be placed to allow for optimal suture passing and cuff manipulation, as well as for lateral row anchor fixation if this technique is to be used. The standard lateral working portal is placed 1 to 2 cm lateral to the lateral border of the acromion, in line with the junction of the anterior one-third and posterior two-thirds of the acromion. This placement should allow for adequate subacromial work, cuff manipulation, suture passing, and repair of a typical supraspinatus tear. If a larger tear is encountered, we prefer 2 lateral working portals—an anterolateral working portal and a posterolateral viewing portal (Figure 11-6). In this configuration, the anterolateral portal is modified to be just anterior to the standard lateral working portal, and the posterolateral portal is made just posterior to the junction of the anterior two-thirds and posterior one-third of the acromion.

Diagnostic Glenohumeral Arthroscopy

Diagnostic shoulder arthroscopy is started from the posterior portal. An anterior working portal is established, and a 7.0-mm cannula is introduced into the glenohumeral joint. Systematic diagnostic arthroscopy is thoroughly performed, noting any intra-articular pathology. Specific attention

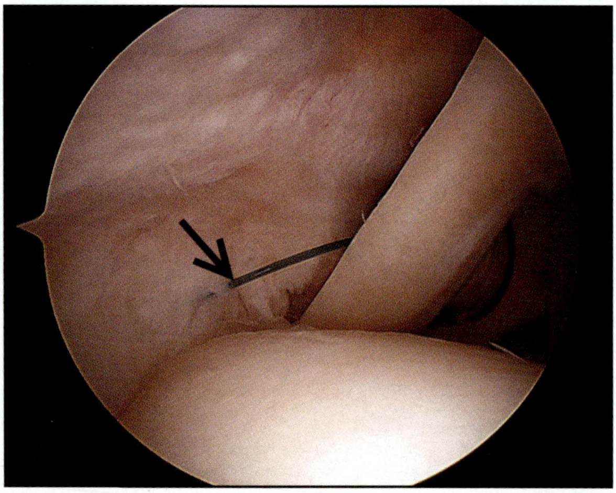

Figure 11-6. Left shoulder in the beach chair position. Arrow demonstrates a suture percutaneously placed through the partial-thickness tear and retrieved out the anterior portal. (Courtesy of Columbia Center for Shoulder, Elbow and Sports Medicine.)

is given to associated biceps tendon pathology (tenosynovitis, partial tears, near-complete tears), labral tears, and rotator cuff tears. Biceps tendon management will be discussed in detail elsewhere, but we prefer an open subpectoral biceps tenodesis for tendons that require surgical treatment. We rarely perform concurrent labral repairs in patients primarily being managed with rotator cuff tears due to the concern of increased stiffness and poorer patient outcomes.

Partial-Thickness Tears

If a partial-thickness tear is identified, a marking suture is placed to facilitate identification from the subacromial space. A spinal needle is percutaneously placed just adjacent to the anterolateral acromion, and a 1-0 suture is passed through the spinal needle into the glenohumeral joint. The marking suture is then retrieved via the anterior portal (Figure 11-7). Evaluation from the subacromial space will then determine if the tear communicates with the bursal surface.

Full-Thickness Tears

Determination of full-thickness tears from the glenohumeral joint is critical. An assessment of the size of the tear, tendon retraction, and possible adhesions are all performed from the glenohumeral joint (Figure 11-7A). The surgeon should also identify synovitis and ablate this with cautery to further assist in pain relief for the patient.

Diagnostic and Therapeutic Subacromial Arthroscopy

The arthroscope is then introduced into the subacromial space. A midlateral or anterolateral working portal is established, dependent on the features described above. A 5.5-mm full-radius shaver is then introduced into the subacromial space, and a thorough bursectomy is performed.

Rotator Cuff Tear Configuration Identification

With a preliminary bursectomy performed, it is critical to identify the rotator cuff and localize any tear(s). The cuff can be dynamically evaluated by internally and externally rotating the shoulder to improve visualization of the posterior and anterior rotator cuff, respectively. The marking suture, if placed, can also assist in identification and localization of the tear, and further bursectomy can be performed to improve visualization. When the tear has been localized, it is critical to appreciate the configuration of the tear by viewing from the posterior and the anterolateral portals (Figures 11-7B and C).

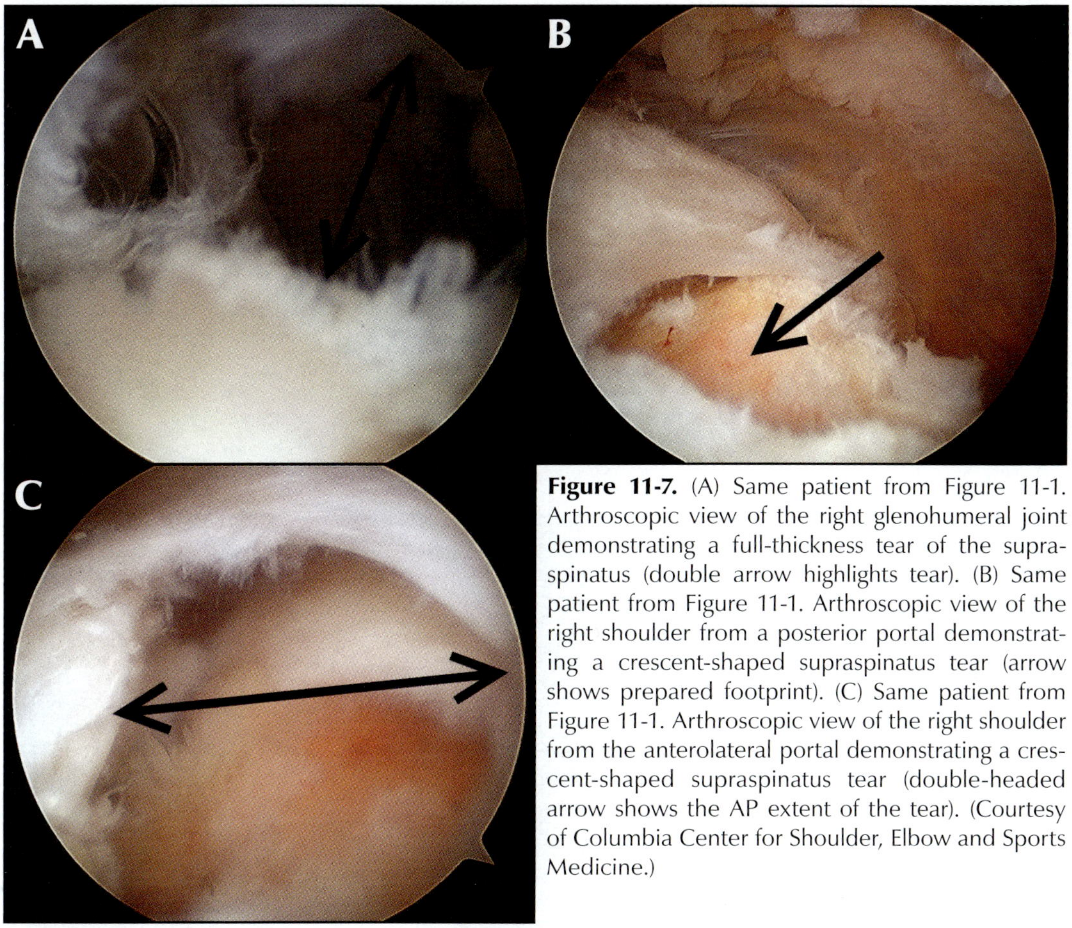

Figure 11-7. (A) Same patient from Figure 11-1. Arthroscopic view of the right glenohumeral joint demonstrating a full-thickness tear of the supraspinatus (double arrow highlights tear). (B) Same patient from Figure 11-1. Arthroscopic view of the right shoulder from a posterior portal demonstrating a crescent-shaped supraspinatus tear (arrow shows prepared footprint). (C) Same patient from Figure 11-1. Arthroscopic view of the right shoulder from the anterolateral portal demonstrating a crescent-shaped supraspinatus tear (double-headed arrow shows the AP extent of the tear). (Courtesy of Columbia Center for Shoulder, Elbow and Sports Medicine.)

With larger tears, we then proceed to make an additional posterolateral portal. If the tear is smaller, however, the additional posterolateral portal is typically not necessary. Any remaining bursa in the subacromial space and subdeltoid recess is resected with the shaver and radiofrequency device with care being taken to avoid damage to the subdeltoid fascia.

We prefer a double-row suture bridge reconstruction for most tears as it is reproducible, recreates the anatomy of the rotator cuff footprint, and has favorable biomechanical properties. The steps that we use for this transosseous-equivalent technique are 1) cuff and footprint preparation; 2) medial row anchor placement; 3) suture passage; 4) suture tying; and 5) lateral row anchor placement with suture bridge configuration.

Cuff and Footprint Preparation

While viewing from the posterior portal, a 5.5-mm full-radius shaver is introduced into the subacromial space. Any devitalized cuff tissue at the tear edge is gently débrided to a margin of healthy cuff tissue. The cuff footprint is identified, and the cortical bone of the exposed greater tuberosity is gently débrided (see Figure 11-7B). A formal trough is not made, however. If the rotator cuff has any adhesions (subacromial, glenohumeral, side to side), then these need to be released at this time, and cuff mobility is assessed. Tension-free anatomic mobilization must be assured prior to beginning the repair.

Figure 11-8. Same patient from Figure 11-1. Arthroscopic view of the right shoulder from the posterolateral portal showing placement of a spinal needle to place the anchor (AC, articular cartilage; AL, anterolateral cannula). (Courtesy of Columbia Center for Shoulder, Elbow and Sports Medicine.)

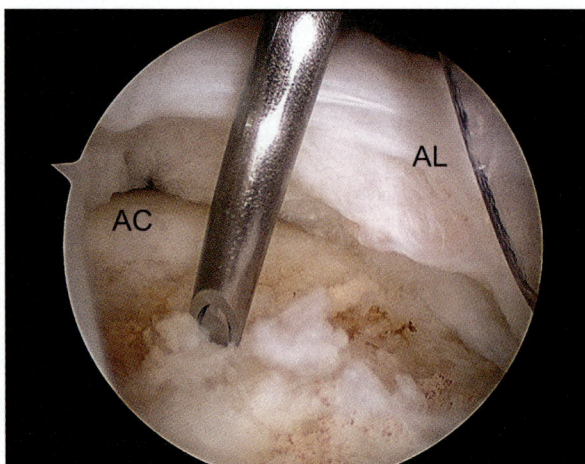

Figure 11-9. Same patient from Figure 11-1. Arthroscopic view of the right shoulder demonstrating using a scalpel in the same angle as the spinal needle to introduce the anchor. (Courtesy of Columbia Center for Shoulder, Elbow and Sports Medicine.)

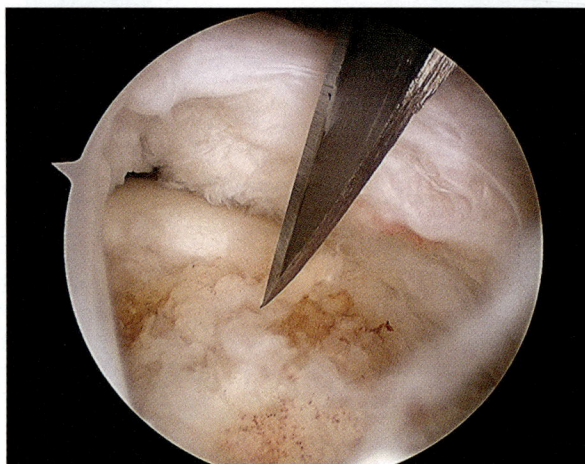

Medial Row Suture Anchor Placement

First, the correct position for percutaneous medial row suture anchor placement is determined with a spinal needle. This is typically done off the anterolateral acromion and can be made either viewing from the posterior or anterolateral cannula. The needle is manipulated and repositioned as necessary to achieve the preferred position and trajectory for placement in the medial footprint (Figure 11-8). Using the same trajectory as the spinal needle, a small stab incision using an 11 blade scalpel is made just lateral to the lateral border of the acromion (Figure 11-9). Through this stab incision, the awl for the suture anchor is introduced into the subacromial space. The guide hole for the anchor is then made with an awl at the junction of the articular cartilage and the bony footprint. The suture anchor is then placed into the hole to the appropriate depth (Figure 11-10). This process is then repeated with the placement of a second suture anchor (for large and massive tears, a third medial row anchor may be necessary). Ideally, the same incision used for the first anchor can be used for placement of the second anchor. However, if necessary for placement of the second anchor, a second percutaneous incision can be used.

We use an anchor that has 2 different color sutures to facilitate suture management (Figure 11-11). At this point, we remove the striped black-and-white suture from the anteromedial anchor and the blue suture from the posteromedial anchor (alternatively, these sutures can be used for additional medial row fixation if desired). Furthermore, the sutures from both anchors are left in the percutaneous incision and are not shuttled into the cannulae to avoid suture management

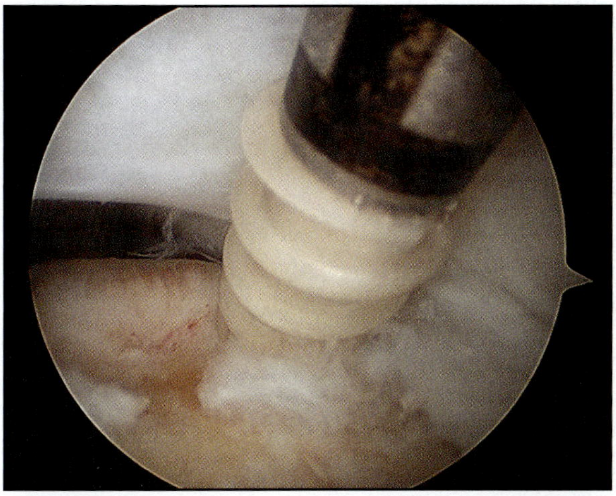

Figure 11-10. Same patient from Figure 11-1. Arthroscopic view of the right shoulder from the posterolateral portal showing placement of the anteromedial suture anchor. (Courtesy of Columbia Center for Shoulder, Elbow and Sports Medicine.)

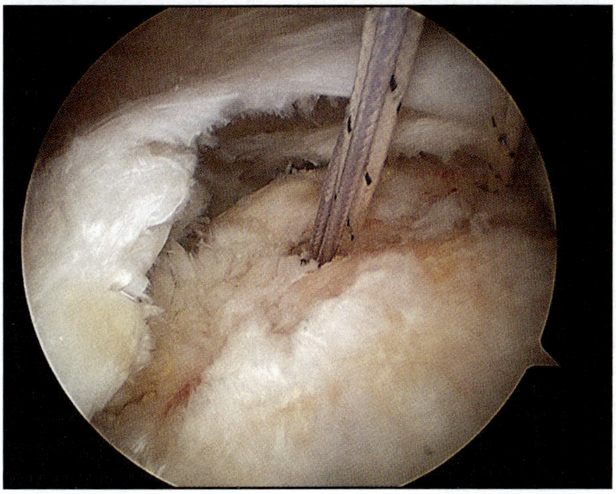

Figure 11-11. Same patient from Figure 11-1. Arthroscopic view of the right shoulder from the anterolateral portal after placement of anteromedial and posteromedial suture anchors. (Courtesy of Columbia Center for Shoulder, Elbow and Sports Medicine.)

issues. When placing the medial row anchors, always keep in mind where they are being placed to minimize the likelihood of developing a dog-ear. Viewing from the posterolateral portal is helpful to identify where the 4 anchors will ultimately go (2 medial row and 2 lateral row).

Suture Passage and Management

Suture passage and management are critically important, and adherence to the following steps will facilitate these steps in the procedure. First, plan out suture passing to maximize footprint restoration and to minimize dog-ear formation. Knowledge of the footprint anatomy helps to determine where the medial row sutures will be placed. Sutures can either be passed from the anterolateral portal with an antegrade device or from Neviaser's portal with a retrograde device. Given that the typical medial-lateral supraspinatus insertion is 14 to 16 mm, many commercially available devices will deliver the suture at this level. We prefer to use a lateral-based device such as a Scorpion (Arthrex, Naples, FL) or an RP 360 (Stryker, Mahwah, NJ).

First, a blue suture from the anteromedial anchor is retrieved out the anterolateral cannula and loaded into the suture passer. Insert the loaded passer into the subacromial space, grasp the rotator cuff in the desired location of the first stitch of the repair, and pass the blue suture through the rotator cuff (Figure 11-12). From the anterior portal, insert a suture-grasping tool, and shuttle the suture out through the anterior cannula. This process is then repeated using the second blue suture, passing it in a mattress-type fashion (Figure 11-13). A second mattress suture configuration

Figure 11-12. Same patient from Figure 11-1. Arthroscopic view of the right shoulder from the anterolateral portal after passing of the first blue suture from the anteromedial anchor. (Courtesy of Columbia Center for Shoulder, Elbow and Sports Medicine.)

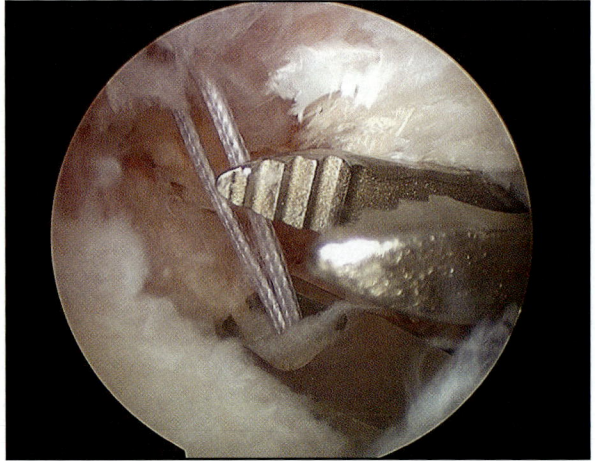

Figure 11-13. Same patient from Figure 11-1. Arthroscopic view of the right shoulder from the anterolateral portal after placement of both blue sutures in mattress fashion from the anteromedial anchor. (Courtesy of Columbia Center for Shoulder, Elbow and Sports Medicine.)

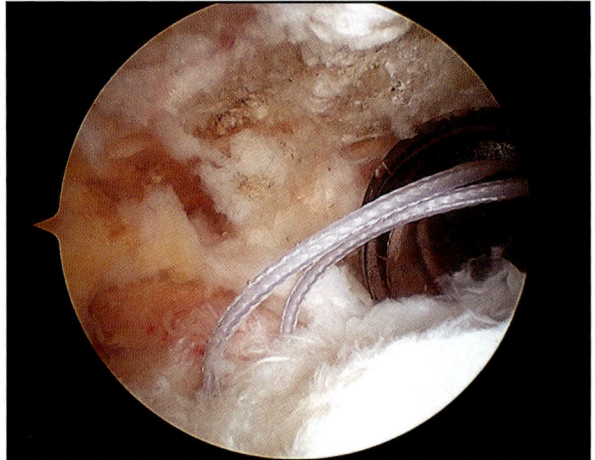

Figure 11-14. Same patient from Figure 11-1. Arthroscopic view of the right shoulder from the posterior portal after passage of the white and black sutures from the posteromedial anchor. (Courtesy of Columbia Center for Shoulder, Elbow and Sports Medicine.)

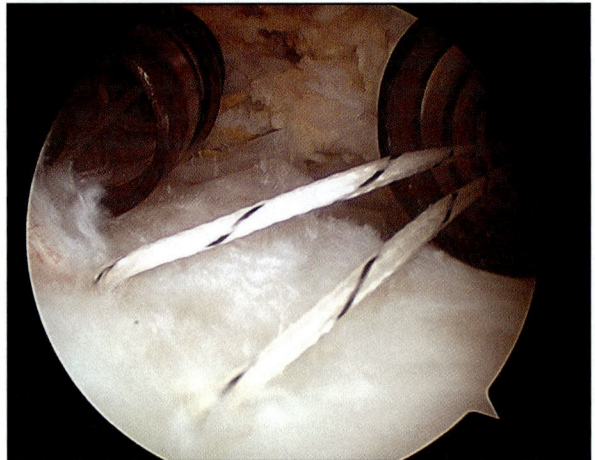

is placed using the white and black striped sutures from the posterior anchor (Figure 11-14). For a tear of this size, typically one mattress stitch for each anchor is all that is required. The additional suture pair in each medial row anchor can be used to augment the repair construct depending on the tear configuration and required construct, although we typically remove it as demonstrated in this case.

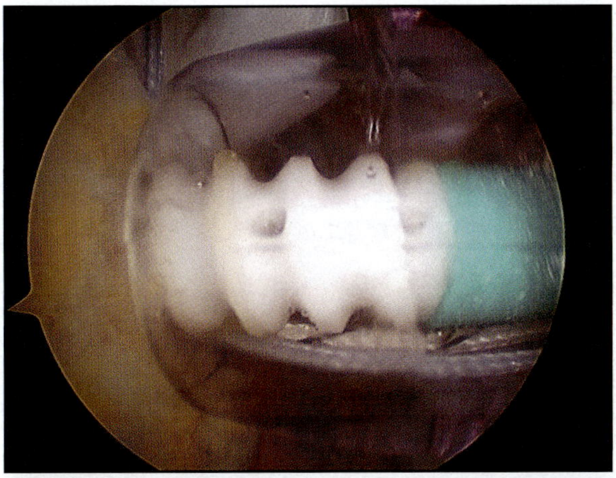

Figure 11-15. Same patient from Figure 11-1. Arthroscopic view of the right shoulder from the posterior portal showing lateral row anchor ready for insertion. (Courtesy of Columbia Center for Shoulder, Elbow and Sports Medicine.)

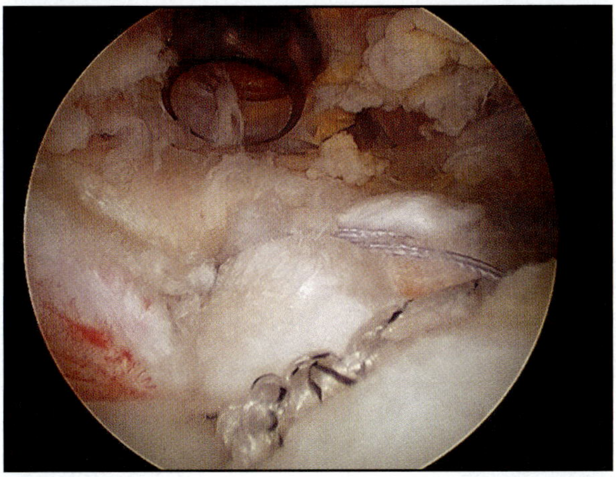

Figure 11-16. Same patient from Figure 11-1. Arthroscopic view of the right shoulder from the posterior portal showing completed double-row suture bridge rotator cuff repair. (Courtesy of Columbia Center for Shoulder, Elbow and Sports Medicine.)

Knot Tying

The next step is arthroscopic knot tying. Using a posterior viewing portal, the anteromedial anchor blue sutures are retrieved out the anterolateral portal. An arthroscopic knot of the surgeon's choice is then tied. Although there are a multitude of arthroscopic knots described, we prefer a simple knot consisting of 2 half hitches thrown in the same direction followed by 4 alternating half hitches. With the last half hitch, the post is flipped to enhance knot security. For our repair construct, the sutures are not cut, as they will be used in the lateral fixation.

Lateral Row Anchors/Fixation

The final step in our arthroscopic repair is the placement of lateral cuff fixation. Our device of choice is the SwivelLock (Arthrex). To use this anchor, a single suture strand from both the anterior and posterior mattress stitch is shuttled to the lateral anchor. The lateral cannula is then directed to the proximal lateral aspect of the proximal humerus to the location of lateral anchor placement. This location had previously been gently débrided of bursal tissue. The entry awl is then used to create the entry hole, and then the SwivelLock is inserted into the pilot hole as the appropriate tension is drawn on the sutures from the medial row (Figure 11-15). The SwivelLock is then secured in the pilot hole, and the insertion device is removed. The suture strands are then cut using an arthroscopic knot cutter. This process is repeated using the remaining 2 suture strands from the anterior and posterior anchors. This completes the repair of the rotator cuff (Figures 11-16 and 11-17).

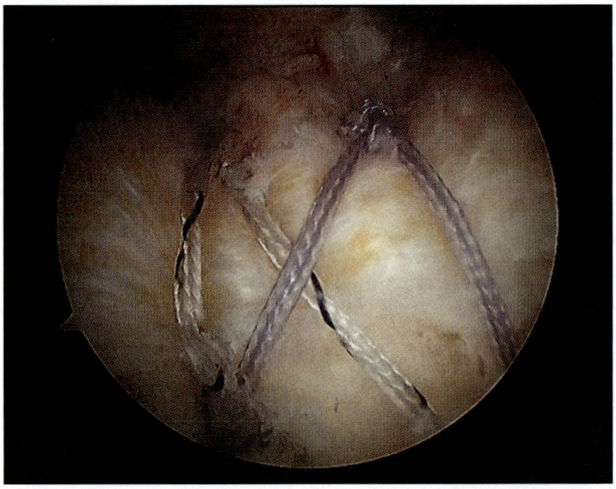

Figure 11-17. Same patient from Figure 11-1. Arthroscopic view of the right shoulder from the anterolateral portal showing completed double-row suture bridge rotator cuff repair. (Courtesy of Columbia Center for Shoulder, Elbow and Sports Medicine.)

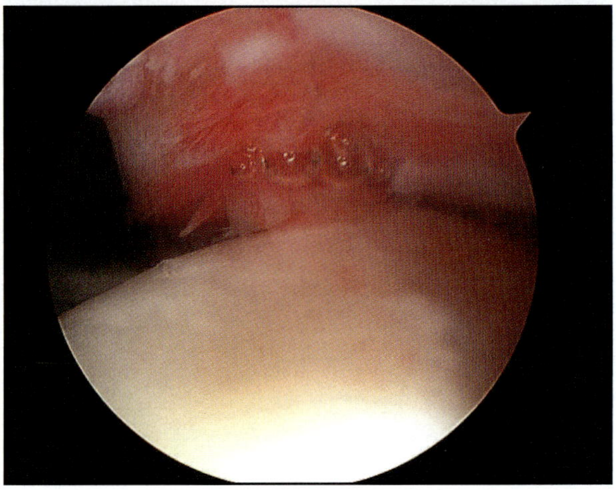

Figure 11-18. Same patient from Figure 11-1. Arthroscopic view of the right shoulder of the glenohumeral joint demonstrating a "synovitis sign"—synovitis on the undersurface of the rotator cuff is lateralized with the anatomic restoration of the previously medially displaced rotator cuff. (Courtesy of Columbia Center for Shoulder, Elbow and Sports Medicine.)

Final Check

The arthroscope should always be placed back in the glenohumeral joint after the cuff has been repaired. We look for the "synovitis sign" to confirm the repair while viewing in the glenohumeral joint (Figure 11-18). By lateralizing the rotator cuff, synovitis on the undersurface of the previously medially displaced rotator cuff is now apparent and signifies anatomic restoration. Cautery is then used to ablate the synovitis to confirm anatomic restoration of the rotator cuff to the footprint (Figure 11-19).

Upon completion of the repair, any subacromial decompression or distal clavicle excision that had not been accomplished previously is completed. The subacromial space is irrigated, and the arthroscope is removed. All portals are closed with interrupted stitches with 4-0 bioabsorbable sutures and steri-strips. A sterile dressing is applied, and the patient is placed in a sling that holds the arm in slight abduction and external rotation to decrease tension on the repair.

POSTOPERATIVE MANAGEMENT

A patient's postoperative rehabilitation program should be customized to his or her individual clinical situation.[42] There exists a delicate balance between immobilizing the shoulder to allow for

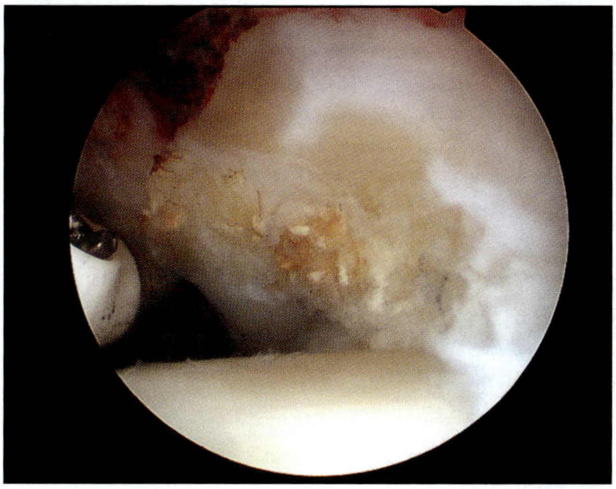

Figure 11-19. Same patient from Figure 11-1. Arthroscopic view of the right shoulder of the glenohumeral joint demonstrating anatomic rotator cuff repair. (Courtesy of Columbia Center for Shoulder, Elbow and Sports Medicine.)

sufficient tendon-to-bone healing and mobilizing the shoulder to prevent postoperative stiffness. However, there is a growing body of literature that suggests that stiffness is a complication that can be effectively overcome and not compromise long-term results.[43,44] Thus, we err on immobilizing the patient in the immediate postoperative period to protect the repair and encourage sufficient healing. We typically immobilize the patient in a sling for the first 4 to 6 weeks following repair. During this period, no shoulder range of motion is allowed. However, the patient is instructed to perform elbow, wrist, and finger range-of-motion exercises.

At 4 to 6 weeks postoperatively, formal physical therapy begins. The initial phase of therapy is designed to begin to restore passive range of motion while placing minimal strain on the repair tissue. This program is progressively expanded to include active-assisted and eventually active range-of-motion exercises over the next 6 weeks. During this period, no strengthening exercises are included.

The final phase focuses on building strength through the progressive use of therabands, weights, and pulleys to strengthen the cuff musculature and dynamic stabilizers of the shoulder. This phase also typically takes 6 weeks. The ultimate goal of the rehabilitation program is restoration of functional range of motion and strength. The program is tailored to the patient's individual clinical situation and can be adjusted to include sport- and/or activity-specific exercises and training.

RESULTS

Open repair has historically been the gold standard for the operative treatment of rotator cuff tears.[38,41,45,46] However, as arthroscopic techniques have been refined, arthroscopic repairs are becoming the treatment of choice for many surgeons. As more and more surgeons adopt arthroscopic repairs into their practice, research investigating arthroscopic repairs has exploded as surgeons begin to study the timing of repair, repair construct, evidence of tendon healing, and other relevant questions. To date, multiple questions remain, and repair of rotator cuff tears will continue to be an area of intense study in the future.

CONCLUSION

Full-thickness tears of the supraspinatus tendon are a common problem in the shoulder, with an increasing prevalence with age. The clinical manifestations of supraspinatus tears are highly variable; some tears can be asymptomatic with little or no functional consequence for the patient, while others can be profoundly painful and debilitating. Thus, discerning the optimal management of supraspinatus tears can be complicated. Multiple factors must be considered when evaluating a patient with a full-thickness supraspinatus tear. A patient's clinical history, physical examination, and imaging studies must all be considered when recommending a patient for nonoperative or operative treatment. With appropriate indications and well-executed plans, both operative and nonoperative management strategies can effectively relieve pain and restore optimal function to patients with full-thickness supraspinatus tears.

PEARLS

- It is critical to discern an acute from chronic tear based upon a patient's history.
- In the patient's physical exam, examination of passive range of motion must be examined with the patient upright and supine. Symmetry or discrepancies between upright and supine range of motion can discern between painful guarding and adhesive capsulitis.
- The use of selective injection of local anesthetic into the subacromial space can aid in the diagnosis of subacromial bursitis and impingement.
- MRI is the imaging modality of choice for the shoulder and must be viewed systematically. Each plane of imaging is ideal for viewing specific characteristics of rotator cuff pathology.
- Small modifications from standard posterior, anterior, and lateral arthroscopic portals greatly facilitate the ease of rotator cuff repair.
- Areas of cuff with a partial-thickness tear that are suspicious for a full-thickness tear can be tagged with a prolene suture for easier identification from the subacromial space.
- The rotator cuff must be viewed from the lateral portal to fully characterize and define the specific tear configuration and pattern.
- Subtle differences exist among techniques, but the critical steps for arthroscopic rotator cuff repair are the same: cuff and footprint preparation, anchor placement, suture passage, suture tying, and SwivelLock placement.
- A patient's postoperative rehabilitation program must be customized to his or her specific situation. Err toward the side of immobilization for the first 4 to 6 weeks; immobilization protects the repair and enhances tendon-to-bone healing, and resultant stiffness can be effectively managed.

REFERENCES

1. Curtis AS, Burbank KM, Tierney JJ, Scheller AD, Curran AR. The insertional footprint of the rotator cuff: an anatomic study. *Arthroscopy*. 2006;22(6):609, e1.
2. Dugas JR, Campbell DA, Warren RF, Robie BH, Millett PJ. Anatomy and dimensions of rotator cuff insertions. *J Shoulder Elbow Surg*. 2002;11(5):498-503.
3. Minagawa H, Itoi E, Konno N, et al. Humeral attachment of the supraspinatus and infraspinatus tendons: an anatomic study. *Arthroscopy*. 1998;14(3):302-306.
4. Roh MS, Wang VM, April EW, Pollock RG, Bigliani LU, Flatow EL. Anterior and posterior musculotendinous anatomy of the supraspinatus. *J Shoulder Elbow Surg,* 2000;9(5):436-440.
5. Ruotolo C, Fow JE, Nottage WM. The supraspinatus footprint: an anatomic study of the supraspinatus insertion. *Arthroscopy*. 2004;20(3):246-249.
6. Volk AG, Vangsness CT Jr. An anatomic study of the supraspinatus muscle and tendon. *Clin Orthop Relat Res*. 2001;384:280-285.
7. Sher JS, Uribe JW, Posada A, Murphy BJ, Zlatkin MB. Abnormal findings on magnetic resonance images of asymptomatic shoulders. *J Bone Joint Surg Am*. 1995;77(1):10-15.
8. Teefey SA, Rubin DA, Middleton WD, Hildebolt CF, Leibold RA, Yamaguchi K. Detection and quantification of rotator cuff tears. Comparison of ultrasonographic, magnetic resonance imaging, and arthroscopic findings in seventy-one consecutive cases. *J Bone Joint Surg Am*. 2004;86-A(4):708-716.

9. Tempelhof S, Rupp S, Seil R. Age-related prevalence of rotator cuff tears in asymptomatic shoulders. *J Shoulder Elbow Surg*. 1999;8(4):296-299.

10. Yamaguchi K, Ditsios K, Middleton WD, Hildebolt CF, Galatz LM, Teefey SA. The demographic and morphological features of rotator cuff disease. A comparison of asymptomatic and symptomatic shoulders. *J Bone Joint Surg Am*. 2006;88(8):1699-1704.

11. Yamaguchi K, Tetro AM, Blam O, Evanoff BA, Teefey SA, Middleton WD. Natural history of asymptomatic rotator cuff tears: a longitudinal analysis of asymptomatic tears detected sonographically. *J Shoulder Elbow Surg*. 2001;10(3):199-203.

12. Wolf BR, Dunn WR, Wright RW. Indications for repair of full-thickness rotator cuff tears. *Am J Sports Med*. 2007;35(6):1007-1016.

13. Misamore GW, Ziegler DW, Rushton JL 2nd. Repair of the rotator cuff. A comparison of results in two populations of patients. *J Bone Joint Surg Am*. 1995;77(9):1335-1339.

14. Pai VS, Lawson DA. Rotator cuff repair in a district hospital setting: outcomes and analysis of prognostic factors. *J Shoulder Elbow Surg*. 2001;10(3):236-241.

15. Gerber C, Hersche O, Farron A. Isolated rupture of the subscapularis tendon. *J Bone Joint Surg Am*. 1996;78(7):1015-1023.

16. Gerber C, Krushell RJ. Isolated rupture of the tendon of the subscapularis muscle. Clinical features in 16 cases. *J Bone Joint Surg Br*. 1991;73(3):389-394.

17. Hertel R. Lag signs. *J Shoulder Elbow Surg*. 2005;14(3):343; author reply 343-344.

18. Hertel R, Ballmer FT, Lombert SM, Gerber C. Lag signs in the diagnosis of rotator cuff rupture. *J Shoulder Elbow Surg*. 1996;5(4):307-313.

19. Neer CS 2nd. Anterior acromioplasty for the chronic impingement syndrome in the shoulder: a preliminary report. *J Bone Joint Surg Am*. 1972;54(1):41-50.

20. Neer CS 2nd. Impingement lesions. *Clin Orthop Relat Res*. 1983;173:70-77.

21. Hawkins RJ, Kennedy JC. Impingement syndrome in athletes. *Am J Sports Med*. 1980;8(3):151-158.

22. Jobe FW, Jobe CM. Painful athletic injuries of the shoulder. *Clin Orthop Relat Res*. 1983;173:117-124.

23. Cadet ER, Hsu JW, Levine WN, Bigliani LU, Ahmad CS. The relationship between greater tuberosity osteopenia and the chronicity of rotator cuff tears. *J Shoulder Elbow Surg*. 2008;17(1):73-77.

24. Chaipat L, Palmer WE. Shoulder magnetic resonance imaging. *Clin Sports Med*. 2006;25(3):371-386, v.

25. Sanders TG, Miller MD. A systematic approach to magnetic resonance imaging interpretation of sports medicine injuries of the shoulder. *Am J Sports Med*. 2005;33(7):1088-1105.

26. Balich SM, Sheley RC, Brown TR, Sauser DD, Quinn SF. MR imaging of the rotator cuff tendon: interobserver agreement and analysis of interpretive errors. *Radiology*. 1997;204(1):191-194.

27. Ferrari FS, Governi S, Burresi F, Vigni F, Stefani P. Supraspinatus tendon tears: comparison of US and MR arthrography with surgical correlation. *Eur Radiol*. 2002;12(5):1211-1217.

28. Quinn SF, Sheley RC, Demlow TA, Szumowski J. Rotator cuff tendon tears: evaluation with fat-suppressed MR imaging with arthroscopic correlation in 100 patients. *Radiology*. 1995;195(2):497-500.

29. Goutallier D, Postel JM, Bernageau J, Lavau L, Voisin MC. Fatty muscle degeneration in cuff ruptures. Pre- and postoperative evaluation by CT scan. *Clin Orthop Relat Res*. 1994;304:78-83.

30. Deutsch A, Altchek DW, Veltri DM, Potter HG, Warren RF. Traumatic tears of the subscapularis tendon. Clinical diagnosis, magnetic resonance imaging findings, and operative treatment. *Am J Sports Med*. 1997;25(1):13-22.

31. Shubin Stein BE, Ahmad CS, Pfaff CH, Bigliani LU, Levine WN. A comparison of magnetic resonance imaging findings of the acromioclavicular joint in symptomatic versus asymptomatic patients. *J Shoulder Elbow Surg*. 2006;15(1):56-59.

32. Williams GR Jr, Rockwood CA Jr, Bigliani LU, Iannotti JP, Stanwood W. Rotator cuff tears: why do we repair them? *J Bone Joint Surg Am*. 2004;86-A(12):2764-2776.

33. Kim HM, Dahiya N, Teefey SA, Keener JD, Galatz LM, Yamaguchi K. Relationship of tear size and location to fatty degeneration of the rotator cuff. *J Bone Joint Surg Am*. 2010;92(4):829-839.

34. Kim HM, Dahiya N, Teefey SA, et al. Location and initiation of degenerative rotator cuff tears: an analysis of three hundred and sixty shoulders. *J Bone Joint Surg Am*. 2010;92(5):1088-1096.

35. Yamanaka K, Matsumoto T. The joint side tear of the rotator cuff. A followup study by arthrography. *Clin Orthop Relat Res*. 1994;304:68-73.

36. Schaefer O, Winterer J, Lohrmann C, Laubenberger J, Reichelt A, Langer M. Magnetic resonance imaging for supraspinatus muscle atrophy after cuff repair. *Clin Orthop Relat Res*. 2002;403:93-99.

37. Neer CS 2nd, Craig EV, Fukuda H. Cuff-tear arthropathy. *J Bone Joint Surg Am*. 1983;65(9):1232-1244.

38. Cofield RH, Parvizi J, Hoffmeyer PJ, Lanzer WL, Ilstrup DM, Rowland CM. Surgical repair of chronic rotator cuff tears. A prospective long-term study. *J Bone Joint Surg Am*. 2001;83-A(1):71-77.

39. Feng S, Guo S, Nobuhara K, Hashimoto J, Mimori K. Prognostic indicators for outcome following rotator cuff tear repair. *J Orthop Surg (Hong Kong)*. 2003;11(2):110-116.

40. Hattrup SJ. Rotator cuff repair: relevance of patient age. *J Shoulder Elbow Surg*. 1995;4(2):95-100.

41. Romeo AA, Hang DW, Bach BR Jr, Shott S. Repair of full thickness rotator cuff tears. Gender, age, and other factors affecting outcome. *Clin Orthop Relat Res.* 1999;367:243-255.
42. Koo SS, Burkhart SS. Rehabilitation following arthroscopic rotator cuff repair. *Clin Sports Med.* 2010;29(2):203-211, vii.
43. Huberty DP, Schoolfield JD, Brady PC, Vadala AP, Arrigoni P, Burkhart SS. Incidence and treatment of postoperative stiffness following arthroscopic rotator cuff repair. *Arthroscopy.* 2009;25(8):880-890.
44. Parsons BO, Gruson KI, Chen DD, Harrison AK, Gladstone J, Flatow EL. Does slower rehabilitation after arthroscopic rotator cuff repair lead to long-term stiffness? *J Shoulder Elbow Surg.* 2010;19(7):1034-1039.
45. Bigliani LU, Cordasco FA, McIlveen SJ, Musso ES. Operative treatment of failed repairs of the rotator cuff. *J Bone Joint Surg Am.* 1992;74(10):1505-1515.
46. Galatz LM, Griggs S, Cameron BD, Iannotti JP. Prospective longitudinal analysis of postoperative shoulder function: a ten-year follow-up study of full-thickness rotator cuff tears. *J Bone Joint Surg Am.* 2001;83-A(7):1052-1056.

Please see video on the accompanying Web site at
http://www.slackbooks.com/rotatorcuffvideos

CHAPTER 12

DOUBLE-ROW ARTHROSCOPIC REPAIR OF ROTATOR CUFF INJURIES

Drew Lansdown, MD; Abbas Kothari, BS; and C. Benjamin Ma, MD

Rotator cuff injuries can be a common cause of shoulder pain and disability, particularly in older patients. One study reports the overall prevalence of rotator cuff tears to be 23.1 to 49.4%.[1] The etiology of rotator cuff tears can be degenerative or traumatic.

While mini-open rotator cuff repairs have good clinical success, arthroscopic rotator cuff repairs have gained significant popularity due to their lower morbidity. Reproducing the suturing techniques of an open or mini-open repair proved to be a difficult technical challenge in arthroscopy. While open rotator cuff repairs have focused on using better tissue-holding suture configurations, such as modified Mason-Allen stitches or transosseous suture repairs, arthroscopic repair has focused on single-row fixation with suture anchors in its initial technique development. While the initial reports on subjective outcomes following rotator cuff repairs approached 90% to 95% satisfaction, radiographic and objective evaluation following arthroscopic rotator cuff repairs have shown failures of up to 90% with larger tears.[2,3] Our field began to evaluate the differences between open and arthroscopic rotator cuff repairs. While the majority of the procedure was equivalent with a mini-open or arthroscopic repair, most investigators attributed the high rate of retears to be secondary to the weaker fixation achieved with a single-row repair.

In 2003, Lo and Burkhart first formally described the use of an arthroscopic double-row rotator cuff repair technique.[4] This method uses 2 sets of suture anchors in the humeral head to reattach the supraspinatus tendon.[4] The medial row is placed adjacent to the articular cartilage, and a second set is placed at the lateral aspect of the footprint of the supraspinatus tendon on the greater tuberosity. This technically demanding procedure may offer a stronger fixation and also better restoration of the tendon footprint on the greater tuberosity.

Prior to the description of a double-row repair, it was shown that a single row of suture anchors reconstructs a supraspinatus footprint that is approximately 67% of the original insertion.[5] Cadaveric and in vivo studies that have examined the supraspinatus coverage following double-row repair show that the normal anatomy of the rotator cuff is restored.[5-7] A double-row suture anchor repair restores at least 100% of the native supraspinatus footprint.[6,7]

Ma CB, Feeley BT, eds.
*Basic Principles and Operative Management
of the Rotator Cuff (pp 181-190)*
© 2012 SLACK Incorporated

Numerous researchers have evaluated the biomechanical properties of the double-row repair, and the majority of evidence supports the hypothesis that a double-row repair offers biomechanical advantages over the single-row repair. In one cadaveric study, the double-row repair proved to have a significantly higher tensile load to fail when compared with simple suture repair.[8] This general observation has been confirmed with other cadaveric studies as well, with superior tensile load to failure. Double-row fixation has also demonstrated better cyclic loading patterns when compared to single row-repair and transosseous repair. In a test-to-failure of cyclic loading at 180 N, the transosseous repair failed at an average of 75 cycles, and the single-row repair failed at 798 cycles. No rotator cuff repaired with the double-row method failed before reaching 5000 cycles.[9] Additionally, the strain across the repaired tendon is lower for double-row fixation. Table 12-1 provides a summary of selected studies that have examined the biomechanical properties of the double-row repair.[8-12]

The purpose of this chapter is to describe the surgical technique of the double-row suture anchor repair for a rotator cuff tear. A brief discussion of the results of several clinical trials comparing single- and double-row fixation follows the description of the procedure. A video of the procedure accompanies this chapter.

SURGICAL TECHNIQUE

Perioperative Care

Patient Positioning

For this technique, we will describe the surgical technique of double-row fixation in the beach chair position. Upon induction of anesthesia, the patient is placed in the beach chair position. A beach chair positioner or a full-length bean bag can be used. The advantage of the beach chair positioner is that it can provide great access to the operative shoulder. However, the positioner works best with patients within the range of normal body habitus. Smaller patients with narrow shoulders or tall and large patients may not fit into the positioner. A full-length bean bag can also be used. It can accommodate all patients but does require some experience for positioning. The bean bag should be positioned so that it extends all the way to the level of the top of the head. The bean bag is inflated with the operative shoulder exposed and the head supported. The patient and the bean bag are then shifted to the edge of the operating table to expose the shoulder and scapula area. A sterile arm positioner is extremely helpful for shoulder arthroscopy. The arm should be distracted inferiorly and anteriorly to open up the subacromial space.

Portal Placement

Optimal port placement allows for safe and effective visualization of key structures throughout the operation. We place the posterior viewing portal in the "high lateral" position. The portal is placed more superior and lateral than the standard posterior portal in the soft spot on the shoulder. The high lateral portal is placed in line with the lateral edge of the acromion and just inferior to the posterolateral corner of the acromion. The reason for a high lateral portal is because most of the work for arthroscopic rotator cuff repairs will be in the subacromial space. Placing the portal more superior and laterally allows for better visualization of the greater tuberosity and the rotator cuff tendon. If a standard posterior portal is used, the retracted rotator cuff tendon will be in the way during and following repair. A second anterior working portal is placed just lateral to the coracoid to facilitate intra-articular shoulder work for labral débridement or probing of the biceps tendon. This is also used as an accessory portal when performing suture shuttling for the repair. A standard lateral portal is used for acromioplasty and as the instrument portal. This portal should accommodate a larger-size cannula to allow easy instrument passage. Knot tying and suture shuttling will be performed using the lateral portal. We commonly use separate stab incisions for anchor placement. When using separate incisions for anchor placement, it will allow you to manage the sutures a bit easier, especially with double-row rotator cuff repairs.

		Table 12-1. Selected Studies of Biomechanical Properties of Double-Row Fixation		
Author	Journal	Suture Configuration Tested	Testing Methods	Findings
Kim et al[11]	AJSM 2006	SR DR	Cyclic loading from 10 to 180 N for 200 cycles Load to failure	1. Gap formation significantly smaller in DR versus SR 2. Initial strain over repair significantly lower in DR 3. Ultimate load of failure decreased by 48% in DR
Ma et al[8]	JBJS 2006	Two-simple Massive cuff Arthroscopic Mason-Allen DR	Cyclic loading from 5 to 100 N for 50 cycles Load to failure	1. DR had highest ultimate load to failure of 287 N, significantly greater than massive (250 N), modified Mason-Allen (212 N), and two-simple (191 N) 2. Peak-to-peak elongation was 1.4 mm for SR, 1.5 for arthroscopic Mason-Allen, 1.1 mm for massive cuff, and 1.1 for DR
Mazzocca et al[12]	AJSM 2005	SR Diamond DR Mattress double anchor Modified mattress double anchor	Cyclic loading to 100 N for 3000 cycles Load to failure	1. Significantly larger footprint in all DR repairs compared to SR 2. No difference in load to failure or displacement in any of the repairs 3. Failure occurred for SR at 287 N, diamond at 305 N, mattress double anchor at 256 N, and modified mattress double anchor at 289 N
Meier and Meier[9]	AJSM 2006	Transosseous SR DR	Cyclic loading from 5 to 180 N for 5000 cycles	1. Transosseous repair failed at 75 cycles and SR at 798 cycles 2. No failures of the DR repairs at 5000 cycles
Smith et al[10]	JBJS 2006	SR DR	Cyclic loading at 40 to 50 N for 10 cycles, then increased max load by 50 N every 10 cycles until failure	1. Gap formation similar between SR and DR (3.2 versus 2.7 mm) 2. Ultimate cyclic failure load was 224 N for SR and significantly higher at 320 N for DR

SR = single row; DR = double row

Diagnostic Arthroscopy

Diagnostic arthroscopy is performed using the posterolateral viewing portal (Figure 12-1). Depending on the size of the rotator cuff tendon tear, diagnostic arthroscopy can begin in the standard fashion by going through the infraspinatus tendon and evaluating the intra-articular structures. If the tendon tear is larger or retracted, it is best to begin the diagnostic arthroscopy in the subacromial space. You can then enter through the tear into the intra-articular portion to perform

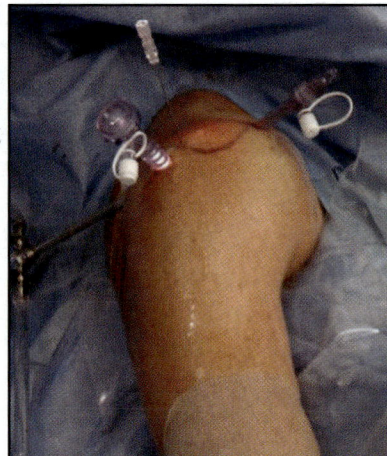

Figure 12-1. Posterior viewing portal. Midlateral working portal that is established with a larger cannula for suture-passing equipment. Anterior suture management portal that is established with a smaller portal for suture management. Anchors are placed through stab incisions localized using spinal needle, usually along the edge of the acromion. No cannula is needed.

your intra-articular evaluation. This technique will allow you not to put another hole through the infraspinatus tendon for the larger size tear. You can get a very thorough diagnostic evaluation of the joint without further injuring the rotator cuff tendons. The size of the rotator cuff tear can be easily assessed with a diagnostic arthroscopy. Other important structures, such as the biceps tendon, the labrum, and the articulating surfaces of the glenoid and humerus, should be inspected for additional pathology. It is also important to have a thorough evaluation of the subscapularis tendon and its insertion. It is not uncommon to miss the subscapularis tendon tear during routine arthroscopic rotator cuff repairs. This will lead to continued discomfort and failure of the surgical repair. The arm should be internally rotated to allow adequate visualization of the entire lesser tuberosity. A clue to subscapularis tendon disruption is the loss of the attachment of the superior glenohumeral ligament or subluxation or dislocation of the biceps tendon.

Subacromial Decompression and Acromioplasty

We commonly perform subacromial decompression and acromioplasty at the time of rotator cuff repair. The amount of acromion resection or need for coracoacromial (CA) ligament repair will depend on the shape of the acromion. A lateral portal is established to have good height relative to the acromial spur. The portal should be placed so that the height is along the same level of the resection level. A coagulation device is first used to isolate the acromion and release the CA ligament through the lateral portal. The anterior and lateral edge of the acromion is released, and acromioplasty is performed to coplane the acromion. A generous bursectomy is also performed to ensure good visualization using a mechanical shaver. We start at the posterior gutter, then move to the lateral gutter and finally to the anterior gutter. The edge of the CA ligament is also débrided. Most of the bleeding vessels are located at the posteromedial aspect near the acromial spine. This is the last area where we perform the bursectomy, and hemostasis should be achieved immediately. The radiofrequency ablation device is passed through the lateral portal to coagulate and remove the involved bursa. A thorough bursectomy is important to identify the tear and facilitate suture passage. It is important to realize that the medial row of the double-row repairs are more medial than standard single-row repairs, and it is important that the bursa is removed up to the musculotendinous junction of the rotator cuff tendons.

Release of Rotator Cuff Tendons

The tendon edges and the greater tuberosity are cleared of adhesions using a shaver or a coagulation device. It is important to recognize the tear pattern of the rotator cuff tendon. Crescent tears can be repaired easily using a double-row rotator cuff repair technique. For L-shaped, reverse L-shaped, or U-shaped tears, margin convergence stitches should be placed first prior to the double-row construct. Most tendons are adequately released when the subacromial space is cleared.

Figure 12-2. Medial suture anchor placement. Anchor is placed over the medial aspect of the greater tuberosity, just lateral to the articular cartilage.

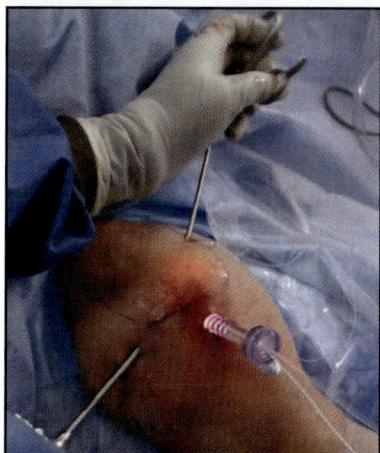

Figure 12-3. The shoulder is viewed through the posterolateral viewing portal. The lateral working portal is the larger portal that enables suture-passing devices to go in. Sutures are retrieved individually after each pass through the anterior portal.

At times, further release is needed on the undersurface of the tendon. A radiofrequency device or a dissecting device can be used to release the adhesion between the supraspinatus, infraspinatus, and the glenoid fossae. One should be careful not to dissect too medially, especially for the infraspinatus tendon because of the traversing suprascapular nerve.

Anchor Placement

If the tear is amenable to a double-row repair, the first row of anchors is placed medially, just lateral to the articulating surface of the humeral head (Figure 12-2). A spinal needle is used to guide the anchor to a "dead-man's angle" on the greater tuberosity. A stab incision is made along the spinal needle, and the anchor is introduced through the stab incision to the greater tuberosity.

Medial Row Anchors

- The anchors are placed percutaneously through the stab incisions. The most anterior anchor is placed first. The reason behind the sequence is that, while viewing from the posterior aspect of the shoulder, the view is clear when you place suture in an anterior-to-posterior fashion. Following anchor placement, the individual sutures are retrieved through the lateral portal for suture shuttling.
- We usually use a suture-passing device to pass horizontal mattress suture constructs through the medial edge of the tendon.
- Sutures are placed approximately 15-mm medial to the tendon edge.
- The sutures that are placed through the tendon are retrieved through the anterior portal that is placed just superior to the CA ligament and under the acromion (Figure 12-3).
- We start with the most anterior suture first, then move to the posterior aspect of the rotator cuff tendon. As the arthroscope is in the posterior viewing position, it is helpful to place the most anterior sutures first so that it does not affect visualization. After the first set of sutures

Figure 12-4. The lateral row anchors are placed through the same stab incision and are placed at the lateral aspect of the greater tuberosity.

Figure 12-5. The lateral row sutures are placed in a simple knot fashion (white). The blue sutures are the medial row sutures that were placed first in a horizontal mattress configuration. These were retrieved through the anterior portal.

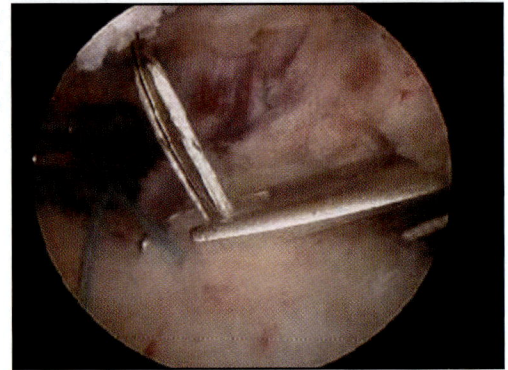

are all passed through as horizontal mattress configuration, the more posterior anchor can be placed, and the same suture passing steps are used. Usually, a more posterior stab incision is used to place the posterior anchor. This can later be used for the lateral row anchors as well.

- As these are all horizontal mattress suture configurations, all of the limbs are retrieved through the anterior portal. These can be clamped together prior to the lateral row sutures.

Lateral Row Anchors

- The lateral row anchors can be placed through the same stab incision for the medial row anchors (Figure 12-4).
- These will be simple suture constructs, and only one limb is passed through the lateral edge of the tendon.
- The sutures are retrieved through the lateral working portal and are passed through the tendon using a suture-passing device.
- The sutures are usually placed 8- to 10-mm away from the edge of the tendon (Figure 12-5).
- Again, the most anterior edge suture is placed first to allow for better visualization.
- If 2 anchors are used in the lateral row, a separate stab incision is used for the more posterior anchor placement. This will allow the sutures to be separated from the first anchor and will allow easier suture management.

Suture Tying

- After all sutures are passed through the tendon, the lateral row is tied down first, prior to the medial row.
- This will allow the tendon to be repaired to the edge of the greater tuberosity first, and then the medial row is tied down to ensure better coverage of the footprint.
- The lateral row simple sutures are tied first, starting from the most posterior set, moving anteriorly. Again, this will allow better visualization because the arthroscope is in the posterior viewing portal.

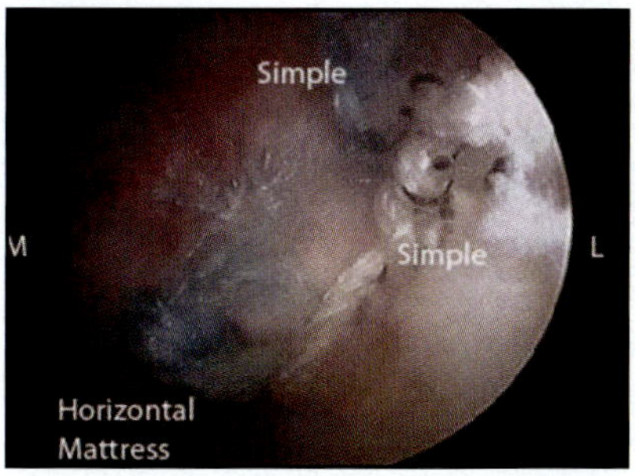

Figure 12-6. Double-row finished product.

- Most of the time, visualization is more difficult after the lateral row sutures are tied down and the medial row is untied. The tendon is brought laterally, and it is important to have a high lateral portal to enable good visualization.
- After the lateral rows are tied, the medial rows are then tied down, from posterior to anterior fashion again. The medial row will allow the tendon to be repaired down along the entire tuberosity. As the medial row is being tied down, visualization improves as the tendon is repaired down to the greater tuberosity, and more space is available in the subacromial area (Figure 12-6).

Postoperative Protocol

Our standard rotator cuff protocol focuses on controlling pain and minimizing swelling to facilitate early passive motion of the shoulder. Patients are kept in a shoulder immobilizer with an abduction pillow continuously for 6 weeks postoperatively. After 2 weeks, patients begin passive motion, avoiding external rotation beyond the neutral position. Active motion begins 6 weeks postoperatively, with low-resistance strengthening exercises along with gradually increasing passive external rotation. Resistive strengthening with weights is allowed at 12 weeks postoperatively, and full normal activities can be resumed at 18 weeks postoperatively with the supervision of a physical therapist.

RESULTS

While the biomechanics of a double-row repair are significantly superior to single-row repairs, the clinical results are lacking. Prospective trials that have evaluated double-row repairs exclusively have shown very good subjective and objective outcome measures, with excellent results in up to 90% of patients.[13-15] These good results, however, are also seen in single-row repairs, regardless of the integrity of the rotator cuff. An assessment of cuff tear rate by ultrasonography showed that 83% of shoulders had an intact repair at 2 years and that those patients with larger preoperative tears were more likely to have a failed repair.[15] In a prospective nonrandomized study, 19 of 31 patients who had a double-row repair attained anatomic healing, while 14 of 35 of those who had a single-row repair showed anatomic healing.[16] Magnetic resonance imaging (MRI) and computed tomography (CT) at follow-up have shown improved tendon healing in patients who have undergone a double-row repair compared to single row.[13,16]

The evidence to support a double-row repair has been less conclusive in prospective randomized controlled trials. The biomechanical benefits of cadaveric studies have not translated into an improvement in patient outcomes. Most evidence points to equivalent outcomes for double- and single-row repairs at a follow-up of 2 years, as measured by Constant and University of California Los Angeles (UCLA) scores.[16-21] Objective clinical measurements, such as range of motion and strength, have also been equivalent between these 2 types of repairs. Table 12-2 summarizes multiple different clinical trials of differing strengths of evidence.

TABLE 12-2. CLINICAL STUDIES EXAMINING THE OUTCOMES OF PATIENTS TREATED WITH DOUBLE-ROW FIXATION

AUTHOR	JOURNAL	STUDY DESIGN	NUMBER OF PATIENTS	FINDINGS
Huijsmans et al[15]	JBJS 2007	Nonrandomized retrospective review of DR fixation	264	1. Pain score improved from 7.4 preoperatively to 0.7 postoperatively 2. 90.9% had excellent or good outcome 3. Constant score increased by 25.4, from 54.9 preoperatively to 80 postoperatively 4. Ultrasound showed 83% had intact rotator cuffs
Lafosse et al[13]	JBJS 2007	Nonrandomized consecutive series of DR repair	105	1. Constant score improved 37 points—from 43 preoperatively to 80 postoperatively 2. Failure of 12 in 105
Sugaya et al[14]	JBJS 2007	Cohort of DR fixation	86	1. All outcome measures improved significantly: UCLA—14.5 pre-operatively, 32.9 postoperatively; ASES—42.3 preoperatively, 94.3 postoperatively 2. 17% had a retorn cuff
Charousset et al[16]	AJSM 2007	Prospective, nonrandomized study of SR and DR fixation	76 (35 SR, 31 DR)	1. No significant difference in Constant score between the 2 groups 2. Significantly more patients with DR repair had anatomic healing as assessed by CT arthrography—19 versus 14 patients
Burks et al[19]	AJSM 2009	Prospective randomized controlled trial	40	1. No difference in any postoperative measures, strength, or range of motion 2. No significant difference on MRI of footprint, tendon thickness, or tendon signal
Franceschi et al[17]	AJSM 2007	Randomized controlled trial	60 (30 SR, 30 DR)	1. No statistically significant difference in range of motion or UCLA scores 2. MRA showed intact cuff in 14 patients with SR and 18 with DR
Grasso et al[18]	*Arthroscopy* 2009	Randomized controlled trial	80 (40 SR, 40 DR)	1. No significant difference in any outcome measures 2. Univariate and multivariate analyses performed and age, gender, and baseline strength affected outcome

(continued)

TABLE 12-2 (CONTINUED). CLINICAL STUDIES EXAMINING THE OUTCOMES OF PATIENTS TREATED WITH DOUBLE-ROW FIXATION

Author	Journal	Study Design	Number of Patients	Findings
Koh et al[21]	*Arthroscopy*, 2011	Randomized controlled trial	62 (31 SR, 31 DR)	1. No significant difference in outcome measures 2. There were 6 full-thickness and 1 partial-thickness retears in DR group, and 4 full-thickness and 11 partial-thickness retears in SR, but this was not a significant difference
Park et al[20]	AJSM, 2008	Cohort study with first group with SR, second with DR	78 (40 SR, 38 DR)	1. No significant difference overall in Constant scores or function 2. For patients with initial tear greater than 3 cm, all outcome measures were significantly better for DR group

SR = single row; DR = double row

One explanation for the equivocal results in most prospective randomized trials is that the superiority of the double-row repair may only be seen in larger rotator cuff tears. Several randomized trials included patients with cuff tears less than 3 cm, and the results of these studies could be skewed given the smaller rotator cuff tears. A subgroup analysis in one trial addressed this question and suggested that there was an improvement in outcome metrics for patients with rotator cuff tears larger than 3 cm who had a double-row repair.[20] Patients with large cuff tears are historically most susceptible to retear in the postoperative period, but the double-row repair showed significantly improved outcome metrics. A subsequent randomized controlled trial to look exclusively at tears of 2 to 4 cm was unable to demonstrate that a double-row repair offered a benefit in this set of patients.[21] There is, however, some evidence to support the double-row repair in the setting of large cuff tears that are greater than 3 cm.[20]

The clinical role for the double-row repair of a rotator cuff tear has yet to be established. Biomechanical testing has shown that there is a superior biomechanical advantage to this method, but the clinical benefits have yet to be determined. However, further clinical evaluation is needed to determine its actual benefit.

REFERENCES

1. Reilly P, Macleod I, Macfarlane R, Windley J, Emery RJ. Dead men and radiologists don't lie: a review of cadaveric and radiological studies of rotator cuff tear prevalence. *Ann R Coll Surg Engl.* 2006;88(2):116-121.
2. Gartsman GM, Khan M, Hammerman SM. Arthroscopic repairs of full-thickness tears of the rotator cuff. *J Bone Joint Surg Am.* 1998;80(6):832-840.
3. Galatz LM, Ball CM, Teefey SA, Middleton WD, Yamaguchi K. The outcome and repair integrity of completely arthroscopically repaired large and massive rotator cuff tears. *J Bone Joint Surg.* 2004;86A(2):219-224.
4. Lo IKY, Burkhart SS. Double-row arthroscopic rotator cuff repair: re-establishing the footprint of the rotator cuff. *Arthroscopy.* 2003;19(9):1035-1042.
5. Apreleva M, Ozbaydar M, Fitzgibbons PG, Warner JJ. Rotator cuff tears. *Arthroscopy.* 2002;18(5):519-526.
6. Meier SW, Meier JD. Rotator cuff repair: the effect of double-row fixation on three-dimensional repair site. *J Shoulder Elbow Surg.* 2006;15(6):691-696.

Figure 13-1. The lateral suture fixation anchor is placed approximately 1 cm distal-lateral to the footprint edge, creating an obligatory compression vector over the tendon (arrows). This can improve load to failure, gap resistance, and footprint contact.

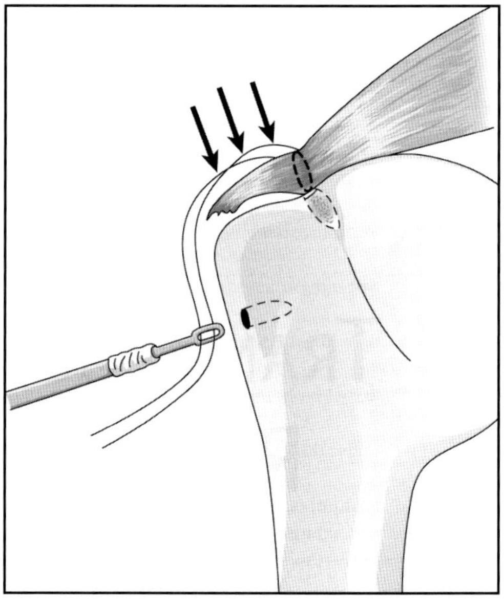

Figure 13-2. Schematic for 2 testing methods. Testing with a fixed humerus distributes stress more equally between anterior and posterior tendon regions. The supraspinatus tendon in neutral rotation (left schematic) is just posterior to the center of humeral head rotation. Rotation creates differential stress between anterior and posterior tendon regions. Up arrows represent tension, and the down arrow represents compression. Strain, tension, and gap are accentuated at the anterior tendon with external rotation (A, anterior tendon region; P, posterior tendon region).

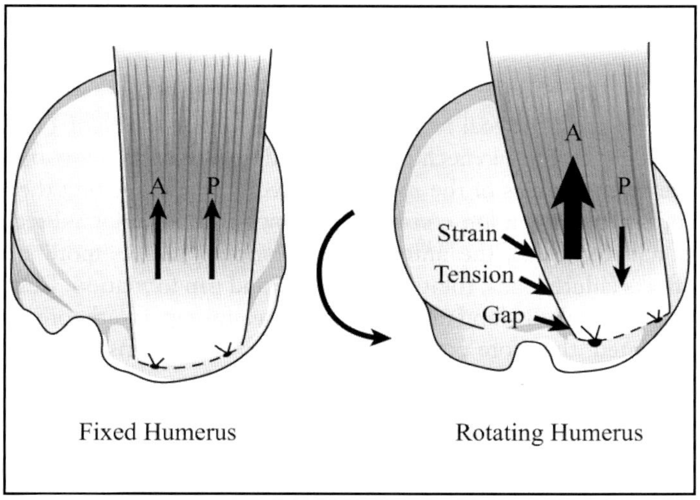

improved footprint contact is critical to successful repair. Compared to a double-row technique using 4 isolated points of fixation, the TOE repair has been shown to provide both a higher ultimate load and energy absorbed to failure, with no more gap formation.[13,14]

As its name implies, one fundamental function for the rotator cuff includes rotation. The anterior and posterior subregions of the supraspinatus have different functional roles; with the humerus internally or externally rotated, the anterior region internally or externally rotates the humerus, respectively, based on the fact that the anterior region is off-set from the center of humeral rotation.[15,16] The posterior subregion was found to only externally rotate the humerus. Importantly, the anterior subregion tendon is cord-like compared to the strap-like posterior tendon; the muscle-to-tendon cross-sectional area ratio is approximately 3 times more anteriorly.[17,18] This has implications after repair. In a study comparing testing methods, rotation was found to accentuate anterior tendon strain and gap formation when allowing for dynamic external rotation compared to testing with the humerus fixed in space (Figure 13-2); relatively low loads to better replicate the postoperative setting were employed.[19] In the rotation group, all tendons failed anteriorly first, involving the cord-like region.

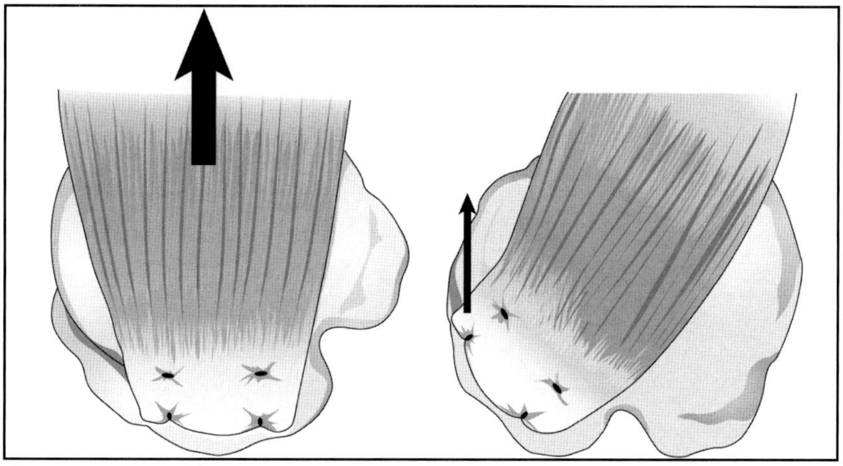

Figure 13-3. Double-row repair in neutral (left) and external (right) rotation. The arrows represent force vectors. The arrow on the right represents the force vector experienced by the posterolateral suture anchor; with rotation, load sharing is diminished and may predispose each anchor to sequential isolated failure.

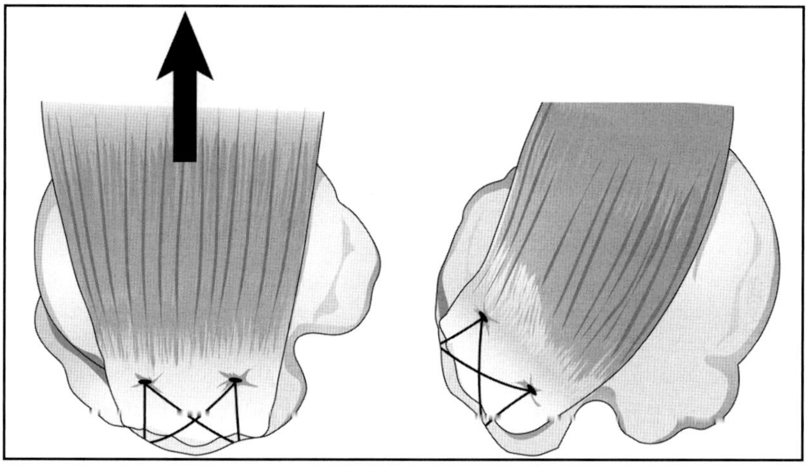

Figure 13-4. TOE repair in neutral (left) and external (right) rotation. The arrow represents the supraspinatus force vector. Because of the interconnectivity between fixation implants, the load is shared with external rotation across the construct.

Another study using a humerus rotation model, comparing the TOE repair to a "standard" double-row technique using 4 isolated points of fixation, found a significantly higher yield load with the TOE repair.[13] The yield load is the maximal load that can be withstood without creating permanent repair deformations. The improved loading characteristics are thought to be attributed to the improved load-sharing ability of the TOE repair ("interconnectivity" between anchor points; Figures 13-3 and 13-4).[13,14,20] However, although there were no differences with respect to gap formation between constructs, the TOE repair exhibited more gap formation anteriorly through the "cord" region.[13] The difference on average was less than 1 mm; however, this raises the question, "Should additional anterior fixation be employed?" For all constructs, the anterior region failed first, suggesting an area of the repair that is most vulnerable postoperatively. Notably, suture configuration has been shown to provide additional load capacity and should be considered in this context.[21,22]

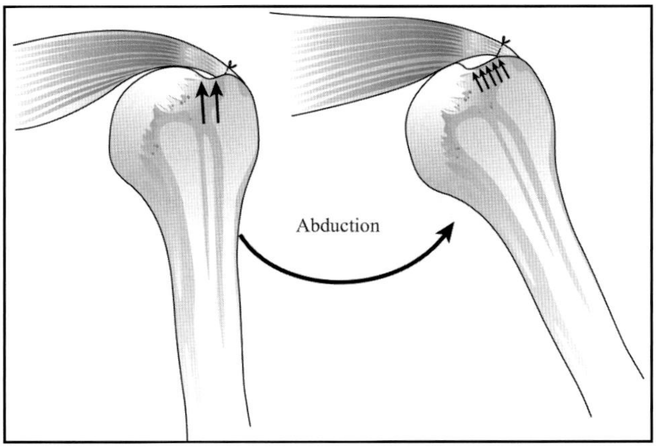

Figure 13-5. Schematic depicting the effect of abduction on footprint contact. Arrowheads represent the area of no contact at 0 degrees of abduction. With abduction, arrows represent a decreased area of contact.

Abduction

The effect of rotation on footprint contact has also been evaluated. The TOE repair was found to have improved contact characteristics when compared to single-row and double-row techniques using isolated suture anchors.[8] Notably, at 60 degrees internal humeral rotation, abducting the humerus 30 degrees (from 0 degrees) significantly decreased contact for the double-row repair using isolated suture anchors; the TOE repair did not show this decrease (Figure 13-5). This raises a question when considering that 60 degrees internal humeral rotation with 0 to 30 degrees abduction represents a postoperative sling position. The TOE repair had better footprint contact dimensions compared to the other techniques at each level of humeral abduction (0 degrees, 30 degrees, 60 degrees). Importantly, abducting the humerus has been shown to decrease repair tension, which has been shown to adversely affect healing.[23-25] With abduction negatively affecting footprint contact, while positively affecting tendon tension, there appears to be competing variables. This highlights the fact that each patient and tear pattern must be individualized, not only during repair, but afterward with a coordinated physical therapy regimen.

Tendon contact with pressurization from tendon-bridging sutures can prevent fluid extravasation. One study has directly shown that this pressurization limits synovial fluid from potentially compromising the tendon-bone interface when comparing a TOE repair to a double-row technique using suture anchors without tendon-bridging sutures.[26] Furthermore, a "wedge effect" has been described whereby, as the tendon is loaded, the tendon-bridging sutures actually provide more compression (a "self-reinforcing" repair). In addition to protecting the tendon-bone interface from extraneous fluid, this also can improve TOE repair loading characteristics (Figure 13-6).[27]

The benefits of concepts including interconnectivity (load-sharing capacity) and gap resistance created by footprint-restoring tendon compression (from distal-lateral lateral fixation on the greater tuberosity) have been confirmed in subsequent studies. Other studies have biomechanically compared the TOE repair using various knot configurations with satisfactory results.[28,29] While additional tendon suture passes will enhance repair-loading capacity and gap resistance, this must also be weighed against additional suture management and potential operating room time. Notably, medial row knots have been shown to be biomechanically favorable compared to a knotless medial row.[30] Failure at the medial row (muscle-tendon junction) has been reported.[31,32] Biomechanically, given that the knots are medial and a certain amount of lateral tissue is a prerequisite for a successful repair, if failure occurs, it is often obligatory in this region at the muscle-tendon junction. This is despite the fact that the medial tendon[33] and medial footprint[34] have both been shown to be biomechanically advantageous compared to the lateral soft tissue and bone, respectively. This highlights the need for careful patient selection when deciding upon the optimal repair—for example, the medial row should not incorporate tissue at, or medial to, the rotator cable when potentially at the expense of tension overload (tension being assessed intraoperatively after mobilization [see below]). The question is not single-row versus double-row (which technique), but more, when and in which patients should a double-row (TOE) repair be performed (Table 13-1)?

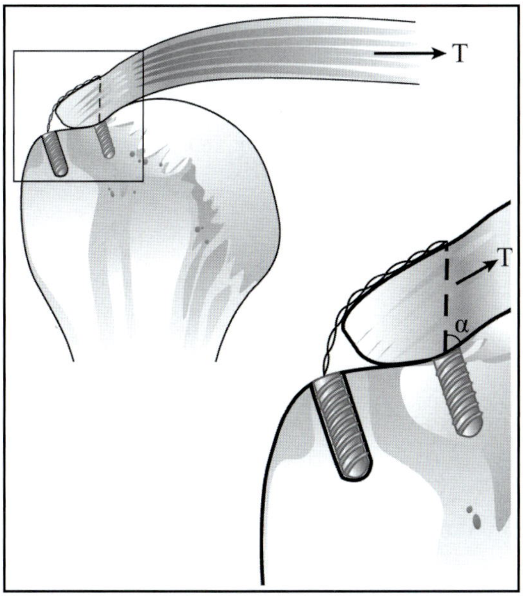

Figure 13-6. After loading the tendon: Wedge effect of FiberChain (Arthrex, Naples, FL) on tendon. As the load (T) increases, the angle (α) decreases, wedging the tendon more tightly between the bridging sutures and the bone.

TABLE 13-1. OUTCOMES

	LEVEL OF EVIDENCE	N	COHORT	AVERAGE AGE (YEARS)	FOLLOW-UP	RESULT
Frank et al (2008)[36]	IV	25	TOE	57.1 (44 to 74)	Minimum 12 months	88% healing rate; successful outcomes measures
Pennington et al (2010)[37]	III	132	TOE versus SR	54 (SR) 55 (TOE)	12 and 24 months	No overall outcomes differences; TOE with significantly more supraspinatus strength at 24 months; TOE with significantly improved healing for tears 2.5 to 3.5 cm
Voigt et al (2010)[32]	IV	51	TOE versus historical control	62 (37 to 76)	Median of 24 months	No overall outcomes differences; significantly improved outcomes measures; retears in 28.9% at 12 months; retear did not mean clinical failure; patient age >60 found to influence tendon healing
Duquin et al (2010)[38]	Review	1252	DR including TOE versus SR	60 (SR) 58 (DR)	15 months to 10 years	DR with lower retear rates for tears >1 cm

SR = single-row; DR = double-row; MRI = magnetic resonance imaging

In summary, the benefits of the TOE repair include the following:

- The relative technical ease given the number of tendon suture passes (essentially a single-row repair medially without additional tendon suture passes required for lateral fixation)[20]
- Obligatory suture compression vector over the tendon[7,12,20]
- The repair does not rely upon the lateral tendon tissue (which tends to be relatively weak)[14,33]
- There is less local implant burden within the greater tuberosity as the lateral row is placed distal-lateral (versus on top of the tuberosity)[34]
- Interconnectivity for improved load-sharing[13,14,35]
- Improved contact with rotation and abduction compared to standard double-row techniques using isolated fixation points[7,8]
- Gap-formation resistance[13,14]
- Protection against synovial fluid extravasation[8,26]
- A self-reinforcing wedge effect (tendon-loading creates tendon compression via tendon-bridging sutures)[27]

SURGICAL MANAGEMENT

Positioning

We prefer the lateral position. However, for this technique, beach chair positioning is not precluded. Ultimately, the surgeon's preference should dictate patient positioning. If concomitant labral work is expected, the lateral position may be preferable.

Surgical Technique

A standard posterior portal is made to access the glenohumeral joint. Using needle localization, an anterior portal is made, typically placed 1-cm lateral to the coracoid process. However, this can be cheated superiorly in expectation of using this same portal for the anteromedial anchor (Figure 13-7). Standard intra-articular diagnostic arthroscopy is performed. Superior capsular releases may be performed at this time using a heat probe.

The arthroscope is then directed to the subacromial space from the posterior position. Using needle localization, an anterolateral portal is established. The needle should localize the anterior half of the greater tuberosity and should allow access to the distal-lateral tuberosity in expectation of lateral row fixation. It should not be placed too distal, as the tuberosity can inhibit or block suture-passing instruments. Bursectomy is performed far laterally, in expectation of providing exposure for the lateral row, which is placed distal-lateral to the footprint.

Success also depends on adequate visualization. This requires careful posterolateral portal placement for the arthroscope when mobilizing the tear and performing repair. Needle localization can help with placement prior to committing the incision. In the lateral position, the arthroscope is moved to the posterolateral position. When needle localizing this area, while the arthroscope is posterior in the subacromial space, care must be taken to not place this incision too close to the anterolateral portal—this would crowd-out the superior accessory portal area, which could make suture anchor advancement for the medial row unnecessarily difficult (placement of the superior accessory portal is described below).

The tear must be carefully characterized. Also, the tear must have enough medial-to-lateral mobility to reach beyond the middle of the footprint, at minimum; otherwise, the repair may be overtensioned, and the TOE repair should not be pursued further. If tendon mobility is limited, then the benefit of tendon compression with sutures is precluded. In other words, there must be tendon lateral to the medial row in order to gain a significant advantage offered by the TOE construct. Once the tendon is deemed suitable for a TOE repair with sufficient medial-to-lateral tendon excursion, anterior-to-posterior trial reductions must be performed. This allows the surgeon

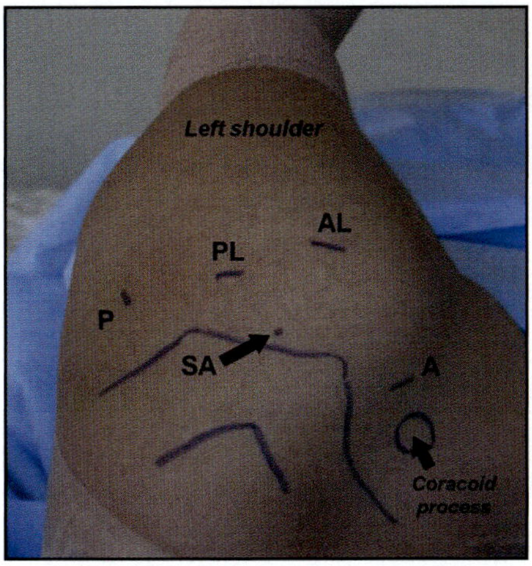

Figure 13-7. Shoulder set-up with left shoulder in the lateral position. Except for the posterior portal, all other portals can be needle localized during the procedure to optimize portal position (P, posterior portal; PL, posterolateral; AL, anterolateral; A, anterior; SA, superior accessory). (Reprinted with permission of Maxwell C. Park, MD.)

to identify where the sutures should be passed to avoid redundancies or "dog ears." A grasper can be used to mark or "crimp" the area of tendon in expectation of suture passing—the grasper should trial-mobilize the tendon to the point where the anchors will be placed and the crimp marks leave an objective reference point for suture passing for the medial row.

The superior accessory portal is also needle localized. Typically centered between the anterolateral and posterolateral portals, it is localized adjacent to the acromion. It is helpful to aim for the anterolateral cannula when localizing. The needle should be able to approach the medial row at a "dead-man's angle." Although rarely necessary, the arm can be slightly adducted to better reach this area by removing weights from the arm positioner (10 pounds are placed on the abduction arm, and 5 pounds are placed on the adduction arm—by removing the 10-pound weight, the arm moves into relative adduction [approximately 30 to 40 degrees from the starting position]). Notably, while this same portal may be used for both posteromedial and anteromedial anchor placement, the anterior portal (used originally for the rotator interval cannula) may be used for the anteromedial anchor. This may facilitate suture management by obligatorily separating the sutures between the 2 medial anchors.

The posteromedial anchor is typically placed first—there are at least 2 reasons why this may be advantageous. The posterior tissue is generally easier to mobilize, as tears often progress from anterior to posterior over time. Also, the posterior soft tissue tends to collapse more readily as it absorbs water over the duration of the procedure. The anchor is then placed, keeping in mind that the infraspinatus does not attach adjacent to the articular cartilage[1]—only the supraspinatus attaches along the "sulcus." The tendon is trial-reduced, and crimp marks are left with a grasper. A suture passer is used to pass a medial mattress suture configuration based on the trial reduction. The suture passes are 7-mm apart anterior to posterior. A nonsliding knot is preferred, although not mandatory, as this is less traumatic to the tendon tissue.[39] This also ensures that the suture limbs are satisfactory in length. The suture limbs are then retrieved out the posterior portal.

The same steps are taken for the anteromedial anchor, which can be passed through the superior accessory portal or the anterior portal. The anchor is placed adjacent to the articular margin sulcus, typically no less than 5-mm posterior to the biceps tendon. Trial reduction is performed again. This cannot be overemphasized to avoid malreductions or dog ears. The cord of the supraspinatus should be palpated during trial reduction, and attempts to visualize the cord thickening should be made. The tendon is crimped to mark the area for suture passing. After knot tying, the anterior-most suture limb is retrieved out the anterior portal. The posterior suture limb remains within the anterolateral working portal, and the posterior-most suture limb from the posteromedial anchor is then retrieved through this working portal.

These suture limbs are then incorporated into a suture-fixation implant, tensioned, and fixed to a point approximately 1-cm distal-lateral to the footprint edge—and generally placed in line with the posteromedial anchor. This distal-lateral fixation point provides an obligatory tendon-bridging compression vector over the tendon.[20] Trial reductions with the sutures are performed prior to implant advancement to optimize the amount of suture over the repaired tendon. During bursectomy, the lateral bursa should have been cleared in expectation of working in this area, distal-lateral to the footprint. The assistant should maintain the cannula over this area, flush to bone, up until the surgeon is ready to advance the suture-fixation implant.

The anterior-most suture limbs from each anchor are then retrieved through the working portal, and the above steps, adhering to the same concepts, are repeated for the anterolateral fixation point.

The above method highlights the basic steps for successful repair using single-loaded anchors. Applying the above principles will allow the ability to use more sutures for repair as deemed necessary. The accompanying video to this chapter shows repairs that add additional FiberTape (Arthex, Naples, FL) to the repair construct.[40]

POSTOPERATIVE MANAGEMENT AND REHABILITATION

Progressive range-of-motion exercises are initiated within 1 week. Progressive resistive exercises are held for 10 to 12 weeks postoperatively, based on clinical progress with pain and range of motion.

POTENTIAL COMPLICATIONS

Tendon tension overload is avoided by confirming proper medial-to-lateral tendon mobility. Tendon malreduction is avoided by anterior-to-posterior trial reductions prior to suture passing through the tendon.

PEARLS AND PITFALLS

- Needle localize all portals; otherwise, visualization and tendon preparation can be adversely affected.
- Ensure the working portal is centered on the tuberosity edge or it may be overly difficult to reach superiorly (the tendon) or distal-laterally (the lateral row).
- Pass sutures at least 10-mm medial to the tendon edge; otherwise, there may not be sufficient lateral tendon to compress, thus precluding a primary benefit of the TOE repair.
- Trial-reduce and mark the tendon, or malreductions (dog ears) may result, thus limiting the amount of tendon available for tendon compression and footprint restoration.
- Incorporate the anterior cord of the supraspinatus in order to take advantage of the anatomy, improving fixation and potentially optimizing function.

REFERENCES

1. Curtis AS, Burbank KM, Tierney JJ, et al. The insertional footprint of the rotator cuff: an anatomic study. *Arthroscopy.* 2006;22(6):603-609.
2. Dugas JR, Campbell DA, Warren RF, et al. Anatomy and dimensions of rotator cuff insertions. *J Shoulder Elbow Surg.* 2002;11(5):498-503.
3. Minagawa H, Itoi E, Konno N, et al. Humeral attachment of the supraspinatus and infraspinatus tendons: an anatomic study. *Arthroscopy.* 1998;14(3):302-306.
4. Bisson LJ, Manohar LM. A biomechanical comparison of transosseous-suture anchor and suture bridge rotator cuff repairs in cadavers. *Am J Sports Med.* 2009;37(10):1991-1995.

5. Kim DH, ElAttrache NS, Tibone JE, et al. Biomechanical comparison of a single-row versus double-row suture anchor technique for rotator cuff repair. *Am J Sports Med.* 2006;34(3):407-414.

6. Ma CB, Comerford L, Wilson J, et al. Biomechanical evaluation of arthroscopic rotator cuff repairs: double-row compared with single-row fixation. *J Bone Joint Surg.* 2006;88A(2):403-410.

7. Park MC, ElAttrache NS, Tibone JE, et al. Part I: footprint contact characteristics for an arthroscopic transosseous-equivalent rotator cuff repair technique. *J Shoulder Elbow Surg.* 2007;16(4):461-468.

8. Park MC, Pirolo JM, Park CJ, et al. The effect of abduction and rotation on footprint contact for single-row, double-row, and transosseous-equivalent rotator cuff repair techniques. *Am J Sports Med.* 2009;37(8):1599-1608.

9. Waltrip RL, Zheng N, Dugas JR, et al. Rotator cuff repair: a biomechanical comparison of three techniques. *Am J Sports Med.* 2003;31(4):493-497.

10. Apreleva M, Ozbaydar M, Fitzgibbons PG, et al. Rotator cuff tears: the effect of the reconstruction method on three-dimensional repair site area. *Arthroscopy.* 2002;18(5):519-526.

11. Meier SW, Meier JD. Rotator cuff repair: the effect of double-row fixation on three-dimensional repair site. *J Shoulder Elbow Surg.* 2006;15(6):691-696.

12. Park MC, Cadet ER, Levine WN, et al. Tendon-to-bone pressure distributions at a repaired rotator cuff footprint using transosseous suture and suture anchor fixation techniques. *Am J Sports Med.* 2005;33(8):1154-1159.

13. Park MC, Idjadi JA, ElAttrache NS, et al. The effect of dynamic external rotation comparing 2 footprint-restoring rotator cuff repair techniques. *Am J Sports Med.* 2008;36(5):893-900.

14. Park MC, Tibone JE, ElAttrache NS, et al. Part II: biomechanical assessment for a footprint-restoring arthroscopic transosseous-equivalent rotator cuff repair technique compared to a double-row technique. *J Shoulder Elbow Surg.* 2007;16(4):469-476.

15. Gates JJ, Gilliland J, McGarry MH, et al. The influence of distinct anatomic subregions of the supraspinatus on humeral rotation. *J Orthop Res.* 2010;28(1):12-17.

16. Ihashi K, Matsushita N, Yagi R, et al. Rotational action of the supraspinatus muscle on the shoulder joint. *J Electromyogr Kinesiol.* 1998;8:337-346.

17. Roh MS, Wang VM, April EW, et al. Anterior and posterior musculotendinous anatomy of the supraspinatus. *J Shoulder Elbow Surg.* 2000;9(5):436-440.

18. Volk AG, Vangsness CTJ. An anatomic study of the supraspinatus muscle and tendon. *Clin Orthop Relat Res.* 2001;384:280-285.

19. Park MC, Jun BJ, Park CJ, et al. The biomechanical effects of dynamic external rotation on rotator cuff repair compared to testing with the humerus fixed. *Am J Sports Med.* 2007;35(11):1931-1939.

20. Park MC, ElAttrache NS, Ahmad CS, et al. "Transosseous-equivalent" rotator cuff repair technique. *Arthroscopy.* 2006;22(12):1360, e1361-1365.

21. Ma CB, MacGillivray JD, Clabeaux J, et al. Biomechanical evaluation of arthroscopic rotator cuff stitches. *J Bone Joint Surg.* 2004;86-A(6):1211-1216.

22. MacGillivray JD, Ma CB. Technical note: an arthroscopic stitch for massive rotator cuff tears: the Mac stitch. *Arthroscopy.* 2004;20(6):669-671.

23. Gimbel JA, Van Kleunen JP, Lake SP, et al. The role of repair tension on tendon to bone healing in an animal model of chronic rotator cuff tears. *J Biomech.* 2007;40(3):561-568.

24. Hatakeyama Y, Itoi E, Pradhan RL, et al. Effect of arm elevation and rotation on the strain in the repaired rotator cuff tendon. *Am J Sports Med.* 2001;29(6):788-794.

25. Zuckerman JD, LeBlanc JM, Choueka J, et al. The effect of arm position and capsular release on rotator cuff repair. *J Bone Joint Surg.* 1991;73-B(3):402-405.

26. Ahmad CS, Vorys GC, Covey A, et al. Rotator cuff repair fluid extravasation characteristics are influenced by repair technique. *J Shoulder Elbow Surg.* 2009;18(6):976-981.

27. Burkhart SS, Adams CR, Burkhart SS, et al. A biomechanical comparison of 2 techniques of footprint reconstruction for rotator cuff repair: the SwiveLock-FiberChain construct versus standard double-row repair. *Arthroscopy.* 2009;25(3):274-281.

28. Pauly S, Kieser B, Schill A, et al. Biomechanic comparison of 4 double-row suture bridging rotator cuff repair techniques using different medial-row configurations. *Arthroscopy.* 2010;26(10):1281-1288.

29. Spang JT, Buchmann S, Brucker PU, et al. A biomechanical comparison of 2 transosseous-equivalent double-row rotator cuff repair techniques using bioabsorbable anchors: cyclic loading and failure behavior. *Arthroscopy.* 2009;25(8):872-879.

30. Busfield BT, Glousman RE, McGarry MH, et al. A biomechanical comparison of 2 technical variations of double-row rotator cuff fixation: the importance of medial-row knots. *Am J Sports Med.* 2008;36:901-906.

31. Cho NS, Yi JW, Lee BG, et al. Retear patterns after arthroscopic rotator cuff repair: single-row versus suture bridge technique. *Am J Sports Med.* 2010;38(4):664-671.

32. Voigt C, Bosse C, Vosshenrich R, et al. Arthroscopic supraspinatus tendon repair with suture-bridging technique. *Am J Sports Med.* 2010;38(5):983-991.

33. Wang VM, Wang FC, McNickle AG, et al. Medial versus lateral supraspinatus tendon properties: implications for double-row rotator cuff repair. *Am J Sports Med.* 2010;38(12):2456-2463. Epub 2010 Oct 7.

34. Kirchhoff C, Braunstein V, Milz S, et al. Assessment of bone quality within the tuberosities of the osteoporotic humeral head: relevance for anchor positioning in rotator cuff repair. *Am J Sports Med*. 2010;38(3):564-569.

35. Kulwicki KJ, Kwon YW, Kummer FJ. Suture anchor loading after rotator cuff repair: effects of an additional lateral row. *J Shoulder Elbow Surg*. 2010;19(1):81-85.

36. Frank JB, ElAttrache NS, Dines JS, et al. Repair site integrity after arthroscopic "transosseous-equivalent/suture-bridge" rotator cuff repair. *Am J Sports Med*. 2008;36:1496-1503.

37. Pennington WT, Gibbons DJ, Bartz BA, et al. Comparative analysis of single-row versus double-row repair of rotator cuff tears. *Arthroscopy*. 2010;26(11):1419-1426.

38. Duquin TR, Buyea C, Bisson LJ. Which method of rotator cuff repair leads to the highest rate of structural healing? A systematic review. *Am J Sports Med*. 2010;38(4):835-841.

39. Kowalsky MS, Dellenbaugh SG, Erlichman DB, et al. Evaluation of suture abrasion against rotator cuff tendon and proximal humerus bone. *Arthroscopy*. 2008;24(3):329-334.

40. Bisson LJ, Manohar LM. A biomechanical comparison of the pull-out strength of no. 2 FiberWire suture and 2-mm FiberWire tape in bovine rotator cuff tendons. *Arthroscopy*. 2010;26(22):1463-1468.

***Please see video on the accompanying Web site at
http://www.slackbooks.com/rotatorcuffvideos***

CHAPTER 14

BIOLOGIC AUGMENTATION OF ROTATOR CUFF REPAIR

Fernando Contreras, MD and Scott A. Rodeo, MD

Despite the improved biomechanical performance of newer methods to repair rotator cuff tears, incomplete or failed healing of the repaired tendon occurs in approximately 20% to 25% of patients, with higher failure rates in patients with increased tear size, chronic tears, and older age, among other factors.[1] Because of the relatively high failure rate of surgical repair, there is a great interest in developing methods to improve rotator cuff tendon healing. It has been recognized that novel methods are needed to improve the biology of rotator cuff tendon repair. Strategies such as the use of osteoinductive cytokines, bone morphogenetic protein-12 (BMP-12), stem cells, or transcription factors have been tested and shown to have beneficial effects in preclinical studies. The manipulation of factors known to inhibit healing, such as inflammatory cells, inflammatory mediators, and matrix metalloproteinases, as well as the mechanical load on the healing tendon-bone interface, also provide opportunities to improve healing.[2]

BIOLOGY OF AUGMENTATION STRATEGIES

Rotator cuff healing occurs by formation of reactive scar tissue rather than regeneration of a histologically normal insertion site.[2] In normal bone-to-tendon healing, the healed tendon attachment site has little resemblance to the native insertion site; instead of the 4 distinct zones of the normal insertion, the bone and tendon are joined by a layer of fibrovascular scar tissue containing type III collagen.[3,4] Specifically, the zone of calcified cartilage does not reform.[5] The resulting attachment site likely has inferior material properties compared to the original insertion site and may contribute to the substantial number of repair failures.[6] Methods of biologic augmentation aim to improve the structure and composition of the healing tendon attachment site.

The potential techniques of biologic augmentation of rotator cuff repair can be broadly divided in 3 groups: tendinous augmentation with cellular components, acellular extracellular matrix (ECM) augmentation, and the addition of growth factors.[6]

Ma CB, Feeley BT, eds.
*Basic Principles and Operative Management
of the Rotator Cuff (pp 201-214)*
© 2012 SLACK Incorporated

Tendon Augmentation With Cellular Components

Allogeneic or autogenic tendon grafts have been proposed to augment deficient or attenuated tendon tissue. A tendon graft may also decrease the tension between the repaired tendon and bone. Additionally, they may provide a scaffold to support the reparative process and may also provide a source of donor cells.[6] A study using allograft tendon for the reconstruction of massive rotator cuff tears showed improvement that was comparable to those patients treated with acromioplasty and débridement without reconstruction. However, the authors found complete radiographic failure of the repair in the 15 cases available for magnetic resonance imaging (MRI) follow-up and reported one case of infection and one case of presumed acute rejection.[7] They concluded that allograft tendon should not be used for the repair of massive or otherwise irreparable rotator cuff tears.

The tenotomized biceps tendon has also been proposed as a source for autograft augmentation in massive rotator cuff repairs. A retrospective review of open and arthroscopic repair of massive rotator cuff tears with biceps augmentation showed a statistically significant improvement in pain at rest and during exercise, range of motion, strength, and outcome scores compared to the preoperative status. There was no statistically significant difference between open and arthroscopic procedures.[8] Another retrospective review showed that patients who underwent biceps augmentation had greater strength and a lower structural failure rate than those without augmentation. However, there was no difference in pain, range of motion, or clinical outcome at 12 months postoperatively.[9]

Extracellular Matrix Augmentation

An acellular ECM can act as a bridge between the shortened tendon and bone, with its matrix providing a scaffold for cellular ingrowth and new matrix formation.[10] These augmentations are currently available in 3 forms: xenograft, allograft, and synthetic matrices.

Xenogeneic Extracellular Matrices

Xenograft ECMs have been developed from various sources, such as porcine small intestine submucosa (SIS) (Restore Orthobiologic Implant [DePuy Orthopedics, Warsaw, IN], CuffPatch [Biomet, Warsaw, IN]), fetal bovine dermis (TissueMend [Stryker, Mahwah, NJ]), or porcine dermis (Zimmer Collagen Repair Patch [Zimmer Inc, Warsaw, IN]). Restore is supplied as a disk composed of 10 layers of porcine SIS. The SIS is disinfected with peracetic acid and ethanol and does not contain any viable cells. The SIS ECM contains predominately type I collagen, fibronectin, chondroitin sulfate, heparin, heparin sulfate, hyaluronan, and growth factors (such as basic fibroblast growth factor [FGF-2], transforming growth factor-beta [TGF-ß], and vascular endothelial growth factor [VEGF]). To produce the Restore implant, 10 individual layers are oriented at approximately 20 degrees relative to each other and are laminated together under a vacuum press. Restore is not artificially cross-linked. The implant is packaged dry and is nominally 0.8 to 1 mm thick.[11]

Porcine SIS is considered an acellular, strong, biocompatible tissue scaffold that can act as an ECM to potentially improve repair tissue formation.[12] Animal studies have shown the potential of porcine SIS to induce regeneration of a tendon-bone junction after complete resection of the infraspinatus tendon in dogs, with a strength that is similar to that of a reimplanted native tendon.[13] Early healing in a sheep model was improved by supplementing the repair with a porcine SIS patch, as compared with the same surgical technique without supplementation. In this study, the stiffness of the repair was significantly higher in the augmentation group.[14] Despite the fact the Restore patch is considered acellular, one study showed that it can in fact contain residual porcine cells after processing. This residual porcine DNA may lead to an immune reaction against the material, which is supported by the observation of an inflammatory reaction characterized by massive lymphocyte infiltration after implantation of the membrane in mice and rabbits.[15]

The clinical application of xenografts in rotator cuff repairs has yielded mixed results.[6] A retrospective study of 11 consecutive open rotator cuff repairs with the Restore patch used as an interpositional or reinforcement graft showed a retear in 10 of 11 cases on postoperative MRI performed

6 to 10 months after surgery.[12] Phipatanakul and Petersen prospectively followed 11 patients with xenograft augmentation of rotator cuff repair for a mean of 26 months, finding that only 33% of the rotator cuff repairs remained intact and reconstitution of tendon tissue was poor in most instances.[16] The authors of these 2 studies recommended against the use of this material for rotator cuff repair, especially massive tears with atrophy. Malcarney and colleagues reported a nonspecific overt inflammatory reaction in the early postoperative period after rotator cuff repair with porcine SIS patch augmentation in 4 of 25 patients (16%).[17] Two-year follow-up on the patients from this study showed inferior results in patients who received the xenograft augmentation, with significantly less strength on lift-off, internal rotation, and adduction compared to controls. Furthermore, the xenograft augmentation group showed more impingement in external rotation, a slower rate of resolution of pain during activities, more difficulty with hand-behind-the-back activities, and less sports participation.[18]

Allogeneic Extracellular Matrices

Allogeneic ECMs have been developed via decellularization of cadaveric material. Two commercially available allogeneic ECMs have been studied to date: Allopatch (from harvested human fascia lata, Musculoskeletal Transplant Foundation, Edison, NJ) and GraftJacket (from human dermal tissue). GraftJacket Regenerative Tissue Matrix is manufactured by LifeCell (Branchburg, NJ) and is distributed by Wright Medical Technology (Arlington, TN). GraftJacket is derived from human allograft skin that is processed with use of a patented technique to remove the epidermis, cells, and cell remnants. The remaining acellular, dermal layer is preserved by a proprietary freeze-drying method, which retains the native extracellular architecture and vascular channels. The matrix contains biochemical components including collagen, elastin, and proteoglycans and is not artificially cross-linked. It is packaged dry. The material is a single layer and is provided in a variety of thicknesses (0.5 to 2 mm) and sizes for targeted surgical indications.[11]

Snyder and colleagues[19] reported on the histologic evaluation of a biopsy specimen obtained 3 months after rotator cuff repair augmentation with GraftJacket matrix. This biopsy was performed during a revision surgery indicated for retear. The analysis showed that the matrix was incorporated into the surrounding tissue, exhibited alignment of collagen fibers, revascularized with numerous blood vessels, repopulated with host cells, and presented little to no inflammatory response. Wong and colleagues have recently reported the results of 45 patients with massive rotator cuff tears treated arthroscopically with GraftJacket allograft with a follow-up of at least 2 years.[20] The mean University of California, Los Angeles (UCLA) score increased from 18.4 preoperatively to 27.5 postoperatively (p<0.001). At the final follow-up, the average Western Ontario Rotator Cuff score was 75.2, and the American Shoulder and Elbow Surgeons score was 84.1. There was one deep wound infection in an immunocompromised patient, which resolved after arthroscopic irrigation and débridement and antibiotic treatment. There have not been any cases of graft rejection in their series.

Synthetic Extracellular Matrices

Because concern remains that allograft materials may create an immunologic reaction and accompanying inflammatory response, there is considerable interest in developing synthetic ECM grafts for surgical use. Several animal studies have investigated the benefit of augmenting rotator cuff repair with synthetic ECMs.[6] Polyglycolic acid, chitin, poly(L-lactide), and polycarbonate polyurethane patches have been tested as augmentation devices in different animal studies, with some showing improved fibrocartilage formation, cell repopulation, collagen fiber alignment, as well as increased strength and stiffness.[21-24]

Addition of Growth Factors

It is conceivable that the composition and structure of the rotator cuff insertion could be reformed following tendon repair if it were possible to recapitulate the events that occur during embryonic development.[25] There are several fundamental reasons why this does not occur during tissue healing in the postnatal organism. These reasons include an abnormal or insufficient expression of genes that direct insertion site formation,[26] insufficient numbers of undifferentiated cells at the healing interface,[27] and mechanical load on the healing tendon.[28]

The presence of inflammation during tendon healing may lead to insufficient or abnormal molecular signals and cell differentiation. The rapid influx of inflammatory cells following rotator cuff tendon repair may result in cellular and molecular signals that lead to fibrosis rather than tissue regeneration. It is known that wounds in the developing fetus heal by tissue regeneration rather than scar formation. The absence of a substantial inflammatory response in fetal wounds is likely an important factor in what has been termed *scarless healing*.[2]

Growth factors play an important role in cell chemotaxis, proliferation, matrix synthesis, and cell differentiation. Several growth factors are upregulated during the rotator cuff healing process. Animal studies have shown the presence of FGF-2, BMPs 12-14, cartilage oligomeric matrix protein, and TGF-β1. Exogenous addition of these factors may augment the healing process.[29]

The clinical application of biologic therapy poses several challenges. First, the most effective growth factor or combination of factors must be determined. Second, the optimum time for growth factor delivery must be clarified. Finally, an optimal delivery vehicle should be developed.[29] This carrier vehicle should ideally provide sustained release of a relevant cytokine(s), it should serve as a scaffold to support the reparative response, and it must be amenable to placement through an arthroscopic approach.

Osteoinductive Factors

Experimental studies have shown that healing between the repaired rotator cuff tendon and bone is dependent on bone ingrowth. Healing begins with the formation of a fibrovascular interface tissue between the tendon and bone, followed by gradual bone ingrowth into this fibrous interface and then into the tendon, resulting in eventual re-establishment of collagen fiber continuity between the tendon and bone.[30] A study in a sheep model tested an osteoinductive bone protein extract derived from bovine cortical bone including BMP-2-7, TGF-β1-3, and FGF.[30] The experimental animals received the growth factors at the tendon-bone interface using a type I collagen sponge carrier. The 2 control groups consisted of repairs treated with the collagen sponge carrier alone or no implant. MRI, radiographic, histologic, and biomechanical testing were performed at 6 and 12 weeks. The specimens that were treated with the osteoinductive growth factors had significantly greater failure loads at 6 and 12 weeks; however, when the data were normalized by tissue volume, there were no differences between groups. These findings suggest that the growth factor treatment results in formation of poor-quality scar tissue rather than true tissue regeneration. This study was the first to demonstrate the possibility of increasing tissue formation in a tendon-bone gap using a biologic agent.

BMP-12

An animal model has evaluated recombinant human BMP-12 in rotator cuff tendon-to-bone healing. The rhBMP-12 was tested using various delivery vehicles (hyaluronan paste, hyaluronan sponge, type I collagen sponge, and type I/III collagen sponge) using 8 adult sheep per treatment.[31] The sponge carriers had longer rhBMP-12 local retention compared with the buffer or paste carriers, with approximately 50% of the rhBMP-12 still present at 7 days and measurable amounts still present at 21 days. The rhBMP-12 was tested in paste and sponge carriers in the sheep infraspinatus repair model. Four treatment groups with 8 animals each were evaluated: rhBMP-12 in an injectable hyaluronan paste, rhBMP-12 in a hyaluronan sponge, rhBMP-12 in type I/III collagen sponge, and rhBMP-12 in type I collagen sponge. The type I/III collagen sponge was used alone in 10 sheep, and another 14 sheep underwent repair with no implant. The model consisted of complete detachment and subsequent double-row suture reattachment of the infraspinatus tendon to the humerus. The carrier material was placed between the tendon and bone. Radiography, histologic analysis, and biomechanical evaluations were performed at 8 weeks. Ultrasound imaging was performed at 4 and 8 weeks.

The rhBMP-12-treated specimens had significantly increased load to failure and stiffness compared with the animals treated with the sponge alone or without any augmentation. Specimens treated with rhBMP-12 in collagen sponges were 2.7 times stronger than untreated specimens after 8 weeks, whereas those treated with rhBMP-12 in hyaluronan sponges were 2.1 times stronger than untreated specimens. Specimens treated with rhBMP-12 in a hyaluronan paste were similar to untreated specimens, likely due to shorter retention times.[2,31] Ultrasound evaluation demonstrated a gap (10 to 18 mm) between the tendon and the bone in all repair groups. Histologic evaluation found re-establishment of collagen fiber continuity between the bone and the fibrovascular interface scar tissue, with increased glycosaminoglycan content in the rhBMP-12-treated specimens. There was a positive correlation between the glycosaminoglycan content of the repairs and the maximum load.

These results support the potential for BMPs to augment tendon-to-bone healing. Other studies have also shown a positive effect of BMPs on tendon healing,[32,33] as well as a delay in healing when these signaling molecules are absent.[34,35]

Platelet-Derived Growth Factors From Autologous Blood

There has been recent interest in the use of autologous platelet concentrates (platelet-rich plasma, PRP) to improve healing of soft and hard tissues. As a means of growth factor delivery, PRP was first popularized in maxillofacial and plastic surgery in the 1990s. Its use in orthopedics began early in the 2000s as PRP was used with bone grafts to augment spinal fusion and fracture healing.[36] Platelets contain several cytokines that play important roles in initiating the early healing response in connective tissues, including bone and tendon. Cytokines present in platelets include FGF-2, TGF-ß, insulin-like growth factor 1 (IGF-1), IGF-2, VEGF, and platelet-derived growth factor.[37]

Although there are numerous basic science studies, animal studies, and small case reports regarding PRP-related products, there are very few controlled, clinical studies that provide a high level of evidence regarding the potential benefits of PRP. The number of patients in the studies is typically small, and the majority of studies are underpowered. The fundamental problem is the tremendous variability in the different commercially available PRP preparations, with differences in platelet recovery, inclusion of white blood cells, platelet activation, and kinetics of cytokine release from the preparation. Furthermore, there is variability in platelet counts and growth factor content per platelet between different individuals. The majority of reports are anecdotal studies based on small case series. Before adopting PRP into clinical practice, it is important to assess the evidence that supports its safety and efficacy.[38]

Currently, there are several commercial systems to obtain a PRP or "platelet gel" from autologous blood. A simple centrifugation process of autologous blood can be used to form a dense fibrin matrix, which is suturable and can be easily placed directly at the tendon repair site (Figure 14-1).[25] Most systems use calcium chloride and thrombin from human or bovine origin to coagulate the PRP. The use of thrombin may lead to premature platelet activation and degranulation, resulting in immediate release of the cytokines.

An alternative method uses a different strategy that allows the formation of platelets and fibrin into a dense matrix without the use of exogenous thrombin (Cascade Autologous Platelet System, Cascade Medical Enterprises, Wayne, NJ). Calcium chloride is added to initiate the formation of autogenous thrombin from prothrombin during the second centrifugation process, resulting in the formation of a dense fibrin matrix in which intact platelets are trapped. This prevents premature platelet degranulation and ensures platelet integrity. As a result, platelets release growth factors slowly during a 7-day period. The low level of autologous thrombin present in blood achieves a stable fibrin network with no clot retraction.[25,38]

Currently, the majority of orthopedic applications for PRP can be grouped into 4 different categories: chronic tendinopathies, acute ligamentous injuries, muscle injuries, and intraoperative

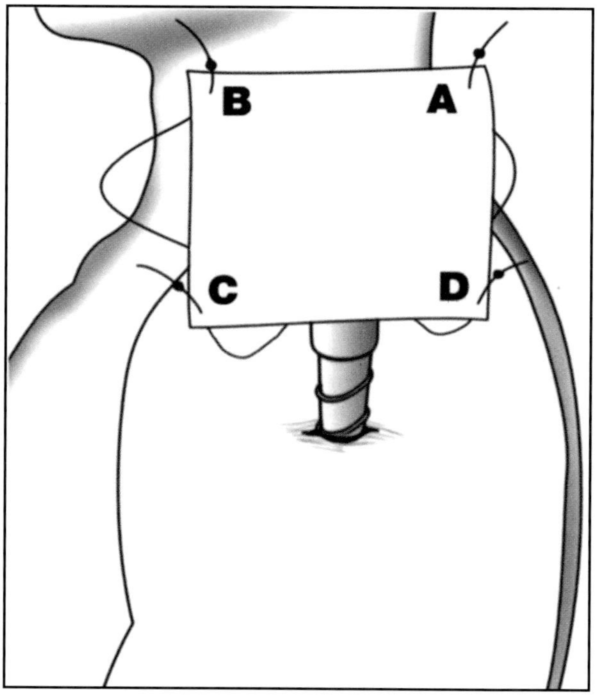

Figure 14-2. STIK sutures with mulberry knots through the ECM patch. (Reprinted from *Arthroscopy*, vol 22, iss 1, Seldes RM, Abramchayev I, Arthroscopic insertion of a biologic rotator cuff tissue augmentation after rotator cuff repair, p 114, Copyright 2006, with permission from Elsevier.)

Four measurements are taken: (1) anterior to posterior adjacent to the medial stump of residual cuff tissue; (2) anterior to posterior at the edge of the articular cartilage; (3) medial to lateral adjacent to the biceps tendon; and (4) medial to lateral adjacent to the posterior edge of residual cuff tissue.

The ECM patch is rehydrated in a sterile solution and is then cut to the proper size as determined by the measurements of the tendon defect. Short-tail interference knotted (STIK) sutures are prepared on the back table by tying mulberry-type knots on the end of a No.2 suture. These STIK sutures are placed around the anterior, medial, and posterior aspect of the graft, 3 mm from the edge and 4 to 5 mm apart using a Keith needle carrying the sutures from top to bottom, leaving the knotted end on the superior surface of the graft (Figure 14-2).

The posterior corner and the anterior edge of the cuff are stabilized using sutures from standard suture anchors. One anchor is inserted into the prepared bone at the posterior edge of the tear and is used to stabilize the posterior corner. The anterior anchor is placed just behind the biceps tendon. Its most anterior suture is passed through the rotator interval tissue or through the adjacent biceps tendon to create a strong anterior edge to anchor the graft. Two separate incisions should be made for these 2 anchors. The midlateral cannula is located just lateral and midway between these 2 anchors and will be used for suture management.

Suture passing should be done in a consistent, sequential manner. The ECM patch is placed on a moistened towel clamped around the arm adjacent to the lateral cannula. It is oriented so that the posterior edge of the graft faces the cannula when sewing to the posterior edge, then turned so that the medial edge faces the cannula when sewing to the medial stump, and the anterior edge faces the cannula when sewing to the anterior cuff and biceps tendon. Suturing should begin posterior, proceed along the medial edge, and finish with the anterior sutures.

The middle suture from the posterior anchor is passed first through the cuff tissue. It is retrieved out the lateral cannula and passed from bottom to top through the corresponding corner of the graft using a straight Keith needle. A STIK suture is tied in the top end of the suture, and the other end of the suture is pulled to remove the slack. Suture shuttles of different angles are used to pass

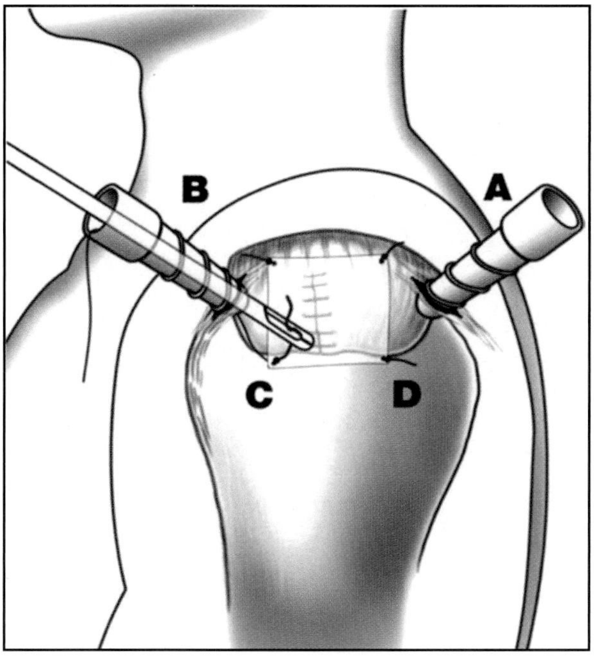

Figure 14-3. ECM patch at the repair site. (Reprinted from *Arthroscopy*, vol 22, iss 1, Seldes RM, Abramchayev I, Arthroscopic insertion of a biologic rotator cuff tissue augmentation after rotator cuff repair, p 114, Copyright 2006, with permission from Elsevier.)

the remaining STIK sutures. All stitching and shuttling is done through the posterior or anterior portals. The shuttle is grasped through the lateral portal, taking care to always stay anterior to the previous suture. The STIK sutures are loaded outside the lateral portal and pulled back through the lateral cannula and cuff.

The graft is folded so that the STIKs are on the inside of the roll and the medial edge faces the lateral cannula. Using a "push-pull" technique, the graft is inserted down the lateral cannula. The graft is pushed with a grasper while the free ends of the STIK sutures that are stored inside the posterior and anterior cannulas are pulled. Tensioning of the STIKs removes slack and causes the graft to unfold inside the joint (Figure 14-3).

The knotted end of the anterior STIK and the corresponding free end of one of the sutures are retrieved into the anterior cannula. Standard knot tying is done, and the process is repeated along the anterior, medial, and finally the posterior edges until all of the STIKs are secure. Finally, the 2 STIKs from the suture anchors are tied to secure the corners of the graft to the anchor sites. A standard single-row technique is used to repair the lateral edge of the graft to the prepared bone in the tuberosity, using the remaining suture from each suture anchor. Additional suture anchors are inserted as needed to achieve an adequate apposition of the graft to the footprint.

Application of Platelet-Rich Plasma

A PRFM is recommended because this preparation is firm enough to hold a suture. A standard suture anchor repair technique is used. After the anchor is placed, one of the anchor sutures is brought through an 8-mm cannula. The PRFM is threaded onto this suture using a free needle (Figure 14-4A). The PRFM implant is then pushed down the suture through the cannula so that the PRFM is adjacent to the bone attachment site (Figures 14-4B and C). The diaphragm on the cannula must first be removed to allow the PRFM implant to pass easily through the cannula and to prevent damaging the PRFM implant. Once the implant is down to bone, the end of the suture is then passed through the tendon in the desired fashion, using standard suture-passing instruments and techniques. Either simple or mattress sutures may be used. The sutures are then tied, trapping the PRFM implant between the tendon and bone (Figure 14-5).

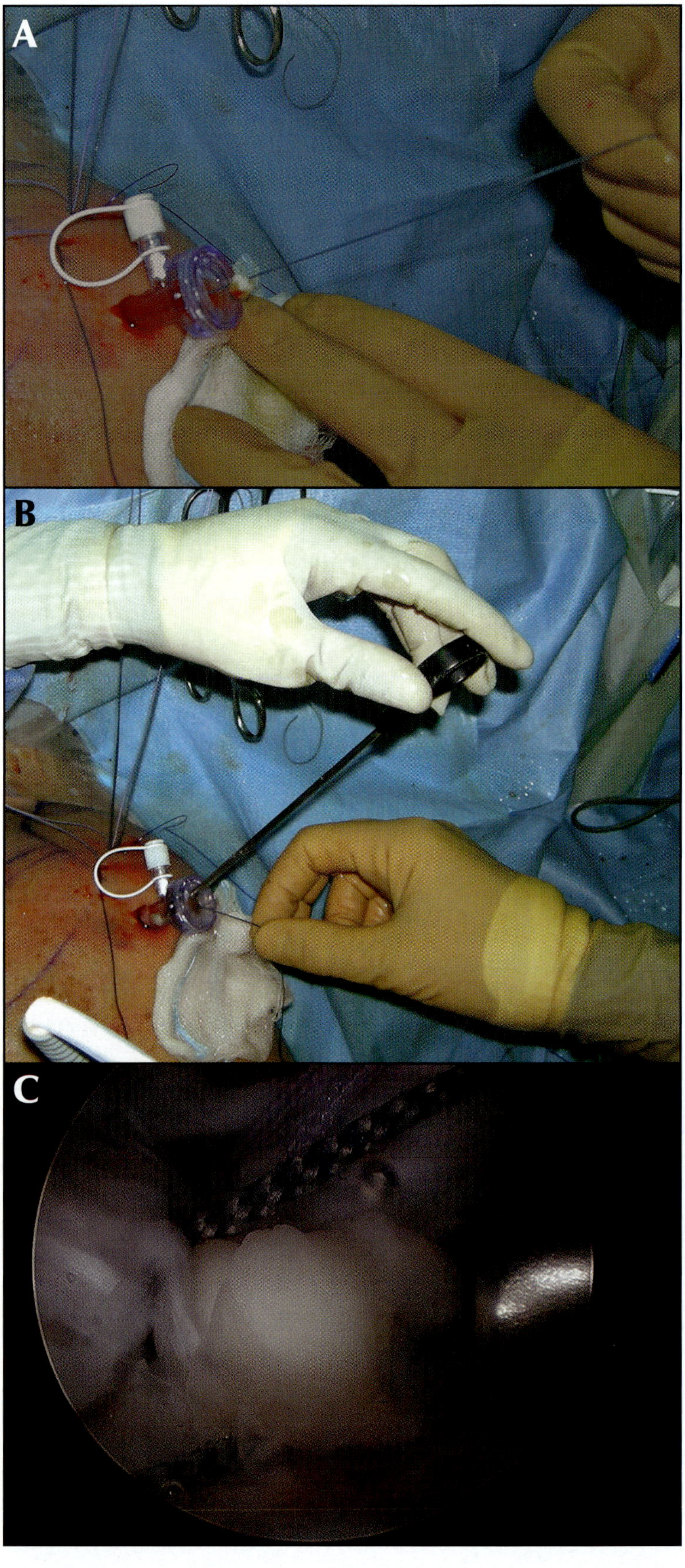

Figure 14-4. (A) PRFM preparation threaded with suture. (B) PRFM preparation brought through the 8-mm cannula with a knot pusher. (C) PRFM delivered at repair site.

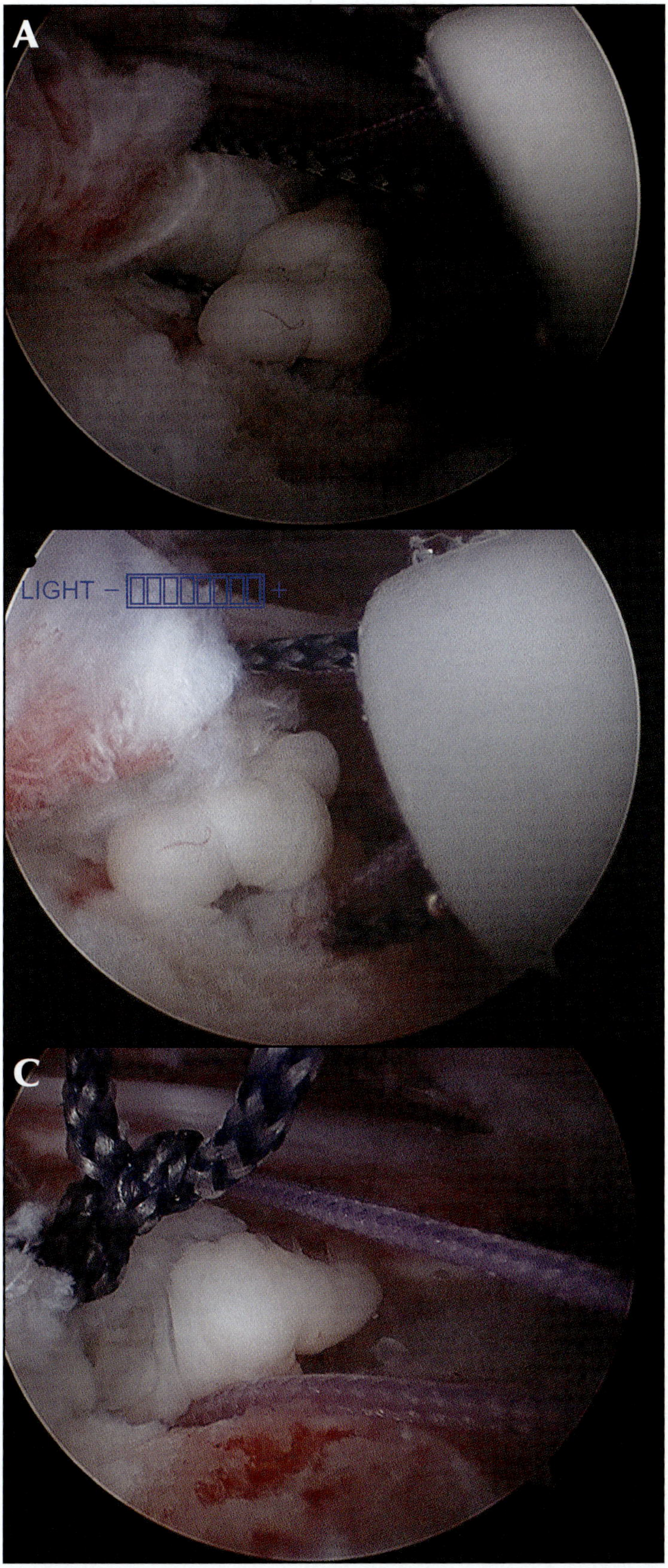

Figure 14-5. (A) PRFM at repair site. (B and C) PRFM trapped at repair site after tying the sutures in the anchor.

Postoperative Management and Rehabilitation

Biologic augmentation techniques are typically used for repairing larger, chronic, or retracted tears. Thus, a conservative postoperative protocol is typically recommended. The operative extremity is supported in a sling for 6 weeks, removing it daily to perform Codman's and pendulum exercises. Only passive motion is recommended for the first 6 weeks, starting with elevation in the plane of the scapula and then progressing to active-assisted motion at the 6-week point. Formal therapy begins at 4 to 6 weeks. The initial goal is to re-establish scapular plane elevation and moderate external rotation. Progressive strengthening begins at 12 weeks.

REFERENCES

1. Duquin TR, Buyea C, Bisson LJ. Which method of rotator cuff repair leads to the highest rate of structural healing? A systematic review. *Am J Sports Med.* 2010;38(4):835-841.
2. Kovacevic D, Rodeo SA. Biological augmentation of rotator cuff tendon repair. *Clin Orthop Relat Res.* 2008;466(3):622-633.
3. Galatz LM, Sandell LJ, Rothermich SY, et al. Characteristics of the rat supraspinatus tendon during tendon-to-bone healing after acute injury. *J Orthop Res.* 2006;24(3):541-550.
4. Rodeo SA, Arnoczky SP, Torzilli PA, Hidaka C, Warren RF. Tendon-healing in a bone tunnel. A biomechanical and histological study in the dog. *J Bone Joint Surg Am.* 1993;75(12):1795-1803.
5. Gerber C, Schneeberger AG, Perren SM, Nyffeler RW. Experimental rotator cuff repair. A preliminary study. *J Bone Joint Surg Am.* 1999;81(9):1281-1290.
6. Cheung EV, Silverio L, Sperling JW. Strategies in biologic augmentation of rotator cuff repair: a review. *Clin Orthop Relat Res.* 2010;468(6):1476-1484.
7. Moore DR, Cain EL, Schwartz ML, Clancy WG Jr. Allograft reconstruction for massive, irreparable rotator cuff tears. *Am J Sports Med.* 2006;34(3):392-396.
8. Rhee YG, Cho NS, Lim CT, Yi JW, Vishvanathan T. Bridging the gap in immobile massive rotator cuff tears: augmentation using the tenotomized biceps. *Am J Sports Med.* 2008;36(8):1511-1518.
9. Cho NS, Yi JW, Rhee YG. Arthroscopic biceps augmentation for avoiding undue tension in repair of massive rotator cuff tears. *Arthroscopy.* 2009;25(2):183-191.
10. Adams JE, Zobitz ME, Reach JS Jr, An KN, Steinmann SP. Rotator cuff repair using an acellular dermal matrix graft: an in vivo study in a canine model. *Arthroscopy.* 2006;22(7):700-709.
11. Derwin KA, Baker AR, Spragg RK, Leigh DR, Iannotti JP. Commercial extracellular matrix scaffolds for rotator cuff tendon repair. Biomechanical, biochemical, and cellular properties. *J Bone Joint Surg Am.* 2006;88(12):2665-2672.
12. Sclamberg SG, Tibone JE, Itamura JM, Kasraeian S. Six-month magnetic resonance imaging follow-up of large and massive rotator cuff repairs reinforced with porcine small intestinal submucosa. *J Shoulder Elbow Surg.* 2004;13(5):538-541.
13. Dejardin LM, Arnoczky SP, Ewers BJ, Haut RC, Clarke RB. Tissue-engineered rotator cuff tendon using porcine small intestine submucosa. Histologic and mechanical evaluation in dogs. *Am J Sports Med.* 2001;29(2):175-184.
14. Schlegel TF, Hawkins RJ, Lewis CW, Motta T, Turner AS. The effects of augmentation with Swine small intestine submucosa on tendon healing under tension: histologic and mechanical evaluations in sheep. *Am J Sports Med.* 2006;34(2):275-280.
15. Zheng MH, Chen J, Kirilak Y, Willers C, Xu J, Wood D. Porcine small intestine submucosa (SIS) is not an acellular collagenous matrix and contains porcine DNA: possible implications in human implantation. *J Biomed Mater Res B Appl Biomater.* 2005;73(1):61-67.
16. Phipatanakul WP, Petersen SA. Porcine small intestine submucosa xenograft augmentation in repair of massive rotator cuff tears. *Am J Orthop (Belle Mead NJ).* 2009;38(11):572-575.
17. Malcarney HL, Bonar F, Murrell GA. Early inflammatory reaction after rotator cuff repair with a porcine small intestine submucosal implant: a report of 4 cases. *Am J Sports Med.* 2005;33(6):907-911.
18. Walton JR, Bowman NK, Khatib Y, Linklater J, Murrell GA. Restore orthobiologic implant: not recommended for augmentation of rotator cuff repairs. *J Bone Joint Surg Am.* 2007;89(4):786-791.
19. Snyder SJ, Arnoczky SP, Bond JL, Dopirak R. Histologic evaluation of a biopsy specimen obtained 3 months after rotator cuff augmentation with GraftJacket Matrix. *Arthroscopy.* 2009;25(3):329-333.
20. Wong I, Burns J, Snyder S. Arthroscopic GraftJacket repair of rotator cuff tears. *J Shoulder Elbow Surg.* 2010;19(2 Suppl):104-109.
21. Derwin KA, Codsi MJ, Milks RA, Baker AR, McCarron JA, Iannotti JP. Rotator cuff repair augmentation in a canine model with use of a woven poly-L-lactide device. *J Bone Joint Surg Am.* 2009;91(5):1159-1171.

22. Funakoshi T, Majima T, Suenaga N, Iwasaki N, Yamane S, Minami A. Rotator cuff regeneration using chitin fabric as an acellular matrix. *J Shoulder Elbow Surg*. 2006;15(1):112-118.

23. Yokoya S, Mochizuki Y, Nagata Y, Deie M, Ochi M. Tendon-bone insertion repair and regeneration using polyglycolic acid sheet in the rabbit rotator cuff injury model. *Am J Sports Med*. 2008;36(7):1298-1309.

24. Cole BJ, Gomoll AH, Yanke A, et al. Biocompatibility of a polymer patch for rotator cuff repair. *Knee Surg Sports Traumatol Arthrosc*. 2007;15(5):632-637.

25. Rodeo SA. Biologic augmentation of rotator cuff tendon repair. *J Shoulder Elbow Surg*. 2007;16(5 Suppl):S191-S197.

26. Thomopoulos S, Hattersley G, Rosen V, et al. The localized expression of extracellular matrix components in healing tendon insertion sites: an in situ hybridization study. *J Orthop Res*. 2002;20(3):454-463.

27. Lim JK, Hui J, Li L, Thambyah A, Goh J, Lee EH. Enhancement of tendon graft osteointegration using mesenchymal stem cells in a rabbit model of anterior cruciate ligament reconstruction. *Arthroscopy*. 2004;20(9):899-910.

28. Thomopoulos S, Williams GR, Soslowsky LJ. Tendon to bone healing: differences in biomechanical, structural, and compositional properties due to a range of activity levels. *J Biomech Eng*. 2003;125(1):106-113.

29. Gulotta LV, Rodeo SA. Growth factors for rotator cuff repair. *Clin Sports Med*. 2009;28(1):13-23.

30. Rodeo SA, Potter HG, Kawamura S, Turner AS, Kim HJ, Atkinson BL. Biologic augmentation of rotator cuff tendon-healing with use of a mixture of osteoinductive growth factors. *J Bone Joint Surg Am*. 2007;89(11):2485-2497.

31. Seeherman HJ, Archambault JM, Rodeo SA, et al. rhBMP-12 accelerates healing of rotator cuff repairs in a sheep model. *J Bone Joint Surg Am*. 2008;90(10):2206-2219.

32. Lou J, Tu Y, Burns M, Silva MJ, Manske P. BMP-12 gene transfer augmentation of lacerated tendon repair. *J Orthop Res*. 2001;19(6):1199-1202.

33. Murray DH, Kubiak EN, Jazrawi LM, et al. The effect of cartilage-derived morphogenetic protein 2 on initial healing of a rotator cuff defect in a rat model. *J Shoulder Elbow Surg*. 2007;16(2):251-254.

34. Nakase T, Sugamoto K, Miyamoto T, et al. Activation of cartilage-derived morphogenetic protein-1 in torn rotator cuff. *Clin Orthop Relat Res*. 2002;399:140-145.

35. Chhabra A, Tsou D, Clark RT, Gaschen V, Hunziker EB, Mikic B. GDF-5 deficiency in mice delays Achilles tendon healing. *J Orthop Res*. 2003;21(5):826-835.

36. Hall MP, Band PA, Meislin RJ, Jazrawi LM, Cardone DA. Platelet-rich plasma: current concepts and application in sports medicine. *J Am Acad Orthop Surg*. 2009;17(10):602-608.

37. Anitua E, Andia I, Ardanza B, Nurden P, Nurden AT. Autologous platelets as a source of proteins for healing and tissue regeneration. *Thromb Haemost*. 2004;91(1):4-15.

38. Foster TE, Puskas BL, Mandelbaum BR, Gerhardt MB, Rodeo SA. Platelet-rich plasma: from basic science to clinical applications. *Am J Sports Med*. 2009;37(11):2259-2272.

39. Randelli PS, Arrigoni P, Cabitza P, Volpi P, Maffulli N. Autologous platelet rich plasma for arthroscopic rotator cuff repair. A pilot study. *Disabil Rehabil*. 2008;30(20-22):1584-1589.

40. Paoloni JA, Appleyard RC, Nelson J, Murrell GA. Topical glyceryl trinitrate application in the treatment of chronic supraspinatus tendinopathy: a randomized, double-blinded, placebo-controlled clinical trial. *Am J Sports Med*. 2005;33(6):806-813.

41. Nassos JT, Chudik SC. Arthroscopic rotator cuff repair with biceps tendon augmentation. *Am J Orthop (Belle Mead NJ)*. 2009;38(6):279-281.

42. Bond JL, Dopirak RM, Higgins J, Burns J, Snyder SJ. Arthroscopic replacement of massive, irreparable rotator cuff tears using a GraftJacket allograft: technique and preliminary results. *Arthroscopy*. 2008;24(4):403-409.e1.

43. Seldes RM, Abramchayev I. Arthroscopic insertion of a biologic rotator cuff tissue augmentation after rotator cuff repair. *Arthroscopy*. 2006;22(1):113-116.

44. Labbe MR. Arthroscopic technique for patch augmentation of rotator cuff repairs. *Arthroscopy*. 2006;22(10):1136.e1-1136.e6.

Please see video on the accompanying Web site at
http://www.slackbooks.com/rotatorcuffvideos

CHAPTER 15

ARTHROSCOPIC TREATMENT OF SUBSCAPULARIS TEARS

Jaicharan J. Iyengar, MD and C. Benjamin Ma, MD

Dysfunction of the subscapularis tendon is a significant source of shoulder pain and concomitant disability that frequently coexists with other sources of intra-articular shoulder pathology.[1,2] Tears of the subscapularis occur less commonly than other tendons of the rotator cuff, with an estimated incidence of 2% in a magnetic resonance imaging (MRI) study of 2167 patients with rotator cuff pathology.[3] The true incidence of subscapularis tears is not known, as the number of unrecognized injuries is likely significant[4] and can be the source of continued pain and disability after a supraspinatus rotator cuff repair. The etiology of subscapularis tears can be traumatic or degenerative, with the latter including tears that are associated with subcoracoid impingement.[5-7] In general, subscapularis tears can be divided into partial, complete, and complete/retracted tears. The biomechanical consequence of a subscapularis tear is loss of the anterior aspect of the transverse plane glenohumeral force couple.[8] This results in unbalanced dynamic forces across the glenohumeral joint and loss of concentricity with attempted shoulder motion.[9]

The clinical manifestation of subscapularis tears includes generalized pain, often localized to the anterior shoulder, and weakness of the shoulder, specifically with respect to overhead movement and active internal rotation of the shoulder.[10] Increased passive external rotation of the affected shoulder compared to the contralateral side may indicate subscapularis insufficiency. Pathology of the long head of the biceps tendon and labral complex is often present with the presentation of subscapularis dysfunction.[11,12] Several clinical tests have been described in the literature to elicit subscapularis pathology, including the lift-off, bear-hug, and belly-press tests.[13-16] MRI examination can help confirm the presence of a tear and provide information related to the location and morphology of the tear, the amount of retraction of complete tears, and associated biceps pathology.[17] MRI also allows a qualitative assessment of fatty infiltration of the subscapularis muscle, an important marker of myotendinous tissue quality.[18] Fatty infiltration is not as common in the subscapularis as much as the supraspinatus and infraspinatus, likely due to its different innervation. Muscle quality is critical in determining which tears can be managed arthroscopically and which require open surgical treatment. Once the diagnosis is made, we favor early repair of subscapularis tears as the natural history of delayed surgical management has been shown to result in

Ma CB, Feeley BT, eds.
*Basic Principles and Operative Management
of the Rotator Cuff (pp 215-222)*
© 2012 SLACK Incorporated

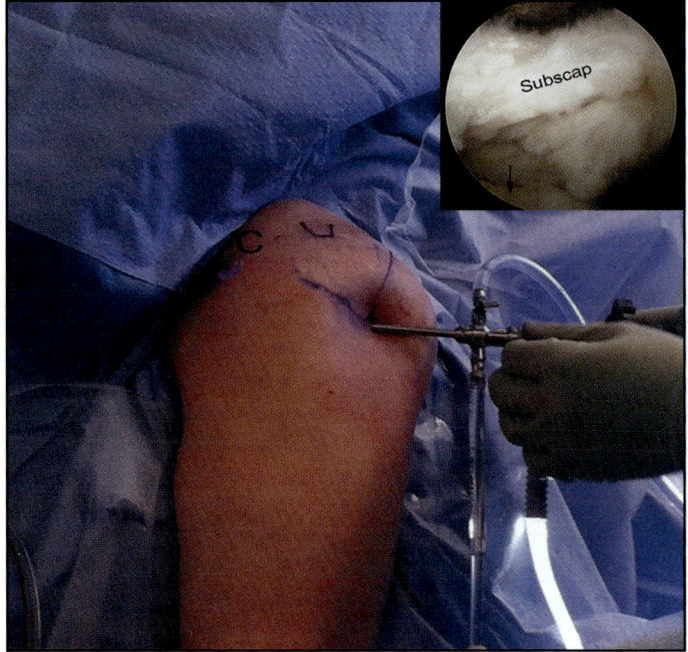

Figure 15-1. Set up for arthroscopic subscapularis repair. Patient is in the beach chair position with a high lateral posterior viewing portal. The coracoid (C) is marked anteriorly. A more medial posterior portal may be used in the repair of an isolated subscapularis tear, but a high lateral portal position is advantageous in the repair of a concomitant supraspinatus tear. The inset shows the arthroscopic view of a subscapularis (Subscap) tear with avulsion off the lesser tuberosity (solid black arrow).

unsatisfactory outcomes.[19] We perform arthroscopic repair of most partial and complete, nonretracted tears. Complete tears with significant retraction that are not amenable to arthroscopic mobilization and repair are treated using open technique.

SURGICAL TECHNIQUE

The patient positioning and surgical preparation for the arthroscopic treatment of subscapularis tears is the same as for standard shoulder arthroscopy in the beach chair position. When positioning the patient for subscapularis repair, we rotate the head toward the contralateral side to open up the anterior aspect of the operative shoulder for instrumentation and to allow for easier passage of the penetrators through the subscapularis. We begin with a thorough arthroscopic examination of the shoulder from a standard posterior viewing portal using a 30-degree arthroscope (Figure 15-1). For an intra-articular subscapularis tendon repair, the posterior portal is created 2-cm inferior to the posterolateral edge of the acromion, optimally centered at the glenohumeral "soft spot." However, if there is a concomitant supraspinatus tear, we use a "high lateral" posterior viewing portal.

The freedom to manipulate the arm to assist in visualization is an advantage of performing subscapularis tendon repair in the beach chair position. The lesser tuberosity can be best viewed by placing the extremity in forward flexion and internal rotation. This position relieves tension on the subscapularis tendon at its insertion and allows visualization of the inferior portion of the lesser tuberosity with a 30-degree arthroscope. A 70-degree arthroscope is sometimes used to better visualize the articular side of the subscapularis tendon at its humeral insertion but is not vital for the procedure. We typically have one available for the procedure but do not use it unless we are unable to fully visualize the relevant anatomy. Humeral avulsion of the superior glenohumeral ligament and coracohumeral (CH) ligament from the superior border of the subscapularis footprint, described as a "comma sign," often corresponds to the retracted edge of the torn subscapularis tendon (Figure 15-2).[20] The presence and absence of the superior glenohumeral ligament is an important marker of biceps stability. The biceps tendon is evaluated to assess its position relative to the subscapularis tendon. Any evidence of anteromedial displacement of the biceps tendon is indicative of biceps subluxation and is treated with concomitant biceps tenodesis.

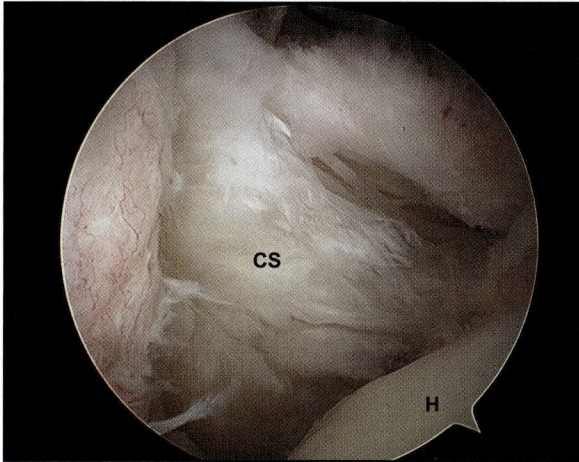

Figure 15-2. The arthroscopic "comma sign" as seen from a posterior portal, which corresponds to humeral avulsion of the superior glenohumeral ligament and CH ligament from the superior border of the subscapularis footprint (CS, comma sign; H, humeral head).

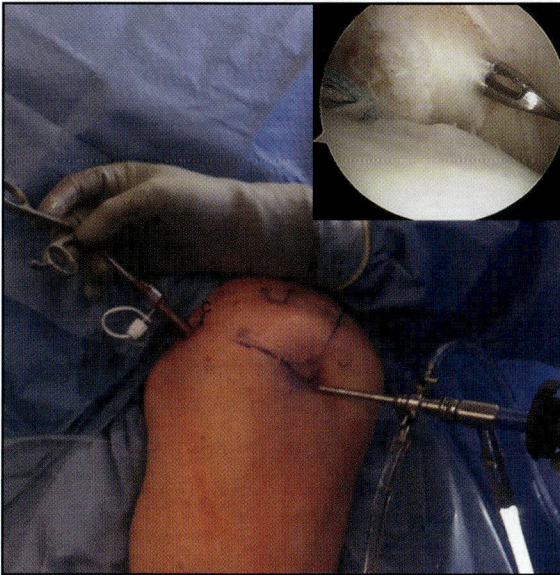

Figure 15-3. Establishment of the anterior portal superior to the subscapularis tendon. An arthroscopic tissue penetrator is seen within the anterior cannula. The inset shows the penetrator passing through the healthy border of the subscapularis tendon.

We next establish an anterior rotator interval portal just lateral to the coracoid that allows access to the lesser tuberosity (Figure 15-3). The coracoid is visualized through the rotator interval, which necessitates soft tissue excision with electrocautery in the interval to allow for arthroscopic access (Figure 15-4). Attention to this portion of the case is critical, as this allows for easier passage of the penetrators during repair and easier suture passage during knot tying.

We routinely perform a coracoplasty at the time of subscapularis repair if there is evidence of subcoracoid impingement. The coracoid tip is cleaned of excess soft tissue and bursa, particularly the posterolateral aspect, which is usually the site of prominence and subscapularis impingement. An arthroscopic burr is used to resect the prominent coracoid; the plane of our resection is oriented parallel to the subscapularis tendon (Figure 15-5). To adequately decompress the anterior tendon interval, we aim to restore a minimum of 6 mm of CH space in the interval.[21]

For an isolated subscapularis tear, we then use the anterior portal to assist with intra-articular arthroscopic mobilization and repair. A spinal needle is used to localize an anterior "percutaneous" incision for optimal trajectory of insertion of suture anchors (Figure 15-6). With this technique, we find it unnecessary to create a second anterior portal for anchor insertion, which can further limit the working space available and complicate suture management. For tears that extend into the

Figure 15-4. Arthroscopic rotator interval release to allow visualization of the coracoid and subscapularis insertion (S, subscapularis).

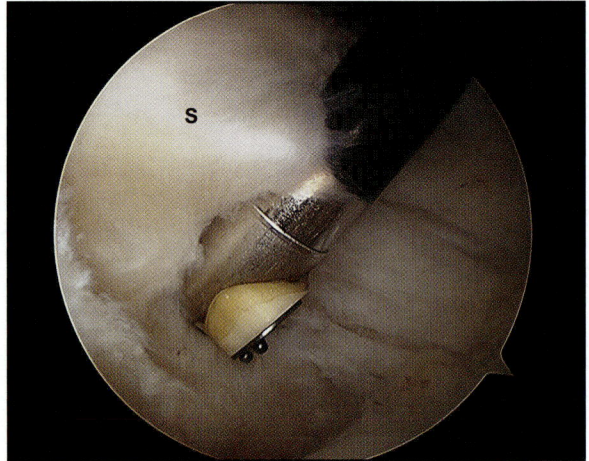

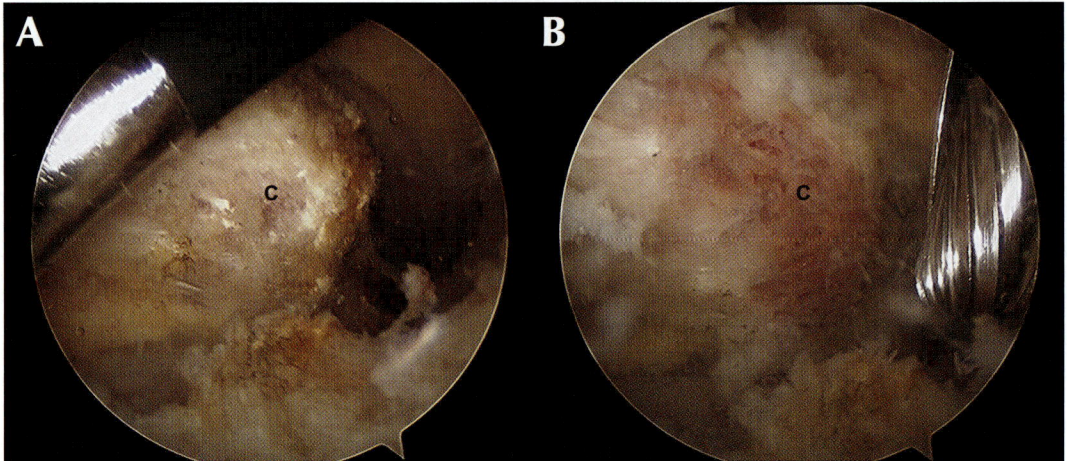

Figure 15-5. Arthroscopic view of the coracoid tip before (top) and after (bottom) coracoplasty. Note that burr width allows us to estimate the width of resection (C, coracoid).

Figure 15-6. Using a spinal needle to achieve optimal trajectory to the bare lesser tuberosity for percutaneous insertion of a suture anchor (S, leading edge of subscapularis; LT, lesser tuberosity).

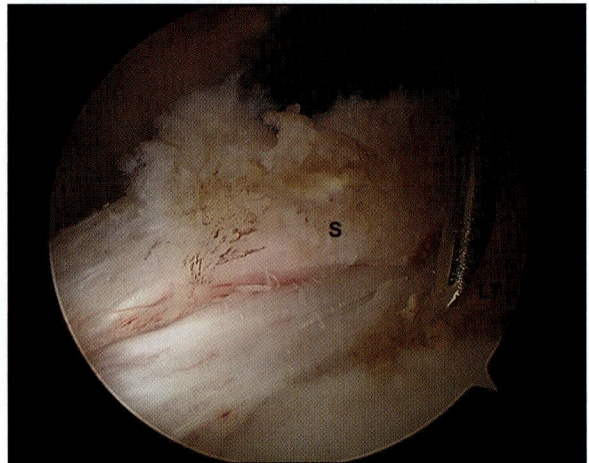

supraspinatus tendon, we will first perform the subscapularis tendon repair through a lateral portal from the subacromial space. We then repair the supraspinatus tendon through the same portal, as described elsewhere in this text.

Once we have defined the morphology, tissue quality, and amount of medial retraction of the subscapularis tear, we then proceed with arthroscopic repair. We insert an arthroscopic forceps into the anterior interval portal and grasp the free edge of the subscapularis tendon to mobilize it laterally while performing the repair. Alternatively, a traction suture can be placed medial to the free edge to allow one to mobilize the tendon with gentle traction during the repair. It is sometimes difficult to recognize the free edge of the subscapularis tendon as there may be fibrous tissue that fills in between the true tendon and the lesser tuberosity. However, the articular surface of the subscapularis tendon will usually have a shiny surface that is distinct from the more lateral tissue that appears frayed and dull. We aim to restore this shiny true intact tendon to its lesser tuberosity footprint. We release the anterior, posterior, and superior aspect of the tendon sharply, using an arthroscopic elevator to allow for minimal tension when approximated to the lesser tuberosity. It is important to avoid blind passage of an elevator along the inferior border of the tendon to minimize the risk of neurovascular injury. Careful dissection needs to be performed anterior to the subscapularis tendon as the upper and lower subscapularis nerves traverse this subcoracoid space. Posteriorly, the middle glenohumeral ligament can be scarred and can resist lateral advancement of the subscapularis tendon. In such cases, it can be helpful to resect the middle glenohumeral ligament to facilitate tendon excursion.

The lesser tuberosity insertion is cleared of soft tissue using arthroscopic electrocautery and a motorized shaver. We favor metal corkscrew anchors for fixation because of the porous bone quality of the lesser tuberosity region. For a superior half subscapularis tendon tear, we insert one double-loaded metal corkscrew anchor into the superior aspect of the lesser tuberosity through the percutaneous incision (Figure 15-7). The superior position of this anchor corresponds to the strongest tendinous attachment of the subscapularis tendon and also the site of origin of most tears.[22] For a full-thickness subscapularis tendon tear, we will use 2 or 3 double-loaded metal anchors for repair. We have shown in a biomechanical cadaveric study that suture anchors are comparable to transosseous subscapularis repair in cyclic loading models despite a smaller insertional contact area.[23]

We use an arthroscopic tissue penetrator placed through the anterior working portal to pass the suture through the healthy portion of the superolateral margin of the tendon. We make sure that the penetrator goes through the leading edge of the shiny portion of the subscapularis tendon. The suture is passed twice through the tendon in horizontal mattress fashion to advance the tendon laterally to the footprint (Figure 15-8).

A second suture is passed at the superior edge in simple interrupted fashion to prevent propagation of a retear along the rotator interval and bicipital groove region (Figure 15-9). Once our sutures have been passed through the tendon, we proceed with sequential arthroscopic knot tying from inferior to superior technique to progressively reduce the tendon to the anchor. Throughout the repair process, we continue to maintain lateral traction on the subscapularis tendon and keep the arm in neutral rotation to avoid overtightening the repair.

POSTOPERATIVE PROTOCOL

Our rehabilitation protocol is similar to our standard rotator cuff protocol. The immediate postoperative period is focused on pain and swelling control in preparation for a passive motion program. Patients are kept in a shoulder immobilizer with an abduction pillow continuously for 6 weeks postoperatively. We routinely obtain anteroposterior and axillary radiographs postoperatively to assess suture anchor placement. At 2 weeks postoperatively, we transition our patients to gentle passive motion, avoiding external rotation beyond the neutral position, and active elevation of the arm.

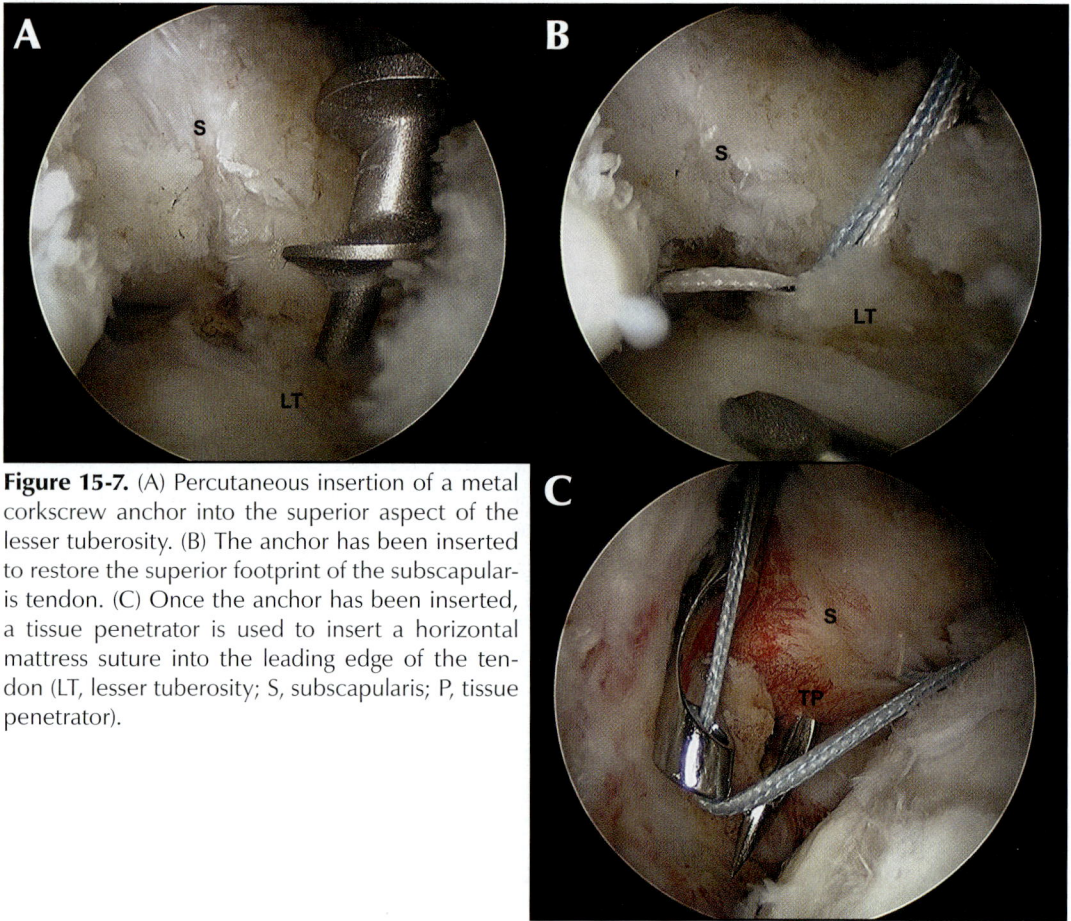

Figure 15-7. (A) Percutaneous insertion of a metal corkscrew anchor into the superior aspect of the lesser tuberosity. (B) The anchor has been inserted to restore the superior footprint of the subscapularis tendon. (C) Once the anchor has been inserted, a tissue penetrator is used to insert a horizontal mattress suture into the leading edge of the tendon (LT, lesser tuberosity; S, subscapularis; P, tissue penetrator).

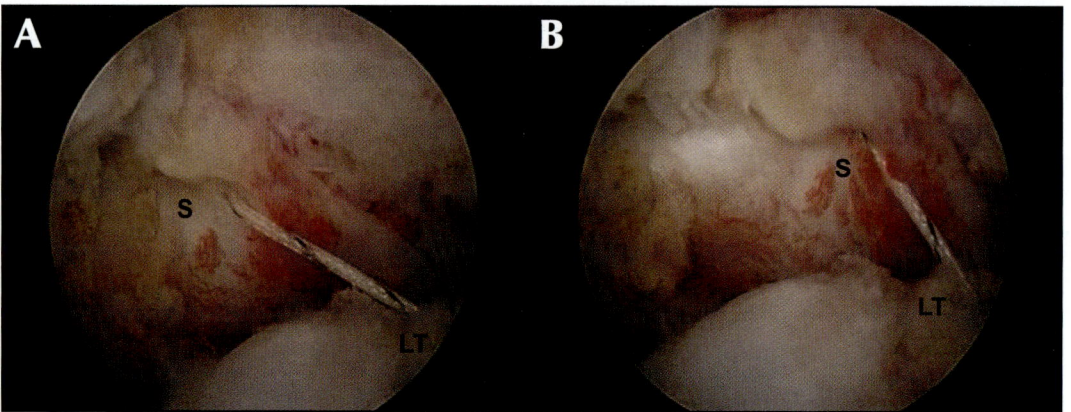

Figure 15-8. The subscapularis tendon is seen (A) before and (B) after advancing the leading edge to its reduced position at the lesser tuberosity footprint (LT, lesser tuberosity; S, subscapularis).

Active motion is started at 6 weeks, with gradual progression of passive external rotation stretching and low-resistance rotator cuff strengthening. Resistive strengthening with weights is restricted until 12 weeks postoperatively. At 18 weeks, we allow patients to gradually return to full, unrestricted activities under the supervision of their physical therapist.

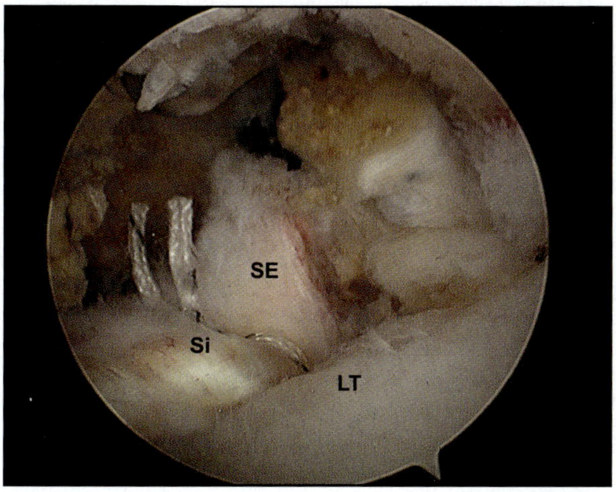

Figure 15-9. Once the initial horizontal mattress suture through the anchor has been tied down (top), a second suture is placed at the superolateral margin of the tendon in simple interrupted fashion to complete the repair (bottom) (LT, lesser tuberosity; SE, superior edge of repaired subscapularis; Si, simple interrupted suture).

RESULTS

Despite the abundance of literature on the treatment of rotator cuff disease, the results of arthroscopic management of subscapularis tears are relatively sparse. Burkhart and Tehrany reported the early results of 25 arthroscopic subscapularis repairs at an average follow-up of 10.7 months using the University of California, Los Angeles (UCLA) shoulder outcome score. In their series, the average UCLA score improved from 10.7 preoperatively to 30.5 postoperatively, with 92% of patients achieving good-excellent results.[14] Bennett reported on a prospective cohort of patients with isolated subscapularis tears at 2 and 4 years postoperatively and found that the outcomes were maintained over time.[12] Regardless of the treatment method employed, it has been shown in several studies that acute management of subscapularis tears is superior to chronic management—the latter being associated with tendon degeneration and fatty infiltration of the muscle belly.[19] For this reason, we favor acute treatment of subscapularis tendon injuries once the diagnosis is made. There is also an association between concomitant rotator cuff pathology involving the posterosuperior cuff and poorer outcomes when compared with isolated subscapularis repair.

REFERENCES

1. Gerber C, Hersche O, Farron A. Isolated rupture of the subscapularis tendon. *J Bone Joint Surg Am*. 1996;78(7):1015-1023.
2. Sakurai G, Ozaki J, Tomita Y, Kondo T, Tamai S. Incomplete tears of the subscapularis tendon associated with tears of the supraspinatus tendon: cadaveric and clinical studies. *J Shoulder Elbow Surg*. 1998;7(5):510-515.
3. Li XX, Schweitzer ME, Bifano JA, Lerman J, Manton GL, El-Noueam KI. MR evaluation of subscapularis tears. *J Comput Assist Tomogr*. 1999;23(5):713-717.
4. Lyons RP, Green A. Subscapularis tendon tears. *J Am Acad Orthop Surg*. 2005;13(5):353-363.
5. Deutsch A, Altchek DW, Veltri DM, Potter HG, Warren RF. Traumatic tears of the subscapularis tendon. Clinical diagnosis, magnetic resonance imaging findings, and operative treatment. *Am J Sports Med*. 1997;25(1):13-22.
6. Ferrick MR. Coracoid impingement. A case report and review of the literature. *Am J Sports Med*. 2000;28(1):117-119.
7. Peidro L, Serra A, Suso S. Subcoracoid impingement after ossification of the subscapularis tendon. *J Shoulder Elbow Surg*. 1999;8(2):170-171.
8. Burkhart SS. Reconciling the paradox of rotator cuff repair versus debridement: a unified biomechanical rationale for the treatment of rotator cuff tears. *Arthroscopy*. 1994;10(1):4-19.
9. Perry J. Anatomy and biomechanics of the shoulder in throwing, swimming, gymnastics, and tennis. *Clin Sports Med*. 1983;2(2):247-270.
10. Gerber C, Krushell RJ. Isolated rupture of the tendon of the subscapularis muscle. Clinical features in 16 cases. *J Bone Joint Surg Br*. 1991;73(3):389-394.

11. Tung GA, Yoo DC, Levine SM, Brody JM, Green A. Subscapularis tendon tear: primary and associated signs on MRI. *J Comput Assist Tomogr.* 2001;25(3):417-424.

12. Bennett WF. Subscapularis, medial, and lateral head coracohumeral ligament insertion anatomy. Arthroscopic appearance and incidence of "hidden" rotator interval lesions. *Arthroscopy.* 2001;17(2):173-180.

13. Barth JR, Burkhart SS, De Beer JF. The bear-hug test: a new and sensitive test for diagnosing a subscapularis tear. *Arthroscopy.* 2006;22(10):1076-1084.

14. Burkhart SS, Tehrany AM. Arthroscopic subscapularis tendon repair: technique and preliminary results. *Arthroscopy.* 2002;18(5):454-463.

15. Greis PE, Kuhn JE, Schulltheis J, Hintermeister R, Hawkins R. Validation of the lift-off test and analysis of subscapularis activity during maximal internal rotation. *Am J Sports Med.* 1996;24(5):589-593.

16. Tokish JM, Decker MJ, Ellis HB, Torry MR, Hawkins RJ. The belly-press test for the physical examination of the subscapularis muscle: electromyographic validation and comparison to the lift-off test. *J Shoulder Elbow Surg.* 2003;12(5):427-430.

17. Pfirrmann CW, Zanetti M, Weishaupt D, Gerber C, Hodler J. Subscapularis tendon tears: detection and grading at MR arthrography. *Radiology.* 1999;213(3):709-714.

18. Ticker JB, Warner JJ. Single-tendon tears of the rotator cuff. Evaluation and treatment of subscapularis tears and principles of treatment for supraspinatus tears. *Orthop Clin North Am.* 1997;28(1):99-116.

19. Warner JJ, Higgins L, Parsons IM IV, Dowdy P. Diagnosis and treatment of anterosuperior rotator cuff tears. *J Shoulder Elbow Surg.* 2001;10(1):37-46.

20. Lo IK, Burkhart SS. The comma sign: an arthroscopic guide to the torn subscapularis tendon. *Arthroscopy.* 2003;19(3):334-337.

21. Richards DP, Burkhart SS, Campbell SE. Relation between narrowed coracohumeral distance and subscapularis tears. *Arthroscopy.* 2005;21(10):1223-1228.

22. Halder A, Zobitz ME, Schultz E, An KN. Structural properties of the subscapularis tendon. *J Orthop Res.* 2000;18(5):829-834.

23. Wheeler DJ, Garabekyan T, Lugo R, et al. Biomechanical comparison of transosseous versus suture anchor repair of the subscapularis tendon. *Arthroscopy.* 2010;26(4):444-450.

Please see video on the accompanying Web site at
http://www.slackbooks.com/rotatorcuffvideos

CHAPTER 16

MANAGEMENT OF THE BICEPS TENDON IN THE SETTING OF ROTATOR CUFF TEARS

John-Paul H. Rue, MD, CDR, USN; Jonathan F. Dickens, MD, CPT, USA; and Kelly G. Kilcoyne, MD, CPT, USA

Pathology of the long head of the biceps tendon is most commonly associated with additional shoulder injury, including rotator cuff disease and labral tears. Although the biomechanical function of the long head of the biceps tendon in the shoulder remains controversial, the anatomy of the biceps, specifically as it relates to the rotator cuff, is well-defined. While numerous physical exam tests have been described to localize and identify biceps pathology, arthroscopy remains the gold standard for diagnosis and treatment. Treatment is dictated by multiple factors including patient age and activity level, biceps pathology, and associated injuries. Surgical options include débridement, tenotomy, tenodesis, and superior labrum anterior to posterior (SLAP) repair. Regardless of the surgical procedure, outcomes of the operative treatment of biceps pathology are overall successful with high patient satisfaction.

EPIDEMIOLOGY

The mechanical effects of the rotator cuff and long head of the biceps tendon are age-related and frequently occur together. In a study of 151 cadaveric shoulder dissections, no degenerative changes were noted in the biceps tendon in specimens younger than 60 years old.[1] In a prospective arthroscopic evaluation of the biceps tendon in 200 patients undergoing surgery for chronic rotator cuff disease, Murthi and colleagues[2] demonstrated that 63% of biceps tendons had histological evidence of chronic inflammation, and only 18% were free of disease.[2] A normal biceps tendon was found in 25% of cases with an arthroscopically evaluated normal rotator cuff tendon, in 16% of patients with a partial-thickness rotator cuff tear, and in only 11% of patients with a full-thickness rotator cuff tear. Similarly, Chen and colleagues[3] arthroscopically evaluated 122 complete rotator cuff tears and found biceps pathology in 76% of patients with tendinitis in 46%, subluxation in 8%, dislocation in 10%, partial tears in 12%, and a complete tear in 5% of patients.[3] There is a strong association between rotator cuff and biceps tendon pathology, with the likelihood and severity of disease increased in an older patient population and those with more severe rotator cuff tears.

Ma CB, Feeley BT, eds.
*Basic Principles and Operative Management
of the Rotator Cuff (pp 223-242)*
© 2012 SLACK Incorporated

Figure 16-1. The attachment of the long head of the biceps tendon on the superior labrum is variable but most frequently is located on the posterosuperior labrum.

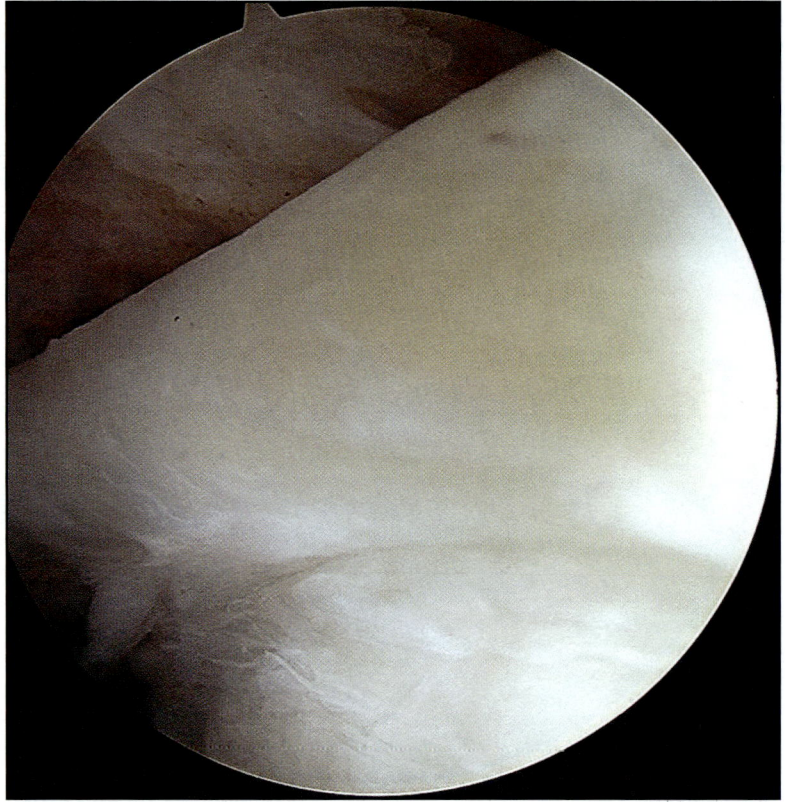

ANATOMY

The long head of the biceps tendon is 1 of only 2 intra-articular tendons in the human body. The long head of the biceps tendon originates from the supraglenoid tubercle and superior glenoid labrum in approximately 30% of cases, sometimes appearing bifurcated.[4] It originates only from the glenoid labrum in 50% of cases and from the supraglenoid tubercle in the remaining 20% of cases.[4] The anterior to posterior distribution of the long head of the biceps tendon attachment to the labrum is also variable, most commonly originating entirely from the posterosuperior labrum (Figure 16-1).[5] The tendon is 9-cm long and is enveloped by a synovial membrane within the shoulder joint, making it intracapsular but extrasynovial.[4] This tubular sleeve allows for excursion of the tendon during abduction and adduction of the arm.[6]

The biceps traverses the anterosuperior portion of the humeral head at an angle of 30 to 40 degrees from its origin to the bicipital groove.[7] The bicipital groove is formed by the lesser tuberosity medially and the greater tuberosity laterally. The tendon enters the bicipital groove in the interval between the subscapularis and supraspinatus known as the rotator cuff interval (Figure 16-2). The rotator cuff interval is the triangular area between the anterior edge of the supraspinatus superiorly, the superior border of the subscapularis tendon inferiorly, and the coracoid process medially. The rotator interval contains the long head of the biceps tendon and the coracohumeral (CH) ligament. The superior glenohumeral ligament, which originates from the anterosuperior labrum, crosses the floor of the rotator cuff interval. At the entrance of the bicipital groove, the superior glenohumeral ligament blends with the CH ligament, forming a reflection pulley that encloses and stabilizes the long head of the biceps tendon. The pulley is reinforced by fibers from the transverse band of the rotator cuff, in addition to fibers from the subscapularis and supraspinatus.[8] The transverse ligament, once thought to be a discrete structure, is now known to be composed of fibers from

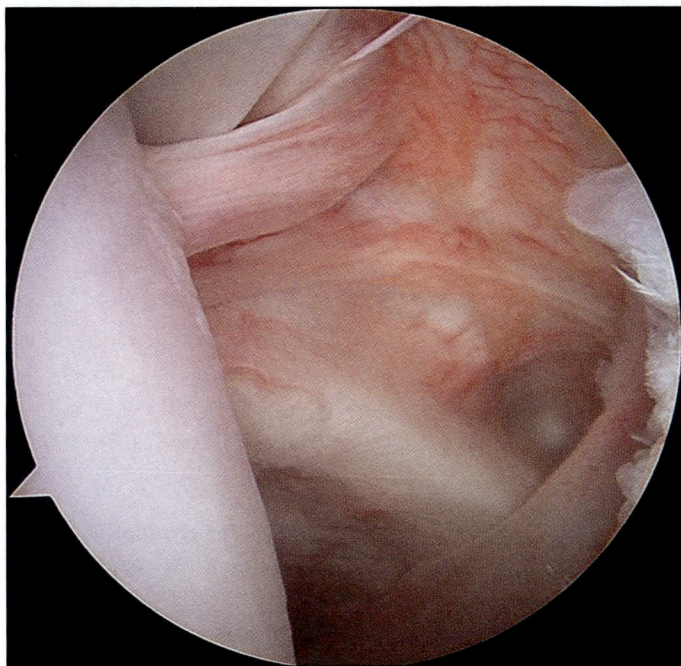

Figure 16-2. The long head of the biceps tendon along with the CH ligament traverse within the rotator interval bordered by the supraspinatus and subscapularis.

the subscapularis and supraspinatus.[9] Originally thought to be the main stabilizer of the long head of the biceps tendon in the bicipital groove, the transverse ligament has been shown to be too weak to stabilize the long head of the biceps tendon in the groove and is sometimes entirely absent.[10]

The long head of the biceps tendon exits the bicipital groove at the level of the humeral neck, becoming musculotendinous near the deltoid insertion. It joins the short head of the biceps distally to form a common tendon before inserting onto the radial tubercle. The long head of the biceps tendon is innervated by the musculocutaneous nerve and is vascularized by contributing branches of the suprascapular, anterior humeral circumflex, and deep brachial arteries.

BIOMECHANICS

It is generally agreed that the long head of the biceps tendon acts as an elbow flexor and a strong supinator of the forearm. However, the function of the proximal biceps in the shoulder remains a controversial topic. Depending on the type of study performed, the range of function proposed for the long head of the biceps tendon ranges from action as a shoulder depressor, stabilizer, to a passive role. To analyze the proposed function of the biceps in the literature, it is best to categorize the studies into anatomic studies, biomechanical studies, and electromyographic (EMG) studies. Unfortunately, conflicting evidence is found not only between the different categories of studies, but even among studies of similar design.

In an analysis of changes in superior translation of the humeral head in patients with documented loss of the proximal biceps, Warner and McMahon[11] found between 2 and 6 mm of superior translation of the humeral head on anteroposterior radiographs in varying degrees of humeral abduction. They concluded that the long head of the biceps tendon acts as a stabilizer of the humeral head in the glenoid during shoulder abduction in the scapular plane. In their analysis of 5 patients undergoing arthroscopy for shoulder pathology, Andrews et al[12] noted that electrical stimulation of the biceps muscle resulted in the tendon becoming taut with the superior portion of the labrum being raised off the glenoid. Additionally, the humeral head was noted to be compressed into the glenoid.[12] Based on this finding and computer-assisted analysis of the throwing mechanism, the authors concluded that the biceps plays an important role in deceleration of the elbow during the follow-through phase of throwing and also provides stability to the glenohumeral joint during acceleration and follow-through phases of throwing. In contrast, Lipmann[13] concluded that the biceps played a minimal active role in producing motion at the shoulder joint based on his own intraoperative observations of the biceps sliding passively in its groove during shoulder movement.

Cadaveric studies, though arguably limited in the reproduction of normal shoulder physiology, have also attempted to evaluate the role of the long head of the biceps tendon in the shoulder. A cadaveric study by Kumar et al[14] used 15 freely hanging shoulder specimens to analyze upward migration of the humeral head when applying different tension to the long and short head of the biceps both before and after division of the long head of the biceps tendon. When the long head of the biceps tendon was cut with both heads under tension, the authors found significant upward migration of the humeral head. As a result, the authors argue the importance of the long head of the biceps tendon as a stabilizer of the humeral head during elbow flexion and forearm supination.[14] In contrast to the argument for the long head of the biceps tendon preventing superior migration of the humeral head, Soslowsky et al argue the biceps is the most efficient stabilizer to inferior subluxation in their own cadaveric model.[15]

To further complicate the analysis of the function of the long head of the biceps tendon in the shoulder, there is even conflicting evidence amongst similar EMG studies. A study that recorded the EMG activity in the long and short heads of the biceps during a range of shoulder flexion and abduction found that both heads were active during shoulder flexion and abduction, regardless of the position of the elbow.[16] In contrast to this study, Levy et al[17] found no electrical activity in the long head of the biceps tendon during flexion and abduction of the shoulder. A possible explanation for this difference may be that, in the former study, subjects were placed in a brace locked in neutral forearm rotation with the elbow free during testing. Levy's subjects were placed in a brace that neutralized elbow and forearm motion during testing.

PHYSICAL EXAM

Patients with biceps pathology may present with a complaint of chronic pain in the anterior shoulder, with or without distal radiation. However, especially if the patient has additional shoulder pathology, he or she may complain of a more nonspecific shoulder pain. These patients could have isolated biceps, rotator cuff, labral pathology, or any combination of these injuries. After an appropriate history is taken, a complete physical exam of the shoulder, including evaluation of the rotator cuff tendons, biceps tendon, and labrum, is paramount. It is most often the examiner's overall impression of the entire clinical picture, including the history and entire shoulder physical exam, that provides the best predictor of the underlying pathology. While there are many described tests specific to the biceps, the available literature on the sensitivity and specificity of these tests suggests they may be somewhat insensitive and relatively nonspecific.

Patients with biceps pathology will often have point tenderness in the bicipital groove. The biceps tendon can be palpated directly anteriorly with the arm in 10 degrees of internal rotation, with the elbow flexed (Figure 16-3).[18] The point tenderness will persist as the examiner moves the patient's arm through internal and external rotation, which can help distinguish it from anterior shoulder pain that is commonly associated with rotator cuff disorders. Additional tests used to help isolate lesions in the biceps include the Yergason sign,[19] Speed test,[20] and biceps instability test.[21]

The Yergason sign is elicited with the patient's elbow flexed to 90 degrees with the forearm pronated (Figure 16-4). The examiner holds the patient's wrist to resist active supination. A positive test localizes pain to the bicipital groove with this resisted supination.[19] While this test isolates the biceps tendon, it has been shown to have only 43% sensitivity, with moderate specificity of 79%, and a 63% accuracy value.[22]

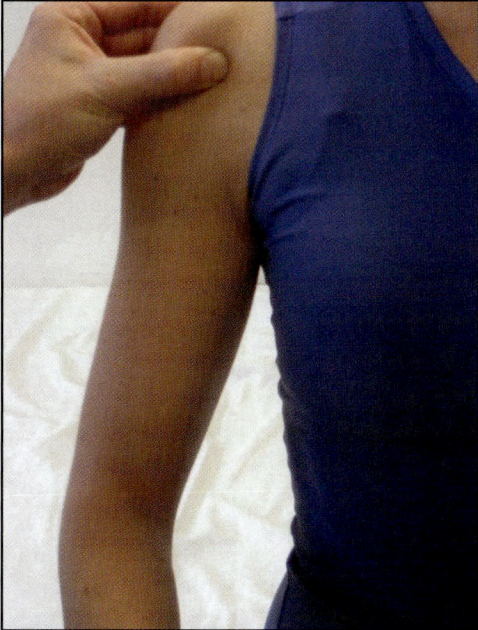

Figure 16-3. Palpation of the biceps tendon in the bicipital groove may elicit point tenderness.

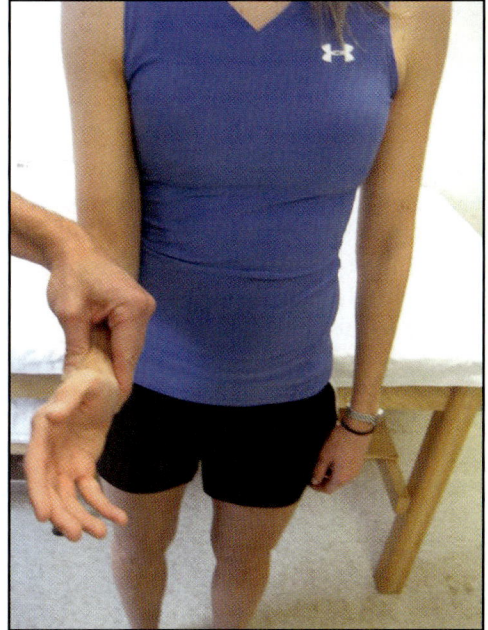

Figure 16-4. The Yergason test performed by resisting active supination with the elbow in 90 degrees of flexion is positive when proximal biceps pain is generated.

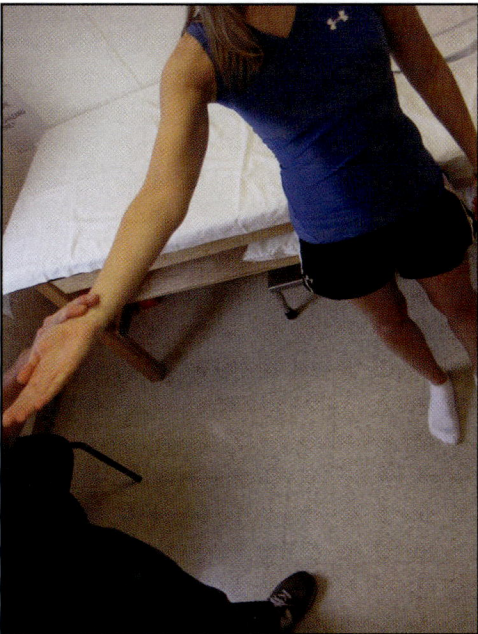

Figure 16-5. The Speed test performed with the elbow extended and forearm supinated by resisting active shoulder forward flexion against resistance.

In the Speed test, the patient flexes the shoulder against resistance with the elbow extended and the forearm supinated (Figure 16-5). A positive test localizes pain to the bicipital groove.[20] The sensitivity of the Speed test is low, 32% in some studies, with a specificity of 75% and an accuracy value of 56%.[22] As a result of the low sensitivity and specificity, little diagnostic information is gained based on the Speed test alone.

The biceps instability test allows for assessment of dislocation or subluxation of the biceps tendon from the groove. The examiner places the patient's arm in full abduction and external rotation. The arm is then slowly brought to the patient's side in the plane of the scapula. Instability of the tendon provokes a palpable and sometimes audible clicking, as it is forcibly subluxed or dislocated from the bicipital groove.[21]

In addition to these tests, selective injections can be used to evaluate pathology of the biceps. Patients with rotator cuff tendinitis will have some relief with a subacromial anesthetic injection, while patients with biceps pathology will typically have more relief with an intra-articular injection. If suspicion for biceps pathology remains despite no pain relief from an intra-articular injection, the biceps sheath can be selectively injected, taking care not to inject the tendon itself.

As a result of the number of tests available to evaluate the biceps tendon, associated pathology, and the lack of sensitivity and specificity of provocative tests, arthroscopy remains the gold standard for the identification of biceps pathology.

PATHOLOGY

Injury to the long head of the biceps tendon can occur as a result of tendon degeneration or tendon instability and from disorders at its origin.[23] While isolated pathology of the long head of the biceps tendon can occur, it most frequently coexists with additional shoulder pathology, including rotator cuff tears, labral tears, and acromioclavicular arthritis.

Although tendon deterioration is often referred to as tendinitis, on a microscopic level, it is often more degenerative than inflammatory.[23] Claessens and Snoeck[24] showed that microscopic changes include atrophy of collagen fibers, fibrinoid necrosis, and proliferation of fibrocytes, along with irregular collagen fiber patterns and fissuring of the tendon. Biceps tendinitis is often subdivided into primary and secondary. Primary tendinitis is due to pathology of the tendon sheath, while secondary tendinitis results from associated pathology, including adjacent osseous, ligamentous, and muscular structures.[25]

Primary biceps tendinitis is characterized by thickening of the transverse ligament and sheath, resulting in stenosis and narrowing of the tendon underneath the sheath, analogous to de Quervain's tenosynovitis in the hand.[26] In their review of 21 patients with chronic bicipital pain attributed to biceps tendinitis, Post and Benca[27] found inflammatory changes of the biceps tendon within the groove alone. These changes can be seen arthroscopically when the portion of the tendon within the groove is pulled with an instrument into the field of view and is referred to as the lipstick sign (Figure 16-6). While tendinitis or degeneration of the biceps tendon does occur in isolation, it is estimated to account for only 5% of cases of biceps tendinitis.[28]

More commonly, secondary biceps tendinitis occurs as a result of the pathology of adjacent structures and the intimate anatomical relationship between the biceps and rotator cuff.[2,20,29-31] In his review of 50 shoulders in patients with rotator cuff impingement, Neer[32] found that one-third of these patients had abnormalities of the biceps tendon at the time of surgery. He concluded that the proximity of the long head of the biceps tendon to the critical area of impingement resulted in the concomitant biceps pathology. Others have reported that between 49% and 70% of patients with clinical evidence of impingement syndrome will have biceps tendon pathology, with as many as 40% requiring biceps tenodesis.[2,31] Chen and colleagues[3] found that 76% of complete rotator cuff tears had associated pathology of the long head of the biceps tendon. Gill and colleagues[33] demonstrated that, in 85% of cases with partial tears of the long head of the biceps tendon, there was concomitant rotator cuff pathology. Thus, as a result of the close anatomic relationship between the rotator cuff and the biceps, the long head of the biceps tendon is subject to the same mechanical abutment and subsequent pathology as the tendons of the rotator cuff.[32,34]

Instability of the long head of the biceps tendon within the groove can result in tendon subluxation, dislocation, or even complete displacement. As with biceps tendinitis, biceps instability is

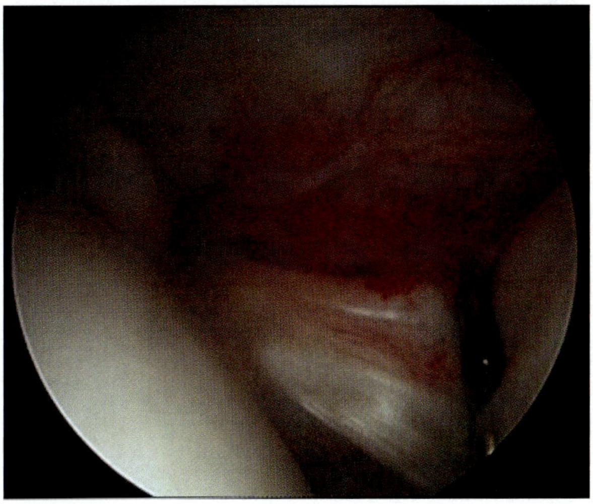

Figure 16-6. The lipstick sign. Biceps tendinitis visualized as increased erythema and injection seen after retracting the intertubercular portion of tendon into the joint.

often related to rotator cuff pathology. Instability of the biceps tendon is often secondary to loss of the soft tissue restraint of the rotator cuff from a result of degeneration. In a retrospective review of 71 cases of dislocation or subluxation of the long head of the biceps tendon, Walch and colleagues[31] found that 35% of subluxations occurred with partial tearing of the subscapularis, and 70% occurred with tears of the supraspinatus. Complete dislocation of the tendon from the groove occurred in 65% of these cases, with only 2 of these having an intact subscapularis. Further emphasizing the importance of the location of the long head of the biceps tendon in the rotator interval, Habermeyer and colleagues[8] describe a spectrum of pathology that starts with lesion of the pulley system (see anatomy section for components), leading to subluxation of the biceps and, ultimately, to anterior shoulder instability. A prospective evaluation of 89 patients with an arthroscopically diagnosed lesion of the biceps pulley found that 89% of patients also had involvement of the LBH including synovitis, subluxation, dislocation, and partial or complete tearing.

Disorders of the long head of the biceps tendon at its origin include rupture and SLAP. The majority of long head of the biceps tendon ruptures are a result of previous degeneration or impingement. Neer[35] believed that repetitive impingement of the biceps against the anterior edge of the acromion, especially when the arm is raised, was the main source of biceps pathology. He also found that tears of the supraspinatus occur before the biceps ruptures at a ratio of 7:1.[35] While traumatic rupture of a previously normal long head of the biceps tendon is uncommon, it has been described.[11] It most commonly occurs after a powerful supination force, after powerful deceleration of the forearm as experienced during pitching, or after a fall onto an outstretched hand.

Snyder et al's[36] original classification of SLAP lesions included 4 types. Type I SLAP lesions are characterized by fraying and degeneration of the superior labrum. Type II lesions have detachment of the superior labrum and biceps tendon from the glenoid rim. Type III lesions have an intact biceps anchor with a bucket-handle tear of the superior labrum. Type IV lesions have displacement of the bucket-handle tear into the biceps tendon. Types II and IV, representing 55% and 10% of SLAP lesions, respectively, in his series, involve the biceps tendon or anchor. It is worth noting that, overall, SLAP lesions are relatively uncommon, occurring in only 6% of shoulder arthroscopies in Snyder's original series.

TREATMENT CONSIDERATIONS AND OUTCOMES

Although the pathology of the long head of the biceps tendon and the treatment of its lesions are the source of significant attention in the literature, there continues to be extensive debate regarding the function, pathology, and optimal treatment of these lesions. The treatment of biceps pathology in the setting of associated rotator cuff disease is not well-studied and continues to be a source of much controversy.

Nonoperative Treatment

Nonoperative treatment of disorders involving the long head of the biceps tendon with concomitant rotator cuff pathology is primarily directed toward treatment of the rotator cuff. Nonoperative treatment generally includes rest, nonsteroidal anti-inflammatory drugs (NSAIDs), local steroid injections, and physical therapy. NSAIDs are the cornerstone of nonoperative management and should be used at anti-inflammatory doses to achieve maximal benefit. Therapeutic benefits of anti-inflammatory medications are maximized when taken over a sustained period of time, even after the resolution of pain, to ensure the inflammatory process is resolved.

Local steroid injections are important adjuvants in cases of refractory pain that does not improve after 6 weeks of nonoperative treatment. Steroid injections may be performed intra-articularly, in the subacromial space, or directly into the biceps tendon sheath. Direct tendon sheath injections have been suggested when subacromial injections have failed.[20,37] Serial hydrocortisone injections into the substance of the tendon effectively relieved bicipital tenosynovitis in 55% of patients in one series.[38] Concern for atrophic tendon changes with intratendinous steroid injections have led to recommendations for injections within the sheath, under the transverse humeral ligament, but avoiding intrasubstance injection.[39] Using this technique, good to excellent results have been reported in 74% of patients.[39,40]

Spontaneous rupture of the long head of the biceps tendon, usually the result of a chronic process, may be treated nonoperatively, especially in the elderly, with satisfactory results. Although associated with a cosmetic defect, the intact brachialis limits any noticeable loss of flexion strength at the elbow, and supination strength is decreased approximately 10%.[41] Mariani and colleagues[42] compared early tenodesis to nonsurgical treatment following traumatic rupture of the long head of the biceps tendon. There was no statistically significant difference in elbow flexion strength. The operative group had an 8% loss in supination strength compared to a 21% loss in strength in the nonoperative group. Residual pain was minimal in both groups, and the nonsurgical cohort returned to work and activity sooner than the surgical group.[42] Others have reported, especially in younger patients, that nonoperative treatment may lead to a more profound loss of supination and flexion strength up to 23% and 29%, respectively. Additionally, there is a higher incidence of cramping pain in the biceps in up to 30% of cases.[43,44] Generally, nonoperative treatment of a rupture of the long head of the biceps tendon is employed in older or less active individuals while early tenodesis is recommended for younger patients.

Tenotomy

Controversy exists in the decision to perform tenodesis or tenotomy. Tenotomy is currently the more popular procedure and has the advantages of being technically easier to perform with easier and less demanding rehabilitation and no need for immobilization in cases of isolated biceps tenotomy (Figure 16-7).[25] The major disadvantages of tenotomy are cramping and weakness with repetitive vigorous exercise, as well as a Popeye deformity.

The literature regarding biceps-related pain following simple tenotomy is variable. Kelly and colleagues[45] reviewed the results of 40 patients at a minimum 2-year follow-up who underwent biceps tenotomy. Only 9 of 40 patients underwent isolated tenotomies, while 5 also underwent rotator cuff repair, and 8 underwent acromioplasty. Postoperatively, 37.5% had biceps-related muscle pain, and 70% were noted to have a Popeye deformity. Relief of biceps tenderness within the biceps groove was successful in 95% of patients, and 68% of patients reported good or excellent results. No patients older than 60 years reported biceps-related symptoms, while 100% of patients younger than 40 years reported persistent biceps symptoms. Two of the 5 patients who had a rotator cuff repair reported poor results.[45]

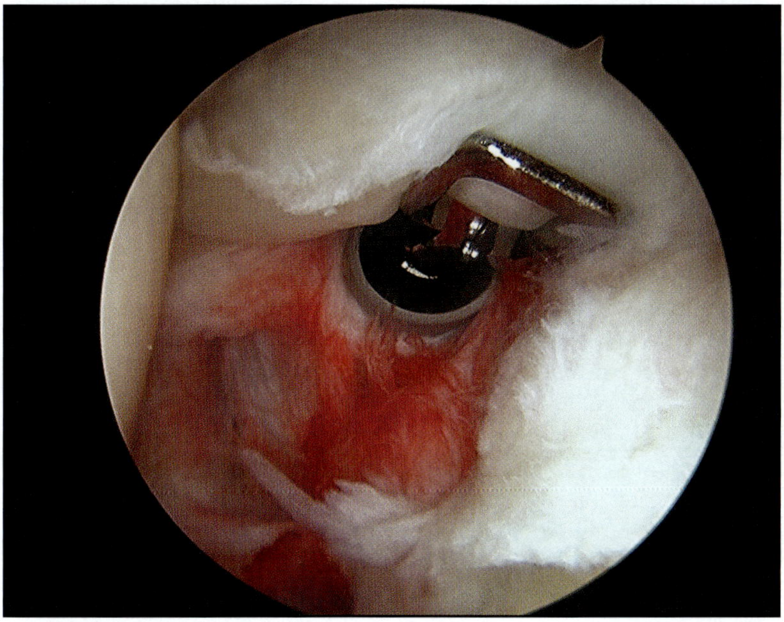

Figure 16-7. Biceps tenotomy performed to relieve refractory proximal biceps tendinitis in a 55-year-old laborer.

Others have reported good results following biceps tenotomy. Gill and colleagues[33] evaluated 30 consecutive biceps tenotomies in patients with a mean age of 50 years after an average follow-up of 19 months. Impingement was associated with 4 cases, and a supraspinatus tear was diagnosed in 12 of 30 shoulders. Only 5 patients had isolated biceps tendinitis. The mean postoperative American Shoulder and Elbow Surgeons (ASES) score was 81.8, and 97% returned to their previous level of sport. There were 4 (13.3%) unacceptable results due to cosmetic deformity (1), residual subacromial impingement (2), and residual shoulder pain (1).[33] Walch and colleagues[46] reviewed 307 arthroscopic biceps tenotomies in patients with full-thickness rotator cuff tears that were deemed irreparable or the patient was not willing to participate in rehabilitation after rotator cuff repair. After a mean 57-month follow-up, 87% of patients were satisfied with their results. The authors report that 50% of patients had an associated Popeye deformity, but no patients characterized their result as fair or poor based on cosmesis. Despite the subjective improvements in pain, radiographic evidence of glenohumeral arthritis progressed in 29% of patients.[46]

Tenodesis

Tenodesis can be performed open or arthroscopically; above, within, or below the bicipital groove; and with soft-tissue or osseous fixation devices. The advantages of biceps tenodesis are improved cosmesis, restoration of strength, and less cramping bicipital pain. Biceps tenodesis is associated with prolonged postoperative immobilization, longer rehabilitation, increased cost, tenodesis failure, and potential neurovascular damage resulting from a more technically demanding procedure.

Biceps tenodesis has commonly been performed using the open keyhole technique as described by Froimson and O[47] or an open or arthroscopic tenodesis technique as described by Mazzocca and colleagues[48] and Romeo and colleagues,[49] respectively. Biomechanical studies evaluating the strength of different tenodesis fixation devices have demonstrated that the interference screw has the greatest initial fixation strength.

The keyhole technique, described in 1974 for the treatment of biceps rupture, instability, and tendinitis, has shown predictably good results. In the original series, Froimson and O[47] reported that 12 shoulders after 24 months all had satisfactory results. The authors noted that patients receiving treatment for biceps pathology often had associated rotator cuff disease. Berlemann and Bayley[50] reviewed the results of 15 shoulders that underwent biceps tenodesis using the keyhole technique at a mean 7-year follow-up. All but one patient had rotator cuff pathology ranging from inflammation to complete tears. The authors reported good to excellent results in approximately 70% of patients after a midterm follow-up. Authors in favor of the keyhole tenodesis cite avoidance of hardware, no medial dissection, removal of the inciting proximal biceps tendon, and relative stability of the fixation allowing early gentle range of motion of the shoulder and elbow as advantages to the procedure.

Other authors have suggested incorporating the biceps tenodesis into the arthroscopic rotator cuff repair by placing a rotator cuff suture through the long head of the biceps tendon. Checchia and colleagues,[51] in 14 patients with a mean age of 71 years, demonstrated 93% good and excellent outcomes after a mean 32 months. Although one patient developed a Popeye deformity, the patient still had a good clinical outcome. One clinical failure was noted, despite evidence of an intact tenodesis and rotator cuff repair. The authors concluded that simultaneous arthroscopic biceps tenodesis can be incorporated into a rotator cuff repair with successful clinical outcomes.

Outcomes following open subpectoral biceps tenodesis have demonstrated the most favorable outcomes with and without concomitant rotator cuff pathology. Mazzocca and colleagues[52] reviewed the results of 50 patients with a mean age of 50 years at 29 months after open biceps tenodesis using an interference screw. The study included 31 patients with lesions of the rotator cuff at the time of arthroscopy who were treated with a single-row repair (17, 55%), double-row repair (6, 19%), subacromial decompression (7, 23%), and margin convergence sutures (1, 3%) for a revision rotator cuff repair. All patients reported relief of their biceps pain, and all had good or excellent clinical outcomes. The mean ASES score and simple shoulder test for patients with and without cuff pathology was significantly improved from baseline; however, the scores were significantly better in patients without a rotator cuff tear (ASES 89.2, simple shoulder test 10.6) compared to patients with a cuff tear (ASES 78.0, simple shoulder test 8.8). There was one case of fixation failure leading to a Popeye deformity. Similarly, Nho and colleagues[53] evaluated the complications following 353 open subpectoral biceps tenodesis. The incidence of complications was 2%. Two patients (0.57%) had persistent bicipital pain, 2 patients (0.57%) had failure of fixation resulting in a Popeye deformity, 1 patient (0.28%) developed a deep wound infection, and 1 patient (0.28%) developed a musculocutaneous neuropathy.[53] These results demonstrate that open subpectoral biceps tenodesis is a reliable and effective procedure for the treatment of bicipital pain in the setting of concomitant shoulder pathology and has few complications.

The location of the tenodesis, within the intertubercular groove or in a subpectoral location, is another source of debate. While some authors have demonstrated good outcomes with proximally based tenodesis of the long head of the biceps tendon,[27,54] others have cited persistent biceps tenderness or rupture as a cause of failure in this location.[50,55,56] In a retrospective review of 188 patients at a mean age of 51 years, the following revision rates were reported: proximal arthroscopic tenodesis, 35.7%; proximal open tenodesis with an intact sheath, 12.5%; proximal open tenodesis, 0%; tenotomy, 8.7%; and distal open tenodesis, 2.7%. The overall revision rate for all proximal techniques, including tenotomy, was 12%, which was significantly more than 2.7% in the open distal subpectoral tenodesis technique.[57] Subpectoral tenodesis, therefore, is less likely to be associated with residual tendinitis than proximal or intertubercular tenodesis.

Despite advances in shoulder arthroscopy, the choice between arthroscopic and open biceps tenodesis remains controversial. Concerns for arthroscopic tenodesis include potential failure to transpose the tendon outside of the potentially inflamed bicipital groove, increased technical difficulty, and suggested higher failure rates compared to the open subpectoral biceps tenodesis.[48,52,53,58] Based on the current literature, open subpectoral biceps tenodesis is favored over arthroscopic tenodesis due to the reliable anatomic tenodesis placement, ease of the procedure, and strength of the fixation with interference screws.

Tenodesis Versus Tenotomy

There are few studies that directly compare biceps tenotomy and tenodesis. Osbahr and colleagues[59] retrospectively reviewed 160 patients following biceps tenotomy or tenodesis. A tenodesis was performed in younger, more physically active patients with an associated rotator cuff tear. The authors found no significant difference between the groups with regard to pain, muscle spasm, or cosmetic deformity after a mean 20 months in the tenodesis group or 23 months in the tenotomy group.[59] Comparing the results of arthroscopic biceps tenotomy versus arthroscopic tenodesis using a suture anchor in patients with rotator cuff tears, Koh and colleagues[58] demonstrated less cosmetic deformity in the tenodesis cohort. The authors noted a Popeye deformity in 4 (9%) patients in the tenodesis group compared to 11 (27%) in the tenotomy group. There were no significant differences between the groups with respect to muscle cramping or ASES scores.

Boileau and colleagues[55] reported the results of arthroscopic biceps tenotomy or tenodesis for the treatment of anterior shoulder pain in massive and irreparable rotator cuff tears. No associated acromioplasty was performed, and after a mean 35-month follow-up, no difference was noted with respect to Constant scores (tenotomy—61, tenodesis—73), muscular cramps (tenotomy—21%, tenodesis—9%), or pain in the bicipital groove (tenotomy—46%, tenodesis—30%) between the groups. The tenotomy group was significantly more likely to develop a Popeye deformity compared to the tenodesis group (62% versus 3%).

Although there is ongoing debate about the appropriate treatment of biceps lesions in the setting of rotator cuff pathology, both tenodesis and tenotomy have been reported to produce favorable clinical results.[2,29,52,53,60,61] High-demand patients and those younger than 50 years benefit from the improved function and cosmesis of a biceps tenodesis. Patients older than 55 to 60 years are less likely to notice a cosmetic deformity, functional deficit, or muscular cramping and, thus, may be better served with a tenotomy, allowing early range of motion with minimal morbidity. Older patients with massive irreparable rotator cuff tears or those not wishing to comply with postoperative rehabilitation may benefit from biceps tenotomy to relieve anterior shoulder pain.

Biceps Instability

Subluxation or dislocation of the biceps tendon is frequently associated with a rotator cuff tear, particularly involving the subscapularis tendon as well as the rotator interval. Habermeyer and colleagues[4] first described the progressive damage to the pulley system, which may be traumatic or degenerative in nature and ultimately lead to biceps instability.[4] Disruption of this pulley system occurs in a stepwise fashion, initiated by an articular-sided supraspinatus tear, leading to a tear of the superior glenohumeral ligament, followed by medial subluxation of the biceps tendon, and then partial articular-sided subscapularis tear. Repetitive subluxations further damage the subscapularis tendon and ultimately lead to frank biceps tendon dislocation.[62,63] The biceps most frequently dislocates medially, although lateral dislocation has been reported.[64] Generally, the long head of the biceps tendon will dislocate deep to the subscapularis; however, in the setting of a full-thickness subscapularis tear, the long head of the biceps tendon may be superficial to the tendon.

The recognition of biceps tendon instability and associated rotator cuff pathology, especially subscapularis tears, is essential for the appropriate treatment of these lesions. Instability of the biceps tendon is strongly associated with the size of the rotator cuff tear. Lafosse and colleagues[65] arthroscopically evaluated 200 consecutive patients undergoing rotator cuff repair. When the long head of the biceps tendon was stable, 70% of the rotator cuff tendons were normal; however, when the long head of the biceps tendon was unstable, 85% of the rotator cuff tendons had pathologic changes.

Treatment options for biceps instability include tenotomy, tenodesis, or reconstruction of the stabilizing structures in addition to addressing the concomitant rotator cuff pathology. Bennett[63] described arthroscopic reconstruction of the biceps pulley in 18 patients with a mean age of 66 years. Postoperatively, 1 patient (6%) had a traumatic rupture of the long head of the biceps

rotator cuff. Patients who receive a biceps tenodesis are generally placed in a sling for 2 weeks followed by gentle range of motion of the shoulder. Resisted active elbow flexion and forearm supination are withheld for 6 weeks. For patients who undergo a SLAP repair, the arm is immobilized for 6 weeks in a sling. During the first 6 weeks, passive rotation with the arm at the side and forward elevation to 90 degrees are allowed. After 6 weeks, progressive active assisted and passive elevation are allowed in a supervised physical therapy setting. Strengthening of the rotator cuff is begun at 12 weeks.

AUTHORS' PREFERRED TECHNIQUE: OPEN SUBPECTORAL TENODESIS

In our relatively young and active patient population, we prefer to use an open subpectoral biceps tenodesis, as described by Mazzocca and colleagues.[48] We prefer open tenodesis to arthroscopic because arthroscopic tenodesis does not completely remove diseased tendon from the bicipital groove. Open subpectoral tenodesis places the biceps in its natural anatomic position deep to the pectoralis tendon, maintaining the natural muscle resting length of the long head of the biceps tendon while removing the diseased tendon from the bicipital groove, avoiding a cosmetic defect.

Operating Room Setup

We prefer beach chair positioning for ease of access to the medial arm as well as more uninhibited arm and shoulder motion during the case. Standard preoperative antibiotics are administered. A complete physical exam of the shoulder, assessing for any range-of-motion restrictions or abnormal translation, is performed after induction of general anesthesia or administration of a regional block.

Adequate access to the anterior and posterior shoulder is ensured, and the arm is draped free in approximately 30 to 60 degrees of forward flexion, 30 degrees of abduction, and 20 degrees of internal rotation. While a commercial arm holder such as the Spider arm positioner (Tenet Medical, Calgary, Alberta) can be used, we prefer to keep the arm and shoulder free by placing the arm on a padded Mayo stand. This allows for adequate internal rotation of the arm when making the initial incision as well as allowing full external rotation of the arm during the procedure.

We have found it helpful to mark the planned tenodesis incision while marking the shoulder landmarks and portal incisions, prior to the start of the case. In the event of a prolonged shoulder arthroscopy prior to the start of the tenodesis, the arm can become swollen and distorted with fluid, making palpation of anatomic landmarks more difficult. Marking the incision prior to the start of the case alleviates any possibly confusion. After marking the planned incision, we also administer local anesthetic with epinephrine to the site for subcutaneous hemostasis and perioperative analgesia. This is especially important if using a regional block, as this area represents T1 dermatome distribution and is not routinely anesthetized with a standard interscalene block.

Arthroscopic Evaluation

A standard posterior portal is established, and an initial evaluation of the biceps tendon is made. After an anterior portal is established, a complete arthroscopic examination of the glenohumeral joint is performed, with specific attention to the labrum and rotator cuff. This includes using a probe or other arthroscopic instrument (via the anterior portal) to pull the more distal biceps out of the bicipital groove and into view to assess for any inflammatory changes (lipstick sign) or decreased mobility. The biceps anchor is evaluated, as is the tendon within the rotator interval. The supraspinatus, subscapularis, and CH ligament are assessed for associated pathology.

After complete arthroscopic evaluation, an arthroscopic cutting device or thermal ablator is placed through the anterior portal to tenotomize the biceps tendon at it base. We routinely smooth and contour the remaining superior labrum. The arthroscope is then placed into the subacromial

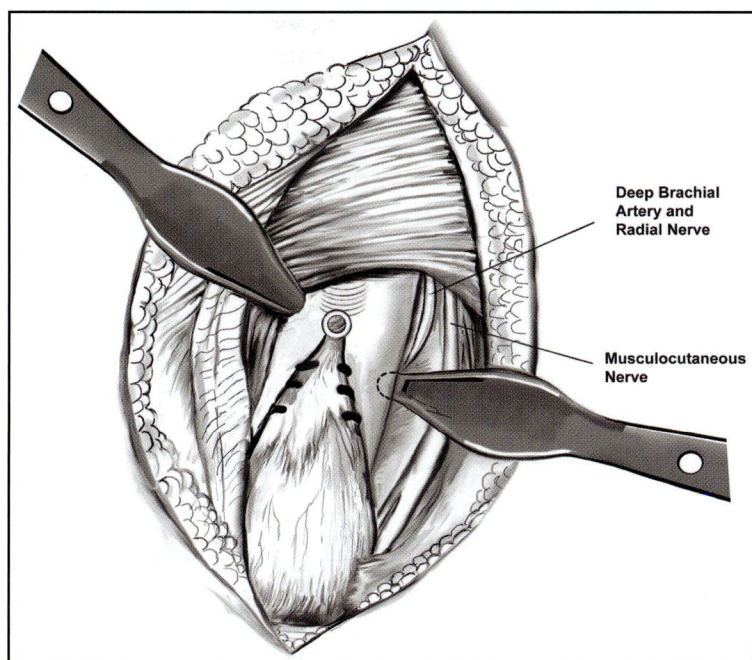

Figure 16-8. Schematic representation of at-risk structures in open subpectoral biceps tenodesis. Deep placement of the medial retractor with the arm in an internally rotated position places the musculocutaneous nerve and radial nerve at risk.

space to assess the bursal side of the rotator cuff, and a subacromial decompression is typically performed at the surgeon's discretion based on patient indications. The arthroscope can then be removed from the shoulder. We do not close the portals until the completion of the tenodesis in the event of any difficulty in delivering the proximal biceps tendon into the tenodesis incision. This can sometimes occur as a result of an incomplete arthroscopic release of the biceps anchor, adhesions within the bicipital groove, or loose bodies obstructing the bicipital groove. Leaving the portals open allows repeat arthroscopic evaluation of the joint, anchor, and tendon if needed.

Tenodesis

Before making an incision for the tenodesis, palpate the pectoralis major tendon, internally and externally rotating the arm if necessary to help localize it. An approximately 3-cm incision is then made on the medial aspect of the arm, 1-cm superior to the inferior border of the pectoralis tendon, and 2-cm below the inferior border, with the arm internally rotated. A more medial incision within the axilla is described, but we prefer a more anterior incision as we find it provides more direct access to the biceps tendon, with fewer neurovascular structures encountered during the approach. Sharp dissection and electrocautery are used in combination, as needed, to expose the fascia of the pectoralis major, coracobrachialis, and long head of the biceps tendon. The fascia of the biceps and coracobrachialis is incised, and blunt dissection is used to identify the underlying long head of the biceps tendon. Again, palpation of the inferior border of the pectoralis tendon often reveals the fusiform long head of the biceps tendon deep to it. A blunt Hohmann retractor is placed into the pectoralis major tendon, staying in close contact with the lateral aspect of the humerus, to retract the pectoralis both proximal and lateral. Medially, the coracobrachialis and short head of the biceps are gently retracted medially with a blunt chandler, being mindful of the musculocutaneous nerve. The proximity of the musculocutaneous nerve to the tenodesis site and medial retractor make this a vulnerable structure during open subpectoral biceps tenodesis (Figure 16-8). In a recent cadaveric study performed by the authors (unpublished) to assess the proximity of neurovascular structures in the arm during this procedure, the mean distance from the medial retractor to the musculocutaneous nerve was 2.9 mm ± 1.4 mm, and in 18% of specimens (of 17 total) the nerve was in direct contact with the retractor. Deep medial retractors and excessive medial retraction should be avoided to prevent iatrogenic injury to the musculocutaneous nerve. External rotation of the arm significantly increased the distance of the musculocutaneous nerve from the tenodesis site by 11.3 mm. This increased distance with external rotation is the reason we prefer the free Mayo stand instead of an arm holder, as we have found arm holders to limit external rotation of the arm.

With appropriate exposure, a right-angle clamp can be placed deep to the previously cut long head of the biceps tendon and can be used to pull the tendon out of the proximal groove and into the field. The proximal portion of the tendon is measured for diameter, and a holding-stitch, typically a Krackow locking stitch, is placed in the 15 mm of tendon proximal to the musculotendinous junction using a No. 2 FiberWire (Arthrex, Naples, FL). This allows maintenance of the biceps normal relationship under the pectoralis tendon, with the musculotendinous junction of the biceps beneath the inferior border of the pectoralis major tendon, and ensures appropriate tensioning of the tendon. The remaining tendon is excised and routinely sent to pathology as a specimen for documentation purposes. A bone tunnel is then made in the humerus at the inferior border of the pec tendon using a guidewire and the appropriately sized reamer. We typically use an 8.5-mm reamer for an 8-mm diameter tendon, rather than using an 8-mm reamer and tapping prior to screw insertion because we have often found it difficult to initiate screw purchase with line-to-line sizing, despite tapping, due to hard cortical bone. The tunnel is kept unicortical and is typically 15 to 17 mm deep. We then irrigate the tunnel to clear any loose bone or debris. The tunnel can be measured using a depth gauge, but we typically use either an 8 x 12 mm PEEK or Bio-Tenodesis screw (Arthrex, Naples, FL).

One limb of the suture (holding stitch) that was placed in the tendon is now passed through a cannulated screwdriver with the screw in place. Placing a snap on the end of this limb allows easy tensioning while placing the interference screw. The 15 mm of tendon that was previously stitched is now placed in the bone tunnel, and the screw is tensioned. After tensioning, the screw should sit flush with the bone tunnel. The screwdriver can then be removed, and the 2 sutures' limbs can now be tied (providing both suture anchor stability and interference fit). The bicep is then assessed for appropriate tension and relationship relative to the pectoralis tendon. The long head of the biceps tendon should now rest in a location similar to its anatomic location, with the musculotendinous junction just deep to the inferior border of the pectoralis major tendon.

The wound is then irrigated and closed in a layered fashion. We close the deep fascia with interrupted 2-0 Vicryl (Ethicon, Inc, Somerville, NJ) and then run a 3-0 Monocryl (Ethicon, Inc) for the subcuticular closure. The skin closure, while seemingly trivial, is important as bandages often come loose and fall off repeatedly given the proximity of the incision to the axilla. Steri-strips are then used to reinforce the closure, and a 4 x 4-inch tegaderm is used as a bandage.

Postoperative management is most often dictated by procedures performed in conjunction with biceps tenodesis (ie, rotator cuff repair). However, when done in isolation, the arm is placed in a sling postoperatively for approximately 4 weeks, during which passive glenohumeral, elbow, and wrist range of motion is initiated and progresses to active-assisted and active range of motion. Strengthening activities are restricted for approximately 6 weeks and then gradually introduced and advanced.

Pearls and Pitfalls

- Drape the arm free and use a padded Mayo instead of an arm holder to allow adequate external rotation during the case.
- Inject the tenodesis incision site with local anesthetic prior to the start of the case whether under general anesthesia or a local block.
- Draw the planned tenodesis incision prior to the start of the case as the shoulder's anatomic landmarks may become distorted after shoulder arthroscopy.

- Internally rotate the arm to draw the incision.
- Externally rotate the arm during the case to increase distance from the medial retractor to the musculocutaneous nerve.
- If it is difficult to deliver the proximal biceps tendon into wound, stop! The proximal tendon may be incompletely released or obstructed in the bicipital groove and may tear if pulled too hard.
- The tenodesed long head of the biceps tendon should rest in a location similar to its anatomic location, with the musculotendinous junction just deep to the inferior border of the pectoralis major tendon.

REFERENCES

1. Petersson CJ. Degeneration of the gleno-humeral joint. An anatomical study. *Acta Orthop Scand.* 1983;54(2):277-283.
2. Murthi AM, Vosburgh CL, Neviaser TJ. The incidence of pathologic changes of the LHB tendon. *J Shoulder Elbow Surg.* 2000;9(5):382-385.
3. Chen CH, Hsu KY, Chen WJ, Shih CH. Incidence and severity of biceps long head tendon lesion in patients with complete RTC tears. *J Trauma.* 2005;58(6):1189-1193.
4. Habermeyer P, Kaiser E, Knappe M, Kreusser T, Wiedemann E. [Functional anatomy and biomechanics of the long biceps tendon]. *Unfallchirurg.* 1987;90(7):319-329.
5. Demondion X, Maynou C, Van Cortenbosch B, Klein K, Leroy X, Mestdagh H. [Relationship between the tendon of the LHB brachii muscle and the glenoid labrum]. *Morphologie.* 2001;85(269):5-8.
6. Hoppenfeld S, DeBoer P, Hutton R. *Surgical Exposures in Orthopaedics: the Anatomic Approach.* 2nd ed. Philadelphia, PA: J.B. Lippincott Co; 1994:xviii.
7. Sethi N, Wright R, Yamaguchi K. Disorders of the LHB tendon. *J Shoulder Elbow Surg.* 1999;8(6):644-654.
8. Habermeyer P, Magosch P, Pritsch M, Scheibel MT, Lichtenberg S. Anterosuperior impingement of the shoulder as a result of pulley lesions: a prospective arthroscopic study. *J Shoulder Elbow Surg.* 2004;13(1):5-12.
9. Gleason PD, Beall DP, Sanders TB, et al. The transverse humeral ligament: a separate anatomical structure or a continuation of the osseous attachment of the RTC? *Am J Sports Med.* 2006;34(1):72-77.
10. Meyer AW. Spolia anatomica. *J Anat Physiol.* 1914;48(Pt 2):107-173.
11. Warner JJ, McMahon PJ. The role of the LHB brachii in superior stability of the glenohumeral joint. *J Bone Joint Surg Am.* 1995;77(3):366-372.
12. Andrews JR, Carson WG Jr, McLeod WD. Glenoid labrum tears related to the LHB. *Am J Sports Med.* 1985;13(5):337-341.
13. Lippmann RK. The frozen shoulder. *Surg Clin North Am.* 1950;31(2):367-383.
14. Kumar VP, Satku K, Balasubramaniam P. The role of the long head of biceps brachii in the stabilization of the head of the humerus. *Clin Orthop Relat Res.* 1989;244:172-175.
15. Soslowsky LJ, Malicky DM, Blasier RB. Active and passive factors in inferior glenohumeral stabilization: a biomechanical model. *J Shoulder Elbow Surg.* 1997;6(4):371-379.
16. Sakurai G, Ozaki J, Tomita Y, Nishimoto K, Tamai S. Electromyographic analysis of shoulder joint function of the biceps brachii muscle during isometric contraction. *Clin Orthop Relat Res.* 1998;354:123-131.
17. Levy AS, Kelly BT, Lintner SA, Osbahr DC, Speer KP. Function of the LHB at the shoulder: electromyographic analysis. *J Shoulder Elbow Surg.* 2001;10(3):250-255.
18. Matsen FA 3rd, Kirby RM. Office evaluation and management of shoulder pain. *Orthop Clin North Am.* 1982;13(3):453-475.
19. Yergason RM. Supination sign. *J Bone Joint Surg Am.* 1931;13:160.
20. Neviaser RJ. Lesions of the biceps and tendinitis of the shoulder. *Orthop Clin North Am.* 1980;11(2):343-348.
21. Abbott L, Saunders JB. Acute traumatic dislocation of the tendon of the LHB brachii. A report of six cases with operative findings. *Surgery.* 1939;6:817-840.
22. Holtby R, Razmjou H. Accuracy of the Speed's and Yergason's tests in detecting biceps pathology and SLAP lesions: comparison with arthroscopic findings. *Arthroscopy.* 2004;20(3):231-236.
23. Eakin CL, Faber KJ, Hawkins RJ, Hovis WD. Biceps tendon disorders in athletes. *J Am Acad Orthop Surg.* 1999;7(5):300-310.
24. Claessens H, Snoeck H. Tendinitis of the LHB brachii. *Acta Orthop Belg.* 1972;58(1):124-128.
25. Barber FA, Field LD, Ryu RK. Biceps tendon and superior labrum injuries: decision making. *Instr Course Lect.* 2008;57:527-538.
26. Lapidus PW, Guidotti FP. Local injections of hydrocortisone in 495 orthopedic patients. *Ind Med Surg.* 1957;26(5):234-244.

CHAPTER 17

OPEN ROTATOR CUFF REPAIR

Zakary A. Knutson, MD and Edward V. Craig, MD

Tears of the rotator cuff are a very common source of pain and dysfunction in the shoulder. Because of this, surgical repair of full-thickness rotator cuff tears is one of the most commonly performed orthopedic surgical procedures. During the past few years, treatment methods have evolved from an open acromioplasty and repair, which involves takedown of the anterior deltoid muscle, to an arthroscopic-assisted mini-open procedure intended to spare the deltoid, to an all-arthroscopic repair technique.[1] Recent literature reports that each of these techniques is successful in treating the pain and dysfunction associated with full-thickness rotator cuff tears. However, even with the trend toward most rotator cuff repairs being treated with the all-arthroscopic technique, literature does not support it as the superior operation in all circumstances.[2-5] Open and mini-open techniques are very useful in the treatment of massive tears or tears involving multiple tendons, including the subscapularis, that may require significant soft-tissue releases, marginal convergence, augmentation with an allograft matrix, tendon transfers, or implant insertion. Because of the similarities, and in some cases superiority, in outcomes between arthroscopic and open rotator cuff surgery, open techniques remain important in the armamentarium of surgical treatment of rotator cuff tears. In the absence of clear-cut superiority of one method over another, surgeon choice, experience, and technical facility all play a role in the decision about which direction the surgical repair should take. An adequate acromioplasty, secure repair of tendon to bone, adequate protection postoperatively, and surgeon-directed rehabilitation remain the hallmark of successful rotator cuff surgery, whichever method the surgeon uses to address the pathology.

INDICATIONS

The primary indication for repair of full-thickness rotator cuff tears is pain. Strength and motion may be regained postoperatively as well but in a less predictable pattern. There are multiple factors that may affect their return, including rotator cuff tendon and muscle quality, periscapular and

Ma CB, Feeley BT, eds.
*Basic Principles and Operative Management
of the Rotator Cuff (pp 243-254)*
© 2012 SLACK Incorporated

deltoid muscle function, patient conditioning, other comorbidities, and patient access to rehabilitation tools. Therefore, surgical repair is infrequently indicated in patients with signs of muscle weakness, documented cuff tear, and no pain. Recent literature has brought to light some of the risks of progression of full-thickness tears in size, which may in turn cause them to become symptomatic over time and be associated with changes in tendon and muscle quality, which make the tear more difficult to repair. Thus, it seems appropriate to counsel patients on the risks of observation versus surgical treatment at the time of diagnosis. For younger patients (younger than 60 years old), and particularly those with clear evidence of an acute traumatic tear, the indication to treat them surgically is significantly clearer. Younger patients, and those with traumatic tears, tend to have better quality tissues, muscles that can be reapproximated to their anatomic position, and more predictably restored anatomy and function.

A consistent algorithm is followed for each patient in whom a rotator cuff repair is planned. Diagnostic arthroscopy with treatment of all intra-articular pathology, characterization of the rotator cuff tear, and subacromial decompression is done for each patient. At the point of characterization of the tear, if it is felt that successful and anatomic repair of the tear can be performed arthroscopically without compromise of the repair quality, an arthroscopic repair is performed. If the tear cannot be predictably treated with arthroscopic repair methods alone, a mini-open approach is performed with repair performed under direct visualization. Deltoid takedown and subsequent repair may be done when further visualization is necessary, such as may be the case in subscapularis repair or treatment of massive and retracted repairs with augmentation devices. Deltoid detachment and repair is performed routinely if it is the surgeon's choice to perform both anterior acromioplasty and cuff repair by open method.

CONTRAINDICATIONS

Patients must have sufficient symptoms and loss of function to warrant the risk of surgery. Infection, neurologic injury, arthrofibrosis, chronic pain, and failure of repair of either cuff or deltoid are all possible complications of repair, and the patient should have a strong understanding of the associated risks. Patients also must be able to function after the repair and comply with the restrictions required to protect the repair. Patients who have concomitant lower extremity injuries requiring crutches, who do not have sufficient help at home to function with the use of only one arm, or who for other reasons cannot participate in the necessary rehabilitation program should consider treatment other than surgery. For other patients, it may not be possible to take the time away from work to address a rehabilitation program and focus on regaining the motion and strength necessary for a successful repair. Finally, medical comorbidities such as cardiovascular risk, smoking history, diabetes, neurological conditions such as Parkinson's disease, and infection history are always considered in advice given to patients about risk/reward of surgery.

SURGICAL MANAGEMENT

Positioning

Prior to positioning, the desired form of anesthesia is induced. In most patients, regional anesthesia in the form of an interscalene block is sufficient. If there is need for increased patient relaxation or if patient comfort issues are a concern, general anesthesia may be used.

While arthroscopic procedures on the shoulder can be performed in the lateral decubitus position, the beach chair position seems preferable for all arthroscopic decompression and rotator cuff procedures because of ready convertibility to open surgery without patient repositioning. When positioning, be sure that the patient's head is well secured in a neutral position and that the seat

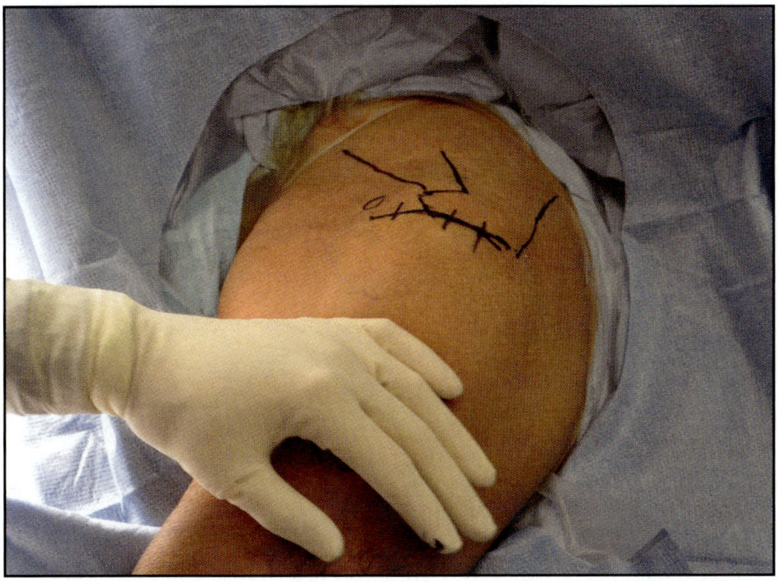

Figure 17-1. A transverse incision is made centered over the anterior edge of the acromion to allow access anteriorly if necessary. The incision is made along Langer's lines to form a more cosmetic scar. The authors feel that the transverse incision prevents dimpling of the skin through scar attachment to the deltoid.

is in an appropriate amount of Trendelenburg to prevent slouching during the procedure. Bony prominences are well-padded, including the peroneal nerves. The patient is placed in the appropriate amount of flexion to make the acromion parallel to the ground for anatomic referencing during surgery. The head should be tilted away from the operative shoulder slightly to allow maximal working room. A small bump, such as a rolled up surgical towel, is positioned behind the medial border of the scapula to stabilize it, holding the shoulder girdle in a more lateralized position and preventing sliding during surgery. The shoulder is prepped and draped with the entire arm free to allow ease of manipulation. The hand and forearm are secured in a sterile limb positioner to allow secure abduction and rotational control during surgery and to minimize the need for a surgical assistant.

Surgical Technique

After positioning, standard portal sites including an anticipated lateral portal are infiltrated with a 1:500,000 concentration of epinephrine to minimize bleeding. The posterior portal is established, and diagnostic arthroscopy is performed. Intra-articular pathology is treated as necessary, particularly that relating to the biceps tendon or labrum. The rotator cuff tear is identified at this point and is marked with a suture if necessary. The arthroscope is then placed into the subacromial space, and the lateral portal is made under needle localization. We position the arm and the lateral portal in conjunction with each other to allow maximum ease of access and visualization. The lateral portal is usually located in line with the posterior edge of the clavicle and at the juncture of the anterior third and posterior two-thirds of acromion. Next, a horizontal incision is made in anticipation of the possible need for extension in mini-open surgery. An expeditious subacromial decompression is performed using arthroscopic techniques. After decompression, when a maximal view of the nature and size of the rotator cuff tear is obtained, the decision is quickly made whether to proceed with open or arthroscopic repair. Prior to the conclusion of arthroscopy and mini-open approach, a tag/traction stitch can be passed arthroscopically through the cuff and brought out of the lateral portal to aid in localization and control of the cuff, particularly if it has retracted.

The skin incision is made as an extension of the lateral portal and is centered directly over it. The incision can be extended anteriorly to the coracoid if necessary for a more extensile approach, but usually 3 to 4 cm is sufficient. The horizontal incision more closely follows Langer's lines and is thus more cosmetic (Figure 17-1). We have also seen a pattern of dimpling of the skin associated with scarring of the vertical incision to the deltoid that is not seen with the horizontal incision.

Figure 17-2. A nonabsorbable suture is placed at the inferior edge of the deltoid split. This prevents propagation of the split during retraction and in turn protects the axillary nerve.

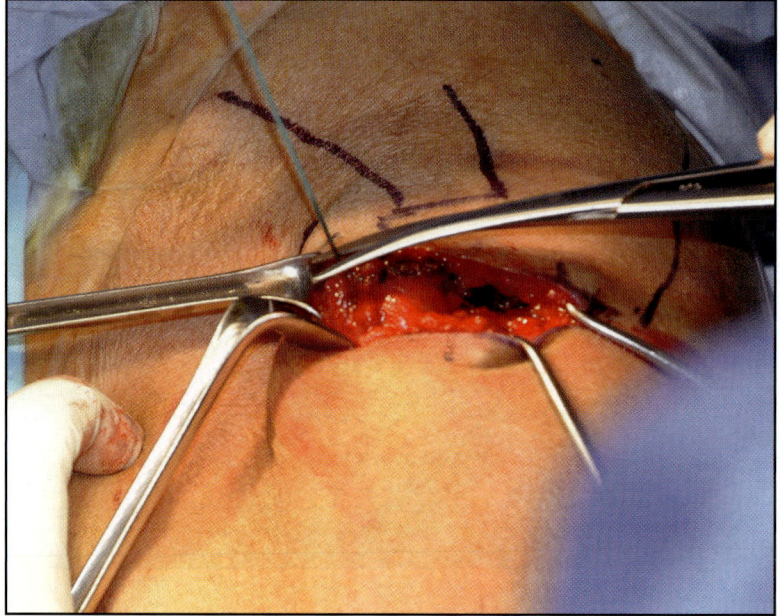

Full-thickness flaps are then made down to the deltoid fascia where the previous portal hole should be visible. The deltoid fibers are then split bluntly from the lateral edge of the acromion to a length of approximately 5 cm. A suture is placed at the bottom of the split to prevent propagation during retraction, which may put the axillary nerve at risk (Figure 17-2). Maintaining the fascia over the edge of the deltoid split is also important for later strength of repair. Adhesions often exist under the deltoid and beneath the acromion and coracoids, which can be removed with blunt finger dissection or a sponge.

Self-retaining retractors are then placed for deltoid retraction, which exposes the remaining bursal tissue over the rotator cuff. At this point, a small amount (1 to 2 mm) of deltoid attachment to the acromion can be released by electrocautery or subperiosteal dissection. The acromioplasty can be palpated through the wound to determine if an adequate resection has been performed. Further bony resection can be done if necessary. Visible remaining bursal tissue is removed sharply with scissors or a rongeur, exposing the underlying rotator cuff. The arm is rotated to position the rotator cuff tear for a point of maximal visualization and manipulation and help using the limb positioner. Extension and internal rotation maximize posterior cuff exposure, abduction and external rotation maximize subscapularis exposure, and longitudinal traction frequently is helpful for complete supraspinatus exposure. Downward traction using the limb positioner also increases visualization in the subacromial space.

The next step is to gain control of the torn rotator cuff for mobilization and subsequent advancement through the use of traction stitches. The stitch previously placed arthroscopically can make this step easier, as the first is frequently the most difficult. Absorbable braided sutures are used, and enough are placed to allow adequate tendon traction and reduction of the cuff to the humeral footprint (Figure 17-3). Sutures seem preferable to clamps for traction, as they are less damaging to an already compromised tendon.

If retraction and muscular atrophy prevent a tension-free reduction of the rotator cuff to its anatomic footprint, then soft-tissue releases may provide additional ability to mobilize the tendon. With tension on the rotator cuff, an elevator or blunt instrument is used to break up adhesions to the superior capsule. This is done by passing the instrument both intra-articularly and extra-articularly along the cuff surface and by gently releasing any bands of tissue tethering the rotator cuff to the acromion, coracoid, acromioclavicular (AC) joint, or deltoid. The coracohumeral (CH) ligament

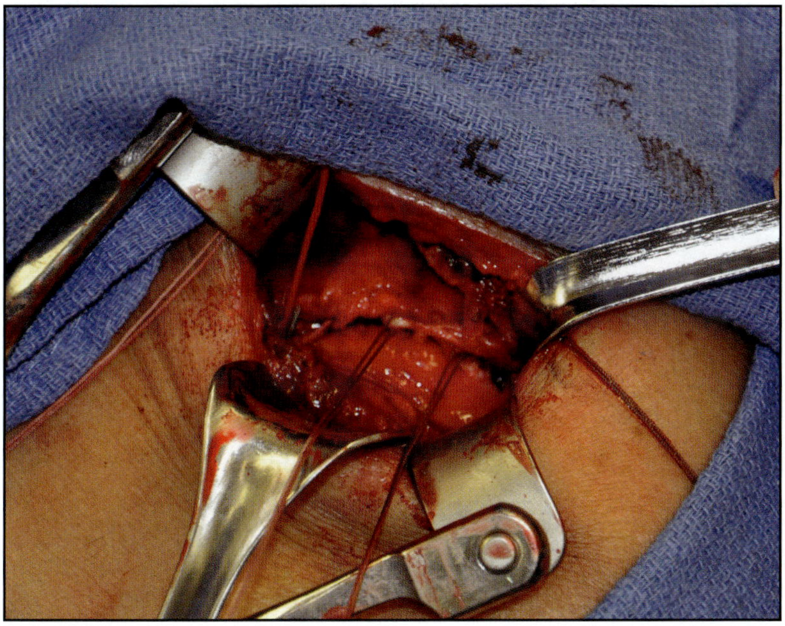

Figure 17-3. Braided suture is placed along the edge of the tendon to allow provisional reduction of the rotator cuff to its footprint. This allows characterization of the size and shape of the tear. Soft-tissue releases can be performed at this point for less mobile and retracted tears if necessary.

and rotator interval tissues, a common source of tethering, can be released sharply with scissors or cautery. Releases are considered complete when the rotator cuff can be reduced to its footprint without tension, although this will depend on the degree of retraction and adequacy of tissue for repair. Assessment of the shape of the tear and the possible need for marginal convergence techniques to reapproximate anatomy are considered.[6,7]

Preparation of the tendon for repair is then begun with a judicious freshening up of the rotator cuff tendon edge. Care must be made in decision making about how much tendon edge should be resected, as excessive removal of tissue can make anatomic reapproximation difficult. The humeral footprint is cleared of soft tissues using a rongeur, and gentle rasping of the bony surface is done to create a bleeding surface for tendon healing. Care should be taken not to be too aggressive with this maneuver, as removal of the cortical surface can compromise bony fixation of tendon to bone.

There are multiple effective techniques for bringing the torn tendon back to bone, with several fixation devices and suture configurations. For rotator cuff tears of most sizes, a double-row repair appears to give secure fixation while maximizing contact surface for healing. The repair is done with the arm in adduction to prevent over-tensioning of the rotator cuff. A repair done in abduction may be at risk when the arm is repositioned to the side. One effective method of double-row repair is to place a medial row consisting of double-loaded 4.5-mm suture anchors with nonabsorbable sutures placed at the anatomic neck, adjacent to the articular surface. The sutures are passed in a horizontal mattress configuration through a medial portion of the tendon, slightly lateral to the myotendinous junction (Figure 17-4). The sutures are tied but not cut, and then they are secured to the humerus at the lateral row with either bone tunnels or a knotless anchor device. Care is made to place the second row lateral enough to avoid possible fracture of the tuberosity. Other common double-row techniques secure the tendon in a mattress fashion, while adding additional security through bone tunnels that emerge from the greater tuberosity (Figure 17-5). The double-row technique creates a large footprint for tendon healing. After completion of the repair, the arm is brought into flexion and external rotation to ensure that the repair is strong enough to withstand passive motion exercises in the initial postoperative period.

Closure is begun after copious irrigation to remove all bony debris from tunnel drilling and/or acromioplasty. Any deltoid taken off of the acromion should be carefully reapproximated to the edge of the acromion. Starting medially at the AC joint using the superior capsular structures of

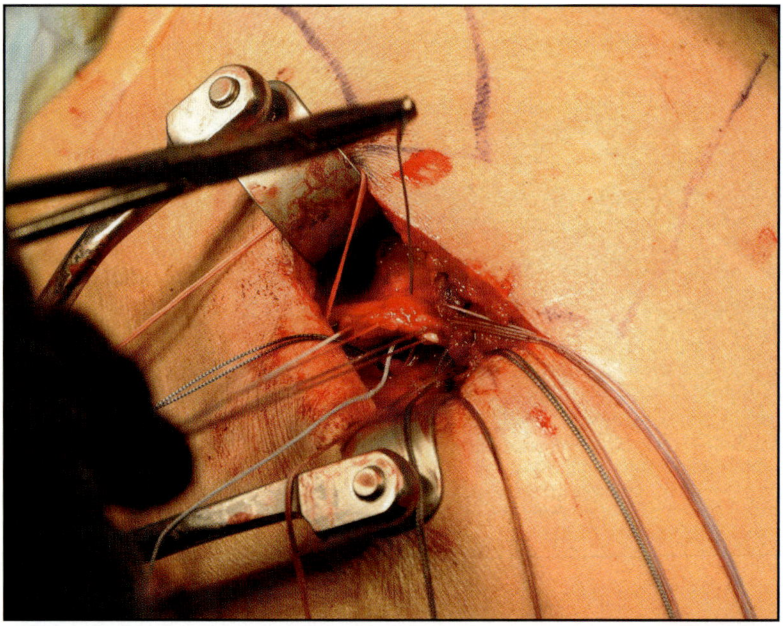

Figure 17-4. With reduction of the rotator cuff being held by the provisional sutures, single- or double-loaded suture anchors are placed along the anatomic footprint of the rotator cuff. Sutures are passed through the rotator cuff in horizontal mattress configuration at the medial edge of where the rotator cuff will attach to bone.

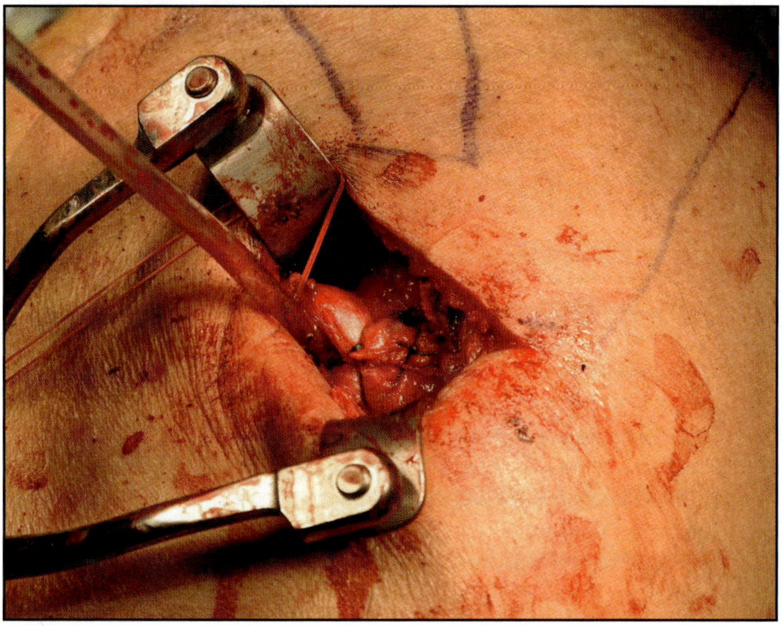

Figure 17-5. Once the medial row is tied down to bone, the second or lateral row of the rotator cuff repair is secured with a nonabsorbable suture that is passed through bone tunnels by a needle. This can be achieved with a simple suture configuration. The goal of the lateral row is to create a broad surface attachment of the rotator cuff for tendon to bone healing.

the joint and both the deep and superficial fascia of the deltoid gives a strong and accurate starting point for repair (Figure 17-6). The deltoid repair is performed from medial to lateral, and the deltoid fascia can be secured back both to its soft tissue point of division as well as the trapezius insertion. Nonabsorbable sutures should be used, and small bone tunnels may be necessary to ensure a secure repair (Figure 17-7). Meticulous closure of the deltoid is vital after an open approach, as deltoid dehiscence can be problematic for satisfactory patient outcome, even following successful healing of the cuff tissue itself. Superficial closure is done in 2 layers, with careful reapproximation of the dermis and a "water tight" seal. Dressings are placed, and the arm is secured in a sling with an abduction pillow to take stress off of the repair. For larger tears, revision cases, and in those in whom augmentation devices or tendon transfers are added, an abduction brace that brings the arm into approximately 45 degrees of abduction may be considered.[8,9]

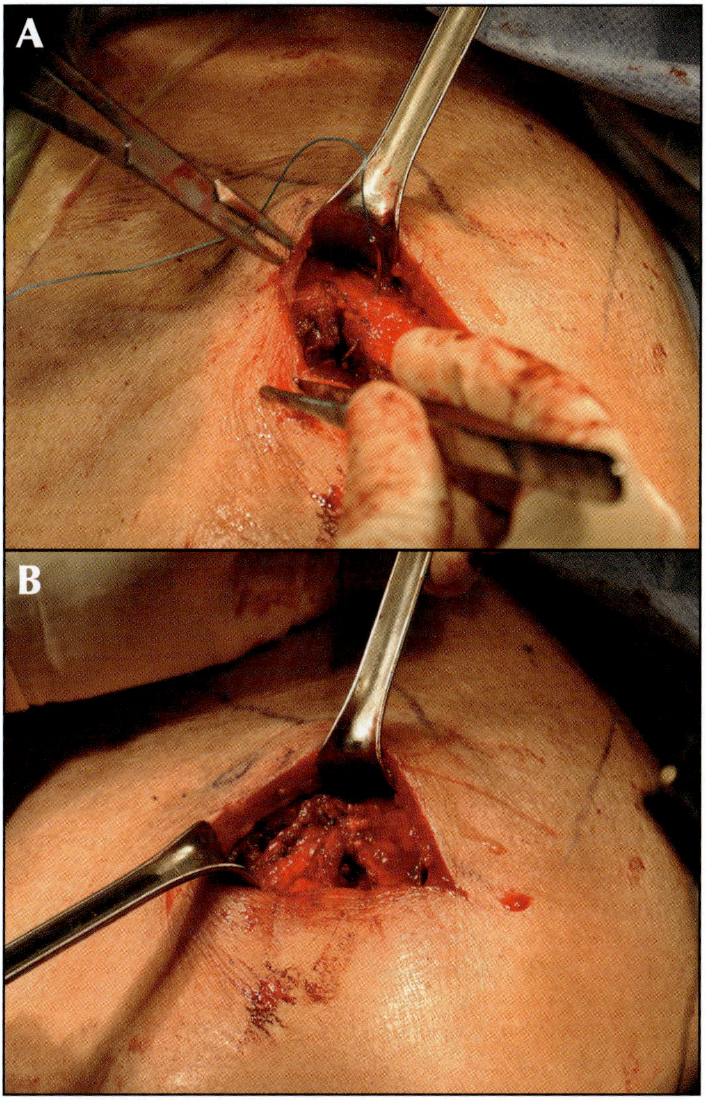

Figure 17-6. (A) The deltoid repair is performed in a medial to lateral direction, with the corner of the AC joint being used as an anatomic landmark. (B) The deltoid is then captured by nonabsorbable suture with full-thickness bites incorporating both the deep and superficial deltoid fascia. Careful repair must be done to avoid partial or complete deltoid dehiscence.

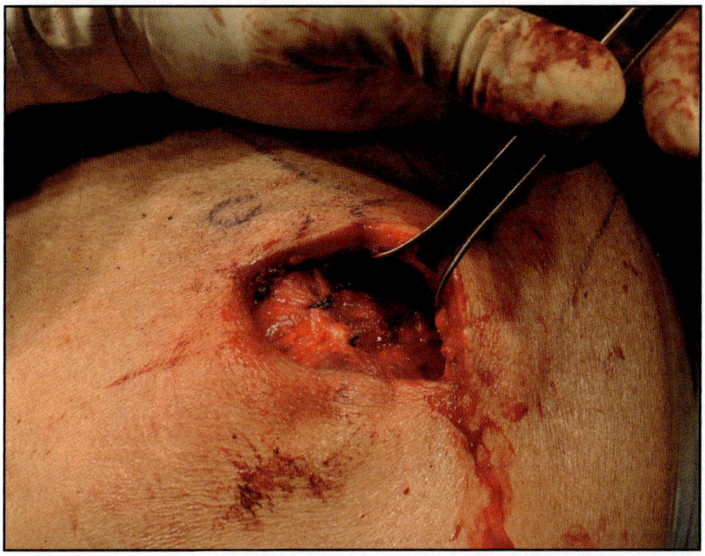

Figure 17-7. Nonabsorbable sutures are used through bone tunnels in the acromion if necessary to ensure a strong repair.

Postoperative Management and Rehabilitation

An individualized approach is taken for each patient based on multiple factors, including quality of tissue (tendon and bone), quality of repair, concomitant procedures performed, adequacy of deltoid, and the patient's ability to understand and comply with postoperative protocols. The more that a repair is felt to be at risk of failure, the less aggressive the rehabilitation regimen becomes. In general, the larger the tear and the poorer the quality of tissue, the longer the time before initiating postoperative rehabilitation. Both before and after deltoid closure, the arm can be taken through a passive range of motion, and an assessment can be performed as to the amount of safe arm motion that can be permitted passively before there is tension on the repair. This will be individualized both according to the patient and according to repair. For instance, subscapularis repair is put under more tension in external rotation and abduction, while supraspinatus repairs are under the most tension in internal rotation and extension. For standard repairs, a passive motion-only protocol is begun, which entails passive supine flexion to 90 degrees and external rotation to 30 degrees. Therapy is begun on postoperative day 1 with strict guidance by a therapist. It is vital that a trusting relationship is formed between the patient and physical therapist, as a lack of understanding of restrictions can compromise the repair.[10] Patients should be cautioned that any active use of the shoulder can put the repair at risk.

It may be useful to the surgeon to end the operative report with general plans for rehabilitation, such as which motions should be added when and when active motion can be begun. The advantage of this is that rehabilitation can be considered at the time when repair and tissue quality is fresh in the surgeon's mind and can be a useful addition if the operative report is given to the therapist. Recall of intraoperative details is frequently difficult with the passage of time.

Patients with smaller tears who are able to participate well in the rehabilitation program are taught circular Codman exercises, which entail standing upright with the waist bent at 90 degrees. Clockwise and counterclockwise circles are made with the shoulder. More complicated exercises include the use of pulleys for forward elevation. This particular exercise is frequently delayed, as patients often have difficulty keeping this exercise a purely passive one. Another effective exercise to regain flexibility in the frontal plane is to use the nonoperative arm to lift the operative arm. A second assistive exercise, useful in regaining external rotation, involves the use of a broom handle or a golf club to rotate the arm away from the side of the body. Both of these exercises are done with the arm in adduction, and it is imperative that no active motion is performed by the operative extremity. At 3 weeks, assistive internal rotation and extension may be added to the regimen. Passive motion protocols, or assistive motion exercises, are continued for 6 weeks. Scapula and trapezius exercises, if they are done safely without recruiting the cuff muscles, can be begun at any time postoperatively.

From 6 weeks to 12 weeks, active-assistive exercises are continued, the sling is discontinued, light active use of the arm is permitted, and submaximal effort isometric exercises are instituted. Progression to full active use of the arm at 12 weeks is accompanied by the institution of resistive exercises. The goal of this phase is to regain full passive range of motion and to initiate isotonic strengthening exercises below 90 degrees of elevation. Periscapular stabilization exercises are important as well in preparation for rotator cuff strengthening. Following the repair of massive rotator cuff tears, this rehabilitation guideline can be delayed, and passive motion can be carried out for as long as 3 to 4 months from surgery to minimize stress on the repaired tendon.[11]

At 12 weeks, the patient is instructed on the use of elastic bands for strengthening of the anterior deltoid and rotator cuff. The goals of this phase are to restore 5/5 strength of both the rotator cuff and the periscapular musculature as well as normalize the scapulothoracic rhythm. Patients should begin return to activities of daily living with the understanding that it may take months to achieve these goals entirely.

Patient expectations form a very important part of the rehabilitation process after rotator cuff repair. It is helpful to use the time before surgery to explain what is considered a reasonable time frame for recovery, anticipated pain, and return of strength and motion. The most painful time for patients, other than the initial postoperative period, is during stretching in attempts to regain passive motion. It is at this time that patients can become frustrated or fall behind in their rehabilitation, thus leading to stiffness. All patients are weak during the initial strengthening period as they have not been using their deltoid and rotator cuff for weeks to months. It can be expected for patients to require 9 to 12 months to regain 95% of their shoulder strength compared to the other side. Resolution of pain is much more predictable in its pattern and degree of improvement than either motion or strength.

Potential Complications

There are many potential complications associated with rotator cuff surgery. Open and mini-open procedures carry a specific set of risks as well.

Axillary Nerve Injury

The axillary nerve is at risk during aggressive exposure of the rotator cuff during the mini-open approach. The fibers of the nerve course within the deep fascia of the deltoid and can be reliably found approximately 5 cm from the muscular origin off of the acromion. Tension from the self-retaining retractors during the procedure can stretch or even tear the nerve. Careful retractor placement and a stitch in the deltoid to prevent propagation minimize this risk.

Postoperative Deltoid Avulsion

If the deltoid muscle is taken off of the acromion for an open procedure, it is at risk for detachment during the early postoperative period. Meticulous repair combined with strict adherence to the passive motion protocols minimizes this possibility. Loss of the deltoid attachment may result in a cosmetic defect in the form of a divot in the anterior shoulder as well as a functional deficit. The anterior deltoid is a key driving force in elevation of the shoulder, especially shoulders with compromised rotator cuff musculature. Most commonly however, only a very small portion of the repair fails. This can be left alone if an otherwise successful repair and decompression have been performed, as it is unlikely to cause clinical deficits.

Postoperative Stiffness

Although not specific to open rotator cuff surgery, postoperative stiffness can be a significant problem and a source of poor clinical outcome. Stiffness may be difficult to predict; is often difficult to treat once established; and may be minimized by the combination of patient understanding, adequate postoperative pain control, early initiation of safe exercises, and effective communication between surgeon and therapist, if one is used, or between surgeon and patient, if a therapist is not involved in postoperative care. If a patient is felt to be stiff during the follow-up period or if there is anything impeding the planned rehabilitation (pain, apprehension, etc), a long discussion is had with the patient to ensure effective exercises are being performed. Frequently, more aggressive passive motion with a physical therapist can restore motion. Manipulation under anesthesia is not typically performed because of potential impact on the repaired tendon.

It should be noted that some patients are more at risk for postoperative stiffness, including those with diabetes, those who have had preoperative stiffness, and those in whom passive motion has not been obtained at the time of surgery.

OUTCOMES

Open and mini-open rotator cuff repairs remain the gold standard for the treatment of full-thickness rotator cuff tears. Baysal and colleagues evaluated 84 shoulders clinically after mini-open rotator cuff repair.[12] They found an overall 96% satisfaction rate with statistically significant improvements in external rotation and several outcomes measures, including American Shoulder and Elbow Surgeons (ASES) scores and Western Ontario Rotator Cuff scores. Shinners and colleagues reported similar results with the arthroscopically assisted mini-open rotator cuff repair.[13] Forty-one shoulders at an average of 36 months postoperatively in relatively young patients (average age 51) were evaluated. All patients had an improvement in their pain and function scores with 93% being rated as good or excellent. Fealy and colleagues evaluated the use of a double-row fixation technique using the arthroscopically assisted mini-open approach in 75 shoulders that had large tears (3 to 5 cm).[14] At 24 months follow-up, there was 92.6% subjective satisfaction with 93% reporting that they would undergo the procedure again. No comparison was made to a single-row technique. In each of the aforementioned studies, rotator cuff tear size did not significantly affect patient outcomes.

Mohtadi and colleagues published one of the few randomized clinical trials concerning open and arthroscopically assisted mini-open rotator cuff repairs.[15] Either a traditional open acromioplasty with rotator cuff repair or an arthroscopic acromioplasty with mini-open rotator cuff repair was carried out on patients who were then followed for 2 years. Outcomes were reported, using the Rotator Cuff Quality of Life Index, ASES score, Shoulder Rating Questionnaire, and Functional Shoulder Elevation Test. At 3 months postoperatively, the mini-open group was noted to be statistically superior to the open group. However, at an average of 28 months follow-up, there was no clinical difference in outcome measures between the open and mini-open groups.

Multiple studies have been performed comparing open and arthroscopic techniques both by clinical and radiographic outcome. Bishop and colleagues evaluated rotator cuff integrity 1 year after repair in patients repaired with both mini-open and all-arthroscopic techniques.[16] When stratified according to the size of the tear, for tears measuring less than 3 cm in size, 74% remained intact in the open group and 84% in the arthroscopic group, which was not a significant difference statistically. However, for tears larger than 3 cm in size, 64% of the open group and only 24% of the arthroscopic group remained intact, which was significant. Verma and colleagues evaluated arthroscopic and mini-open repairs at a minimum 24-month follow-up with ultrasound.[17] Twenty-four percent of all-arthroscopic and 27% of mini-open repairs showed recurrent defects at that time, which was not significant. Regardless of the type of repair, those patients with an original tear size larger than 3 cm were 7 times more likely to have a recurrent defect at follow-up. Those with recurrent defects were also significantly weaker statistically in elevation and external rotation compared to those without defects.

Morse and colleagues performed a meta-analysis of the literature between 1966 and July 2006 to review both arthroscopic and mini-open rotator cuff repairs.[18] With inclusion criteria of only level 1 to 3 studies, minimum 1-year follow-up, with an average of 2 years, and 1 to 4 validated functional outcome scores, only 5 studies were identified. From these studies, no significant difference in functional outcomes scores or complications was able to be ascertained between the mini-open and arthroscopic groups.

Kim and colleagues looked at outcomes from mini-open versus arthroscopic rotator cuff repair performed after a failed attempt at an all-arthroscopic repair.[19] Seventy-six shoulders underwent an initial attempt at arthroscopic rotator cuff repair for medium- to large-sized tears. If the surgeon was unable to successfully complete the repair arthroscopically, then the repair was converted to mini-open, and the repair was completed. At a mean follow-up of 39 months, there was statistical improvement in both groups and no difference between the 2 in UCLA and ASES scores. Between both groups, those with larger tears showed less predictable return of motion and strength. The authors concluded that intraoperative conversion of an attempted all-arthroscopic repair to a mini-open repair did not affect patient outcome.

Churchill and colleagues evaluated the costs of both arthroscopically assisted mini-open procedures and all-arthroscopic rotator cuff repairs and compared the number amount in low, intermediate, and high-volume facilities.[20] Mini-open repairs were noted to be significantly faster (average 10 minutes faster) and less expensive (average approximately $1000 per case) than all-arthroscopic repairs, with high-volume centers noted to be the most expensive.

CONCLUSION

Open cuff repair, accompanied by either arthroscopic or open acromioplasty, continues to be an effective management strategy for those tendon repairs not amenable to all-arthroscopic techniques. Patients are instructed that the tear will be evaluated arthroscopically, and in most cases the bony work will be performed arthroscopically. If the tear is amenable, an all-arthroscopic repair is done. However, each patient understands that conversion to an open procedure is an option if it is felt that a mini-open approach will result in a more effective repair.

PEARLS AND PITFALLS

Pearls

- When placing the patient in the beach chair position, be sure to place a small towel bump at the medial border of the scapula. This keeps the shoulder girdle from sliding medially during the procedure, stabilizes the scapula, and increases the working room.
- Make the lateral portal incision horizontal. This follows Langer's lines and thus is more cosmetic. A horizontal incision is also preferable in case the shoulder is opened to prevent dimpling of the skin.
- Before conclusion of the arthroscopy, pass a single suture through the cuff arthroscopically and bring it out of the lateral portal to act as a traction stitch when localizing and gaining control of the rotator cuff.
- During the deltoid split, place a nonabsorbable retaining suture in the deltoid fascia approximately 4 to 5 cm from the acromion. This prevents propagation of the split and possible harm to the axillary nerve.
- After open procedures in which the anterior deltoid is taken down, repair the deltoid from medial to lateral. Start at the base of the AC joint, and use the superior capsule for a strong soft tissue structure to sew to.
- Use the arm positioned to your advantage. Internally or externally rotate the arm to give the best possible view and access to the cuff.
- Once the shoulder is open, palpate the undersurface of the acromion and AC joint to ensure adequacy of acromioplasty, AC joint coplaning, or resection.
- The rotator cuff, when torn, retracts to predictable positions. The supraspinatus usually is pulled medially by the CH ligament and scars to coracoid. Release of rotator interval thus aids in mobilization.
- The infraspinatus often is pulled inferiorly by the teres minor. Thus, direction of mobilization of the supraspinatus is usually medial to lateral, while mobilization of the infraspinatus is inferior to superior.

Pitfalls

- Do not repair the rotator cuff with the arm in an abducted position. This frequently leads to failure when the arm is brought to the side.
- When identifying the rotator cuff, make sure that you differentiate between the rotator cuff and remaining bursal tissue, which can be quite thickened in some patients. Bursa usually scars to deltoid and thus frequently does not rotate, while cuff tendon moves with arm rotation.
- Do not mobilize patients with massive rotator cuff tears too quickly. Their tissues are often of lesser quality than those tissues with smaller tears and have been proven to retear more often as well. We will maintain patients in a passive motion protocol for 3 months if needed.

- Do not forget to counsel your patients preoperatively about expected outcomes and a timeline for recovery. It frequently takes 1 year to maximize the result, and pain relief is often more predictable than motion and strength, particularly with large tears.
- Do not take too long to do the bony work/subacromial decompression. The tissues become swollen and boggy, which limits the ability to see even in the mini-open procedure. An expeditious acromioplasty is your best friend, whether arthroscopic or open repair of the cuff is performed.

REFERENCES

1. Dunn WR, Schackman BR, Walsh C, et al. Variation in orthopaedic surgeons' perceptions about the indications for rotator cuff surgery. *J Bone Joint Surg Am.* 2005;87(9):1978-1984.
2. Sauerbrey AM, Getz CL, Piancastelli M, Iannotti JP, Ramsey ML, Williams GR Jr. Arthroscopic versus mini-open rotator cuff repair: a comparison of clinical outcome. *Arthroscopy.* 2005;21(12):1415-1420.
3. Warner JJ, Tetreault P, Lehtinen J, Zurakowski D. Arthroscopic versus mini-open rotator cuff repair: a cohort comparison study. *Arthroscopy.* 2005;21(3):328-332.
4. Youm T, Murray DH, Kubiak EN, Rokito AS, Zuckerman JD. Arthroscopic versus mini-open rotator cuff repair: a comparison of clinical outcomes and patient satisfaction. *J Shoulder Elbow Surg.* 2005;14(5):455-459.
5. Nho SJ, Shindle MK, Sherman SL, Freedman KB, Lyman S, MacGillivray JD. Systematic review of arthroscopic rotator cuff repair and mini-open rotator cuff repair. *J Bone Joint Surg Am.* 2007;89(Suppl 3):127-136.
6. Burkhart SS. Arthroscopic treatment of massive rotator cuff tears. *Clin Orthop Rel Res.* 2001;390:107-118.
7. Davidson J, Burkhart SS. The geometric classification of rotator cuff tears: a system linking tear pattern to treatment and prognosis. *Arthroscopy.* 2010;26(3):417-424.
8. Craig EV. Mini-open and open techniques for full-thickness rotator cuff repairs. In: Craig EV, ed. *Master Techniques in Orthopedic Surgery: The Shoulder.* 2nd ed. Philadelphia, PA: Lippincott Williams & Wilkins; 2004:309-340.
9. Wright VJ, Craig EV. Mini-open rotator cuff repair. In: Cole BJ, Sekiya JK, eds. *Surgical Techniques of the Shoulder, Elbow, and Knee in Sports Medicine.* Philadelphia, PA: Saunders; 2008:193-199.
10. Ghodadra NS, Provencher MT, Verma NN, Wilk KE, Romeo AA. Open, mini-open, and all-arthroscopic rotator cuff repair surgery: indications and implications for rehabilitation. *J Orthop Sports Phys Ther.* 2009;39(2):81-89.
11. Masci R, Fives G. Rotator cuff repair: arthroscopic and open. In: Cioppa-Mosca J, Cahill JB, Cavanaugh JT, Corradi-Scalise D, Rudnik H, Wolff AL, eds. *Postsurgical Rehabilitation Guidelines for the Orthopedic Clinician.* St. Louis, MO: Mosby; 2006:497-511.
12. Baysal D, Balyk R, Otto D, Luciak-Corea C, Beaupre L. Functional outcome and health-related quality of life after surgical repair of full-thickness rotator cuff tear using a mini-open technique. *Am J Sports Med.* 2005;33(9):1346-1355.
13. Shinners TJ, Noordsij PG, Orwin JF. Arthroscopically assisted mini-open rotator cuff repair. *Arthroscopy.* 2002;18(1):21-26.
14. Fealy S, Kingham TP, Altchek DW. Mini-open rotator cuff repair using a two-row fixation technique: outcomes analysis in patients with small, moderate, and large rotator cuff tears. *Arthroscopy.* 2002;18(6):665-670.
15. Mohtadi NG, Hollinshead RM, Sasyniuk TM, Fletcher JA, Chan DS, Li FX. A randomized clinical trial comparing open to arthroscopic acromioplasty with mini-open rotator cuff repair for full-thickness rotator cuff tears: disease-specific quality of life outcome at an average 2-year follow-up. *Am J Sports Med.* 2008;36(6):1043-1051.
16. Bishop J, Klepps S, Lo IK, Bird J, Gladstone JN, Flatow EL. Cuff integrity after arthroscopic versus open rotator cuff repair: a prospective study. *J Shoulder Elbow Surg.* 2006;15(3):290-299.
17. Verma NN, Dunn W, Adler RS, et al. All-arthroscopic versus mini-open rotator cuff repair: a retrospective review with minimum 2-year follow-up. *Arthroscopy.* 2006;22(6):587-594.
18. Morse K, Davis AD, Afra R, Kaye EK, Schepsis A, Voloshin I. Arthroscopic versus mini-open rotator cuff repair: a comprehensive review and meta-analysis. *Am J Sports Med.* 2008;36(9):1824-1828.
19. Kim SH, Ha KI, Park JH, Kang JS, Oh SK, Oh I. Arthroscopic versus mini-open salvage repair of the rotator cuff tear: outcome analysis at 2 to 6 years' follow-up. *Arthroscopy.* 2003;19(7):746-754.
20. Churchill RS, Ghorai JK. Total cost and operating room time comparison of rotator cuff repair techniques at low, intermediate, and high volume centers: mini-open versus all-arthroscopic. *J Shoulder Elbow Surg.* 2010;19(5):716-721.

***Please see video on the accompanying Web site at
http://www.slackbooks.com/rotatorcuffvideos***

CHAPTER 18

REHABILITATION OF
ROTATOR CUFF PATHOLOGY

Michael A. Shaffer, PT, ATC, OCS;
Paul J. Pursley, PT, SCS, CSCS; and Brian R. Wolf, MD, MS

Rotator cuff pathology falls along a spectrum of disease from simple irritation of the tendon (tendinitis) to early tendon degeneration (tendinopathy) and finally partial- and full-thickness tearing of the rotator cuff.[1] Full-thickness tears have their own spectrum, ranging from small tears to massive, retracted tears with corresponding muscle atrophy and degeneration. Further complicating matters is the relative lack of correlation between patient symptoms, function, and the degree of structural injury present to the rotator cuff and surrounding tissues.

Any discussion of the treatment of rotator cuff disease requires an appreciation of the natural history. Despite the prevalence of rotator cuff disorders, the natural history of rotator cuff disease is not transparent. Prevailing wisdom suggests rotator cuff disease and tearing correlates with the aging process. Several studies have demonstrated a high prevalence of asymptomatic partial- and full-thickness rotator cuff tears in elderly people using advanced imaging such as ultrasound or magnetic resonance imaging (MRI).[2,3]

Even less is known about what causes some individuals with rotator cuff pathology to become symptomatic. Yamaguchi and colleagues[4] provided insight into the natural history of rotator cuff tears when they performed ultrasound examination of the contralateral shoulder in a group of patients who were already being treated for rotator cuff tears. Based upon ultrasound examination, 40% of the contralateral shoulders presented with a tear of the rotator cuff, yet all were asymptomatic. These patients were followed, revealing 39% of tears progressed in size, and 51% of patients subsequently became symptomatic at an average of 2.8 years later.[4] Finally, a recent study demonstrated there is no difference in shoulder function between a group of patients with an intact rotator cuff and those with an asymptomatic rotator cuff tear based on American Shoulder and Elbow Surgeons scores and Simple Shoulder Tests.[5]

Clearly then, the spectrum of structural injury and range of symptoms makes caring for the individual with rotator cuff disease difficult. The fact that some individuals may have minimal pain and normal function with a full-thickness rotator cuff tear should give the surgeon pause before indiscriminately performing rotator cuff repair. Conversely, untreated tears often increase in size, and many become symptomatic, suggesting early operative repair should be the treatment of choice.

Ma CB, Feeley BT, eds.
Basic Principles and Operative Management
of the Rotator Cuff (pp 255-270)
© 2012 SLACK Incorporated

TABLE 18-1. KEY COMPONENTS OF A PROGRAM FOR SHOULDER IMPINGEMENT/TENDINOPATHY

STRETCHING THE POSTERIOR SHOULDER	Crossed body adduction Sleeper stretch (see Figure 18-1)
ROTATOR CUFF FACILITATION	Elastic resistance (internal rotation, external rotation, unilateral extension, bilateral rowing; see Figure 18-2)
PERISCAPULAR STRENGTHENING	Bilateral rowing (see Figure 18-2)
TRUNK POSITIONING	Verbal cues to minimize flexed trunk, forward head, rounded shoulders positioning
MANUAL TECHNIQUES	Cervical/thoracic spinal mobilizations, glenohumeral mobilizations, passive stretching.

Rehabilitation for rotator cuff disease is an integral part of treatment, whether it is the primary treatment or is done in conjunction with operative intervention. However, given the shifting spectrum of disease and function, the rehabilitation process must be adaptable and appropriate for the underlying diagnosis. This chapter will cover rehabilitation for 3 distinct areas within the spectrum of rotator cuff disease: impingement and/or tendinopathy, nonoperative management of full-thickness tears, and postoperative rehabilitation following rotator cuff repair.

PHYSICAL THERAPY FOR IMPINGEMENT AND/OR ROTATOR CUFF TENDINOPATHY

"Impingement" typically refers to extrinsic irritation of the rotator cuff and subacromial bursa from the overlying coracoacromial arch, specifically the anterolateral acromion and/or the coracoacromial ligament. Symptoms typically include pain with overhead movements as well as painful shoulder extension and internal rotation. Night pain is common, and sleep is frequently affected. An inciting event will be recalled in a portion of cases, but a significant number of patients experience an insidious onset. Patients typically localize their pain to the anterior and lateral aspect of the upper arm, frequently with radiation distally toward the lateral elbow. Descriptions of pain distal to the elbow are not consistent with subacromial pathology. Symptoms below the elbow suggest either cervical nerve root or brachial plexus pathology.

Patients with tendinopathy, such as partial-thickness rotator cuff injuries, typically have similar presenting complaints as those patients with impingement. Partial-thickness tears occur most frequently on the articular side of the rotator cuff and can involve varying percentages of involvement of the rotator cuff footprint attachment at the humeral tuberosities. Rehabilitation is frequently the initial treatment of choice for partial cuff tears that involve less than 30% to 50% of the cuff thickness at the insertion.[6]

Although an individualized rehabilitation plan, established by a rehabilitation professional, may be ideal,[7] there are several universal components to a rehabilitation program that benefit most patients with impingement and/or early rotator cuff tendinopathy (Table 18-1).[8,9] At our institution, we use a largely self-directed program with occasional visits with a therapist for appropriate progressions of the exercise regimen. It would be fairly typical for patients with rotator cuff tendinopathy/impingement to complete physical therapy visits on a weekly or every other week basis for a grand total of 4 to 6 visits. Similar to other authors,[9] we feel that systematically targeting certain key rehabilitation components allows us to adequately address patient needs while being mindful of physical therapy utilization.

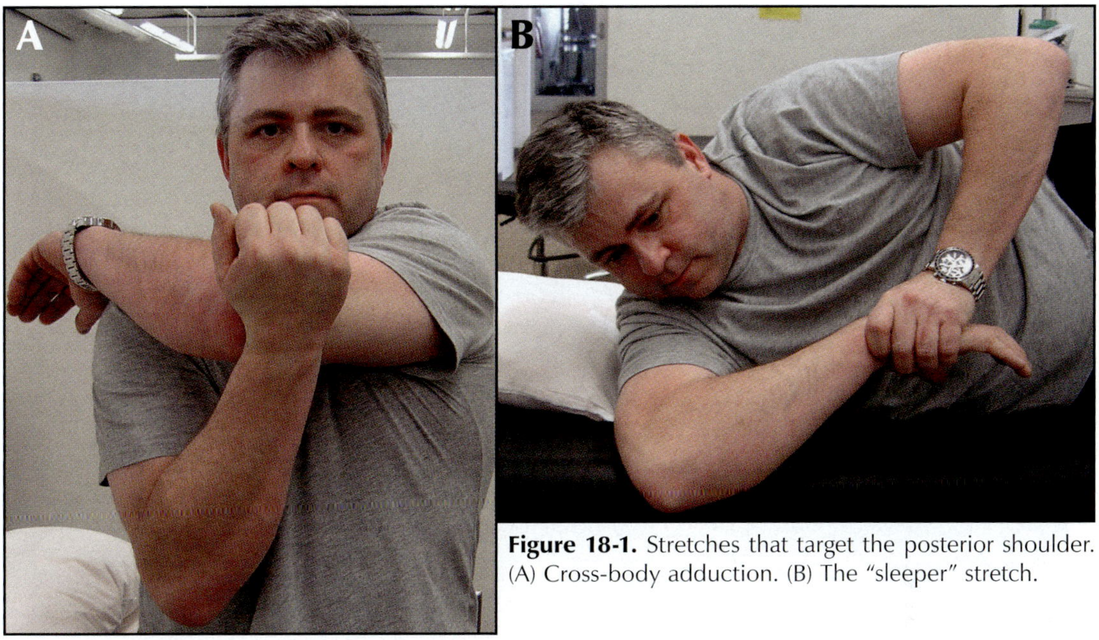

Figure 18-1. Stretches that target the posterior shoulder. (A) Cross-body adduction. (B) The "sleeper" stretch.

There are several active components of rehabilitation, but first and foremost, exacerbating activities such as repetitive overhead motions must be avoided. Patients with impingement/tendinopathy commonly demonstrate posterior shoulder tightness.[10] Maintaining appropriate flexibility of the posterior capsule is vital to avoid obligatory anterosuperior translation of the humeral head.[11] In addition, properly functioning rotator cuff musculature helps to maintain a humeral head centered on the glenoid, thereby minimizing tensile, injurious forces to the rotator cuff tendon. However, a centered humeral head is only possible with a stable scapular base, which in itself requires proper positioning of the thorax and adequate periscapular strength.

Posterior Shoulder Tightness

Tightness of the posterior capsule produces anterosuperior translation of the humeral head[11] and as such is suspected to be a leading cause of subacromial pathology. However, acute changes in posterior shoulder tightness, such as after pitching[12] or stretching,[13] demonstrate that perhaps what has been described as posterior capsular tightness is actually the result of alterations in resting tension in the posterior rotator cuff muscles. Tightness of the posterior shoulder can produce a loss of internal rotation range of motion or a glenohumeral internal rotation deficit. Stretching exercises that target the posterior shoulder are often included in rehabilitation programs for subacromial pathology.[9,14] Reliable methods of assessing and reassessing posterior shoulder stiffness include both cross-body adduction[15,16] and internal rotation. These studies provide clues as to the types of motions and stretches that target the posterior shoulder (Figure 18-1). Cross-body adduction, internal rotation, and full elevation in the sagittal plane produce tightness in the posterior shoulder of a cadaveric specimen with the greatest strain on the posterior capsule occurring with a combination of internal rotation and glenohumeral elevation.[17] However, in a randomized controlled trial, cross-body stretching produced greater gains of posterior shoulder flexibility than a sleeper stretch (glenohumeral internal rotation stretching performed in a side-lying position with the weight of the body providing a stabilizing force for scapular stabilization).[18] As posterior shoulder tightness may be primarily a muscular phenomenon, many clinicians add contract-relax muscle energy techniques to sleeper or cross-body stretches.[19] The resulting improvements in posterior shoulder stiffness have been linked to improvement of patients with impingement[9,14] and other shoulder pathologies.[20]

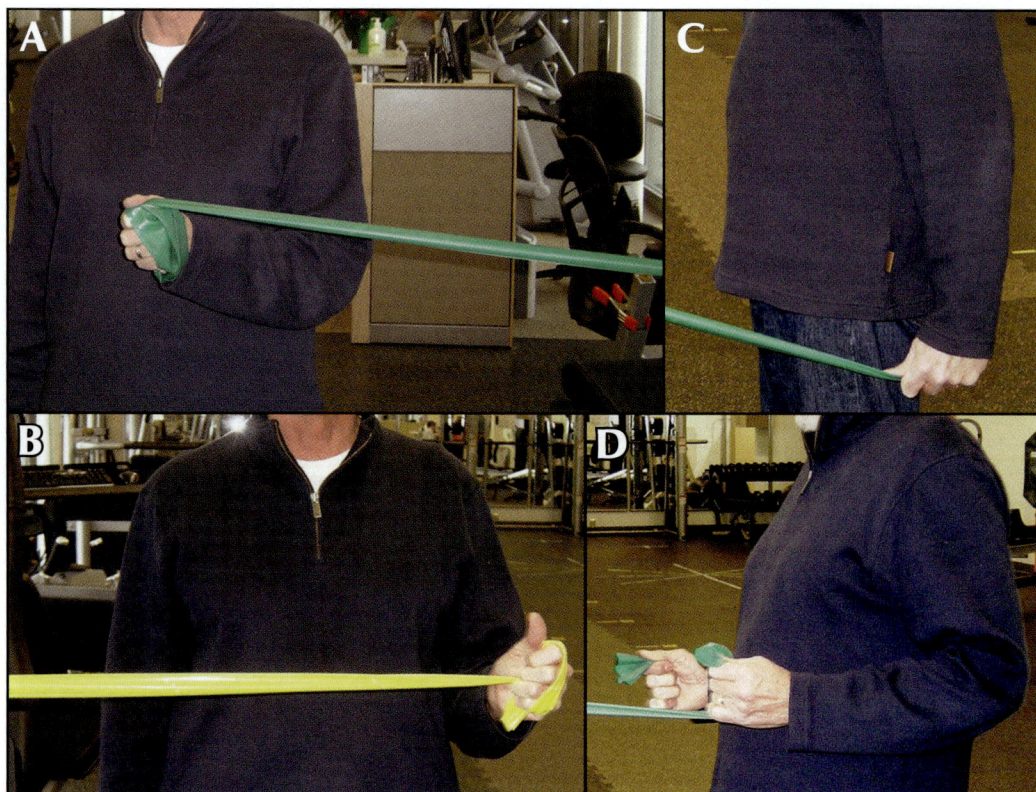

Figure 18-2. Phase 1 elastic resistance exercises. (A) Internal rotation. (B) External rotation. (C) Unilateral extension. (D) Bilateral rowing. The amount of shoulder extension range of motion is limited when these exercises are first performed after rotator cuff repair.

Rotator Cuff Facilitation

Perhaps no topic regarding rehabilitation of the shoulder has been the subject of more scientific inquiry than the maximization of electromyographic (EMG) activity of the rotator cuff musculature. Classic articles[21-23] are part of the training of any rehabilitation practitioner specializing in orthopedic issues. However, the young clinician should be cautioned that maximal activity may not be desirable, particularly in the early stages of rehabilitation. Also, exercises that produce maximal activity of the supraspinatus often include positions above 90 degrees of glenohumeral elevation,[22,24] which decrease subacromial spacing and are therefore inappropriate for the initial stages of rehabilitation when patients still have pain with overhead motions.

For patients with subacromial pathology in particular, the authors prefer to start rotator cuff strengthening with the arm adducted by the side. The first phase of our exercise series includes internal rotation, external rotation, extension, and rowing (Figure 18-2). Although performed with elastic resistance, these exercises generate sufficient activation of the respective rotator cuff muscles to result in a strengthening stimulus,[25] yet all are performed below the impingement zone of elevation (below 90 degrees). Selection of the initial resistance (eg, the color of Theraband [The Hygenic Corporation, Akron, OH]) is made based upon manual muscle examination and observation of patient response. The patient assumes primary responsibility for advancing the resistance of these exercises once he or she has demonstrated that he or she can perform the first phase of exercises with appropriate form and without any adverse reactions. Once the patient is able to perform 3 sets of external rotation with the green band of elastic resistance (approximate midrange for Theraband series, or approximately 3 to 5 lbs of resistance), we believe he or she has sufficient rotator cuff function to safely progress to resisted elevation exercises to shoulder level. Progression to resisted elevation before the patient has re-established appropriate rotator cuff function results in potential over-reliance on the deltoid and superior migration of the humeral head. For patients with mild to moderate subacromial pathology, resisted elevation is added in the scapular plane with the glenohumeral joint externally rotated ("full can"). Evidence suggests "full can" positioning maximizes supraspinatus activity relative to deltoid muscle activity when compared to other forms of resisted elevation.[26] Although elevation in the scapular plane with the shoulder internally rotated (the "empty can" exercise) requires high levels of supraspinatus activity,[22] this exercise should be avoided, particularly for patients with subacromial pathology. Empty can positioning places the greater tuberosity in proximity to the acromion and further encourages anterior tipping of the scapula, which further reduces the clearance of the subacromial space.[27]

Depending upon the patient's needs, resisted elevation may be the final addition to the rehabilitation program. However, if the patient is an overhead athlete or has other high demands, then resisted internal and external rotation can be added in elevated positions. Support under the distal humerus can be added as needed if the patient is initially unable to control shoulder positioning. Nonthrowing athletes, such as contact or collision athletes, may desire to return to weightlifting tasks. In these situations, the first phase of weightlifting involves resisted biceps curls, triceps push downs, and seated rowing. Resisted extension exercises such as "lat pull downs" are introduced next and are typically added before resisted pressing (chest press/bench press) maneuvers. Because the supraspinatus is loaded while the shoulder is in the impingement zone, one of the last progressions is military press or other forms of resisted overhead elevation.

Periscapular Strengthening

The rotator cuff muscles originate off the scapula; therefore, a stable scapular platform is necessary for optimal rotator cuff function. The first phase of periscapular strengthening is resisted retraction. A simple exercise like bilateral rowing is sufficient to activate the scapular retractors,[25] yet can be easily added without approaching the impingement zone. Resisted protraction may be required, but should not be blindly prescribed, as protracted positioning closes the subacromial space while retracted scapular positioning maximizes this space.[28] Therefore, scapular retraction is nearly always promoted for patients with subacromial pathology, but scapular protraction is used only in those athletes who demonstrate winging of the inferior angle of the scapula or who demonstrate other clear indications of serratus anterior dysfunction. Later progressions of scapular retraction often include prone retraction exercises such as "the letter series" or prone "Hughston Clinic" exercises. While these exercises recruit the periscapular and rotator cuff muscles at very high levels,[23,29] many are performed at or above the impingement zone and should therefore be reserved for patients with a full, pain-free range of motion who require very high levels of shoulder strength.

Trunk Positioning

Flexed or kyphotic postures of the thoracic spine make it very difficult to assume the desired retracted scapular position. In addition, flexed trunk and rounded shoulder positioning has been associated with posterior shoulder tightness.[30] Compared to other patients with more advanced rotator cuff disease, patients with impingement and early rotator cuff tendinopathy are often younger and more flexible. Therefore, sometimes simple postural education is sufficient for patients with shoulder impingement.[14] During the early stages of rehabilitation, cues may need to be consistently provided to assume an upright trunk posture when completing resisted rotator cuff or scapular retraction exercises. If simple cueing is not achieving the goal of improved upright posture, then passive thoracic extension stretching or activation of the thoracic erector spinae can be added.

Manual Techniques

Finally, the addition of manual therapies has repeatedly been shown to improve outcomes for patients with impingement when compared to exercise alone.[31-33] Posterior glenohumeral mobilizations[31-33] and/or passive stretching to address posterior tightness are very appropriate additions of manual therapy to an exercise program. Cervical or thoracic mobilizations/manipulations[32] can be added if spinal restrictions are believed to contribute to flexed spine or forward shoulder positioning. Manual techniques such as soft-tissue mobilization and/or passive stretching of the pectoralis minor muscle may also be important adjuncts.

Postoperative Management Following Subacromial Decompression

The majority of patients with impingement and/or tendinopathy respond to the rehabilitation program just described.[9] Arthroscopic subacromial decompression is reserved for those patients with significant, recalcitrant symptoms despite 6 to 12 weeks of rehabilitation. The basic tenets of the nonoperative program hold true for the postoperative condition as well with progression, particularly for overhead elevation range of motion, determined by patient tolerance. Patients typically spend the first 3 to 10 days in a standard sling as needed, removing the sling for pendulum exercises and elbow range of motion. By the third postoperative week, many patients have resumed a large proportion of their preoperative regimen. Patients have typically achieved the goals of subacromial decompression and are discharged from formal physical therapy approximately 6 weeks after surgery.

NONOPERATIVE TREATMENT OF ROTATOR CUFF TEARS

Nonoperative rehabilitation of rotator cuff tears involves 2 relatively distinct groups of patients. The first group involves patients with a repairable injury where either the treating physician or the patient has elected to pursue nonoperative means. This can be a very successful modality for patients with a painful shoulder but who have been able to maintain their function. The second group involves patients who have tears that are not amenable to repair. Despite the evolution of arthroscopic and open techniques allowing for better visualization and mobilization of the rotator cuff, there remains a small number of rotator cuff tears considered irreparable. These tears are often massive in size (>5 cm^2), demonstrate significant retraction, and show evidence of muscular atrophy and fatty degeneration on advanced imaging, such as MRI or ultrasound.

The duration of symptoms before the initiation of treatment can help predict the success of nonoperative treatment. Nearly two-thirds of patients whose duration of pain was less than 3 months were still asymptomatic 7 years after treatment. Conversely, only 56% of patients with symptoms longer than 6 months prior to treatment remained asymptomatic.[34,35] Retrospective studies have been helpful, but are limited in scope. Fortunately, there are several large-scale, prospective, multicenter studies currently in progress that will hopefully address predictors of successful outcome with nonoperative treatment of rotator cuff tears.

Perhaps more so than any other patient cohort with rotator cuff pathology, patients who seek to manage their rotator cuff tear nonoperatively benefit from skilled rehabilitation. Because patients are often unable to reach end ranges independently, one of the foremost goals of rehabilitation is the maintenance of passive range of motion, particularly for forward flexion. The patient should be instructed in the independent exercises of supine elevation or table step backs as will be described in the section of this chapter on rehabilitation after rotator cuff repair. Overhead pulleys are also a nice adjunct for the maintenance of overhead elevation for patients whose rotator cuff tears will be managed nonoperatively. Unlike patients with impingement/tendinopathy or immediately following rotator cuff repair where pain is a primary barrier for overhead elevation, patients with chronic, irreparable rotator cuff tears often have little pain with active-assisted forward flexion. Although

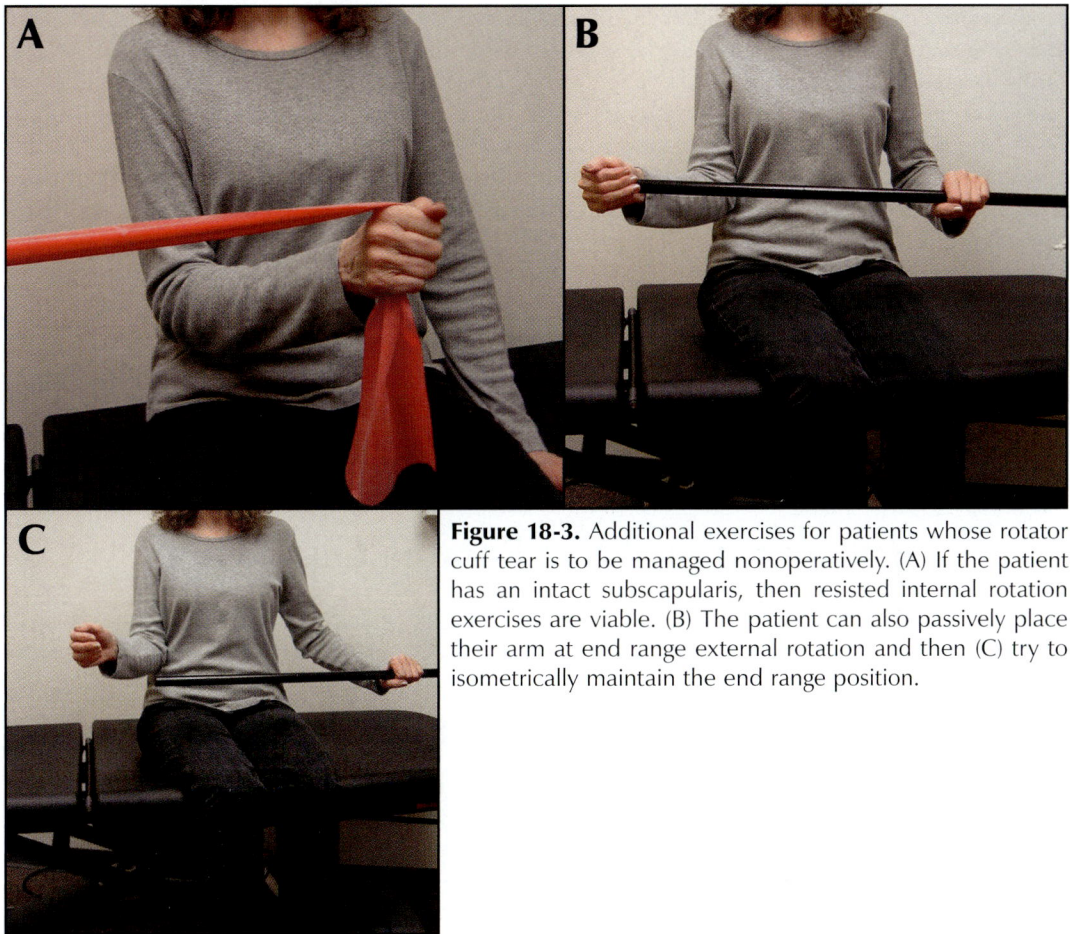

Figure 18-3. Additional exercises for patients whose rotator cuff tear is to be managed nonoperatively. (A) If the patient has an intact subscapularis, then resisted internal rotation exercises are viable. (B) The patient can also passively place their arm at end range external rotation and then (C) try to isometrically maintain the end range position.

overhead pulleys require greater rotator cuff activation than active-assisted supine elevation,[36] because patients with irreparable rotator cuff tears have little pain, these patients are often able to use overhead pulleys to improve or maintain their overhead range of motion.

The hallmark of rehabilitation for patients with conservatively managed rotator cuff tears is to maximize periscapular strength, deltoid function, and strength of the rotator cuff around the area of the tear.[35] As most rotator cuff tears progress according to a predictable pattern (supraspinatus to infraspinatus to subscapularis to teres minor),[37] elevation power is typically most affected. Because the subscapularis is typically spared, most patients with irreparable tears of their rotator cuff can successfully complete resisted internal rotation exercises with the arm by the side (Figure 18-3A). Likewise, resisted shoulder extension is a viable exercise owing to use of the posterior deltoid and triceps muscles. Resisted external rotation, however, may prove quite difficult, particularly if the tear has progressed into the infraspinatus. Patients may be able to perform isometric external rotation against elastic resistance by gradually stepping away from the band. If the patient is profoundly weak, all external resistance is removed, and the patient can attempt simple isometric holds at end range after moving into an externally rotated position with assistance (Figure 18-3B and C).

For the patient with the conservatively managed rotator cuff tear, by far the most challenging part of the rehabilitation process is achieving a meaningful improvement in functional elevation. Due to the loss of power for glenohumeral elevation, it is common for patients with irreparable rotator cuff tears to exhibit significant scapular hiking when attempting to raise their arms. Periscapular strengthening in the form of resisted rowing or, if possible, bilateral-resisted external rotation is a vital component of rehabilitation for patients whose tears will be managed nonoperatively.

However, the most meaningful improvement in overhead elevation often comes from practicing the task against the appropriate amount of resistance. As described by Levy and colleagues,[35] the goal of the progressive elevation protocol ("The Reading Protocol") is to re-educate the anterior deltoid and maximize the function of the remaining rotator cuff musculotendinous complex. The level of resistance the patient feels is determined by the length of the lever arm (the extent to which the elbow is extended) and the patient's posture relative to the line of gravity. Load on the rotator cuff is increased as the elbow is extended and as resisted elevation is progressed from a true supine position to reclining and finally to an upright position.[38,39] In each of these postures, the opposite hand can be used initially as an active assist for elevation. As strength and function improve, the patient can progress the exercise by using progressively less assistance from the opposite upper extremity and using a cane or washcloth for assistance with overhead elevation. Finally, extra resistance in the form of a weight can be added before the patient progresses to the next most upright posture (Figure 18-4A through D). If the patient is having difficulty with elevation in any of these postures, isometric adduction/internal rotation can be added as an attempt to maximize activity of the still intact subscapularis (Figure 18-4E).

REHABILITATION AFTER ROTATOR CUFF REPAIR

The indications for rotator cuff surgery are still somewhat variable and vague.[40-42] Surgical repair of rotator cuff tears using a variety of techniques has produced satisfactory results in the vast majority of patients. Although relatively few studies overall have evaluated the integrity of the rotator cuff after surgery, evidence is mounting that a significant percentage of rotator cuff repairs either fail to heal or retear,[43,44] especially in larger tears (>2 cm).[45-47] Interestingly, in most of these series, patient outcome scores showed significant initial improvement at 12 months despite failure of the repair. Yet, patients with an intact repair tend to have significantly better outcomes than those with a failure to heal or retearing,[43,46] and the outcome of revision surgery is inferior to successful primary repair, with only 69% of patients satisfied.[48] Despite the possibility of retear, rotator cuff repair reliably improves pain, strength, and function of symptomatic patients.[49] Therefore, early operative repair is attempted for any patient younger than 50, with weakness, and/or with relatively acute onset of symptoms. For patients older than 50 years of age, a period of 6 to 12 weeks of physical therapy is recommended. Operative repair is reserved for patients who do not improve with conservative management.[42]

Similar to the management of impingement syndrome, there are several universal themes for the postoperative rehabilitation of patients following rotator cuff repair. However, perhaps more so than for a conservatively managed condition like impingement syndrome, these rehabilitative components can be viewed as stages of postoperative rehabilitation following rotator cuff repair (Table 18-2). Indeed, phase-based progressions of rehabilitation given at distinct postoperative timeframes have yielded results similar to regular, individually based physical therapy following rotator cuff repair.[50]

Protection Phase (0 to 3 Weeks)

The initial stage of rehabilitation is often viewed as simple protection of the repair. Based upon the size of the tear and other intraoperative findings, a choice is made between a standard sling or other mode of support for this period of protection. The structural properties of the healing supraspinatus tendon were improved after strict immobilization versus early activity in an animal model.[51] Although most of the work in this area has been completed in animal models, the consistent superiority of rest on the structural integrity of the repaired supraspinatus has caused some to question whether the initial period of protection should be prolonged.[52-54] In fact, some authors have started to advocate for 6 weeks or more of relative rest,[55] except for those patients who are at risk for developing postoperative stiffness.[56] Patients identified as at risk for stiffness include those with calcific tendinitis or adhesive capsulitis or those patients undergoing only single-tendon

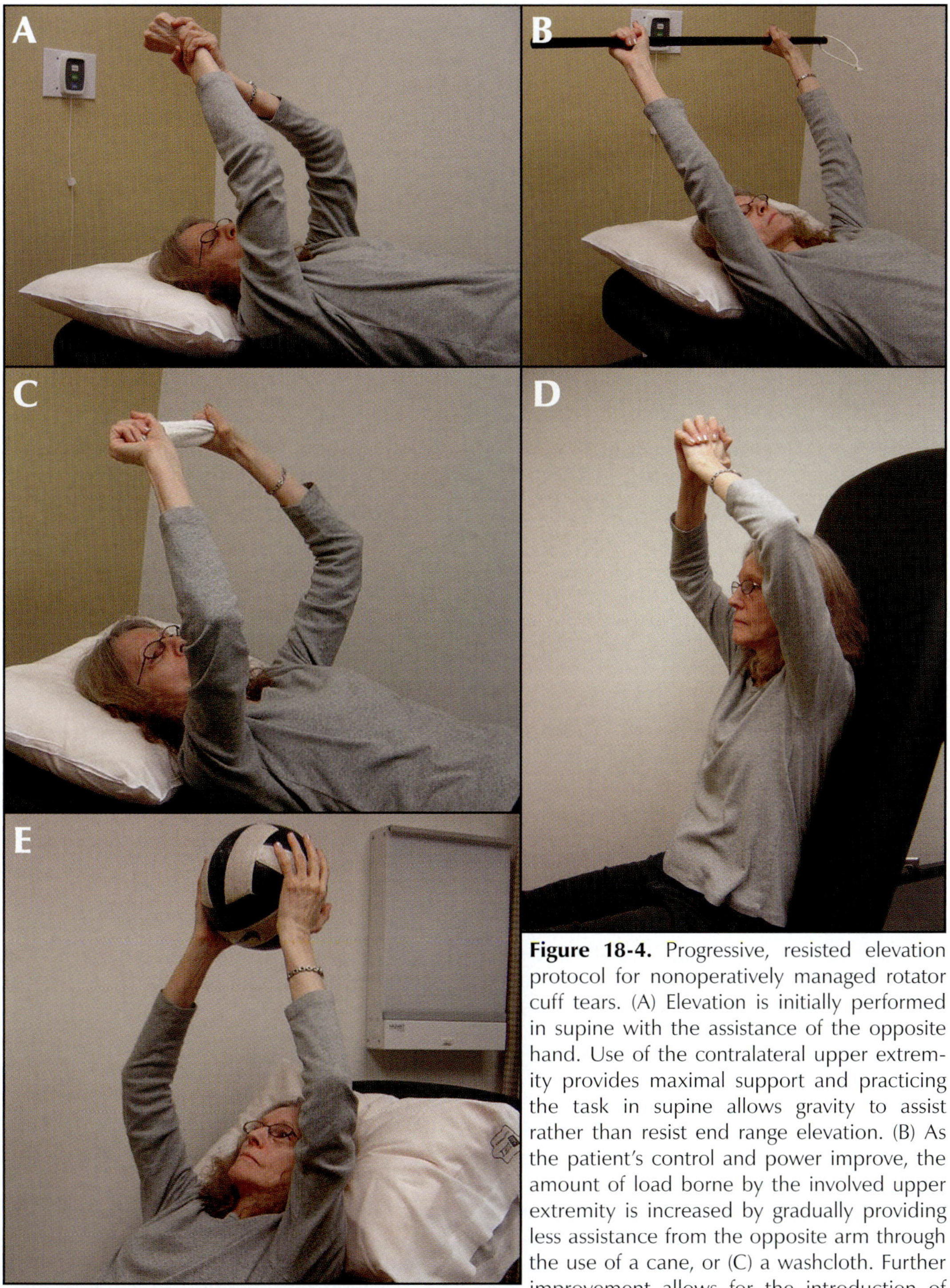

Figure 18-4. Progressive, resisted elevation protocol for nonoperatively managed rotator cuff tears. (A) Elevation is initially performed in supine with the assistance of the opposite hand. Use of the contralateral upper extremity provides maximal support and practicing the task in supine allows gravity to assist rather than resist end range elevation. (B) As the patient's control and power improve, the amount of load borne by the involved upper extremity is increased by gradually providing less assistance from the opposite arm through the use of a cane, or (C) a washcloth. Further improvement allows for the introduction of gravity resisted elevation as the patient moves into first inclined and (D) finally fully upright trunk postures. (E) If the patient is having difficulty elevating against gravity, and if the patient has an intact subscapularis, the patient can adduct/internally rotate against a ball to try to maximize subscapularis function.

TABLE 18-2. PHASES OF POSTOPERATIVE REHABILITATION AFTER ROTATOR CUFF REPAIR

NAME	TIME FRAME	REHABILITATION INTERVENTIONS
Protection phase	0 to 3 weeks	• Instruct to limit use of arm. • Instruct in use of sling. • Instruct in use of cryotherapy. • Instruct in pendulums.
Range-of-motion phase	3 to 6 weeks	• Instruct in active-assisted range of motion—forward flexion and external rotation.
Early strengthening phase	6 to 12 weeks	• Instruct in elastic-resisted internal and external rotation with the arm by the side. • Instruct in elastic-resisted unilateral extension rowing taking care to limit shoulder extension range of motion.
Advanced strengthening phase	12 weeks to 6 months	• Instruct in isotonic (weight) strengthening program. • Instruct in resisted elevation. • Instruct in resisted internal and external rotation in elevated positions.
Return to activity	>6 months	• Finalize independent strengthening program. • Return to sport program. • Gradually return to team activities.

rotator cuff repair or concomitant labral repair.[57] In our practice, the length of the initial period of protection is prolonged for patients with chronic tears, tears repaired under tension, poor quality tissue, or tears larger than 3 cm^2. However, most commonly, this initial period of protection lasts until the patient's first postoperative visit, 10 to 14 days following surgery. To that point, the patient has been completing only very low level exercises, such as pendulum exercises, elbow active range of motion, active scapular retraction, and isometric grip strengthening. There has been some debate whether pendulum exercises are truly sufficiently passive to be added in the rehabilitation of patients immediately following rotator cuff repair. Indeed, a recent study indicates that large arc pendulums may in fact require levels of muscle activation that place the healing rotator cuff at risk.[58] In contrast, small arc pendulum exercises produce only low levels of EMG activation below a threshold considered possibly injurious.[58]

In our multidisciplinary facility, after rotator cuff repair, patients will see the surgeon or physician's assistant as well as a physical therapist on the same day. The first postoperative visit with the medical team serves as a time for suture removal, discussion of intraoperative findings, and medication refills. The initial visit with the rehabilitation specialist focuses on ensuring patient comprehension of postoperative restrictions, the expected goals for each phase of the recovery, and the progression of current range-of-motion exercises.

At the time of the first postoperative visit, most patients following rotator cuff repair have relative control of their pain with daily activities. That is, patients are able to moderate their pain with use of their sling, oral medication, and cryotherapy. Cryotherapy has been shown to reduce temperature in the subacromial space, allowing patients after shoulder surgery to be able to sleep more hours uninterrupted and with less reliance on oral analgesic medications.[59,60]

After this initial visit with the physical therapist, range-of-motion exercises will be performed on a 2 or 3 times daily basis. These exercises should never cause an increase in pain lasting longer than 1 hour after the completion of the program. Pain with duration longer than 1 hour indicates that either the exercises are being done too aggressively or that the patient is not truly performing the exercises passively.

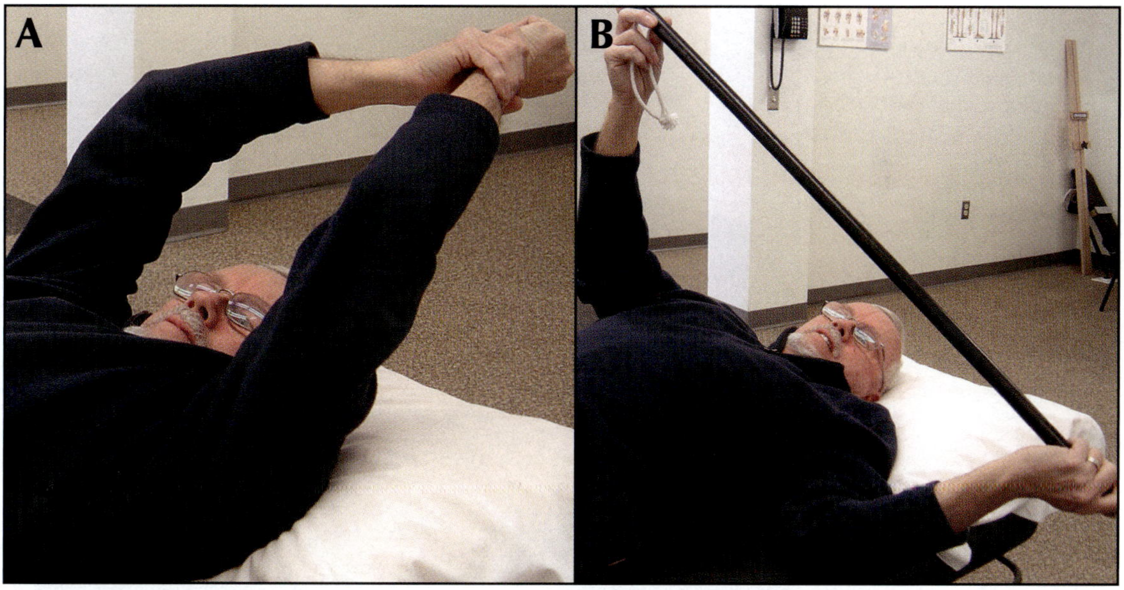

Figure 18-5. Active-assisted range of motion (A) overhead elevation performed with the assistance of the opposite hand and (B) external rotation performed with the assistance of an exercise wand. This exercise should be completed with a pillow under the elbow to limit shoulder extension in the early stages of rehabilitation after rotator cuff repair.

In terms of range-of-motion exercises, patients are instructed in forward flexion with use of the opposite hand and external rotation with an exercise wand (Figure 18-5). Both exercises are added in supine to make use of gravity as an aid rather than resistance during performance of the exercises. Patients are purposely instructed to stretch their arms overhead with their elbows flexed to minimize the lever arms of an extended upper extremity. We expect most patients to be able to achieve at least 80 degrees of passive elevation during this initial postoperative visit and to gain at least 10 degrees of forward flexion and external rotation with completion of these exercises under the supervision of the physical therapist.

Range-of-Motion Phase (3 to 6 Weeks Postoperatively)

If the patient is able to achieve the expected range-of-motion milestones, then the next physical therapy visit can be delayed for 2 to 3 weeks (approximately 3 to 4 weeks postoperatively) at which point the sling can be removed. If the patient is not achieving 80 degrees of elevation and/or the exercises do not produce a 10-degree increase in external rotation range of motion, then the patient is asked to return on a once or twice weekly basis for supervision of his or her range-of-motion exercises and the addition of passive stretching with the therapist as necessary.

Occasionally, patients will be unable to sufficiently relax for supine forward flexion. In these patients, table step backs (Figure 18-6) can be very helpful. To perform the table step back, the patient places his or her hand on an elevated surface and then simply walks backward. As the patient steps or leans back, he or she is, sometimes unknowingly, placing the glenohumeral joint in an elevated position. Although table step backs require essentially the same amount of supraspinatus activation as supine forward flexion,[38] the fact that patients move their bodies versus their injured limbs seems to decrease muscle guarding.[36,38,61]

Early Strengthening Phase (6 to 12 Weeks Postoperatively)

In our practice, the focus remains on passive- or active-assisted exercises until approximately the sixth postoperative week. However, more important than the absolute timeframe, the patient's

Figure 18-6. Table step backs. An alternate method of active-assisted overhead elevation that is particularly helpful for patients who tend to muscle guard.

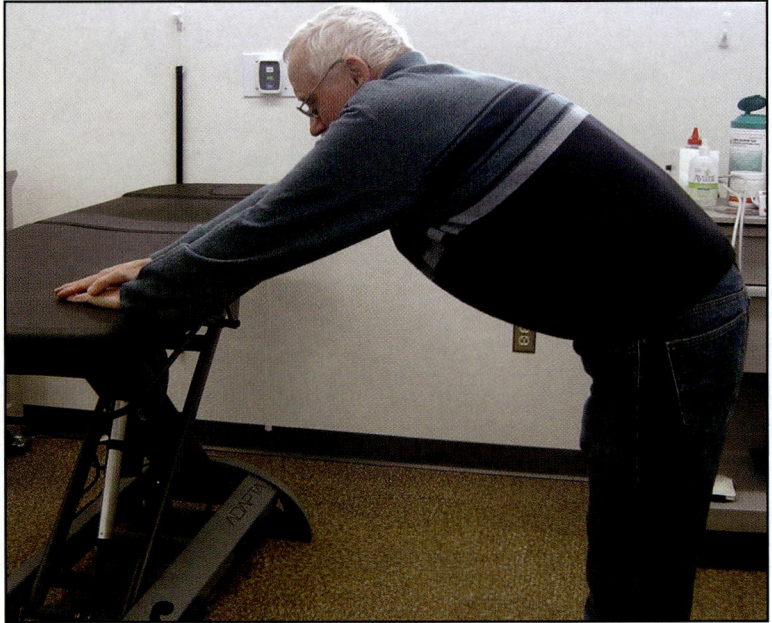

ability to tolerate additional stress on his or her healing rotator cuff is the single most important factor determining progression. Approximately 6 weeks after surgery, we allow the patient to complete supine, overhead elevation range-of-motion activities with an exercise wand and add new stretching exercises (such as active-assisted shoulder extension and cross-body adduction), which put greater tension on the rotator cuff and posterior shoulder tissues. If patients can tolerate these new stresses without any increase in discomfort, then patients will be instructed in elastic resistance exercises. It is our belief that what are commonly termed *stretching* and *strengthening* exercises lie on a continuum of stresses applied to the rotator cuff. With this approach, there is not a definitive point at which "strengthening" exercises become safe, but rather control of symptoms and progressive range of motion increases our confidence that the patient is healing as expected and his or her rotator cuff is ready to withstand additional stresses. It is commonly believed that the moderation of these stresses is the stimulus for laying down additional collagen fibers to help bridge the tissue gap across the rotator cuff repair. EMG activity increases as expected as the patient moves from passive- to active-assisted and active exercises and, finally, to true, resisted motions.[36-38]

Earlier in this chapter, we presented the prolific number of studies that analyze the EMG activity of the rotator cuff muscles with commonly performed rehabilitation exercises. However, particularly for patients following rotator cuff repair, the astute clinician should question whether maximal rotator cuff activity is desirable. Particularly in the early stages of rehabilitation following rotator cuff repair, we purposely select exercises that will not maximally activate the rotator cuff. Instead, we select the lowest level of elastic resistance to start resisted motions. Our phase 1 program consists of resisted internal and external rotation of the glenohumeral joint, shoulder extension allowing for deltoid and triceps substitution, and scapular retraction (see Figure 18-2D). Patients are asked to begin with a single set of 10 for each of these exercises. If the patient is able to perform the exercise with correct form and without any discomfort, the patient is allowed to add a second set and eventually a third set. If the patient still thinks he or she is able to handle additional resistance after completing 3 sets of 10 repetitions, then the next time he or she completes the exercises, he or she is allowed to use the next most resistive level of elastic resistance. Recent evidence has demonstrated that EMG activity is directly related to the perceived exertion levels of patients.[62] Therefore, in our opinion, progressive, self-selected resistance is most appropriate for patients following rotator cuff repair. Although elastic resistance levels can be quite similar to resistance levels with weights,[63]

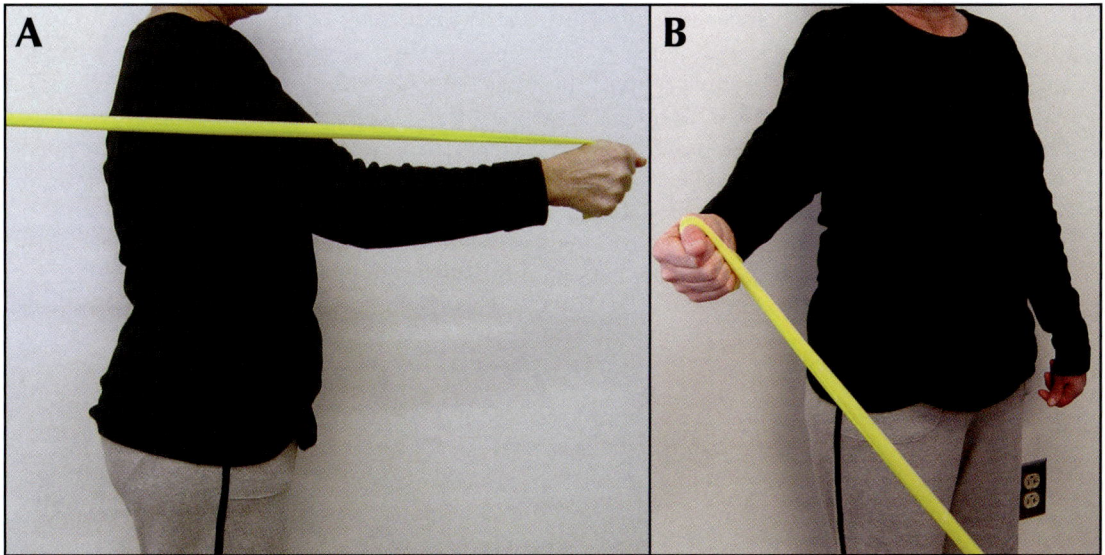

Figure 18-7. Resisted elevation performed with (A) the elbow flexed and (B) the elbow extended. Shortening the lever arm, by flexing the elbow, in the earlier phases of rehabilitation decreases the load on the healing rotator cuff.

we prefer elastic resistance for this population as, in our opinion, elastic resistance is easily progressed and portable and, therefore, is easy to complete on a daily basis. It is our opinion that patients are less likely to "overdo" resisted external rotation in a standing position against elastic resistance versus completing the exercise in side-lying against isotonic, weighted resistance. Other authors feel similarly that elastic resistance is appropriate for patients with postoperative shoulder conditions.[25]

Once the patient is able to complete his or her workout sets of external rotation with sufficient resistance (the green color of Theraband and/or approximately 3 to 5 lbs of resistance),[64] then we believe it is appropriate to consider resisted elevation. Although we believe that patient response to resisted external rotation provides important clues as to patient readiness for resisted elevation, we still suggest that resisted elevation should initially be completed using a flexed elbow to shorten the lever arm, and thereby resultant load, with which the rotator cuff would have to contend (Figure 18-7).[36] As appropriate, the elbow can be extended for resisted elevation exercises. As stated earlier, our preference for true resisted elevation is to be completed in the plane of the scapula with the glenohumeral joint externally rotated (ie, the "full can" exercise). Performing full can elevation allows for a progressive challenge to the rotator cuff yet helps avoid anatomic encroachment within the subacromial space.

Scapular hiking can be a common compensatory pattern when patients lack sufficient strength for glenohumeral elevation. Occasionally, simply making the patient aware of the compensation may improve the pattern. But if the patient "hikes" his or her scapula and is unable to correct this inappropriate pattern after cueing, we suggest the resistance level should be reduced and/or resisted elevation should be postponed until the patient gains additional strength of the external rotators with the arm by the side.

Advanced Strengthening Phase (12 Weeks to 6 Months)

If the patient has been progressing as expected, he or she should have nearly full range of motion by 12 weeks postoperatively and be tolerating a regularly performed home strengthening program. For patients with low demands, this may be the conclusion of their formal rehabilitation. This group of patients with lower demands would simply continue to advance the resistance levels for their home strengthening program, discontinuing the program altogether when they feel they have achieved symmetric shoulder strength. For competitive athletes or laborers, however, a more advanced form of strengthening is required. Twelve weeks after rotator cuff repair, the patient is allowed to return to more aggressive weightlifting activities. As described for the patient with impingement and/or tendinopathy, isotonic exercises typically begin with resisted motions of the elbow as well as seated rowing exercises for the scapular retractors. Although completed overhead, "lat pull down" exercises are added next with cautious progression to resisted chest pressing maneuvers. Overhead pressing ("military press"), the prone "letter" series, and long lever (extended elbow) resisted elevation exercises require high levels of rotator cuff activation and are therefore appropriately reserved for the later stages of rehabilitation in this small subset of patients who will return to high-demand activities.

Return to Activity (>6 Months Postoperatively)

Once the patient demonstrates a tolerance for progressive demand activities, has minimal to no pain, and has full range of motion, the physician may "release" him or her for return to high-demand work or athletic competition. It is important that the athlete or laborer continue regular rotator cuff strengthening and weightlifting for an additional 3 to 6 months after return to activity. Although not the focus of this chapter, baseball players or other overhead athletes who have undergone rotator cuff repair may start a return to throwing or similar program for their particular sport approximately 4 to 5 months after surgery with eventual return to sport between approximately 6 and 9 months postoperatively.

CONCLUSION

Rotator cuff pathology involves a spectrum of disease and a spectrum of patient pain and disability. We divided this chapter into 3 sections to highlight distinct patient types, each presenting the physical therapist and surgeon with a unique challenge and particular focus for the rehabilitation program. To be sure, there are common themes of rehabilitation programs within each subsection. But, it is important that the physical therapist and surgeon work together to provide rehabilitation that is safe, progressive, and tailored to the individual needs of patients with rotator cuff pathology.

REFERENCES

1. Neer CS. Impingement lesions. *Clin Orthop.* 1983;173:70.
2. Sher JS, Uribe JW, Posada A, Murphy BJ, Zlatkin MB. Abnormal findings on magnetic resonance images of asymptomatic shoulders. *J Bone Joint Surg Am.* 1995;77(1):10.
3. Tempelhof S, Rupp S, Seil R. Age-related prevalence of rotator cuff tears in asymptomatic shoulders. *J Shoulder Elbow Surg.* 1999;8(4):296.
4. Yamaguchi K, Tetro AM, Blam O, Evanoff BA, Teefey SA, Middleton WD. Natural history of asymptomatic rotator cuff tears: a longitudinal analysis of asymptomatic tears detected sonographically. *J Shoulder Elbow Surg.* 2001;10(3):199-203.
5. Keener JD, Steger-May K, Stobbs G, Yamaguchi K. Asymptomatic rotator cuff tears: patient demographics and baseline shoulder function. *J Shoulder Elbow Surg.* 2010;19(8):1191-1198.
6. Strauss E, Salata M, Kercher J, et al. The arthroscopic management of partial-thickness rotator cuff tears: a systematic review of the literature. *Arthroscopy.* 2011;27(4):568-580.
7. Fleming J, Seitz A, Ebaugh DD. Exercise protocol for the treatment of rotator cuff impingement syndrome. *J Athl Training.* 2010;45(5):483.
8. Kuhn J. Exercise in the treatment of rotator cuff impingement: a systematic review and a synthesized evidence-based rehabilitation protocol. *J Shoulder Elbow Surg.* 2009;18(1):138.
9. Tate AR, McClure PW, Young IA, Salvatori R, Michener LA. Comprehensive impairment-based exercise and manual therapy intervention for patients with subacromial impingement syndrome: a case series. *J Orthop Sports Phys Ther.* 2010;40(8):474-493.

10. Tyler TF, Nicholas SJ, Roy T, Gleim GW. Quantification of posterior capsule tightness and motion loss in patients with shoulder impingement. *Am J Sports Med.* 2000;28(5):668.

11. Harryman DT, Sidles JA, Clark JM, McQuade KJ, Gibb TD, Matsen FA. Translation of the humeral head on the glenoid with passive glenohumeral motion. *J Bone Joint Surg Am.* 1990;72(9):1334.

12. Reinold M, Wilk K, Macrina L, et al. Changes in shoulder and elbow passive range of motion after pitching in professional baseball players. *Am J Sports Med.* 2008;36(3):523.

13. Laudner K, Sipes R, Wilson J. The acute effects of sleeper stretches on shoulder range of motion. *J Athl Training.* 2008;43(4):359.

14. McClure P, Bialker J, Neff N, Williams G, Karduna A. Shoulder function and 3-dimensional kinematics in people with shoulder impingement syndrome before and after a 6-week exercise program. *Phys Ther.* 2004;84(9):832.

15. Tyler TF, Roy T, Nicholas SJ, Gleim GW. Reliability and validity of a new method of measuring posterior shoulder tightness. *J Orthop Sports Phys Ther.* 1999;29(5):262.

16. Laudner K, Stanek J, Meister K. Assessing posterior shoulder contracture: the reliability and validity of measuring glenohumeral joint horizontal adduction. *J Athl Training.* 2006;41(4):375.

17. Borstad J, Dashottar A. Quantifying strain on posterior shoulder tissues during 5 simulated clinical tests: a cadaver study. *J Orthop Sports Phys Ther.* 2010;41(2):90-99.

18. McClure P, Balaicuis J, Heiland D, Broersma M, Thorndike C, Wood A. A randomized controlled comparison of stretching procedures for posterior shoulder tightness. *J Orthop Sports Phys Ther.* 2007;37(3):108.

19. Moore S, McLoda T, Shaffer MA, Laudner K. The use of muscle energy techniques for stretching the posterior shoulder. *J Orthop Sports Phys Ther.* In submission.

20. Tyler T, Nicholas S, Lee S, Mullaney M, McHugh M. Correction of posterior shoulder tightness is associated with symptom resolution in patients with internal impingement. *Am J Sports Med.* 2010;38(1):114.

21. Moseley JB, Jobe FW, Pink M, Perry J, Tibone J. EMG analysis of the scapular muscles during a shoulder rehabilitation program. *Am J Sports Med.* 1992;20(2):128.

22. Townsend H, Jobe FW, Pink M, Perry J. Electromyographic analysis of the glenohumeral muscles during a baseball rehabilitation program. *Am J Sports Med.* 1991;19(3):264.

23. Blackburn TA, McLeod WD, White B, Wofford L. EMG analysis of posterior rotator cuff exercises. *Athl Train J Nat'l Athl Train Assoc.* 1990;25:40-45.

24. Burke W, Vangsness CT, Powers C. Strengthening the supraspinatus: a clinical and biomechanical review. *Clin Orthop.* 2002;402:292.

25. Hintermeister RA, Lange GW, Schultheis JM, Bey MJ, Hawkins RJ. Electromyographic activity and applied load during shoulder rehabilitation exercises using elastic resistance. *Am J Sports Med.* 1998;26(2):210-220.

26. Reinold MM, Macrina LC, Wilk KE, et al. Electromyographic analysis of the supraspinatus and deltoid muscles during 3 common rehabilitation exercises. *J Athl Train.* 2007;42(4):464-469.

27. Thigpen CA, Padua DA, Morgan N, Kreps C, Karas SG. Scapular kinematics during supraspinatus rehabilitation exercise: a comparison of full-can versus empty-can techniques. *Am J Sports Med.* 2006;34(4):644-652.

28. Solem-Bertoft E, Thuomas KA, Westerberg CE. The influence of scapular retraction and protraction on the width of the subacromial space. An MRI study. *Clin Orthop Relat Res.* 1993;296:99-103.

29. Boettcher CE, Ginn KA, Cathers I. Which is the optimal exercise to strengthen supraspinatus? *Med Sci Sports Exerc.* 2009;41(11):1979-1983.

30. Laudner K, Moline M, Meister K. The relationship between forward scapular posture and posterior shoulder tightness among baseball players. *Am J Sports Med.* 2010;38(10):2106.

31. Kachingwe AF, Phillips B, Sletten E, Plunkett SW. Comparison of manual therapy techniques with therapeutic exercise in the treatment of shoulder impingement: a randomized controlled pilot clinical trial. *J Man Manip Ther.* 2008;16(4):238-247.

32. Bang MD, Deyle GD. Comparison of supervised exercise with and without manual physical therapy for patients with shoulder impingement syndrome. *J Orthop Sports Phys Ther.* 2000;30(3):126.

33. Senbursa G, Baltaci G, Atay A. Comparison of conservative treatment with and without manual physical therapy for patients with shoulder impingement syndrome: a prospective, randomized clinical trial. *Knee Surgery, Sports Traumatology, Arthroscopy.* 2007;15(7):915.

34. Bokor DJ, Hawkins RJ, Huckell GH, Angelo RL, Schickendantz MS. Results of nonoperative management of full-thickness tears of the rotator cuff. *Clin Orthop Relat Res.* 1993;294:103-110.

35. Levy O, Mullett H, Roberts S, Copeland S. The role of anterior deltoid reeducation in patients with massive irreparable degenerative rotator cuff tears. *J Shoulder Elbow Surg.* 2008;17(6):863-870.

36. McCann PD, Wootten ME, Kadaba MP, Bigliani LU. A kinematic and electromyographic study of shoulder rehabilitation exercises. *Clin Orthop Relat Res.* 1993;288:179-188.

37. Patte D. Classification of rotator cuff lesions. *Clin Orthop Relat Res.* 1990;254:81-86.

38. Uhl TL, Muir TA, Lawson L. Electromyographical assessment of passive, active assistive, and active shoulder rehabilitation exercises. *PM R.* 2010;2(2):132-141.

39. Jackins S. Postoperative shoulder rehabilitation. *Phys Med Rehabil Clin N Am.* 2004;15(3):vi, 643-682.

40. Oh LS, Wolf BR, Hall MP, Levy BA, Marx RG. Indications for rotator cuff repair: a systematic review. *Clin Orthop Relat Res.* 2007;455:52-63.

41. Dunn W, Schackman B, Walsh C, et al. Variation in orthopaedic surgeons' perceptions about the indications for rotator cuff surgery. *J Bone Joint Surg Am.* 2005;87(9):1978.

42. Wolf B, Dunn W, Wright R. Indications for repair of full-thickness rotator cuff tears. *Am J Sports Med.* 2007;35(6):1007.

43. Knudsen HB, Gelineck J, Sjbjerg JO, Olsen BS, Johannsen HV, Sneppen O. Functional and magnetic resonance imaging evaluation after single-tendon rotator cuff reconstruction. *J Shoulder Elbow Surg.* 1999;8(3):242.

44. Zanetti M, Jost B, Hodler J, Gerber C. MR imaging after rotator cuff repair: full-thickness defects and bursitis-like subacromial abnormalities in asymptomatic subjects. *Skeletal Radiol.* 2000;29(6):314-319.

45. Franceschi F, Ruzzini L, Longo UG, et al. Equivalent clinical results of arthroscopic single-row and double-row suture anchor repair for rotator cuff tears: a randomized controlled trial. *Am J Sports Med.* 2007;35(8):1254-1260.

46. Gerber C, Fuchs B, Hodler J. The results of repair of massive tears of the rotator cuff. *J Bone Joint Surg Am.* 2000;82(4):505.

47. Thomazeau H, Boukobza E, Morcet N, Chaperon J, Langlais F. Prediction of rotator cuff repair results by magnetic resonance imaging. *Clin Orthop.* 1997;344:275.

48. Djurasovic M, Marra G, Arroyo JS, Pollock RG, Flatow EL, Bigliani LU. Revision rotator cuff repair: factors influencing results. *J Bone Joint Surg Am.* 2001;83-A(12):1849.

49. Jost B, Pfirrmann CW, Gerber C, Switzerland Z. Clinical outcome after structural failure of rotator cuff repairs. *J Bone Joint Surg Am.* 2000;82(3):304.

50. Hayes K, Ginn KA, Walton JR, Szomor ZL, Murrell GA. A randomised clinical trial evaluating the efficacy of physiotherapy after rotator cuff repair. *Aust J Physiother.* 2004;50(2):77-83.

51. Thomopoulos S, Williams GR, Soslowsky LJ. Tendon to bone healing: differences in biomechanical, structural, and compositional properties due to a range of activity levels. *J Biomech Eng.* 2003;125(1):106-113.

52. Thomopoulos S, Williams GR, Gimbel JA, Favata M, Soslowsky LJ. Variation of biomechanical, structural, and compositional properties along the tendon to bone insertion site. *J Orthop Res.* 2003;21(3):413-419.

53. Gimbel JA, Van Kleunen JP, Williams GR, Thomopoulos S, Soslowsky LJ. Long durations of immobilization in the rat result in enhanced mechanical properties of the healing supraspinatus tendon insertion site. *J Biomech Eng.* 2007;129(3):400-404.

54. Peltz CD, Dourte LM, Kuntz AF, et al. The effect of postoperative passive motion on rotator cuff healing in a rat model. *J Bone Joint Surg Am.* 2009;91(10):2421-2429.

55. Koo SS, Burkhart SS. Rehabilitation following arthroscopic rotator cuff repair. *Clin Sports Med.* 2010;29(2):203, 211, vii.

56. Koo SS, Parsley BK, Burkhart SS, Schoolfield JD. Reduction of postoperative stiffness after arthroscopic rotator cuff repair: results of a customized physical therapy regimen based on risk factors for stiffness. *Arthroscopy.* 2011;27(2):155-160.

57. Huberty DP, Schoolfield JD, Brady PC, Vadala AP, Arrigoni P, Burkhart SS. Incidence and treatment of postoperative stiffness following arthroscopic rotator cuff repair. *Arthroscopy.* 2009;25(8):880-890.

58. Long JL, Ruberte Thiele RA, Skendzel JG, et al. Activation of the shoulder musculature during pendulum exercises and light activities. *J Orthop Sports Phys Ther.* 2010;40(4):230-237.

59. Osbahr DC, Cawley PW, Speer KP. The effect of continuous cryotherapy on glenohumeral joint and subacromial space temperatures in the postoperative shoulder. *Arthroscopy.* 2002;18(7):748-754.

60. Singh H, Osbahr DC, Holovacs TF, Cawley PW, Speer KP. The efficacy of continuous cryotherapy on the postoperative shoulder: a prospective, randomized investigation. *J Shoulder Elbow Surg.* 2001;10(6):522-525.

61. Dockery ML, Wright TW, LaStayo PC. Electromyography of the shoulder: an analysis of passive modes of exercise. *Orthopedics.* 1998;21(11):1181-1184.

62. Dark A, Ginn KA, Halaki M. Shoulder muscle recruitment patterns during commonly used rotator cuff exercises: an electromyographic study. *Phys Ther.* 2007;87(8):1039-1046.

63. Andersen LL, Andersen CH, Mortensen OS, Poulsen OM, Bjornlund IB, Zebis MK. Muscle activation and perceived loading during rehabilitation exercises: comparison of dumbbells and elastic resistance. *Phys Ther.* 2010;90(4):538-549.

64. Patterson RM, Stegink Jansen CW, Hogan HA, Nassif MD. Material properties of thera-band tubing. *Phys Ther.* 2001;81(8):1437.

CHAPTER 19

REVISION ROTATOR CUFF REPAIR

Jonathan Gelber, MD; Frank A. Petrigliano, MD; and Seth C. Gamradt, MD

Approximately 200,000 rotator cuff surgeries are performed annually in the United States.[1] The goals of rotator cuff surgery are to eliminate or decrease pain and to restore function and strength to the shoulder. It is commonly thought that the majority of rotator cuff surgeries, whether performed arthroscopically or open, results in clinical success. However, it is also clear that a large percentage of rotator cuff repairs will fail to demonstrate radiographic evidence of healing. Indeed, the incidence of persistent tears or retears following rotator cuff repair can range from 25% to 35% for smaller tears[2-6] to 90% in larger multi-tendon tears.[7,8] Galatz and colleagues[8] found recurrent defects in 17 of 18 large-to-massive rotator cuff repairs 12 months after surgery. Despite these poor radiographic outcomes, 16 of 18 patients improved clinically, and 14 had an American Shoulder and Elbow Surgeons (ASES) score above 90. This chapter discusses the pathophysiology and management of recurrent rotator cuff tears after repair.

A brief analysis of current surgical treatment is necessary to properly discuss the management of recurrent rotator cuff tears. While a radiographically unhealed rotator cuff repair may yield good clinical results in regard to pain relief, there is evidence to suggest that a healed tear results in improved strength and outcome scores compared to tears that did not completely heal. Slabaugh and colleagues performed a systemic review of rotator cuff repairs that had been imaged postoperatively to evaluate structural integrity.[9] In this review, the authors found several studies that concluded that a healed rotator cuff resulted in improved clinical outcome scores, strength, and forward elevation when compared to an unhealed rotator cuff tear. The results of this study must be interpreted with caution as this systematic review represents a compendium of level 4 evidence rather than a summary of strong, evidence-based literature.

Despite limited evidence that complete healing of the rotator cuff is necessary for clinical success, the goal of improving tendon-to-bone healing has prompted advances in surgical technique in an attempt to provide the strongest biomechanical construct for rotator cuff repair. Indeed, both double-row repairs and "transosseous-equivalent" repairs are superior to single-row repairs in cadaveric time-zero biomechanical studies.[10] In addition, there is a trend toward improved tendon healing clinically in double-row repairs.[11-13] However, randomized trials comparing

Ma CB, Feeley BT, eds.
*Basic Principles and Operative Management
of the Rotator Cuff (pp 271-290)*
© 2012 SLACK Incorporated

single-row versus double-row rotator cuff repairs have failed to reveal a significant difference in clinical results.[11,13] Furthermore, double-row repairs may decrease an already tenuous vascular supply to the tendon,[14] and they can fail medial to an intact footprint postoperatively.[15] Finally, other factors aside from tendon-to-bone healing may mitigate ultimate functional outcome, including the degree of atrophy and fatty infiltration of the rotator cuff musculature and the presence of neurologic dysfunction in the setting of massive tears. Undeniably, there remains controversy surrounding the most effective technical manner in which to repair a rotator cuff. Due to the challenging biological environment present in many rotator cuff repairs, it is unlikely that further optimization of the biomechanical strength of repair would completely eliminate the problem of recurrent rotator cuff defects after surgery. While it is unclear why some patients have few symptoms despite recurrence of a rotator cuff defect,[16] it appears that suboptimal biology at the site of repair contributes to failed cuff repair.

Most information about the biology of tendon-to-bone healing comes from animal models that have demonstrated that certain growth factors are critical for both development and repair of the tendon-bone enthesis.[17-19] Tendon healing occurs in 3 phases: inflammation, repair, and remodeling. However, a normal tendon-bone interface is not recreated following rotator cuff repair. Instead of a normal tendon-bone enthesis, a fibrovascular scar is created at the junction of tendon and bone.[17]

Little is known about the biology of rotator cuff repair in humans. Recently, 2 studies using contrast-enhanced ultrasound have provided in vivo data describing human rotator cuff healing. Rudzki and colleagues used ultrasound to demonstrate that patients older than 40 years of age with an asymptomatic shoulder have a decrease in blood supply to the rotator cuff.[20] In a follow-up ultrasound study, Gamradt and colleagues demonstrated that, at 3 months after arthroscopic repair, much of the blood supply to the healing rotator cuff originates from bone and that the healing tendon is relatively avascular.[21] Clearly, further research into the biology of rotator cuff repair is necessary. Efforts to improve blood supply and introduce growth factors to the repair site will be critical to improving healing of the rotator cuff.

Despite a propensity for clinical success in rotator cuff repair, the high rate of persistent and recurrent rotator cuff tears and compromised biology of rotator cuff healing will render a certain subset of patients with persistent symptoms of weakness and pain. Some of these patients will benefit from further surgery, and some will not. This chapter discusses 1) the causes of failure of rotator cuff repair, 2) evaluation of the failed rotator cuff surgery (including history, physical exam, and imaging), 3) indications for revision rotator cuff repair, 4) the author's preferred technique for revision cuff surgery, and 5) the outcomes of published series of revision rotator cuff surgeries.

CAUSES OF FAILURE OF ROTATOR CUFF REPAIR

The evaluation of a patient with failed rotator cuff surgery begins with an attempt to determine the reasons for failure of the initial repair. Determining the cause or causes of a failed rotator cuff surgery will often help determine whether another attempt at repair is warranted. Because failure of rotator cuff repair is multifactorial, a systematic approach to the causes of cuff failure is employed. When discussing causes of failure of anterior cruciate ligament repairs, authors commonly divide causes among 3 categories: biologic, technical, and traumatic.[22] This same strategy can be employed in evaluating the failed rotator cuff repair (Table 19-1). It is important to note multiple factors can often conspire to result in a failure of repair.

Biologic patient-related factors are probably the most important causative factors in the failure of rotator cuff repairs. These factors often include the age of the patient, medical comorbidities, size of tear, chronicity of the tear, and quality of the cuff tissue. Advanced age is associated with decreased healing rates after rotator cuff repair.[2,3,23-27] Age-related degenerative changes coupled with decreased microcirculation of the tendon likely decreases healing potential. Larger size of the

TABLE 19-1. CAUSES OF ROTATOR CUFF REPAIR FAILURE

BIOLOGIC	Patient age Size of tear Fatty infiltration/muscle atrophy Diabetes Nicotine Stiffness
TECHNICAL	Inadequate fixation Inadequate visualization Inadequate mobilization of tear Failure of deltoid repair Improper or aggressive rehabilitation
TRAUMATIC	Early—prior to complete cuff healing Late—failure of a previously well-functioning repair

initial tear is a significant predisposing factor for a recurrent tear.[2,3,5,25-31] Tears involving more than one tendon also have a greater chance for recurrence.[3] Furthermore, increased fatty infiltration of the rotator cuff and severe muscle atrophy are poor prognostic factors in rotator cuff surgery. The Goutallier classification is often used by surgeons to classify the amount of fatty infiltration present on preoperative imaging studies.[32] With current repair techniques, atrophy and fatty infiltration appear to be irreversible despite successful tendon-to-bone healing. In patients with a persistent tear following rotator cuff after repair, atrophy and fatty infiltration as determined by magnetic resonance imaging (MRI) progress significantly more postoperatively than those with a healed repair.[33-35] The amount of fatty infiltration of the rotator cuff increases with the chronicity of the tear. It has been shown that moderate supraspinatus fatty infiltration appears an average of 3 years after onset of symptoms and severe fatty infiltration at an average of 5 years after the onset of shoulder symptoms.[36] Chronicity of the tear affects not only the quality of the muscle, but overall compliance of the musculotendinous unit, resulting in increased tension on the repair site. This has been demonstrated in both clinical studies[37] and in animal models.[38,39] An infraspinatus sheep model illustrated that earlier repair of the tendon results in a more rapid recovery of both muscle function and tendon elasticity and that delayed repairs may not reach the postoperative muscle function that earlier repairs can achieve.[40] Therefore, it is not surprising that some studies have shown that earlier repair after acute rotator cuff injury results in improved clinical results when compared to a delayed repair.[41] Last, medical comorbidities such as diabetes[42-44] and use of tobacco inhibit healing of the rotator cuff.[45,46]

The aforementioned studies outline the pertinent patient-related and biological obstacles that must be overcome for a successful rotator cuff repair, but there is a subset of rotator cuff repairs that fail due to technical errors at the time of surgery. Using a Medicare database, Sherman and colleagues[44] found that surgeon volume was an independent risk factor for reoperation after rotator cuff repair. Rotator cuff repair is technically demanding and requires attention to detail throughout the procedure. This begins with adequate visualization of the tear through an open, mini-open, or arthroscopic approach. In the authors' opinion, the arthroscopic approach is the preferred manner in which to visualize and repair the rotator cuff. The arthroscope can be used to visualize from posterior, lateral, and anterior portals and preserves the deltoid insertion. An open approach is also an excellent manner in which to view and repair the rotator cuff, provided that the deltoid is securely repaired. There are 2 common scenarios in which inadequate visualization may compromise rotator cuff repair. First, large to massive tears are difficult to mobilize and repair through a "mini-open" deltoid splitting approach; in these cases, the small deltoid window is very limiting when compared to open or arthroscopic approaches. Second, arthroscopic repair of large tears can also fail because the operating surgeon failed to expose and visualize the posterior extent of the tear. The clue to this clinical scenario is a postoperative imaging study showing fixation devices present only in the anterior greater tuberosity in a shoulder that clearly had a large to massive tear preoperatively.

Rotator cuff tears result from a combination of intrinsic degeneration of the tendon and from extrinsic mechanical wear secondary to acromial spurs. Failure to perform an adequate acromioplasty can contribute to failure of rotator cuff surgery in those patients with abnormal acromial morphology or calcification of the coracoacromial ligament. Randomized studies have failed to show a consistent clinical benefit from acromioplasty in conjunction with rotator cuff repair. However, untouched acromial spurs, partially resected acromial spurs, and fraying of the coracoacromial ligament indicative of impingement are common findings at the time of revision rotator cuff repair.[47,48] Djurasovic and colleagues[49] found evidence of inadequate acromioplasty at the time of revision surgery in two-thirds of their series of 80 revision rotator cuff repairs.

Mobilization of contracted and adhesed rotator cuff tissue is necessary to facilitate a tension-free repair. Release of adhesions on both the bursal and articular side of the cuff is required in most chronic tears. Inadequate mobilization leads to either an incomplete repair or a repair on tension, which is likely destined to fail. Inadequate fixation of a properly mobilized cuff tendon can also contribute to repair failure. As mentioned previously, there has been a significant increase in the number of rotator cuff fixation options in the past decade. Despite this improvement in technology, knot security, knotless anchor security, suture type, suture configuration, and anchor fixation in bone, all remain potential areas for technical failure. Cummins and Murrell demonstrated that the predominant mode of failure of rotator cuff repair performed with suture anchors is sutures pulling through tendon.[50] The potential for cutout of simple sutures through rotator cuff tissue is one of the main reasons surgeons advocate the use of mattress sutures with linkage between medial and lateral rows if tear configuration and tissue mobility permit.[12]

Last, trauma can play a role in failure of rotator cuff repair. Traumatic injury to the rotator cuff may occur at any time, but 2 clinical scenarios are apparent. An "early" traumatic failure can occur in a patient prior to complete rotator cuff healing. The patient will often report initially doing well prior to an event or setback that the patient attributes to a fall on the arm or aggressive physical therapy. The other clinical scenario is a patient with a "late" traumatic rupture of a previously healed cuff. This type of patient has had a previously well-functioning cuff repair with documented return of strength and range of motion with a new reinjury. A thorough workup including history, physical, and imaging is required to determine which of the aforementioned factors contributed to the failure of the rotator cuff repair and if the patient with failed cuff surgery would benefit from another operation.

EVALUATION OF THE FAILED ROTATOR CUFF SURGERY

History and Physical Exam

A careful history is the key to understanding the potential causes of rotator cuff repair failure and the role of patient expectations. Table 19-2 summarizes the critical points of history taking in a patient with previous rotator cuff surgery. It is important to question the patient as to whether the pain ever improved after the surgery or if it remained constant. All previous surgeries should be documented, and if a previous surgery was performed at an outside institution, the patient's medical records including operative reports, preoperative imaging, and arthroscopic photos, should be acquired and reviewed. It is critical to document the postoperative rehabilitation protocol. The duration of immobilization as well as the duration and type of physical therapy after surgery should be noted.

TABLE 19-2. HISTORY TAKING IN FAILED CUFF REPAIR
Side of injury and dominant extremity
Duration of pain/date of initial injury
Mechanism of injury
Sports/occupation
Complete medical history (systemic disease, diabetes, nicotine)
Location/character of pain
Aggravating/relieving factors
Neurologic symptoms/neck pain
Previous surgery
Where/when
Concomitant procedures
Open or arthroscopic
Pain/strength/motion better or worse after surgery
Any signs of recent or distant infection
Treatment since surgery
Physical therapy
Duration of immobilization
Nonsteroidal anti-inflammatory drugs/narcotics
Postoperative injections

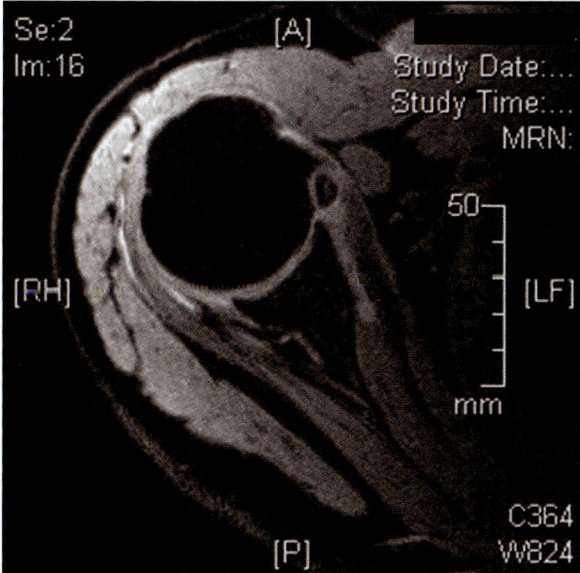

Figure 19-1. MRI illustrating a subscapularis tendon rupture with associated dislocation of the long head of the biceps tendon.

The physical exam should begin with careful inspection of the undraped shoulder, which can be compared to the contralateral shoulder. Any portals or incisions from previous surgeries should be noted and examined for healing, contracture, inflammation, erythema, or tenderness. Deltoid deformity, deltoid atrophy, or rotator cuff atrophy should be noted. Assessment of the long head of the biceps tendon should include inspecting for the Popeye sign. Palpation of the biceps tendon and acromioclavicular (AC) joint is important for surgical planning. Tear of the subscapularis tendon can often result in accompanying dislocation of the long head of the biceps tendon (Figure 19-1).

TABLE 19-3. PLAIN RADIOGRAPHIC FINDINGS IN REVISION ROTATOR CUFF SURGERY

Presence of acromial spur

Presence of inferior AC osteophytes

Status of AC joint (normal, osteoarthritis, resected)

Status of greater tuberosity (previous trough, anchor placement)

Presence of joint space narrowing or osteophytes indicative of osteoarthritis

Assessment of acromiohumeral interval

High-riding humeral head

Figure 19-2. Coronal MRI illustrating a recurrent supraspinatus tear and artifact from indwelling anchor.

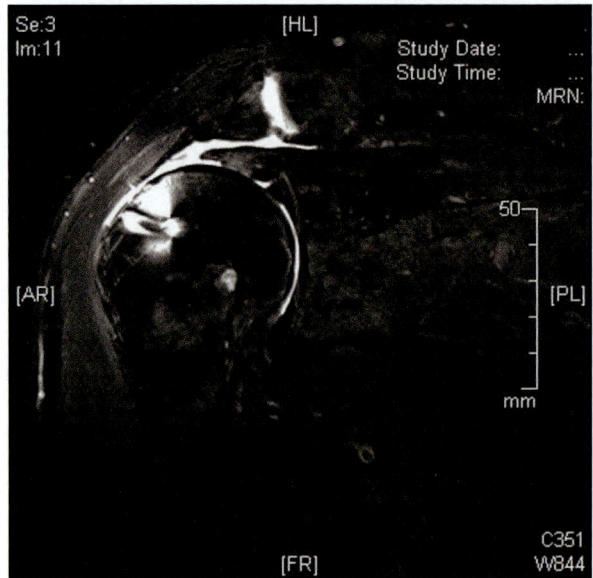

Active and passive shoulder range of motion should be measured, documented, and compared with the contralateral shoulder. Patients with smaller tears often will have preserved range of motion with pain only at the extremes. Patients with large and massive tears will preferentially lose active range of motion. A significant loss of passive range of motion should make the examiner suspect a postoperative adhesive capsulitis or progression to arthritis. Crepitus, stiffness, and pain can be determined during passive range of motion. Muscle strength testing of deltoid, supraspinatus, subscapularis, and external rotation is performed and compared to the contralateral side. The Neer and Hawkins impingement signs are tested. Neurologic testing should include the cervical innervation of the shoulder and arm, and any pain recreated with cervical maneuvers such as the Spurling test must be investigated to rule out other sources of pain.

Imaging of Recurrent Cuff Tears

Plain radiographs are very important in revision rotator cuff surgery. We commonly obtain anteroposterior, Grashey, axillary, and Y view of the affected shoulder and assess them for several factors (Table 19-3). We are especially critical to look for signs of rotator cuff arthropathy (fixed high riding humeral head and arthritis), which are contraindications to revision rotator cuff repair.

While MRI has become the gold standard for imaging the rotator cuff, the diagnostic accuracy of MRI for evaluating the integrity of rotator cuff repair may be diminished. Furthermore, surgical implants such as suture anchors may result in the generation of artifact (Figure 19-2). Despite these limitations, MRI remains the best option to image the postoperative rotator cuff, and we prefer a recent noncontrast MRI to evaluate a patient's shoulder after rotator cuff repair. We always attempt to obtain the patient's MRI from prior to the first surgery for comparison as it aids greatly in determining the mechanism of surgical failure. Gadolinium-enhanced MRI can certainly be used, but it is not routinely necessary. Longobardi and colleagues[51] have demonstrated that MRI is accurate for evaluating the rotator cuff in this setting. Dislocation of the long head of the biceps can provide a clue to a superior edge subscapularis tear that can be difficult to see with MRI. Ultrasound is also effective at determining the integrity of the rotator cuff postoperatively. A retrospective study comparing ultrasound with revision arthroscopic surgical findings resulted in a sensitivity of 91%, specificity of 86%, and accuracy of 89% for detection of postoperative cuff integrity.[52] We feel, however, that ultrasound images are much less useful than MRI images for planning rotator cuff surgery due to the increased detail of MRI and the ability to assess the shoulder in 3 planes. Computed tomography arthrography (CTA) is an excellent imaging modality and provides a detailed evaluation of the rotator cuff. Due to high radiation exposure from this procedure, it has largely been replaced by MRI. CTA is mainly used at our institution in those who have a contraindication to MRI (eg, pacemaker). It is important to obtain adequate imaging prior to planning revision surgery, even if repeat MRI is needed following suboptimal imaging from an outside institution. Proper imaging helps prepare the surgeon and the patient for the procedure and expected outcomes.

Davidson and Burkhart recently published an excellent classification scheme that aids in predicting size and tear pattern on MRI.[28] We try to estimate the repairability of a tear based mainly on 2 factors: the degree of retraction on coronal views and the degree of muscle atrophy on sagittal views through the rotator cuff muscle bellies at the level of the scapula. We evaluate the thickness of the cuff tendon and its proximity to the previous trough or anchor sites in the greater tuberosity. To reattempt rotator cuff repair, we prefer that the rotator cuff tendon be lateral to the glenohumeral joint line on the "worst" coronal cut (the apex of the tear) and that the Goutallier classification be stage 3 or better (muscle equals fat). In a level 4 evidence case series, Burkhart et al suggested that arthroscopic cuff repair can still be successful in the presence of fatty infiltration.[53] Similarly, we do not consider fatty infiltration of the cuff an absolute contraindication to revision cuff surgery.

RESULTS OF REVISION ROTATOR CUFF REPAIR AND INDICATIONS FOR SURGERY

The results of revision rotator cuff surgery are outlined in Table 19-4. Keener and colleagues,[27] Lo and Burkhart,[48] and Piasecki and colleagues[47] have all documented in retrospective case series that arthroscopic revision rotator cuff repair is clinically effective in the majority of cases in improving pain and function. Keener and colleagues[27] published the only series of revision rotator cuff repairs with postoperative ultrasound and found that 7 of 10 one-tendon tears healed and that 3 of 11 two-tendon repairs healed, for an overall 50% retear rate. One of the largest and most important series of revision cuff repairs remains a series of 80 open repairs published in 2001 by the Shoulder Service at Columbia University.[49] These authors found 4 main factors that correlated with a good result: 1) intact deltoid, 2) good rotator cuff tissue, 3) preoperative active elevation past 90 degrees, and 4) only one previous surgery. Despite the fact that many revision repairs are now performed arthroscopically, we feel that these factors identified by Djurasovic and colleagues remain very important at predicting clinical success.

A patient who presents for a second opinion with a painful or failed rotator cuff surgery is often frustrated. He or she has undergone a painful surgery and lengthy rehabilitation, has not regained function, and has not been relieved of pain. To determine if the patient would benefit from further surgery, we consider several factors (Table 19-5).

An optimal candidate for revision rotator cuff repair would be a younger patient with high functional demand, high pain level, a reparable tear without atrophy, good preoperative range of motion, an intact deltoid, and only one surgery. Obviously, these candidates are in the minority. Therefore,

TABLE 19-4. RESULTS OF REVISION ROTATOR CUFF SURGERY

SOURCE	LEVEL OF EVIDENCE	NO. OF SHOULDERS	MEAN AGE (YEARS)	MEAN FOLLOW-UP (MONTHS)	MEAN TIME FROM INITIAL PROCEDURE TO REVISION (MONTHS)	OPEN OR ARTHRO-SCOPIC	OUTCOME MEASURE	RESULTS	FACTORS ASSOCIATED WITH BETTER OUTCOMES
Djurasovic et al[49]	IV (case series)	80	59	49	6.5	Open	Rated as excellent, good, fair, or poor based on pain, range of motion, and function	33% excellent; 25% good; 11% fair, 31% poor	1. Intact deltoid origin prior to revision 2. Good quality tissue at time of revision 3. Preoperative active elevation of >90 degrees 4. Only one prior operative procedure
Bigliani et al[54]	IV (case series)	31	57	75	13	Open	Rated as excellent, good, fair, or poor based on pain, range of motion, and function	19% excellent; 32% good; 23% fair, 26% poor	1. Intact acromion 2. Intact deltoid origin 3. Good quality tissue at time of revision
DeOrio et al[55]	IV (case series)	27	52	64	46	Open	Rated as good, fair, or poor based on pain, motion, strength, the patient's response, and the need for additional surgery	17% good; 25% fair; 58% poor	1. Functioning deltoid 2. Smaller cuff tear found at revision 3. Less tissue needed to close tendon defect
Lo & Burkhart[48]	IV (case series)	14	57.9	23.4	41.4	Arthroscopic	UCLA score	Mean 13.1 preoperatively to mean 28.6 postoperatively	1. Intact deltoid 2. Visualization and classification of all tears (improved with arthroscopy)

(continued)

TABLE 19-4 (CONTINUED). RESULTS OF REVISION ROTATOR CUFF SURGERY

SOURCE	LEVEL OF EVIDENCE	NO. OF SHOULDERS	MEAN AGE (YEARS)	MEAN FOLLOW-UP (MONTHS)	MEAN TIME FROM INITIAL PROCEDURE TO REVISION (MONTHS)	OPEN OR ARTHROSCOPIC	OUTCOME MEASURE	RESULTS	FACTORS ASSOCIATED WITH BETTER OUTCOMES
Neviaser & Neviaser[56]	IV (case series)	50	54.5	30	16.9	Open	Pain, active elevation, patient satisfaction	92% improvement in pain, 8% pain unchanged; 26 patients improved average of 50 degrees, 22 remained unchanged, 2 lost motion; 90% satisfaction rate	1. Intact deltoid 2. Adequate decompression 3. Closure of all defects with tendon-to-bone junctures (by direct repair, interpositional grafting, or local tendon transfers) 4. Avoiding use of weights or resistive exercises during the first 3 months postoperatively
Keener et al[27]	IV (case series)	21	55.6	33	13.5	Arthroscopic	VAS, SST, ASES score	VAS improved from 6.1 to 2.8; SST improved from 5.3 to 8.8; ASES improved from 40.1 to 73.0	1. Younger age 2. Fewer tendons involved 3. Intact repair at time of revision
Piasecki et al[47]	IV (case series)	54	54.9	31.1	N/A	Arthroscopic	VAS, SST, ASES score	VAS improved from 5.17 to 2.75; SST improved from 3.6 to 7.5; ASES improved from 43.8 to 68.1	1. Male gender 2. Only one prior procedure

VAS = Visual Analog Pain Scale; SST = Simple Shoulder Test

> ## TABLE 19-5. IMPORTANT INDICATIONS IN CONSIDERING A PATIENT FOR REVISION ROTATOR CUFF SURGERY
>
> - Functional demands
> - Pain level
> - Repairability of tear (based on recent MRI showing level of muscle atrophy and retraction of tendon)
> - Active range of motion (preoperative forward elevation of less than 90 degrees is a poor prognostic sign)
> - Status of deltoid muscle (a poor deltoid predicts poor results)
> - Number of surgeries (more than one surgery is a poor prognostic sign)
> - Has physical therapy been optimized?

most patients who present with a failed rotator cuff repair are treated nonoperatively. In the case of an elderly patient with a massive recurrent tear with atrophy and moderate pain, we explain to the patient that his or her repair was destined to fail due to the large size of the tear and muscle atrophy and that it is not feasible to again attempt repair. The indications for débridement, latissimus transfer, allograft augmentation, and reverse arthroplasty are beyond the scope of this chapter but are comprehensively reviewed by Bedi and colleagues.[42] In cases that we deem irreparable, a cortisone injection is offered, and we begin another course of rehabilitation for the patient using Levy anterior deltoid strengthening exercises.[57]

Based on the criteria in Table 19-5, if an adequate course of physical therapy fails, we offer revision rotator cuff repair to those patients with painful, full-thickness tears that appear reparable on MRI. Often, the most satisfying revisions are those cases in which technical error or trauma has caused failure of cuff surgery in a patient with good-quality rotator cuff tissue. Reattempting repair on a tear that was borderline reparable at the index surgery due to muscle atrophy is typically unsatisfying.

AUTHORS' PREFERRED TECHNIQUE

One of the most important elements in a successful revision rotator cuff repair is the preoperative discussion with the patient. The surgeon needs to formally educate the patient about his or her condition and set the patient's expectations at a proper level. Patient expectations that are too high can critically doom a surgery to fail. For example, a patient with a massive, retracted recurrent rotator cuff tear that is expecting full, unrestricted return to activity does not have an understanding of the severity of the condition being treated. For this reason, we try to establish realistic expectations in our preoperative discussions. Those patients who are unable to comprehend the severity of the problem, the limited goals of revision surgery, or the myriad potential complications may not be candidates for further intervention.

Dr. Edward Craig and Dr. Robert Bell have both published the content of their preoperative discussion for rotator cuff repair.[58,59] We found these discussions to be excellent and have paraphrased them to a degree with respect to revision cuff surgery in Table 19-6. Additionally, in the preoperative workup, we are certain to evaluate both the AC joint and biceps tendon to determine their contribution to the patient's symptoms. Concomitant biceps tendinitis or AC joint arthrosis is subsequently addressed at the time of revision rotator cuff repair.

Operating Room Setup

We prefer the beach chair position for rotator cuff surgery. It affords several advantages including the effect of gravity opening the subacromial space, easy internal and external rotation of the

TABLE 19-6. PREOPERATIVE PATIENT DISCUSSION OF REVISION ROTATOR CUFF REPAIR

- There is no evidence that full-thickness tears heal without surgery.
- The main reason to have rotator cuff surgery is to improve pain. Added function is an additional benefit, and the shoulder will not likely return to "normal."
- Small tears can enlarge over time and become more difficult to repair.
- Recurrence of rotator cuff repair is very common after repair but is not always associated with a clinical failure. The incidence of recurrent tear increases with tear size.
- The cause of the retear being treated cannot always be determined, but as long as certain criteria are met with respect to repairability, the majority of revision rotator cuff surgeries will result in improved pain and function.
- Revision repairs have a high likelihood of retearing again.
- Some patients with large tears will develop arthritis (rotator cuff tear arthropathy) in the future. It is not clear at this time in which patients this occurs and how long it will take.
- The rehabilitation will consist of 6 weeks of passive range of motion, 6 weeks of active range of motion, and 6 weeks of strengthening. Pain and stiffness can persist for as long as 6 months, and continued improvement can be seen in shoulders until 1 year.
- There is a chance that another attempt at repair of your rotator cuff may not improve pain or function. Because the repair is being performed arthroscopically, there is only a small chance of it being made worse.

arm to view posterior and anterior aspects of the tear, respectively, and easy conversion to open surgery if necessary. Lateral decubitus is a highly effective position for rotator cuff surgery as well, and certainly surgeon preference and familiarity is most critical when selecting surgical position. We also perform the vast majority of revision repairs arthroscopically. We prefer double-row repairs with suture anchors, knot tying, and linkage between the medial and lateral row, if possible. We will not place the cuff on tension to attain a double-row construct; however, in these cases, a single-row repair to the medial aspect of the footprint is performed. While newer knotless designs provide excellent and secure repairs in mobile, crescent-shaped tears, we do not believe that they are not versatile enough to be used effectively in every revision case.

As outlined in Table 19-4, direct comparison of arthroscopic versus open revision repairs in the literature is impossible due to difference in techniques, disparity of patient populations, and inconsistency of tear size. Open repair is certainly an excellent option, but it is at risk of becoming a "lost art." Most critical again is surgeon preference and familiarity. An open revision cuff repair, while perhaps associated with increased early morbidity, will certainly perform as well as an arthroscopic approach as long as the deltoid repair is secure. In large, retracted tears, we do consent the patient for open surgery should it be necessary to convert if the tear cannot be adequately mobilized arthroscopically. We feel that the arthroscopic approach is slightly safer than an open approach because it carries essentially no risk of compromising a functioning deltoid. We do not recommend approaching massive tears through a mini-open approach because the deltoid split becomes very limiting in these cases.

Ultrasound-guided interscalene block is performed by a dedicated regional anesthesiologist. General anesthesia or sedation is induced. We prefer the patient to be sitting in the beach chair position at 60 to 70 degrees using a Maquet table with a beach chair head positioner. The patient is sat up to 30 degrees, and the blood pressure cuff is cycled. If blood pressure is adequate, full beach position is assumed, and the blood pressure is rechecked. We instruct the anesthesiologist to maintain systolic blood pressure between 95 and 110 to ensure cerebral perfusion but avoid subacromial bleeding. The addition of 1 cc of 1:1000 epinephrine per 3000 mL of arthroscopy fluid may also improve hemostasis. We also find that an arthroscopic pump is essential for fluid management in these cases. The pump is initially set to 35 mm Hg and can be intermittently increased via lavage to improve visualization. Adequate access to anterior and posterior shoulder is ensured, and the entire arm is then prepped and placed in a Spider arm positioner (Tenet Medical, Calgary, Alberta).

The Spider arm positioner allows distraction of the subacromial space while allowing near unlimited adjustment of internal and external rotation. The arm is not abducted for the repair so that tension on the repair can be truly assessed. Necessary instruments include a 5-mm cannula, 8.25-mm cannula, suture retriever, arthroscopic grasper, knot pusher, devices for antegrade and retrograde suture passage, and suture anchors of choice for medial and lateral double-row repair. For antegrade suture passage, we prefer the Expressew suture passer (Depuy-Mitek, Raynham, MA) or an equivalent device.

Portals

Portal placement is critical for successful revision arthroscopic rotator cuff repair. We are not influenced by portals created during previous surgery. The posterior viewing portal is higher and more lateral than for cases that are predominately glenohumeral. We prefer this portal to be 1 cm inferior and 1 cm medial to the posterolateral acromion. This is a suboptimal portal for extensive glenohumeral work, but it then allows for a bird's eye view of the tear in the subacromial space. All subsequent portals are then made via spinal needle localization. The other 2 main portals are the anterior portal (localized mid acromion anteriorly) and the lateral portal (localized in the center of the tear laterally). After insertion of the arthroscope, we place a rotator interval portal anteriorly with attention being paid to staying lateral on the skin so the portal functions well later for subacromial arthroscopy.

Diagnostic Arthroscopy, Rotator Cuff Repair, and Associated Procedures

We perform a standard diagnostic arthroscopy, paying close attention to the biceps tendon and subscapularis and assessing the size of the supraspinatus/infraspinatus tear. The glenohumeral portion of the case should be efficient, as much work is to be done in the subacromial space. If indicated, a biceps tenotomy or biceps tenodesis is performed. It is important to discuss the long head of the biceps in every case preoperatively to determine the patient's preference. If a tenodesis is performed, it is done through a mini-open approach distal to the groove as we do not feel that arthroscopic approaches to biceps tenodesis properly address biceps pathology in the groove. The description in this chapter describes a repair of a massive tear with involvement of the subscapularis, supraspinatus, and part of the infraspinatus.

If a subscapularis tear is present, it often involves only the upper half of the tendon and can be repaired with the arthroscope in the glenohumeral joint (Figure 19-3). Subscapularis tendon repair is technically easier in the presence of a supraspinatus tear as the tear is used for the second portal placement. The superolateral border of the subscapularis is localized by finding the medial sling of the biceps (referred to as the "comma" tissue by Burkhart and colleagues[53]). The anterior portal is placed just above the subscapularis and medial to the comma, and the lateral portal is placed through the supraspinatus tear. A traction stitch is placed in the tendon using the Expressew and is placed outside the cannula through the lateral portal. With traction on the tendon through the lateral portal, adhesions are cleared using radiofrequency so that the tendon can easily be reduced to the lesser tuberosity. It is critical to remove soft tissue anterior to the tendon so that sutures can be passed low and medial in the tendon under direct vision. The arthroscope is then driven over the top of the humeral head, and the camera is pointed directly inferiorly to visualize the lesser tuberosity. Occasionally, the 70-degree arthroscope is needed to improve visualization for this step. Modest decortication of the lesser tuberosity is followed by the placement of a double-loaded suture anchor through the anterior portal. The proper angle of insertion of this anchor is to direct the surgeon's hand toward the patient's face. When using an arm positioner, it is sometimes helpful to flex and slightly externally rotate the shoulder to facilitate anchor placement. The Expressew is then used to place a low mattress stitch and a high simple stitch in the subscapularis tendon. Suture passage is accomplished from the lateral portal, passing the limb of suture from posterior to

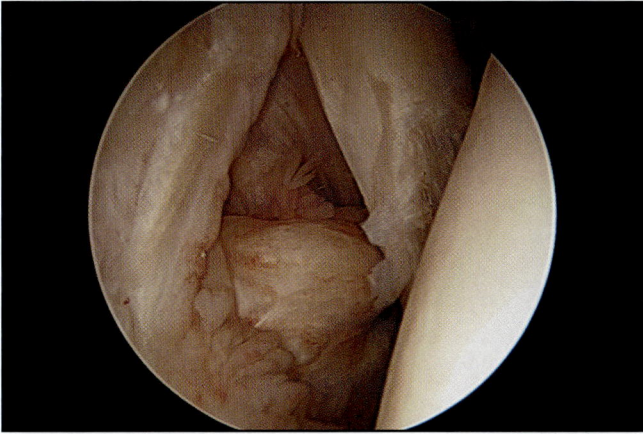

Figure 19-3. A vertical biceps consistent with subscapularis tendon rupture as viewed from a posterior portal.

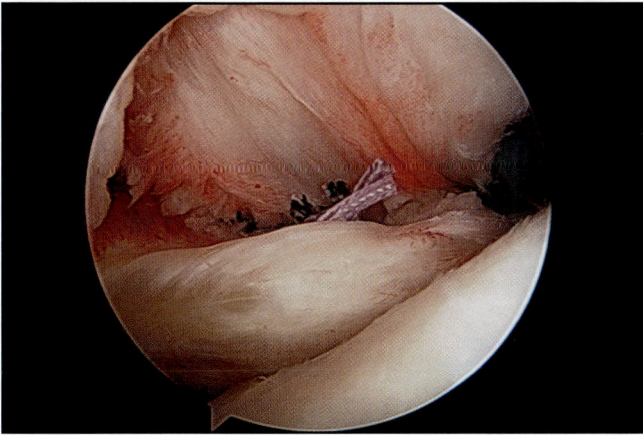

Figure 19-4. Arthroscopic view of a biceps tenotomy and subscapularis tendon repair.

anterior through the tendon and retrieving each limb through the anterior portal. The arm is then internally rotated slightly to decrease tension, and the knots are tied arthroscopically. We prefer to tie arthroscopic knots with half hitches, as we use mostly mattress sutures and therefore rarely use sliding knots (Figure 19-4).

Once the subscapularis repair is complete, we prefer to mobilize the articular side of the supraspinatus/infraspinatus tear while in the glenohumeral joint, as this step is difficult with the arthroscope in the subacromial space (Figure 19-5). Starting anteriorly, we release just above the glenoid in the plane between the labrum and rotator cuff using radiofrequency. Anteriorly, the limit of the release is the coracoid process. We avoid releasing beyond 2 cm medial to the glenoid to avoid injury to the suprascapular nerve. The release is carried as far posteriorly as necessary.

After the articular-sided cuff release, the arthroscope is removed. We then carefully reintroduce the arthroscope into the subacromial space, taking care to stay in the plane above the bursa. A complete subacromial bursectomy is then performed. In the revision setting, due to previous surgical scarring, it is not always easy to discern between rotator cuff and bursal tissue. We identify the rotator cuff anteriorly first and carry the bursectomy posteriorly with the shaver facing away from the rotator cuff. The goal of the bursectomy is 2-fold. First, the entirety of the tear must be visualized; this requires identifying the extent of the tear anteriorly and where the cuff inserts posteriorly on the humeral head. Second, the bursectomy is critical to visualizing stitches that are to be placed in the posterior cuff. After completing the bursectomy and identifying the tear pattern, we develop a plan for fixing the tear arthroscopically. It is helpful to view the tear from at least 2 orthogonal portals to plan the repair (Figure 19-6). We prefer to place the camera in the lateral portal intermittently to garner a "50-yard-line" view of the tear.

Figure 19-5. View of a recurrent tear from the articular surface.

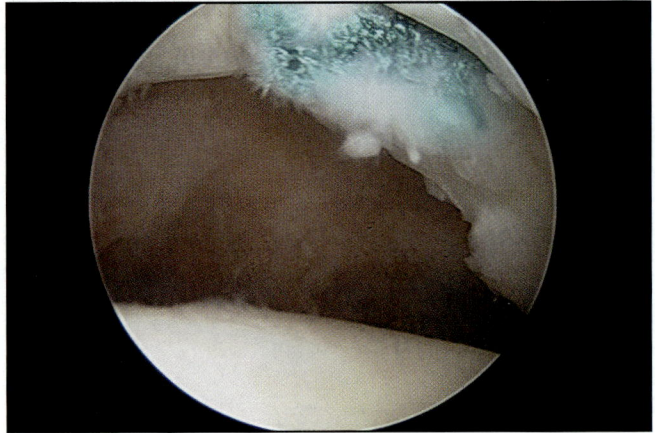

Figure 19-6. A large tear viewed from a posterior portal.

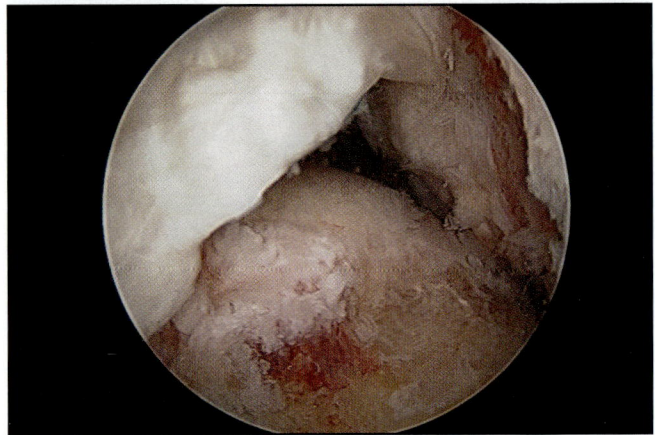

We first assess the mobility of the tear by grasping the rotator cuff from both laterally and anteriorly to test its excursion and the ability to reduce it to the greater tuberosity. Almost invariably in large tears, the tissue is more mobile from posterior to anterior than it is from medial to lateral. A bursal-sided release using radiofrequency is then performed first without traction on the rotator cuff and then again with 2 traction stitches pulling the tendon from medial to lateral. In large tears, an anterior interval slide can be performed. We commonly release back to the scapular spine. During the release, it is common to incite bleeding, especially posterior and medially. If a large bleeder is encountered, it is best to "not leave the scene of the crime," meaning the arthroscope should remain directly at the site of bleeding, and the cautery device is then brought to the scope; this technique avoids high pump pressures and "red-out" situations. Once maximum excursion of the rotator cuff is obtained, we have an assistant hold gentle traction on the rotator cuff during the acromioplasty to perhaps gain some extra excursion of the tendon.

Revision acromioplasty begins by identifying the anterolateral aspect of the acromion with the radiofrequency probe. Soft tissue is stripped off the undersurface of the acromion from anterolateral to medially and posteriorly, exposing the entire anterior acromion and AC joint (Figure 19-7). An oval burr is then used to perform an acromioplasty so that the anterior acromion is flush with the posterior acromion, taking care to spare the deltoid fascia and avoid fluid extravasation (Figure 19-8). The distal clavicle is then resected in standard fashion if necessary.

Once the revision acromioplasty is complete, the anterior cannula (5 mm) and lateral cannula (8.25 mm) are re-established. The greater tuberosity is cleared of soft tissue and then lightly decorticated using a burr. Prior to anchor placement, U-shaped tears and L-shaped tears are first

Figure 19-7. Arthroscopic view of a large, residual acromial spur.

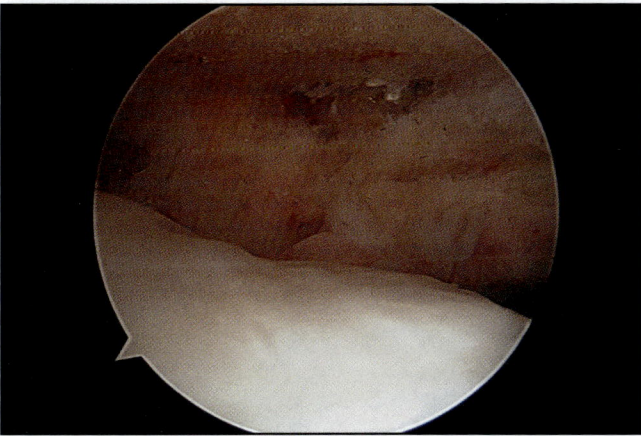

Figure 19-8. A completed acromioplasty.

converted to crescent-shaped tears using margin convergence sutures. We prefer passing margin convergence sutures using 2 individual bites from the Expressew device. The posterior limb of the suture is passed through the anterior cannula and the anterior limb of the suture through the lateral cannula. These knots are tied down immediately, and the tear is reassessed to determine if more margin convergence is needed.

Once the tear has been converted to a crescent-shaped pattern, we begin anchor placement with separate 5-mm stab incisions for each anchor starting posteriorly and working anteriorly. The first anchor is placed through a separate stab incision just off the lateral edge of the acromion. A blunt trocar opens the deltoid slightly, and the anchor is inserted in the posterior aspect of the tear in the medial footprint of the rotator cuff. We almost always use medial footprint anchors. The 2 most common repair types we do are single-row repairs to the medial footprint in shoulders with immobile tissue and double-row repairs in shoulders with adequate cuff. The first 1 or 2 antegrade suture passings are usually performed from the anterior cannula in order to reach the posterior cuff to attain the posterior to anterior mobility that is common in large tears. We use mostly horizontal mattress sutures spaced 5- to 7-mm apart, taking 15- to 18-mm bites of tissue. Once all limbs of suture are passed satisfactorily, the sutures are retrieved out of the separate anchor stab, docking them without confusion until tying. In general, we use one medial row anchor for every 1 to 1.5 cm of tear width. Each successive anchor is placed through a separate stab incision, avoiding suture confusion. Once all medial row sutures have been passed, the medial row is tied arthroscopically from posterior-to-anterior, and the sutures are not cut. It is critical for the knot pusher to recreate the angle of anchor insertion during knot tying to enable close coaptation of tendon

Figure 19-9. View of medial row suture anchors after placement.

Figure 19-10. Lateral view of lateral row anchors.

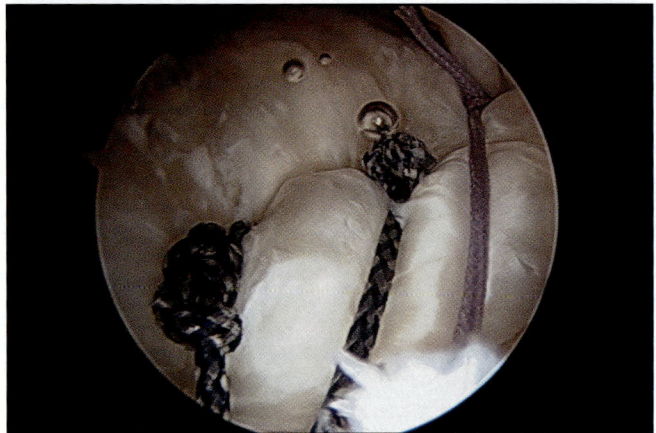

Figure 19-11. Final repair configuration as viewed from a posterior portal.

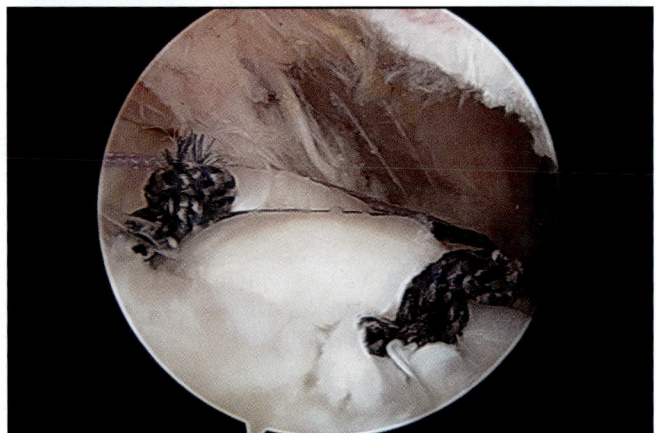

to bone. Once all knots have been tied, the sutures are all retrieved out of the anterior cannula (Figure 19-9). The lateral aspect of the greater tuberosity is then cleared of soft tissue to allow for visualization for placement of the lateral row suture anchors (Figure 19-10). Sutures from the medial row are draped over the cuff edge and secured on tension inside lateral row anchors inserted in standard fashion in the greater tuberosity (Figure 19-11). Choice of implants is not critical. If the repair fails, it is highly unlikely that it will fail due to strength of suture or fixation devices; it will fail due to poor-quality tissue. We will occasionally augment our repair with platelet-rich plasma as per Gamradt and colleagues[60] in cases of diabetes or smoking, although there is no current level 1 evidence to support this use at this time. In addition, the indications for suprascapular nerve decompression deserve further study in this population.

We prefer to close each portal with buried 4-0 Monocryl stitches, mastisol, and steri-strips. This is a very cosmetic closure and saves time in the office avoiding suture removal. An abduction pillow sling and cold therapy device are placed in the operating room. In most cases, we allow immediate shoulder shrugs, distal range of motion, passive forward elevation to 90 degrees, and passive external rotation to neutral. If a tear is particularly large or if tissue quality is poor, we will completely immobilize the shoulder for no longer than 4 weeks. Sling is discontinued, and active range of motion is started at week 6. Very light strengthening can be started at 12 weeks. Patients are advised that pain and stiffness can persist for 6 months and that the shoulder will continue to improve for 1 year.

OUTCOMES AND CONCLUSION

The outcomes of revision rotator cuff repair are summarized in Table 19-4. Note that these studies are disparate with regard to patient population, surgical technique, and outcomes. The only study to critically evaluate the success of revision rotator cuff repair with postoperative imaging was Keener and colleagues,[27] which demonstrated a 50% retear rate despite the use of double-row fixation in most patients. Clinical success can be expected in 40% to 90% of revision rotator cuff repairs. However, there have been no comparative trials in revision rotator cuff surgery to guide optimal treatment. This reflects the overall difficulty of conducting high-level evidence research in this type of patient population. In addition, Yamaguchi[1] recently published the conclusions of an AAOS Clinical Practice Guideline work group on optimizing the management of rotator cuff problems. Despite evaluating more than 4000 published articles, none of the 31 recommendations of the group carried a "strong" grade. Therefore, surgeons are left to draw their own conclusions regarding rotator cuff literature. We believe that, based on clinical experience and critical review of the literature, certain conclusions can be drawn.

- Rotator cuff repair is very likely to be clinically successful when performed well and rehabilitated properly, especially when judged with patient satisfaction outcome scores.
- A healed rotator cuff tendon will likely result in an improved and lasting clinical result. A small tear is much more likely to heal completely when compared to a large tear.
- Recurrent tears will still be present despite optimal mobilization and fixation of the rotator cuff to bone, especially in large tears with retraction and atrophy.
- In cadaveric studies, double-row fixation is superior biomechanically to single-row repair, and there is some evidence that a double-row repair may improve tendon healing, but many tears are not amenable to this type of repair due to tendon retraction and muscle atrophy.
- Failure of rotator cuff repairs is multifactorial with recurrent trauma, technical factors, and biologic (patient) factors all playing a role.
- Revision rotator cuff repair can be a very successful procedure, particularly in those patients who have the following:
  - Minimal muscle atrophy
  - A tendon not retracted past the glenohumeral joint line
  - Preoperative forward elevation of greater than 90 degrees
  - A functioning deltoid
  - Had only one previous surgery
  - No evidence of cuff tear arthropathy (eg, fixed high-riding humeral head)

PEARLS AND PITFALLS

- Patient selection is critical; most failed cuff repairs should be treated nonoperatively. Use strict criteria when deciding to revise a rotator cuff surgery.
- Ensure the patient has realistic goals for surgery, that he or she understands the natural history of rotator cuff disease, and that the repair could fail again.
- Use a high lateral posterior portal for optimal visualization.
- Mobilize the articular side of the rotator cuff while still in the glenohumeral joint.
- Mobilize extensively on the bursal side of the tear using traction stitches to ensure a tension-free repair.
- Assess mobility and tissue quality of each tear, and individualize repair construct for each tear.
- Convert complex tears to simple ones using margin convergence sutures.
- Resist the temptation to do too much; many tears are not completely reparable.

REFERENCES

1. Yamaguchi K. *New Guideline on Rotator Cuff Problems*. AAOS Now, Vol 5. Rosemont, IL: American Academy of Orthopaedic Surgeons; 2011.
2. Gazielly DF, Gleyze P, Montagnon C. Functional and anatomical results after rotator cuff repair. *Clin Orthop Relat Res*. 1994;304:43-53.
3. Harryman DT 2nd, Mack LA, Wang KY, Jackins SE, Richardson ML, Matsen FA 3rd. Repairs of the rotator cuff. Correlation of functional results with integrity of the cuff. *J Bone Joint Surg Am*. 1991;73(7):982-989.
4. Knudsen HB, Gelineck J, Sojbjerg JO, Olsen BS, Johannsen HV, Sneppen O. Functional and magnetic resonance imaging evaluation after single-tendon rotator cuff reconstruction. *J Shoulder Elbow Surg*. 1999;8(3):242-246.
5. Liu SH, Baker CL. Arthroscopically assisted rotator cuff repair: correlation of functional results with integrity of the cuff. *Arthroscopy*. 1994;10(1):54-60.
6. Wulker N, Melzer C, Wirth CJ. Shoulder surgery for rotator cuff tears. Ultrasonographic 3-year follow-up of 97 cases. *Acta Orthop Scand*. 1991;62(2):142-147.
7. Calvert PT, Packer NP, Stoker DJ, Bayley JI, Kessel L. Arthrography of the shoulder after operative repair of the torn rotator cuff. *J Bone Joint Surg Br*. 1986;68(1):147-150.
8. Galatz LM, Ball CM, Teefey SA, Middleton WD, Yamaguchi K. The outcome and repair integrity of completely arthroscopically repaired large and massive rotator cuff tears. *J Bone Joint Surg Am*. 2004;86-A(2):219-224.
9. Slabaugh MA, Nho SJ, Grumet RC, et al. Does the literature confirm superior clinical results in radiographically healed rotator cuffs after rotator cuff repair? *Arthroscopy*. 2010;26(3):393-403.
10. Wall LB, Keener JD, Brophy RH. Double-row vs single-row rotator cuff repair: a review of the biomechanical evidence. *J Shoulder Elbow Surg*. 2009;18(6):933-941.
11. Nho SJ, Slabaugh MA, Seroyer ST, et al. Does the literature support double-row suture anchor fixation for arthroscopic rotator cuff repair? A systematic review comparing double-row and single-row suture anchor configuration. *Arthroscopy*. 2009;25(11):1319-1328.
12. Burkhart SS, Cole BJ. Bridging self-reinforcing double-row rotator cuff repair: we really are doing better. *Arthroscopy*. 2010;26(5):677-680.
13. Duquin TR, Buyea C, Bisson LJ. Which method of rotator cuff repair leads to the highest rate of structural healing? A systematic review. *Am J Sports Med*. 2010;38(4):835-841.
14. Accousti KJ, Gladstone J, Parsons B, Klug R, Flatow EL. In-vivo measurement of rotator cuff perfusion using laser doppler flowmetry. Arthroscopy Association of North America Annual Meeting. San Francisco, CA; 2007.
15. Trantalis JN, Boorman RS, Pletsch K, Lo IK. Medial rotator cuff failure after arthroscopic double-row rotator cuff repair. *Arthroscopy*. 2008;24(6):727-731.
16. Abrams JS. Management of the failed rotator cuff surgery: causation and management. *Sports Med Arthrosc*. 2010;18(3):188-197.
17. Gulotta LV, Rodeo SA. Growth factors for rotator cuff repair. *Clin Sports Med*. 2009;28(1):13-23.
18. Thomopoulos S, Genin GM, Galatz LM. The development and morphogenesis of the tendon-to-bone insertion—what development can teach us about healing. *J Musculoskelet Neuronal Interact*. 2010;10(1):35-45.
19. Galatz LM, Rothermich SY, Zaegel M, Silva MJ, Havlioglu N, Thomopoulos S. Delayed repair of tendon to bone injuries leads to decreased biomechanical properties and bone loss. *J Orthop Res*. 2005;23(6):1441-1447.
20. Rudzki JR, Adler RS, Warren RF, et al. Contrast-enhanced ultrasound characterization of the vascularity of the rotator cuff tendon: age- and activity-related changes in the intact asymptomatic rotator cuff. *J Shoulder Elbow Surg*. 2008;17(1 Suppl):96S-100S.

21. Gamradt SC, Gallo RA, Adler RS, et al. Vascularity of the supraspinatus tendon three months after repair: characterization using contrast-enhanced ultrasound. *J Shoulder Elbow Surg.* 2010;19(1):73-80.

22. Getelman MH, Friedman MJ. Revision anterior cruciate ligament reconstruction surgery. *J Am Acad Orthop Surg.* 1999;7(3):189-198.

23. Boileau P, Brassart N, Watkinson DJ, Carles M, Hatzidakis AM, Krishnan SG. Arthroscopic repair of full-thickness tears of the supraspinatus: does the tendon really heal? *J Bone Joint Surg Am.* 2005;87(6):1229-1240.

24. DeFranco MJ, Bershadsky B, Ciccone J, Yum JK, Iannotti JP. Functional outcome of arthroscopic rotator cuff repairs: a correlation of anatomic and clinical results. *J Shoulder Elbow Surg.* 2007;16(6):759-765.

25. Cole BJ, McCarty LP 3rd, Kang RW, Alford W, Lewis PB, Hayden JK. Arthroscopic rotator cuff repair: prospective functional outcome and repair integrity at minimum 2-year follow-up. *J Shoulder Elbow Surg.* 2007;16(5):579-585.

26. Nho SJ, Brown BS, Lyman S, Adler RS, Altchek DW, MacGillivray JD. Prospective analysis of arthroscopic rotator cuff repair: prognostic factors affecting clinical and ultrasound outcome. *J Shoulder Elbow Surg.* 2009;18(1):13-20.

27. Keener JD, Wei AS, Kim HM, et al. Revision arthroscopic rotator cuff repair: repair integrity and clinical outcome. *J Bone Joint Surg Am.* 2010;92(3):590-598.

28. Davidson J, Burkhart SS. The geometric classification of rotator cuff tears: a system linking tear pattern to treatment and prognosis. *Arthroscopy.* 2010;26(3):417-424.

29. Bishop J, Klepps S, Lo IK, Bird J, Gladstone JN, Flatow EL. Cuff integrity after arthroscopic versus open rotator cuff repair: a prospective study. *J Shoulder Elbow Surg.* 2006;15(3):290-299.

30. Huijsmans PE, Pritchard MP, Berghs BM, van Rooyen KS, Wallace AL, de Beer JF. Arthroscopic rotator cuff repair with double-row fixation. *J Bone Joint Surg Am.* 2007;89(6):1248-1257.

31. Sugaya H, Maeda K, Matsuki K, Moriishi J. Repair integrity and functional outcome after arthroscopic double-row rotator cuff repair. A prospective outcome study. *J Bone Joint Surg Am.* 2007;89(5):953-960.

32. Goutallier D, Postel JM, Bernageau J, Lavau L, Voisin MC. Fatty muscle degeneration in cuff ruptures. Pre- and postoperative evaluation by CT scan. *Clin Orthop Relat Res.* 1994;304:78-83.

33. Gerber C, Schneeberger AG, Hoppeler H, Meyer DC. Correlation of atrophy and fatty infiltration on strength and integrity of rotator cuff repairs: a study in thirteen patients. *J Shoulder Elbow Surg.* 2007;16(6):691-696.

34. Gladstone JN, Bishop JY, Lo IK, Flatow EL. Fatty infiltration and atrophy of the rotator cuff do not improve after rotator cuff repair and correlate with poor functional outcome. *Am J Sports Med.* 2007;35(5):719-728.

35. Liem D, Lichtenberg S, Magosch P, Habermeyer P. Magnetic resonance imaging of arthroscopic supraspinatus tendon repair. *J Bone Joint Surg Am.* 2007;89(8):1770-1776.

36. Melis B, DeFranco MJ, Chuinard C, Walch G. Natural history of fatty infiltration and atrophy of the supraspinatus muscle in rotator cuff tears. *Clin Orthop Relat Res.* 2010;468(6):1498-1505.

37. Hersche O, Gerber C. Passive tension in the supraspinatus musculotendinous unit after long-standing rupture of its tendon: a preliminary report. *J Shoulder Elbow Surg.* 1998;7(4):393-396.

38. Gimbel JA, Mehta S, Van Kleunen JP, Williams GR, Soslowsky LJ. The tension required at repair to reappose the supraspinatus tendon to bone rapidly increases after injury. *Clin Orthop Relat Res.* 2004;426:258-265.

39. Gimbel JA, Van Kleunen JP, Mehta S, Perry SM, Williams GR, Soslowsky LJ. Supraspinatus tendon organizational and mechanical properties in a chronic rotator cuff tear animal model. *J Biomech.* 2004;37(5):739-749.

40. Coleman SH, Fealy S, Ehteshami JR, et al. Chronic rotator cuff injury and repair model in sheep. *J Bone Joint Surg Am.* 2003;85-A(12):2391-2402.

41. Bassett RW, Cofield RH. Acute tears of the rotator cuff. The timing of surgical repair. *Clin Orthop Relat Res.* 1983;175:18-24.

42. Bedi A, Dines J, Warren RF, Dines DM. Massive tears of the rotator cuff. *J Bone Joint Surg Am.* 2010;92(9):1894-1908.

43. Clement ND, Hallett A, MacDonald D, Howie C, McBirnie J. Does diabetes affect outcome after arthroscopic repair of the rotator cuff? *J Bone Joint Surg Br.* 2010;92(8):1112-1117.

44. Sherman SL, Lyman S, Koulouvaris P, Willis A, Marx RG. Risk factors for readmission and revision surgery following rotator cuff repair. *Clin Orthop Relat Res.* 2008;466(3):608-613.

45. Galatz LM, Silva MJ, Rothermich SY, Zaegel MA, Havlioglu N, Thomopoulos S. Nicotine delays tendon-to-bone healing in a rat shoulder model. *J Bone Joint Surg Am.* 2006;88(9):2027-2034.

46. Mallon WJ, Misamore G, Snead DS, Denton P. The impact of preoperative smoking habits on the results of rotator cuff repair. *J Shoulder Elbow Surg.* 2004;13(2):129-132.

47. Piasecki DP, Verma NN, Nho SJ, et al. Outcomes after arthroscopic revision rotator cuff repair. *Am J Sports Med.* 2010;38(1):40-46.

48. Lo IK, Burkhart SS. Arthroscopic revision of failed rotator cuff repairs: technique and results. *Arthroscopy.* 2004;20(3):250-267.

49. Djurasovic M, Marra G, Arroyo JS, Pollock RG, Flatow EL, Bigliani LU. Revision rotator cuff repair: factors influencing results. *J Bone Joint Surg Am.* 2001;83-A(12):1849-1855.

50. Cummins CA, Murrell GA. Mode of failure for rotator cuff repair with suture anchors identified at revision surgery. *J Shoulder Elbow Surg.* 2003;12(2):128-133.

51. Longobardi RS, Rafii M, Minkoff J. MR imaging of the postoperative shoulder. *Magn Reson Imaging Clin N Am.* 1997;5(4):841-859.

52.   Prickett WD, Teefey SA, Galatz LM, Calfee RP, Middleton WD, Yamaguchi K. Accuracy of ultrasound imaging of the rotator cuff in shoulders that are painful postoperatively. *J Bone Joint Surg Am*. 2003;85-A(6):1084-1089.

53.   Burkhart SS, Barth JR, Richards DP, Zlatkin MB, Larsen M. Arthroscopic repair of massive rotator cuff tears with stage 3 and 4 fatty degeneration. *Arthroscopy*. 2007;23(4):347-354.

54.   Bigliani LU, Cordasco FA, McIlveen SJ, Musso ES. Operative treatment of failed repairs of the rotator cuff. *J Bone Joint Surg Am*. 1992;74:1505-1515.

55.   DeOrio JK, Cofield RH. Results of a second attempt at surgical repair of a failed initial rotator-cuff repair. *J Bone Joint Surg Am*. 1984;66:563-567.

56.   Neviaser RJ, Neviaser TJ. Operation for failed rotator cuff repair. Analysis of fifty cases. *J Shoulder Elbow Surg*. 1992;1:283-286.

57.   Levy O, Mullett H, Roberts S, Copeland S. The role of anterior deltoid reeducation in patients with massive irreparable degenerative rotator cuff tears. *J Shoulder Elbow Surg*. 2008;17(6):863-870.

58.   Bell R. Arthroscopic repair of the rotator cuff. In: Craig E, ed. *Master Techniques of Orthopaedic Surgery—The Shoulder*. 2nd ed. Philadelphia, PA: Lippincott; 2004:35-57.

59.   Craig E. Techniques for full thickness rotator cuff repairs. In: Craig E, ed. *Master Techniques of Orthopaedic Surgery—The Shoulder*. 2nd ed. Philadelphia, PA: Lippincott; 2004:309-340.

60.   Gamradt S, Rodeo S, Warren R. Platelet rich plasma in rotator cuff surgery. *Techniques in Orthopaedics*. 2007;22(1):26-33.

***Please see video on the accompanying Web site at
http://www.slackbooks.com/rotatorcuffvideos***

CHAPTER 20

ARTHROSCOPIC MANAGEMENT OF MASSIVE ROTATOR CUFF TEARS

Stephanie H. Hsu, MD, Bob Yin, MD; and William N. Levine, MD

A massive rotator cuff tear has been variably defined as a tear measuring 5 cm or more or as the complete detachment of 2 or more tendons.[1-4] While no study has examined the true prevalence of massive tears, various authors have noted a prevalence of 10% to 40% in individual patient series.[5-8] In general, massive rotator cuff tears can be classified as posterosuperior or anterosuperior depending on which tendons are involved. The more common posterosuperior tears involve the supraspinatus and infraspinatus tendons, with or without involvement of the teres minor tendon.[8] Anterosuperior tears are less common and involve the supraspinatus and subscapularis tendons.[9]

Burkhart's 3-category classification of massive rotator cuff tears (crescent, U-shaped, and L-shaped) is a useful way to conceptualize tear patterns.[2,10] Crescent-shaped tears are not significantly retracted and can be easily reduced to the rotator cuff footprint with minimal tension. U-shaped tears are retracted medially, with the apex of the tear located at the level of the glenoid, thus requiring more advanced techniques, including selective releases and the technique of margin convergence, to advance the cuff to its anatomic insertion site.[11] L-shaped tears are distinguished by a longitudinal tear parallel to the fibers of the rotator cuff tendon with a transverse component at the footprint. Generally, both limbs of the "L" must be addressed for a successful repair. It is useful to classify massive tears into one of these 3 patterns because tear pattern has implications on the surgeon's strategy for cuff mobilization and repair. Conversely, the recognition that the massive tear being treated does not conform to one of these types (the presence of a complex tear pattern) may be equally important for the formulation of a repair strategy.

EVOLUTION IN TREATMENT OF MASSIVE ROTATOR CUFF TEARS

The current state of shoulder arthroscopy has made the majority of massive rotator cuff tears amenable to all-arthroscopic repair. Although the results of open repair of massive tears were favorable,[3,12-14] certain drawbacks of open procedures prompted the evolution of arthroscopic

Ma CB, Feeley BT.
*Basic Principles and Operative Management
of the Rotator Cuff (pp 291-310)*

techniques. A distinct advantage afforded by the arthroscopic approach is superior visualization of the tear from virtually every angle through proper portal placement. The standard anterolateral approach exposed an operative "window" through the deltoid into which the retracted tendon edge must be pulled to anatomically restore the rotator cuff footprint. Furthermore, whereas open repair and the associated subacromial decompression require detachment of the deltoid, arthroscopic treatment allows for preservation of the deltoid attachment to the acromion. Failure of the detached deltoid fibers to heal represents a devastating complication of open repair. Last, arthroscopic procedures involve less soft-tissue dissection, thus minimizing the risk of postoperative stiffness, therefore affording the patient longer postoperative immobilization during which healing may occur without excessive motion at the tendon-bone interface.

Earlier attempts at arthroscopic treatment of massive tears focused on débridement of tears that were considered irreparable.[15] Limited débridement, coupled with partial repair when appropriate, yielded satisfactory results in certain subsets of patients.[16,17] Gradually, there was a move toward arthroscopically assisted "mini-open" procedures where the arthroscope was used to perform decompression and tear characterization, followed by definitive repair performed through a limited open incision.[18] In the past 2 decades, increased understanding of tear pattern, tear mobilization through selective releases, and ideal repair constructs under minimal tension have occurred so that most massive rotator cuff tears can be definitively repaired arthroscopically.[2,18-25]

PATIENT EVALUATION AND SURGICAL INDICATIONS

Patient Presentation

Patients with massive rotator cuff tears often present with pain and decreased shoulder function. In the setting of a massive tear, the patient will often experience difficulty with all overhead activities, often to the point of limited ability to perform activities of daily living. It is important to elicit possible tear chronicity from the patient's history, as chronic tears tend to be retracted and more difficult to repair, resulting in less predictable long-term functional outcomes.

Physical Examination

Upon initial examination, a thorough cervical spine and upper extremity neurologic exam should be performed to rule out cervical spine disease as the cause of the patient's complaints. Once the examiner has localized the pathology to the shoulder, a variety of physical examination maneuvers can effectively characterize the rotator cuff tear. Infraspinatus involvement will result in weakness with external rotation when compared to the unaffected shoulder, and patients may demonstrate an external rotation lag sign, which is an inability to hold the arm in maximum external rotation.[26] This finding would suggest the presence of a posterosuperior tear. The hornblower's sign is a highly sensitive and specific test for a tear of the teres minor.[14] A positive sign is the lack of active external rotation when the arm is held in 90 degrees of abduction. Anterosuperior tears involving the subscapularis will result in variable amounts of weakness with resisted internal rotation, so several tests can be used to more objectively diagnose this tear pattern. With the affected arm in a "behind the back" position, the examiner can perform the lift-off test and the internal rotation lag sign.[27] A positive lift-off test occurs when the patient is unable to lift the affected arm away from the back, and this has been shown by electromyelographic data to correlate with a tear in the lower portion of the subscapularis tendon.[28] The internal rotation lag sign is positive when the patient cannot hold the arm away from the back after the examiner has passively placed it there. The belly-press test can be used to assess the superior portion of the subscapularis.[28] The examiner asks the patient to press on the belly with both hands, and a positive test is observed when the elbow fails to break the plane of the body. A recent report by Barth and colleagues introduced the bear-hug test, which they found to be more sensitive than the belly-press and lift-off tests in a series of patients with arthroscopically

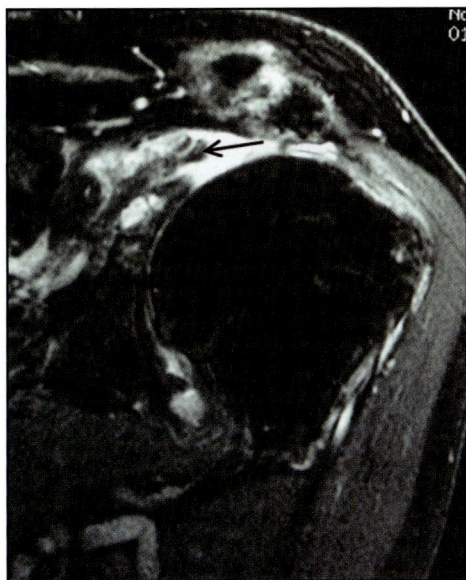

Figure 20-1. Coronal MRI demonstrating massive rotator cuff tear retracted to the level of the glenoid (arrow points to tendon edge). (Courtesy of Columbia University Center for Shoulder, Elbow and Sports Medicine.)

confirmed subscapularis tears.[29] This test is performed by placing the palm of the affected arm on the contralateral shoulder with the fingers fully extended. The test is positive when the patient is unable to hold this position while the examiner pulls on the forearm to exert an external rotation force across the affected shoulder.

Imaging

Massive rotator cuff tears can usually be diagnosed based on history and physical examination alone. Patients can be further evaluated with imaging studies to confirm the diagnosis and characterize the tear. Plain films are needed to evaluate the glenohumeral joint and are useful for detecting chronic changes, such as proximal humeral migration, rotator cuff arthropathy, or glenohumeral osteoarthritis. Cystic changes of the greater tuberosity on radiographs may support the diagnosis, as a recent magnetic resonance imaging (MRI) study showed that anterior greater tuberosity cysts were strongly associated with rotator cuff tears (p<0.001).[30]

Computed tomography (CT) scans are useful to assess rotator cuff atrophy and the degree of fatty infiltration,[31] but in North America, they have largely been replaced by MRI because it can detect these characteristics and additionally characterize the size and location of the tear (Figure 20-1).[8,32] Ultrasonography has been established as a sensitive and specific test in some institutions and is useful for dynamic evaluation of the shoulder during provocative maneuvers,[33-35] but it remains highly operator-dependent, and its widespread use has been hampered by an inferior ability to detect concomitant labral pathology and characterize complex tear patterns when compared with MRI.[36]

Surgical Indications, Contraindications, and Alternatives

The indications for arthroscopic treatment for massive rotator cuff tears include pain, poor shoulder function, and weakness that have failed to respond to nonoperative management. It is important to determine the patient's current and desired functional level so that realistic treatment goals can be established that are satisfactory to both the patient and surgeon.

There are few absolute contraindications to surgical treatment, and these include active infection, medical comorbidities that put the patient at undue risk during surgery, or patients who cannot comply with postoperative immobilization and rehabilitation. Relative contraindications include advanced rotator cuff arthropathy, manifest as proximal humeral migration and

Figure 20-3. Anatomy and portals marked on a right shoulder (A, anterior; P, posterior; AL, antero-lateral; PL, posterolateral; PC, per-cutaneous). (Courtesy of Columbia University Center for Shoulder, Elbow and Sports Medicine.)

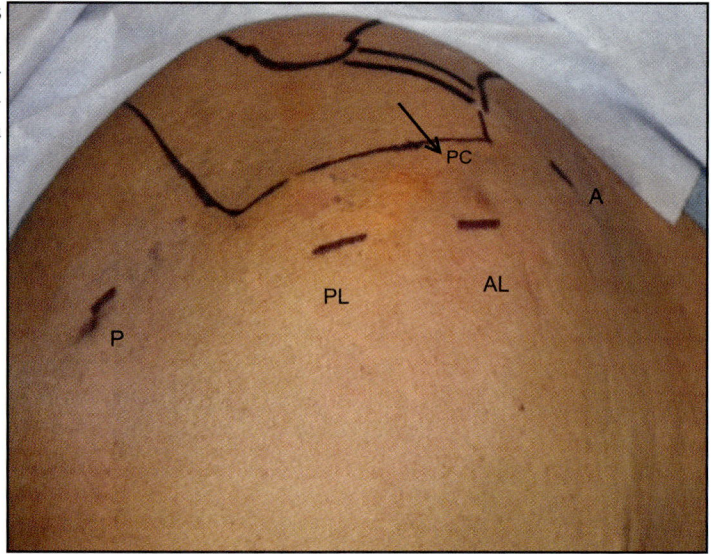

The posterior portal is used routinely to enter the glenohumeral joint. We prefer to attach the arm positioner after intra-articular placement has been confirmed by arthroscopic visualization. An anterior portal, just lateral to the coracoid, is created using an outside-in technique under direct visualization into the rotator interval. A systematic diagnostic arthroscopy is performed, concluding with assessment of the rotator cuff footprint from anteriorly to posteriorly. At this time, capsular adhesions to the rotator cuff over the superior glenoid should be identified and released as they will prevent anatomic mobilization of the rotator cuff to the footprint.

The arthroscope is placed into the subacromial space directly inferior to the acromion. The trocar is then swept medially to far laterally and anteriorly toward the coracoacromial (CA) ligament to break up subacromial and subdeltoid adhesions. An anterolateral portal is placed just anterior to the posterior aspect of the acromioclavicular joint (see Figure 20-3). This is established using a spinal needle for localization, and a fully threaded 7.0-mm cannula is placed to prevent fluid extravasation.

Initially, a 5.5-mm full-radius shaver is used to clear the subacromial bursal veil with the assistance of a cautery device as needed. A thorough bursectomy should be performed to provide excellent visualization and access to the rotator cuff tear. Bleeding is often encountered when resecting bursa or adhesions posteromedially; therefore, cautery may be more effective than a shaver in this area. It is often necessary to expose the scapular spine (Figure 20-4) as an important landmark for delineating the supraspinatus and infraspinatus tendons and to localize the suprascapular nerve (SSN) as it crosses beneath the spine, approximately 2.5 to 3 cm medial to the supraglenoid tubercle above the tendon and 1 cm medial to the posterior glenoid rim below.[43,44] Medial bursectomy is necessary for suture passing during repair. Also, working laterally under the deltoid fascia is necessary to release subdeltoid adhesions and create exposure for a double-row construct over the greater tuberosity. Care must be taken to avoid violating the deltoid fascia as bleeding, fluid extravasation, and functional deltoid complications may occur if the fascia is disrupted. Laterally, the greater tuberosity can impede instrumentation if it has become hypertrophic or if the humeral head has migrated superiorly. A burr can be used to recess the greater tuberosity excrescences to increase working space. We do not perform an acromioplasty or release the CA ligament in the setting of a massive rotator cuff tear to avoid iatrogenic anterosuperior humeral escape in the event of repair failure or an irreparable tear.

For massive rotator cuff tears, we also establish a posterolateral portal, in line with the posterior edge of the acromion and approximately 2 cm lateral, for viewing or instrumentation (see Figure 20-3). This portal allows greater access to the posterolateral shoulder, to facilitate assessment and repair of the posterior rotator cuff.

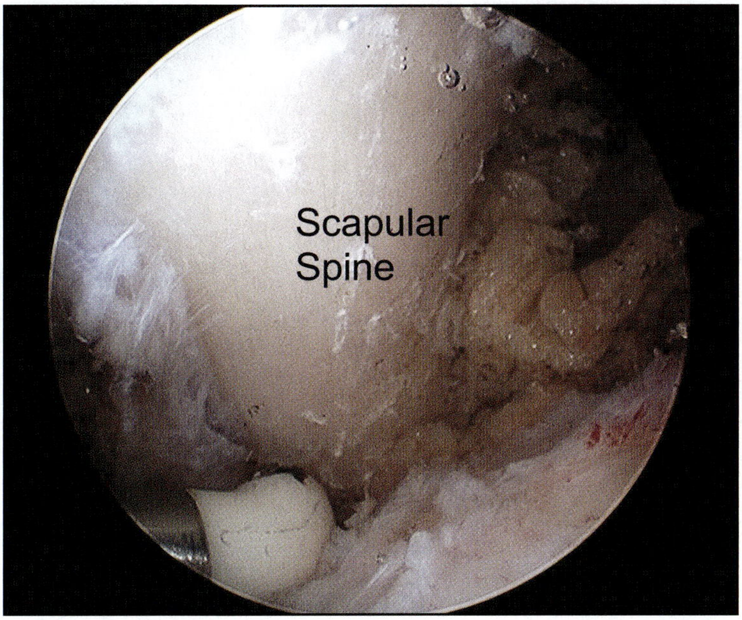

Figure 20-4. Arthroscopic view of a right shoulder demonstrating scapular spine. (Courtesy of Columbia University Center for Shoulder, Elbow and Sports Medicine.)

Assessment of Rotator Cuff Tear Characteristics

Proper visualization and portal placement allow for full assessment of tear size, number of tendons involved, degree of retraction, and tendon quality. This information, together with preoperative knowledge of muscle belly atrophy from sagittal MRI and a familiarity with basic tear geometry patterns as described by Burkhart et al,[19] will allow the surgeon to determine an optimal repair strategy.

The arthroscope can be placed in any of the established portals to view the cuff tear from posteriorly, laterally, or anteriorly. Typically, we start viewing posteriorly but often find that viewing from the anterolateral portal is best for identifying the tear pattern. Then, a tissue grasper is introduced through an alternate portal to assess mobility. Crescent tears have excellent medial to lateral mobility, while U-shaped tears have better anterior to posterior mobility. L- and reverse L-shaped tears also exhibit more mobility in the anterior to posterior direction. A chronic, retracted tear may not demonstrate excursion initially due to scarring, and alternative methods for mobilization will need to be used and are especially helpful when placing the lateral row of a double-row construct.

Techniques for Cuff Mobilization—Glenohumeral and Subacromial

Most massive rotator cuff tears can be mobilized by addressing glenohumeral and subacromial adhesions. First, intra-articular adhesions should be addressed. While viewing from a posterior portal, electrocautery can be introduced from either the anterior or the anterolateral subacromial portal (introduced through the massive cuff defect) and can be used to release all adhesions between the rotator cuff and the labrum, releasing the contracted capsule. Awareness of the SSN medially is essential to avoid iatrogenic damage.

Next, the arthroscope is redirected into the subacromial space, and superior cuff adhesions are released between the rotator cuff and the acromion. If the patient has had prior surgery, the retracted retorn cuff may be adherent to the undersurface of the acromion, and the tendons need to be carefully dissected free. In addition to a thorough bursectomy, rotator cuff tendon adhesions to the deltoid, acromion, or capsule should be released. It is necessary to carefully distinguish true rotator cuff tissue from bursa and adhesions.

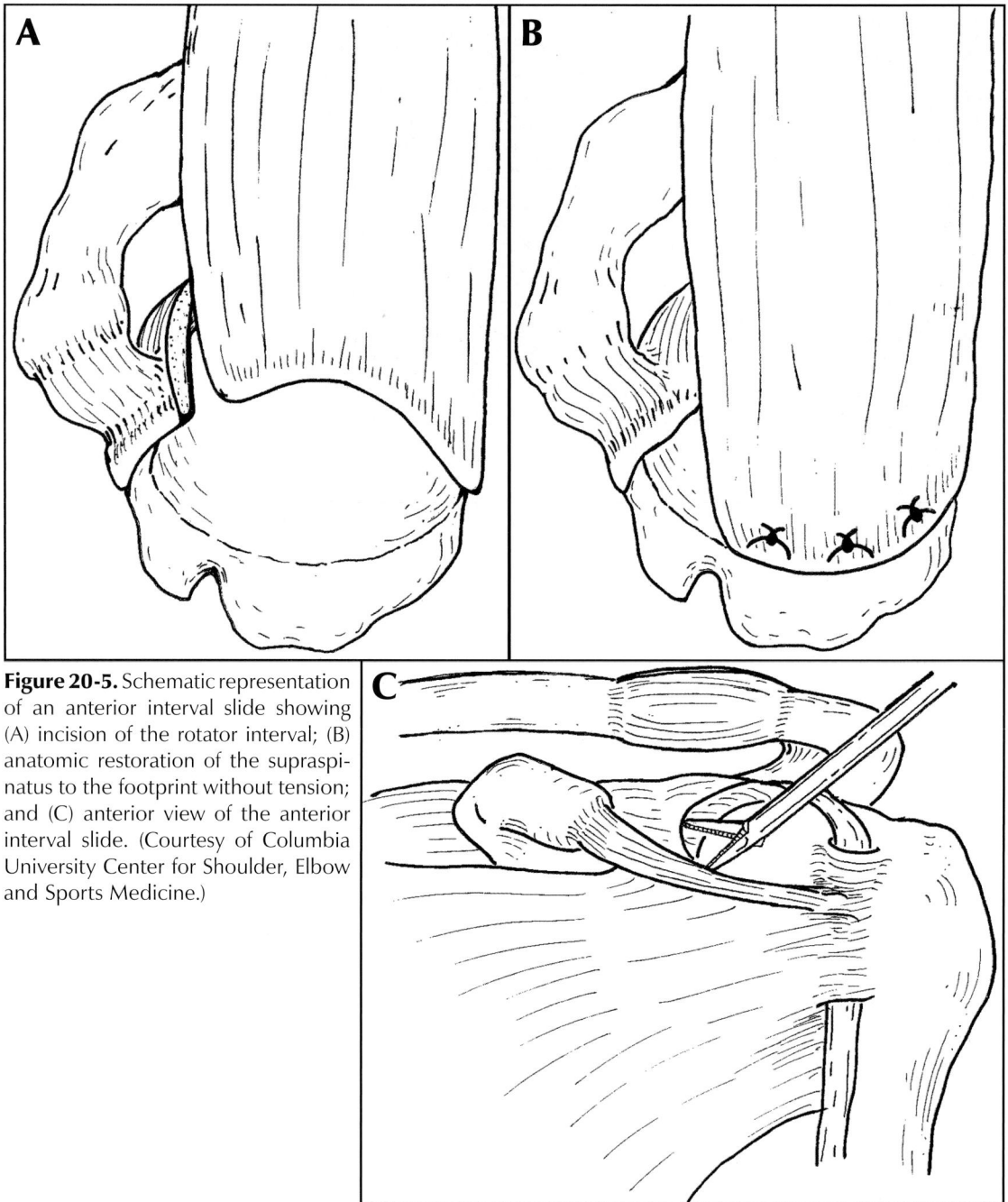

Figure 20-5. Schematic representation of an anterior interval slide showing (A) incision of the rotator interval; (B) anatomic restoration of the supraspinatus to the footprint without tension; and (C) anterior view of the anterior interval slide. (Courtesy of Columbia University Center for Shoulder, Elbow and Sports Medicine.)

Techniques for Cuff Mobilization—Anterior and Posterior Interval Slides

Once primary adhesions are released, cuff mobility is again reassessed. We prefer to view from one of the subacromial portals while using the tissue grasper through the other subacromial portal to pull the tendon edges laterally, posteriorly, and anteriorly.

If the rotator cuff still requires further mobilization, several release options exist. The anterior slide is an arthroscopic technique adapted by Tauro[45] modified from the open anterior interval slide originally described by Cordasco and Bigliani.[46] The anterior slide involves releasing the rotator interval just anterior to the leading edge of the supraspinatus toward the coracoid (Figure 20-5).

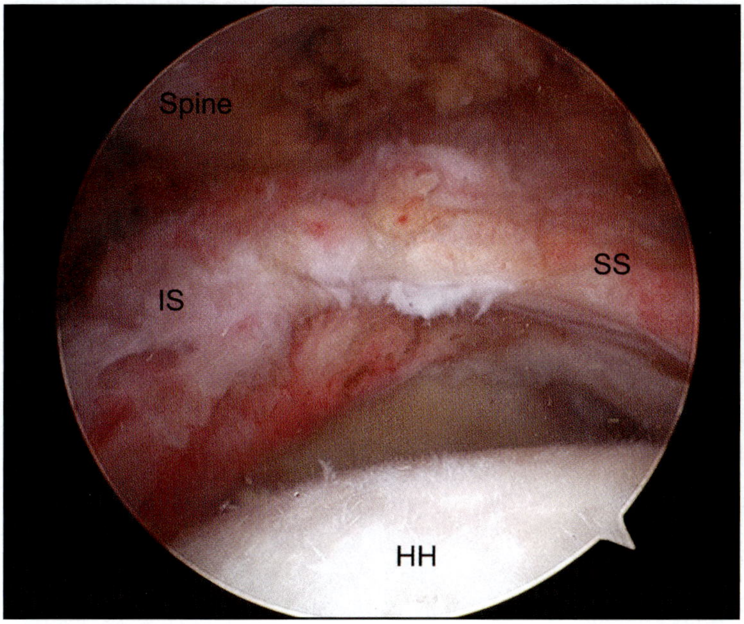

Figure 20-6. Arthroscopic view of a right shoulder from an anterolateral portal demonstrating retracted supraspinatus (SS), infraspinatus (IS) with the scapular spine delineating the 2 retracted tendons. The humeral head (HH) is seen below the tendons. (Courtesy of Columbia University Center for Shoulder, Elbow and Sports Medicine.)

This can be accomplished by viewing from the posterior or posterolateral portal and introducing arthroscopic scissors through the anterolateral portal. The supraspinatus tendon is released by dividing the rotator interval from the lateral free tendon edge medially toward the base of the coracoid. The coracohumeral ligament can be cut or released directly off of the coracoid, as it is often contracted in chronic massive tears. Release of the coracohumeral ligament can be combined with an anterior slide and is referred to as an anterior slide in continuity.[47] This should provide approximately 1 to 2 cm of lateral excursion of the supraspinatus.[25]

A posterior slide technique is also a powerful option to gain tendon excursion. The arthroscopic technique was adapted from the open technique described by Codd and Flatow.[48] For this technique, exposure of the scapular spine is essential. The spine delineates the limits of the supraspinatus and infraspinatus tendons, which can be difficult to distinguish in chronic scarred and retracted tears (Figure 20-6). While viewing from a lateral portal, tension may be held on the tendon using a tissue grasper or traction sutures. Arthroscopic scissors are introduced and kept above the glenoid rim, carefully dividing the supraspinatus and infraspinatus tendons from lateral to medial, keeping in mind that the SSN travels underneath the base of the scapular spine 1 cm medial to the glenoid rim (Figure 20-7). Alone, this can provide enough mobility to bring the tendon edges to the footprint with much less tension. With a combined double interval release (anterior and posterior slide releases), tendon excursion can improve up to 3 to 5 cm (Figure 20-8).

Techniques for Repair

After releases and mobilization are satisfactory, a strategy for suture and anchor placement can be made. Massive rotator cuff tears often require tendon-to-tendon suture techniques and adjustment in the pattern of fixation techniques.

The footprint should be débrided down to bleeding bone in order to enhance tendon healing and is helpful in defining cuff tendon edges.

Crescent-shaped tears usually have good medial to lateral mobility and can be brought back to the footprint by grasping the tendon edges and pulling over laterally through the anterolateral portal. We use a double-row transosseous equivalent suture bridge technique, as biomechanical studies have shown that this construct creates greater tendon-to-bone contact surface area, pressure, and strength of construct.[49-52] To date, long-term studies have not shown a clear advantage of a

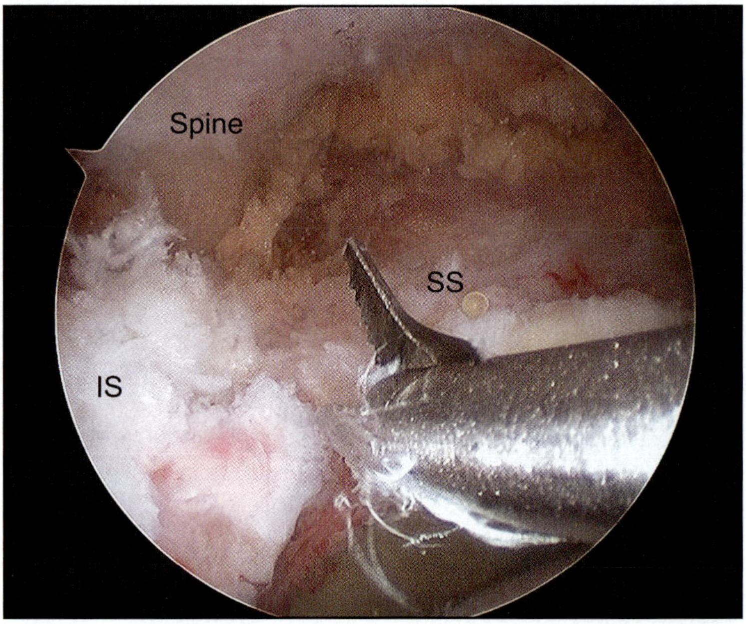

Figure 20-7. Arthroscopic view of a right shoulder from a posterolateral portal with an arthroscopic scissors (from the anterolateral portal) incising the scarred posterior interval between the supraspinatus (SS) and the infraspinatus (IS) using the scapular spine as the road-map. (Courtesy of Columbia University Center for Shoulder, Elbow and Sports Medicine.)

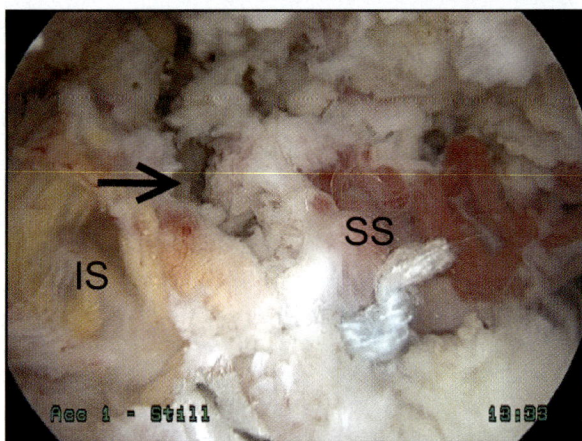

Figure 20-8. Arthroscopic view of a right shoulder from the anterolateral portal following the posterior interval slide. The previously retracted and "irreparable" supraspinatus (SS) and infraspinatus (IS) have been anatomically repaired to the footprint without tension. The arrow delineates the incised interval between the 2 tendons. (Courtesy of Columbia University Center for Shoulder, Elbow and Sports Medicine.)

double-row versus single-row construct in clinical outcomes,[53-56] but we believe that the transosseous suture bridge technique provides the best opportunity for rotator cuff footprint restoration and stability for healing.

For placement of the anchors, the arm is slightly abducted to introduce the anchor at a 45-degree angle. The shoulder is externally rotated for placement more anteriorly in the footprint and is internally rotated for more posterior placement. We use a percutaneous anchor technique. A spinal needle inserted just lateral to the acromion is used for localization and approach angle (Figure 20-9). A percutaneous stab incision is made in line with the fibers of the deltoid. The bone awl and then anchor are introduced though the percutaneous incision. For the medial row, we routinely use 4.5-mm Peek FT (fully threaded) suture anchors (Arthrex, Naples, FL) or 5.5 metal FT anchors (Arthrex) in the rare case of poor bone quality. The anchor is placed just lateral to the articular edge, usually anterior to posterior. We place all of the medial row anchors prior to suture passing and take the sutures out posteriorly for individual management. Ideally, anchors are spaced approximately 5 to 8 mm apart. Depending on our repair strategy, we usually remove 1 of the 2 sutures in the double-loaded anchor, leaving each anchor with alternating colors for easier identification and suture management (Figure 20-10).

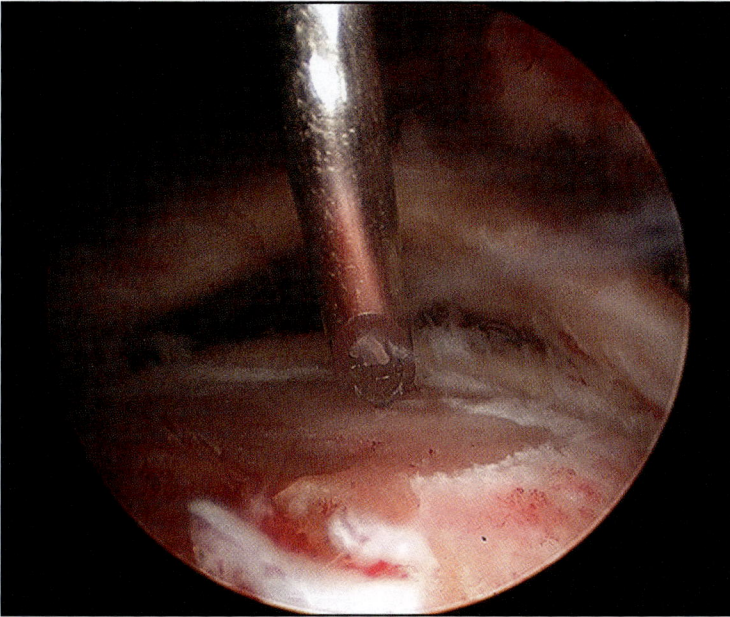

Figure 20-9. Arthroscopic view of a right shoulder from anterolateral portal showing percutaneous localization of the medial anchor placement with a spinal needle. (Courtesy of Columbia University Center for Shoulder, Elbow and Sports Medicine.)

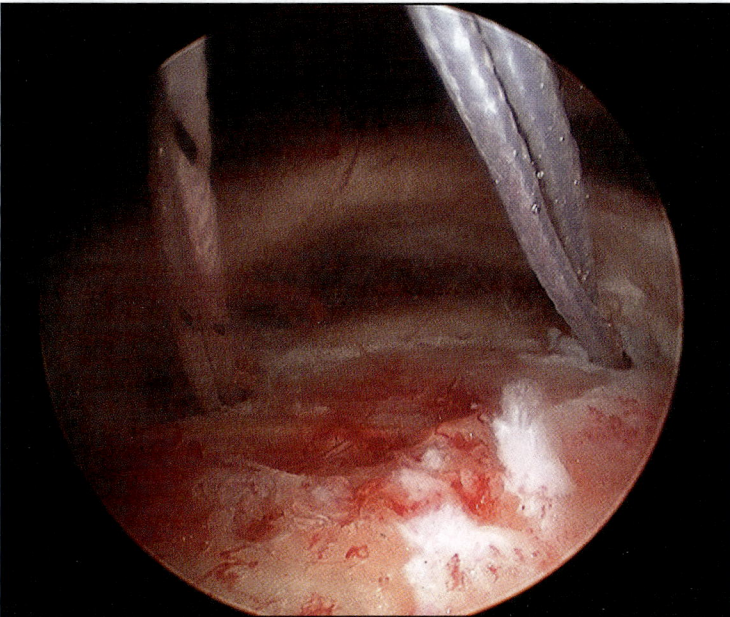

Figure 20-10. Arthroscopic view of a right shoulder from anterolateral portal showing 2 medial row suture anchors placed with the second suture pair removed from each. (Courtesy of Columbia University Center for Shoulder, Elbow and Sports Medicine.)

Options for suture passage include antegrade or retrograde devices. We often use an antegrade suture passing device, such as the Scorpion (Arthrex) or the RP 360 (Stryker, Mahwah, NJ) from the lateral portal that provides the best angle, while viewing from the other subacromial portal or posterior portal. The tendon edge may be grasped and pulled toward the footprint to expose the tendon for suture placement and anatomic approximation. The sutures are passed in a mattress fashion, from anterior to posterior approximately 5- to 10-mm apart and approximately 14- to 16-mm medially from the tendon edge. After each set of sutures is passed, they are taken out through the anterior portal and cannula using a loop grasper.

Figure 20-11. Arthroscopic view of a right shoulder from posterior portal showing a posteromedial striped white and black suture pair temporarily parked in anterior cannula after knot tying. (Courtesy of Columbia University Center for Shoulder, Elbow and Sports Medicine.)

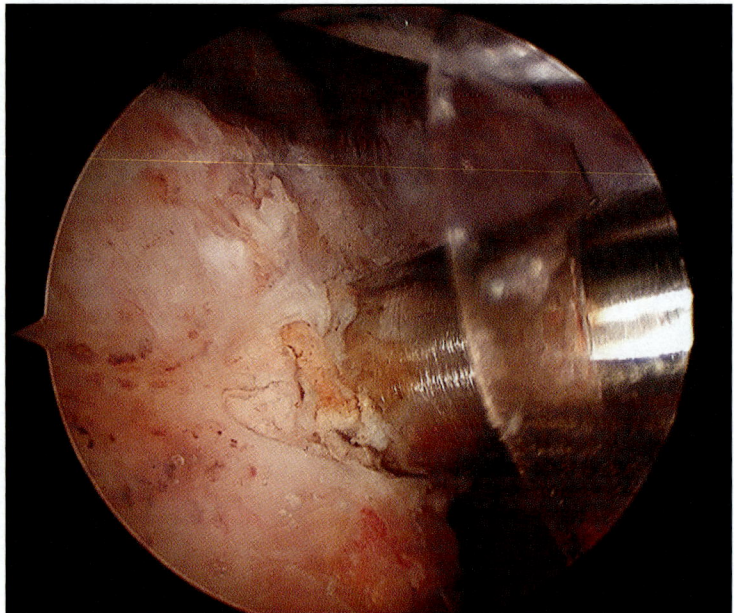

Figure 20-12. Arthroscopic view of a right shoulder from posterior portal showing awl on lateral proximal greater tuberosity in preparation of making a tunnel for lateral row anchor. (Courtesy of Columbia University Center for Shoulder, Elbow and Sports Medicine.)

One set of sutures is then retrieved through the lateral cannula, and a knot is tied using static half hitches. Sutures are not cut at this time. After the knot is tied, the suture ends are taken out through an alternate portal (Figure 20-11). This is repeated for each suture set, creating a horizontal mattress construct, which should perform the majority of tendon reduction to the footprint. To complete the suture bridge technique, one suture from each set is retrieved using the loop grasper out of a lateral cannula. These are threaded through the eyelet tip of the 4.75-mm Swivel Lock or 4.5-mm Push Lock anchor (Arthrex). While viewing from the other lateral portal, an optimal position for the double-row anchor is chosen over the lateral greater tuberosity, remembering to plan for 2 anchors—1 anterior and 1 posterior. The instrumenting cannula is held over the intended site of the lateral row anchor, and the bed is prepared with the awl (Figure 20-12).

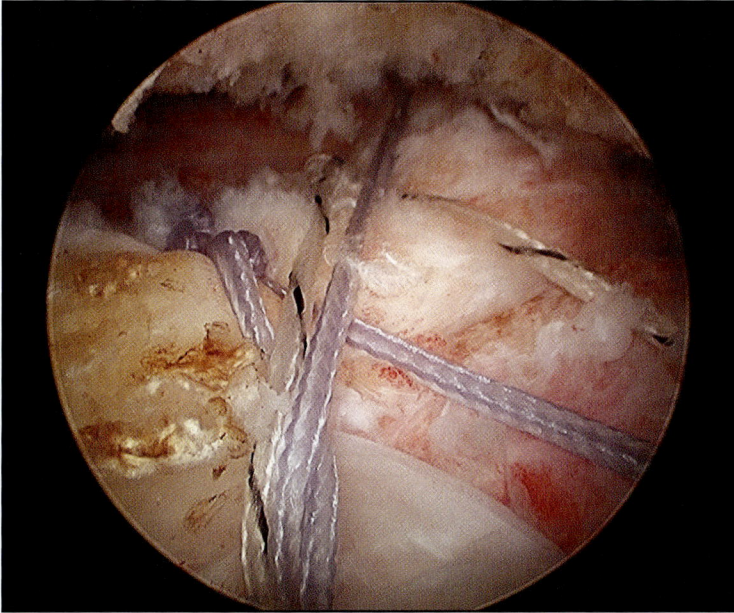

Figure 20-13. Arthroscopic view of a right shoulder from anterolateral portal showing double-row suture bridge construct in this case with 3 medial row anchors given the massive nature of the tear. (Courtesy of Columbia University Center for Shoulder, Elbow and Sports Medicine.)

The anchor is placed, and each suture is evenly tensioned as it passes through the lateral anchor from its respective medial knot. After tensioning the suture, ends are cut at the anchor edge. The remaining sutures from each set are retrieved, and this is repeated. After completion, the tendon should be well-reduced to the footprint in a secure fashion with good apposition of tendon to bone (Figure 20-13).

U-shaped tears are more difficult to manage. Their apex is often retracted farther medially, and there is less medial-to-lateral mobility. Burkhart et al rediscovered the concept of margin convergence,[11] which McLaughlin had described in the 1950s. The tendons are repaired in a side-to-side fashion with free sutures, bringing the longitudinal component of the tear together medially to laterally to transform a U-shaped tear to a crescent-type tear that can be managed with the above techniques (Figure 20-14). This decreases strain on the repair and allows for the repair of medially extending tears that previously may have appeared irreparable.[11]

Passing the sutures through the tendon can be achieved with an antegrade suture passer, or if the space is limited or too medial for an acceptable access from a lateral portal, we also use Suture Lasso retrograde passers (Arthrex). These are oriented in a 90-, 45-, or 25-degree left or right angle. Most often, the 90-degree angle passer can be used through the anterior or posterior portal. Or, in the case of a medially retracted tear, the Banana Suture Lasso (Arthrex) can be used percutaneously through Nevaiser's portal for optimal suture placement. The suture to be passed is taken out through a lateral portal, and the suture lasso is passed through the tendon and wire loop retrieved through the same lateral portal. The suture is passed through the wire loop outside and pulled back in and through the tendon in a retrograde fashion.

L- and reverse L-shaped tears should be repaired using a side-to-side technique for the longitudinal component and then directly to the footprint for the transverse component. L-shaped tears have a split between the supraspinatus and infraspinatus and detachment off the greater tuberosity (Figure 20-15). The longitudinal component of a reverse L-shaped tear extends between the supraspinatus and rotator interval, while the leading edge of the supraspinatus is detached off the greater tuberosity. It is important to repair this leading edge. Chronic tears may be retracted and rotated, changing the appearance of an L-shape to a U-type shape. Therefore, it is important to fully assess both the anterior and posterior leaflets of the tear for difference in mobility.

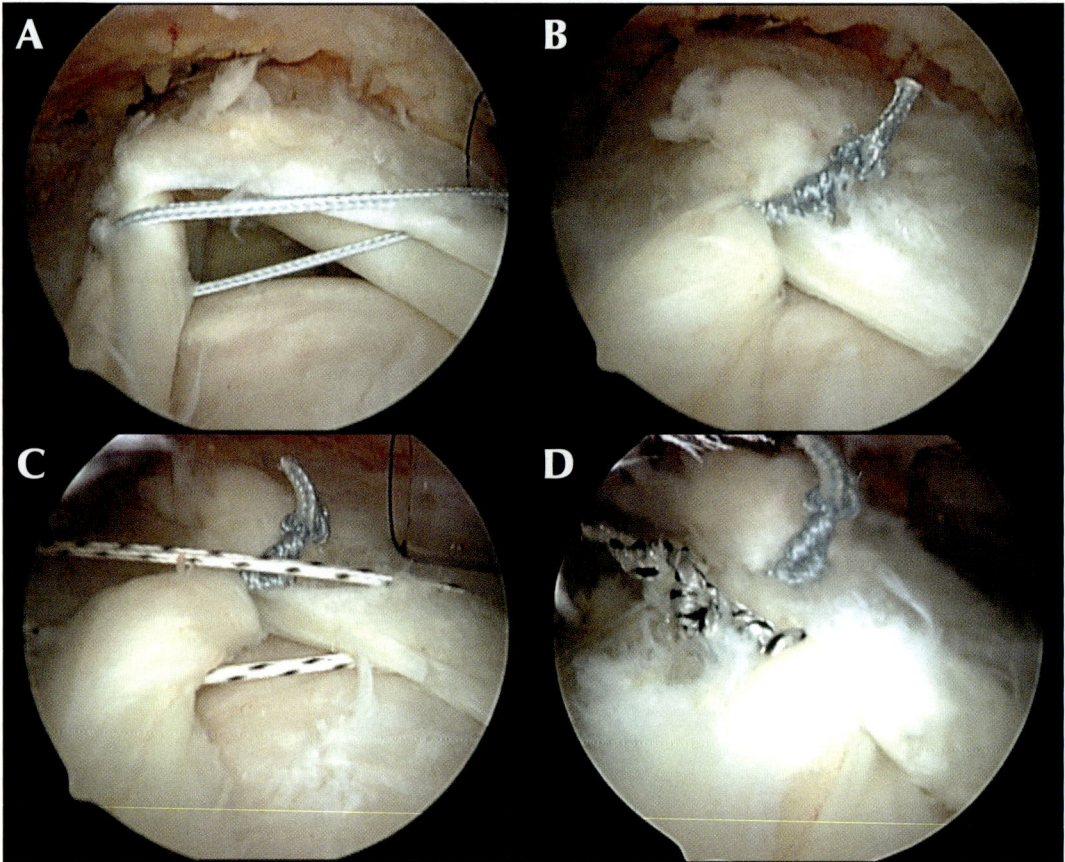

Figure 20-14. Arthroscopic view of a right shoulder from anterolateral portal showing (A) first side-to-side blue #2 nonabsorbable suture is passed; (B) first side-to-side suture is tied, dramatically decreasing the size of the tear; (C) second side-to-side (striped white and black) suture is passed; and (D) second suture is tied, dramatically decreasing the size of the massive tear. (Courtesy of Columbia University Center for Shoulder, Elbow and Sports Medicine.)

Figure 20-15. Arthroscopic view of a right shoulder from anterolateral portal showing a massive L-shaped tear after the supraspinatus (SS) has been anatomically restored to the footprint. Note that the infraspinatus (IS) has likewise been repaired anatomically, and 2 side-to-side sutures have been placed and are ready for tying. (Courtesy of Columbia University Center for Shoulder, Elbow and Sports Medicine.)

Figure 20-16. Arthroscopic view of a right shoulder from posterior glenohumeral portal showing the "synovitis sign"— the previously medially displaced rotator cuff has been anatomically restored laterally, thereby exposing synovitis on the undersurface of the rotator cuff. (Courtesy of Columbia University Center for Shoulder, Elbow and Sports Medicine.)

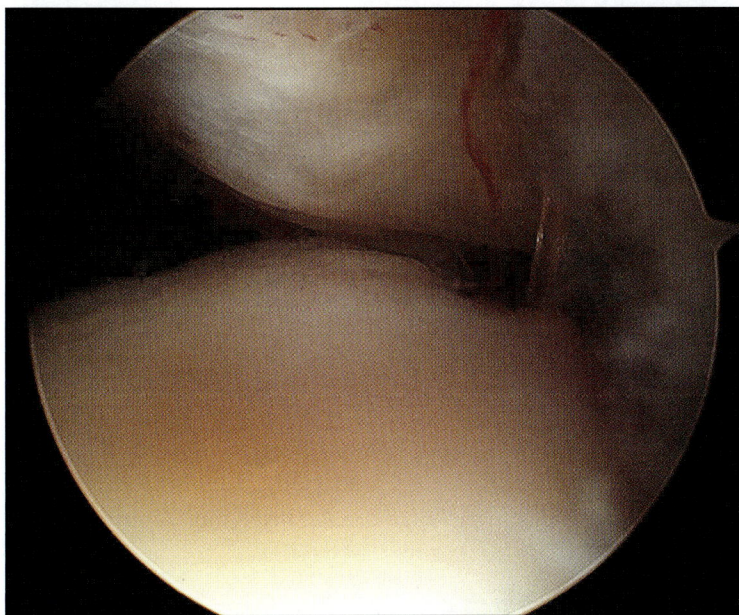

Figure 20-17. Arthroscopic view of a right shoulder from posterior glenohumeral portal showing the anatomic restoration of the rotator cuff to the footprint after ablation of the synovitis. (Courtesy of Columbia University Center for Shoulder, Elbow and Sports Medicine.)

After repair of the tendons is completed, synovitis under the rotator cuff is typically seen in the glenohumeral joint (Figure 20-16). This ensures that the rotator cuff tendons have been restored to the anatomical footprint, as the synovitis was initially hidden medially under the retracted tear. Cautery can be used to ablate the synovitis, demonstrating the anatomic repair of the rotator cuff to the footprint (Figure 20-17).

Retracted and immobile massive tears are the most difficult to define and repair. They often cannot be fully mobilized to the full extent of the footprint and should be repaired medially within 10 mm of the footprint if anatomical reduction is not possible, rather than creating an overtensioned repair construct. A combination of the outlined mobilization techniques should be used to prepare the cuff tear for repair as needed. The number of anchors, suture placement and management, and complexity of tendon reduction to footprint is challenging. This is where balancing force couples is extremely important. If mobilization techniques have been exhausted or tendon quality is poor, a partial repair is acceptable and is preferable to no repair. Restoration of the transverse force couple can provide a functional shoulder if the subscapularis and infraspinatus can both be repaired.[57] Despite all-arthroscopic options, one should be prepared to convert to an open approach if necessary in cases of extended operative time, poor visualization precluding the use of proper repair techniques, or circumstances affecting patient safety.

POSTOPERATIVE MANAGEMENT AND REHABILITATION

Postoperatively, we maintain the patient in a pillow abduction sling. Physical therapy is not started until 6 weeks postoperatively, although patients do perform elbow, wrist, and hand range of motion immediately. Small arc pendulums are allowed. At 6 weeks postoperatively, we begin passive- and active-assisted range of motion with limits based upon the tear pattern and repair. The patient may be progressed to active range of motion in the supine position from 6 to 12 weeks with progression to active motion in the upright position and increased range of motion as symptoms allow. Light strengthening is started at 8 to 12 weeks (Table 20-1).

PEARLS AND PITFALLS

- Establish good visualization and careful portal placement.
- Multiple portals are needed. Be prepared to view from several different portals.
- Expose the scapular spine as a landmark to delineate the supraspinatus and infraspinatus and location of the SSN.
- Do not perform an acromioplasty or CA ligament release, even if it helps visualization, in order to avoid anterosuperior escape if repair fails or is irreparable.
- Always assess the tear configuration before and after mobilization and releases and from multiple viewing portals.
- Anterior work should be approached first, before swelling impedes visualization. Usual order of surgical technique may need to be adjusted for the massive tear.
- Interval slides can be used to increase tendon excursion and mobility in complex retracted tears.
- Knowing how to use different suture passing instruments can assist in placing sutures properly with limited access.
- Do not overtension tendon repairs to footprint as it will increase the chance of repair failure.

REFERENCES

1. Post M, Silver R, Singh M. Rotator cuff tear. Diagnosis and treatment. *Clin Orthop Relat Res*. 1983;173:78-91.
2. Burkhart SS. Arthroscopic treatment of massive rotator cuff tears. *Clin Orthop Relat Res*. 2001;390:107-118.
3. Zumstein MA, Jost B, Hempel J, Hodler J, Gerber C. The clinical and structural long-term results of open repair of massive tears of the rotator cuff. *J Bone Joint Surg Am*. 2008;90(11):2423-2431.
4. Warner JJ, Higgins L, Parsons IM, Dowdy P. Diagnosis and treatment of anterosuperior rotator cuff tears. *J Shoulder Elbow Surg*. 2001;10(1):37-46.
5. Bedi A, Dines J, Warren RF, Dines DM. Massive tears of the rotator cuff. *J Bone Joint Surg Am*. 4;92(9):1894-1908.
6. Ellman H, Hanker G, Bayer M. Repair of the rotator cuff. End-result study of factors influencing reconstruction. *J Bone Joint Surg Am*. 1986;68(8):1136-1144.
7. Ellman H, Kay SP, Wirth M. Arthroscopic treatment of full-thickness rotator cuff tears: 2- to 7-year follow-up study. *Arthroscopy*. 1993;9(2):195-200.

TABLE 20-1. OUTCOMES

Authors and Year	# of Shoulders	Average Age (Range)	Tear Characteristics	Techniques	Average Follow-up in Months (Range)	Outcomes
Lee et al, 2007[58]	71	63 (36 to 86)	21 of 71 tears were massive (>5 cm)	Arthroscopic suture anchor repair, 72% had anterior or posterior interval releases	12 (0.25 to 240)	For massive tears: significant (p<0.01) improvement in ASES, Constant, and Visual Analog Pain Scale scores; modest trends of improvement in strength and ROM (p value 0.11 to 0.38)
Burkhart et al, 2007[39]	22	66.5	22 massive tears with Goutallier stage 3 and 4 fatty degeneration, average	Arthroscopic repair, all single-row, selective releases	39.3 (24 to 60)	Clinical improvement based on ROM, UCLA, and Constant scores in all patients (17 of 17) with fatty degeneration 50% to 75%; improvement in only 2 of 5 patients with fatty degeneration >75%
Lo and Burkhart, 2004[25]	9	67.2	9 massive (>5 cm) retracted immobile tears	All tears required arthroscopic interval slide (anterior, posterior, or both), complete repair in 4 patients, partial repair in 5 patients	17 (10 to 24)	8 of 9 patients satisfied with procedure; UCLA score improved from 10 to 28.3; significant improvements in active FE/ER and strength
Lo and Burkhart, 2004[59]	14	57.9	11 massive (>5 cm) 1 large (3 to 5 cm) 2 medium (2 to 3 cm)	Arthroscopic revision of previous failed rotator cuff repairs	24.3	13 of 14 patients satisfied with procedure; UCLA score improved from 13 to 29; active FE improved from 120 to 153 degrees
Galatz et al, 2004[24]	18	61 (50 to 87)	All involved 2 or more tendons, 15 tears (>3 cm)	Arthroscopic repair, 10 of 18 had biceps tenotomy	36 (24 to 42)	All patients satisfied with procedure although 17 of 18 had recurrent tears by ultrasound; ASES score improved from 48 preop to 80 at 24 months postop; best results seen at 1 year follow-up; ASES scores deteriorated with longer follow-up
Jones and Savoie, 2003[60]	50	61 (41 to 76)	13 massive (>5 cm) 37 large (3 to 5 cm)	Arthroscopic repair with releases	32 (12 to 63)	88% good or excellent outcomes; no significant difference in outcomes for massive and large tear subgroups
Bennett, 2003[21]	37	67.1	37 massive (>5 cm) (29 anterosuperior, 8 posterosuperior)	Arthroscopic repair with capsular release, margin convergence	38 (24 to 48)	95% patients satisfied with procedure; ASES improved from 29 to 85 for anterosuperior tears and from 23 to 77 for posterosuperior tears
Bittar, 2002[20]	74	67 (54 to 82)	74 massive (>5 cm) retracted tears	Arthroscopic repair	60 minimum	By UCLA rating scale: 38% excellent, 45% good, 9% fair, 8% poor results
Burkhart, 2001[2]	13	N/A	13 massive (>5 cm) (2 crescent, 11 U-shaped)	Arthroscopic repair: margin convergence for U-shaped tears, direct repair to bone for crescent	42 (24 to 60)	UCLA improved from 14 to 30; good or excellent outcomes in 92%; massive tears did just as well as smaller tears

NA = not available; ASES = American Shoulder and Elbow Surgeons; ROM = range of motion; FE = forward elevation; ER = external rotation

8.   Harryman DT 2nd, Hettrich CM, Smith KL, Campbell B, Sidles JA, Matsen FA 3rd. A prospective multipractice investigation of patients with full-thickness rotator cuff tears: the importance of comorbidities, practice, and other covariables on self-assessed shoulder function and health status. *J Bone Joint Surg Am*. 2003;85-A(4):690-696.

9.   Warner JJ. Management of massive irreparable rotator cuff tears: the role of tendon transfer. *Instr Course Lect*. 2001;50:63-71.

10.   Burkhart SS. Reconciling the paradox of rotator cuff repair versus débridement: a unified biomechanical rationale for the treatment of rotator cuff tears. *Arthroscopy*. 1994;10(1):4-19.

11.   Burkhart SS, Athanasiou KA, Wirth MA. Margin convergence: a method of reducing strain in massive rotator cuff tears. *Arthroscopy*. 1996;12(3):335-338.

12.   Bigliani LU, Cordasco FA, McIlveen SJ, Musso ES. Operative treatment of failed repairs of the rotator cuff. *J Bone Joint Surg Am*. 1992;74(10):1505-1515.

13.   Rokito AS, Cuomo F, Gallagher MA, Zuckerman JD. Long-term functional outcome of repair of large and massive chronic tears of the rotator cuff. *J Bone Joint Surg Am*. 1999;81(7):991-997.

14.   Gerber C, Fuchs B, Hodler J. The results of repair of massive tears of the rotator cuff. *J Bone Joint Surg Am*. 2000;82(4):505-515.

15.   Rockwood CA Jr, Williams GR Jr, Burkhead WZ Jr. Débridement of degenerative, irreparable lesions of the rotator cuff. *J Bone Joint Surg Am*. 1995;77(6):857-866.

16.   Burkhart SS. Arthroscopic treatment of massive rotator cuff tears. Clinical results and biomechanical rationale. *Clin Orthop Relat Res*. 1991(267):45-56.

17.   Gartsman GM. Massive, irreparable tears of the rotator cuff. Results of operative débridement and subacromial decompression. *J Bone Joint Surg Am*. 1997;79(5):715-721.

18.   Yamaguchi K, Ball CM, Galatz LM. Arthroscopic rotator cuff repair: transition from mini-open to all-arthroscopic. *Clin Orthop Relat Res*. 2001(390):83-94.

19.   Burkhart SS, Danaceau SM, Pearce CE Jr. Arthroscopic rotator cuff repair: analysis of results by tear size and by repair technique-margin convergence versus direct tendon-to-bone repair. *Arthroscopy*. 2001;17(9):905-912.

20.   Bittar ES. Arthroscopic management of massive rotator cuff tears. *Arthroscopy*. 2002;18(9 Suppl 2):104-106.

21.   Bennett WF. Arthroscopic repair of massive rotator cuff tears: a prospective cohort with 2- to 4-year follow-up. *Arthroscopy*. 2003;19(4):380-390.

22.   Yamaguchi K, Levine WN, Marra G, Galatz LM, Klepps S, Flatow EL. Transitioning to arthroscopic rotator cuff repair: the pros and cons. *Instr Course Lect*. 2003;52:81-92.

23.   Ahmad CS, Levine WN, Bigliani LU. Arthroscopic rotator cuff repair. *Orthopedics*. 2004;27(6):570-574.

24.   Galatz LM, Ball CM, Teefey SA, Middleton WD, Yamaguchi K. The outcome and repair integrity of completely arthroscopically repaired large and massive rotator cuff tears. *J Bone Joint Surg Am*. 2004;86-A(2):219-224.

25.   Lo IK, Burkhart SS. Arthroscopic repair of massive, contracted, immobile rotator cuff tears using single and double interval slides: technique and preliminary results. *Arthroscopy*. 2004;20(1):22-33.

26.   Hertel R, Ballmer FT, Lombert SM, Gerber C. Lag signs in the diagnosis of rotator cuff rupture. *J Shoulder Elbow Surg*. 1996;5(4):307-313.

27.   Gerber C, Krushell RJ. Isolated rupture of the tendon of the subscapularis muscle. Clinical features in 16 cases. *J Bone Joint Surg Br*. 1991;73(3):389-394.

28.   Tokish JM, Decker MJ, Ellis HB, Torry MR, Hawkins RJ. The belly-press test for the physical examination of the subscapularis muscle: electromyographic validation and comparison to the lift-off test. *J Shoulder Elbow Surg*. 2003;12(5):427-430.

29.   Barth JR, Burkhart SS, De Beer JF. The bear-hug test: a new and sensitive test for diagnosing a subscapularis tear. *Arthroscopy*. 2006;22(10):1076-1084.

30.   Fritz LB, Ouellette HA, O'Hanley TA, Kassarjian A, Palmer WE. Cystic changes at supraspinatus and infraspinatus tendon insertion sites: association with age and rotator cuff disorders in 238 patients. *Radiology*. 2007;244(1):239-248.

31.   Goutallier D, Postel JM, Bernageau J, Lavau L, Voisin MC. Fatty muscle degeneration in cuff ruptures. Pre- and postoperative evaluation by CT scan. *Clin Orthop Relat Res*. 1994;304:78-83.

32.   Yoo JC, Ahn JH, Yang JH, Koh KH, Choi SH, Yoon YC. Correlation of arthroscopic repairability of large to massive rotator cuff tears with preoperative magnetic resonance imaging scans. *Arthroscopy*. 2009;25(6):573-582.

33.   Teefey SA, Hasan SA, Middleton WD, Patel M, Wright RW, Yamaguchi K. Ultrasonography of the rotator cuff. A comparison of ultrasonographic and arthroscopic findings in one hundred consecutive cases. *J Bone Joint Surg Am*. 2000;82(4):498-504.

34.   Teefey SA, Middleton WD, Bauer GS, Hildebolt CF, Yamaguchi K. Sonographic differences in the appearance of acute and chronic full-thickness rotator cuff tears. *J Ultrasound Med*. 2000;19(6):377-378; quiz 383.

35.   Middleton WD, Teefey SA, Yamaguchi K. Sonography of the rotator cuff: analysis of interobserver variability. *AJR Am J Roentgenol*. 2004;183(5):1465-1468.

36.   Teefey SA, Rubin DA, Middleton WD, Hildebolt CF, Leibold RA, Yamaguchi K. Detection and quantification of rotator cuff tears. Comparison of ultrasonographic, magnetic resonance imaging, and arthroscopic findings in seventy-one consecutive cases. *J Bone Joint Surg Am*. 2004;86-A(4):708-716.

37. Neer CS 2nd, Craig EV, Fukuda H. Cuff-tear arthropathy. *J Bone Joint Surg Am.* 1983;65(9):1232-1244.

38. Goutallier D, Postel JM, Gleyze P, Leguilloux P, Van Driessche S. Influence of cuff muscle fatty degeneration on anatomic and functional outcomes after simple suture of full-thickness tears. *J Shoulder Elbow Surg.* 2003;12(6):550-554.

39. Burkhart SS, Barth JR, Richards DP, Zlatkin MB, Larsen M. Arthroscopic repair of massive rotator cuff tears with stage 3 and 4 fatty degeneration. *Arthroscopy.* 2007;23(4):347-354.

40. Bokor DJ, Hawkins RJ, Huckell GH, Angelo RL, Schickendantz MS. Results of nonoperative management of full-thickness tears of the rotator cuff. *Clin Orthop Relat Res.* 1993;294:103-110.

41. Green A. Chronic massive rotator cuff tears: evaluation and management. *J Am Acad Orthop Surg.* 2003;11(5):321-331.

42. Lee HW. Hypotensive and bradycardic episodes in the sitting position during shoulder arthroscopy using interscalene block: can those be alerted? *Korean J Anesthesiol.* 2010;58(1):1-3.

43. Bigliani LU, Dalsey RM, McCann PD, April EW. An anatomical study of the suprascapular nerve. *Arthroscopy.* 1990;6(4):301-305.

44. Warner JP, Krushell RJ, Masquelet A, Gerber C. Anatomy and relationships of the suprascapular nerve: anatomical constraints to mobilization of the supraspinatus and infraspinatus muscles in the management of massive rotator-cuff tears. *J Bone Joint Surg Am.* 1992;74(1):36-45.

45. Tauro JC. Arthroscopic "interval slide" in the repair of large rotator cuff tears. *Arthroscopy.* 1999;15(5):527-530.

46. Cordasco FA, Bigliani LU. The rotator cuff. Large and massive tears. Technique of open repair. *Orthop Clin North Am.* 1997;28(2):179-193.

47. Edwards TB, Walch G, Sirveaux F, et al. Repair of tears of the subscapularis. Surgical technique. *J Bone Joint Surg Am.* 2006;88 Suppl 1 Pt 1:1-10.

48. Codd T, Flatow EL. Anterior acromioplasty, tendon mobilization, and direct repair of massive rotator cuff tears. In: Burkhead W, ed. *Rotator Cuff Disorders.* Baltimore, MD: Williams and Wilkins; 1996:323-334.

49. Ahmad CS, Stewart AM, Izquierdo R, Bigliani LU. Tendon-bone interface motion in transosseous suture and suture anchor rotator cuff repair techniques. *Am J Sports Med.* 2005;33(11):1667-1671.

50. Park MC, ElAttrache NS, Tibone JE, Ahmad CS, Jun BJ, Lee TQ. Part I: footprint contact characteristics for a transosseous-equivalent rotator cuff repair technique compared with a double-row repair technique. *J Shoulder Elbow Surg.* 2007;16(4):461-468.

51. Park MC, Tibone JE, ElAttrache NS, Ahmad CS, Jun BJ, Lee TQ. Part II: biomechanical assessment for a footprint-restoring transosseous-equivalent rotator cuff repair technique compared with a double-row repair technique. *J Shoulder Elbow Surg.* 2007;16(4):469-476.

52. Park MC, Cadet ER, Levine WN, Bigliani LU, Ahmad CS. Tendon-to-bone pressure distributions at a repaired rotator cuff footprint using transosseous suture and suture anchor fixation techniques. *Am J Sports Med.* 2005;33(8):1154-1159.

53. Grasso A, Milano G, Salvatore M, Falcone G, Deriu L, Fabbriciani C. Single-row versus double-row arthroscopic rotator cuff repair: a prospective randomized clinical study. *Arthroscopy.* 2009;25(1):4-12.

54. Franceschi F, Ruzzini L, Longo UG, et al. Equivalent clinical results of arthroscopic single-row and double-row suture anchor repair for rotator cuff tears: a randomized controlled trial. *Am J Sports Med.* 2007;35(8):1254-1260.

55. Sugaya H, Maeda K, Matsuki K, Moriishi J. Functional and structural outcome after arthroscopic full-thickness rotator cuff repair: single-row versus dual-row fixation. *Arthroscopy.* 2005;21(11):1307-1316.

56. Lafosse L, Brozska R, Toussaint B, Gobezie R. The outcome and structural integrity of arthroscopic rotator cuff repair with use of the double-row suture anchor technique. *J Bone Joint Surg Am.* 2007;89(7):1533-1541.

57. Thompson WO, Debski RE, Boardman ND 3rd, et al. A biomechanical analysis of rotator cuff deficiency in a cadaveric model. *Am J Sports Med.* 1996;24(3):286-292.

58. Lee E, Bishop JY, Braman JP, Langford J, Gelber J, Flatow EL. Outcomes after arthroscopic rotator cuff repairs. *J Shoulder Elbow Surg.* 2007;16(1):1-5.

59. Lo IK, Burkhart SS. Arthroscopic revision of failed rotator cuff repairs: technique and results. *Arthroscopy.* 2004;20(3):250-267.

60. Jones CK, Savoie FH 3rd. Arthroscopic repair of large and massive rotator cuff tears. *Arthroscopy.* 2003;19(6):564-571.

Please see video on the accompanying Web site at
http://www.slackbooks.com/rotatorcuffvideos

CHAPTER 21

Latissimus Dorsi and Teres Major Transfers for Posterosuperior Rotator Cuff Tears

Demetris Delos, MD and Russell F. Warren, MD

Massive Rotator Cuff Tears: Definition, Pathobiology, Pathomechanics

Massive rotator cuff tears have been previously defined either anatomically or by the dimensions of the defect. Gerber et al[1] described massive cuff tears as those that involve at least 2 tendons, whereas DeOrio and Cofield[2] defined them as those in which the length of the greatest diameter of the tear was at least 5 cm. Tauro proposed incorporating both the anteroposterior and mediolateral dimensions in classifying the tear.[3] Despite lack of consensus with respect to definition, massive rotator cuff tears nevertheless present a unique clinical challenge. The tissue is often less compliant and stiffer than normal tendon, which can lead to significant retraction.[4] Atrophy, fibrosis, and fatty infiltration have been shown to occur within the tendon and its associated muscle belly.[1] Reduced cellularity, greater disorganization, decreased collagen content, and poor vascularization also contribute to the difficulties in handling and repairing these types of tears.[4-6]

In addition, shoulder mechanics are often significantly affected. The deltoid and rotator cuff muscles are responsible for maintaining balanced force couples in both the axial and coronal planes. Massive posterosuperior cuff tears involve both the supraspinatus and infraspinatus (rarely, the teres minor), thereby disrupting the force coupling and impairing normal glenohumeral mechanics. This manifests in diminished function and loss of the subacromial space.[7-13]

History and Physical Exam

Patients with massive rotator cuff tears often report pain with daily activities and pain at night. Weakness and range-of-motion limitations can be variable. When evaluating the patient with a possible massive rotator cuff tear, the physical exam should begin with a thorough inspection of

Ma CB, Feeley BT.
*Basic Principles and Operative Management
of the Rotator Cuff (pp 311-322)*
© 2012 SLACK Incorporated

the affected shoulder as well as the contralateral extremity. Patients with massive cuff tears will often demonstrate significant muscular atrophy of the supraspinatus and infraspinatus compared to the unaffected side. Active and passive range of motion should be evaluated, including abduction, external and internal rotation, as well as motion in the plane of the scapula. Posterosuperior cuff tears often manifest in loss of active abduction, forward flexion, and external rotation.[14] Important physical exam findings include the external rotation lag sign, which is associated with massive cuff tears as well as fatty infiltration of the infraspinatus and the hornblower's sign, which is sensitive and specific for massive cuff tears with supraspinatus, infraspinatus, and teres minor involvement.[15] The lift-off and belly-press tests are useful for assessing subscapularis strength.

IMAGING

Plain radiographs are mandatory for evaluating joint morphology and characterizing the joint space, as well as to look for evidence of superior migration (ie, to measure the acromiohumeral distance). A true anteroposterior view of the shoulder, an axillary view, a scapular-Y view, and a supraspinatus outlet view should be obtained. Magnetic resonance imaging (MRI) is critical for evaluating the integrity of the supraspinatus, infraspinatus, teres minor, and subscapularis tendons, as well as the glenohumeral joint articular surface for evidence of early arthritis, which may occur with time following a massive tear. Just as importantly, MRI provides information regarding the degree of muscle atrophy and fatty infiltration.

TREATMENT

Treatment of massive posterosuperior cuff tears should begin with activity modification, anti-inflammatory medications, physical therapy, and corticosteroid injections as needed. Failed nonoperative management is an indication for surgical intervention except in acute massive tears where early repair is indicated for most active patients. This may occur after a shoulder dislocation.

SURGICAL DECISION MAKING

After electing to proceed with operative management, the surgeon must first identify whether the tear is reparable or irreparable. Preoperative factors that have been associated with irreparable massive cuff tears include significant external rotation weakness,[15] significant muscle atrophy and fatty infiltration of the rotator cuff muscles,[1,16] and superior migration of the humeral head.[7,17,18] If the tear is deemed irreparable, salvage treatment with a latissimus dorsi transfer for posterosuperior defects may be an option in patients younger than 50 years of age. First proposed by Gerber et al in 1988,[19] the procedure attempts to close the defect and restore motion by transferring the latissimus dorsi to the greater tuberosity of the humerus. We have modified the technique to include the teres major tendon in the transfer in order to increase the amount of tendon tissue available for coverage of the posterosuperior footprint.[20,21] The latissimus/teres major type of transfer has been used in the past for the treatment of pediatric Erb's palsy with positive clinical results and is supported by biomechanical studies.[22-25]

Our current indications and contraindications for latissimus dorsi transfer are described next.

Indications

- For the primary treatment of massive, irreparable, posterosuperior (ie, supraspinatus and infraspinatus) rotator cuff tears in younger patients (age <50 years) who report pain and functional limitations.

- Patients with limited elevation and external rotation but with an intact subscapularis.
- Younger patients with minimal glenohumeral arthritis.
- As a salvage procedure after failed surgery if the joint is free of arthritis and the patient's young age precludes a reverse prosthesis. For elderly patients who have failed prior surgery, a reverse prosthesis usually affords a more predictable outcome.

Contraindications

- Lack of motivation on the part of the patient to undergo the procedure and participate in the associated rehabilitation.
- Patients with an overall poor general fitness level, morbid obesity, and extremes of age.
- Female patients with poor shoulder function and generalized muscle weakness prior to surgery (greater likelihood of having a poor clinical result).[26]
- Patients with subscapularis tendon tears, deltoid dysfunction, and shoulder stiffness tend to have poorer outcomes.[27]
- Patients with glenohumeral arthritis and cuff tear arthropathy (recommend reverse arthroplasty procedure).
- Patients with chronic pseudoparesis of elevation that is not painful and who demonstrate anterosuperior subluxation with escape of the humeral head on attempted elevation will require a reverse total shoulder prosthesis.[28]

SURGICAL MANAGEMENT

Patient Positioning

The patient is placed in the lateral decubitus position with the affected side facing upward, ensuring that all bony prominences are well-padded. The torso is stabilized with a sandbag, and the limb and hemithorax are draped free within the sterile field. The operative extremity is prepped and is maintained in a limb holder—we typically use the Spider limb positioner (Smith & Nephew, Andover, MA) at approximately 60 degrees of abduction. We have found the limb holder extremely useful, as it allows for manipulation and stabilization of the limb throughout the procedure and can accommodate both internal and external rotation.

Surgical Technique

In the original description by Gerber and colleagues,[19] only the latissimus dorsi is transferred during the procedure. We, however, prefer harvesting both the latissimus dorsi and the teres major rather than the latissimus dorsi tendon alone because this increases the surface area of tendon tissue available for restoring the rotator cuff footprint at the greater tuberosity. Furthermore, including the teres major in the transfer does not significantly affect the dissection and approach.

Approach to the Rotator Cuff

Two incisions are required for the procedure—one to approach the rotator cuff and the other to harvest the latissimus dorsi and teres major. We begin with a standard open approach to the rotator cuff (Figure 21-1). A vertical incision, originating at the anterolateral edge of the acromion and extending inferiorly for approximately 5 cm is made. The anterior deltoid raphe is identified and split bluntly. Dissection should not proceed further distal than 5 cm from the acromion, for this will put the anterior distribution of the axillary nerve at risk.

Using sharp dissection, the anterior portion of the deltoid is released from the acromion, and an acromioplasty is performed as needed. Next, the rotator cuff tendons are evaluated, with careful inspection of the subscapularis. Using a grasper, an attempt is made to mobilize the retracted tendon toward its insertion in order to determine if a tension-free primary repair is possible. This

Figure 21-1. Incisions for the latissimus transfer. (A) The superior incision is a vertical (as described in the text) or saber-type incision (as pictured here) just lateral to the acromion in order to expose the anterosuperior rotator cuff. The deltoid is released partially from the acromion, and the rotator cuff tear is confirmed to be irreparable. (B) The second incision is made in line with the latissimus along the posterolateral border of the muscle. (Reprinted with permission of Julianne Ho.)

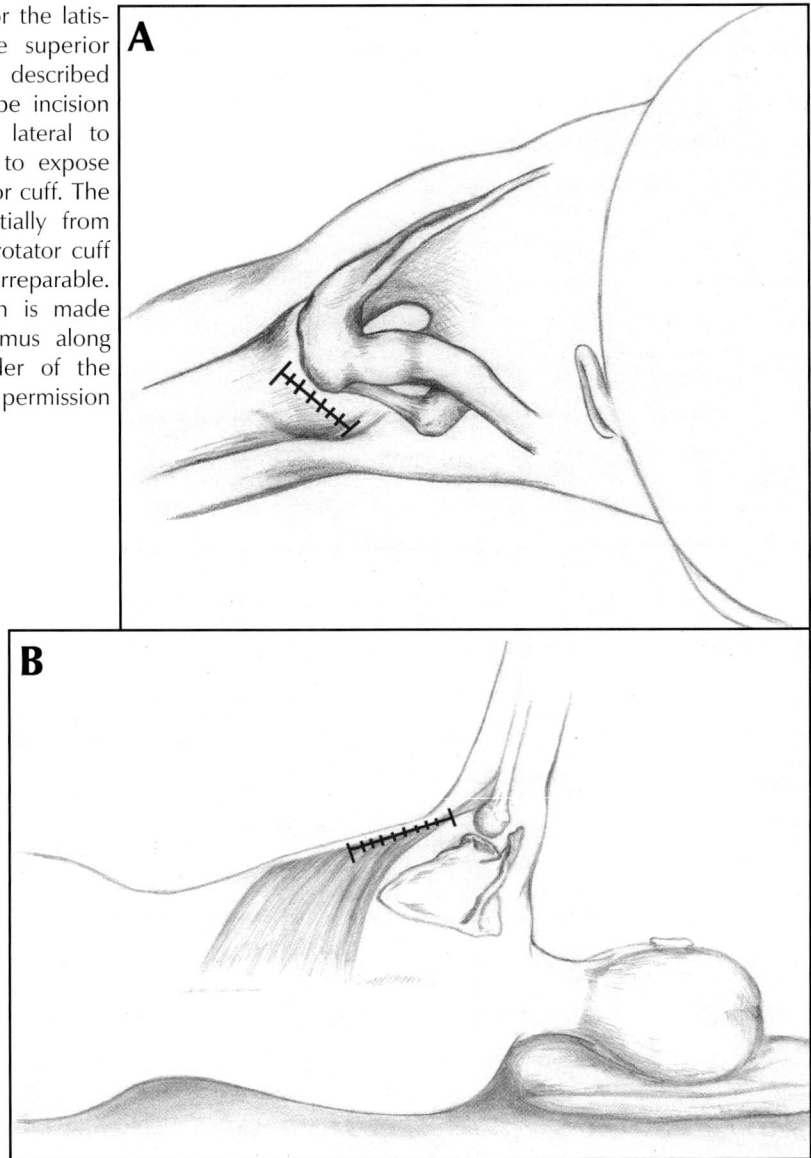

may require releasing the coracohumeral ligament and capsule, as well as performing a lysis of adhesions. Only after it has been determined that a primary repair of the rotator cuff tendon cannot be performed satisfactorily do we proceed with harvesting the latissimus dorsi and teres major tendons for transfer. In patients with prior failed surgery, the latissimus dorsi and teres major are harvested first, and the cuff is exposed afterward. A partial repair is completed if possible.

Posterior Axillary Approach

Attention is then turned to the posterior aspect of the affected shoulder. A 15-cm long incision along the lateral border of the latissimus dorsi is made, continuing proximally to the posterior border of the axilla (see Figure 21-1). The latissimus dorsi muscle belly is identified and carefully dissected free in a proximal direction. The neurovascular structures on the undersurface of the muscle are carefully protected throughout.

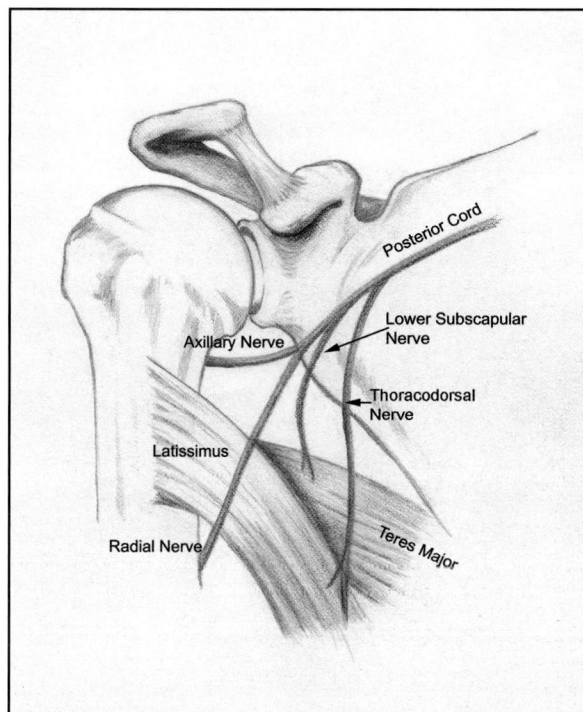

Figure 21-2. Anatomy of the latissimus and teres muscle and tendon. Knowledge of the anatomy of the radial and axillary nerves is important in order to avoid injury to these nerves. (Reprinted with permission of Julianne Ho.)

Next, the tendinous portions of the latissimus dorsi and teres major are identified and traced laterally to their insertions on the anteromedial humerus.

At this point, it is important that the humerus is maximally internally rotated in the limb-holding device in order to deliver the tendons into the surgical field and minimize the risk of neurovascular injury. We have previously demonstrated that by maximally internally rotating the extremity, an additional 1.9 cm of latissimus dorsi and teres major tissue can be exposed as compared to when the humerus is in the neutral rotation position.[20,21]

Using the posterior axillary approach as described above, a palpable band of variable thickness can be identified just anterior to the insertion of the latissimus dorsi tendon. This band is actually the proximal portion of the intermuscular septum between the anterior and posterior compartments of the arm. We use it as an important anatomic landmark when performing tenotomy of the latissimus dorsi tendon. By releasing the tendon off the bone posterior to this septum, one can avoid injury to the radial nerve.

Tenotomy of the latissimus tendon and teres major tendon is performed at the insertion sites on the humerus (Figure 21-2). In our previous cadaveric study, we noted that the average width of the latissimus dorsi tendon at its insertion site is 3.1 cm (range, 2.4 to 4.8 cm), and the average length of the tendinous portion is 8.4 cm (range, 6.3 to 10.1 cm). The average width of the teres major tendon at its insertion site is 4.0 cm (range, 3.3 to 5.0 cm), and the average length is 3.9 cm (range, 3.3 to 4.6 cm).[20] Subsequently, the tendons and muscle bellies are mobilized from the chest wall. Tagging sutures are placed through the tendon substance. By applying tension to the tagging sutures, the anterior and superior borders of the latissimus dorsi and teres major tendons and their lateral muscle bellies are dissected free from the chest wall (Figure 21-3). Excursion must be enough to reach the posterolateral border of the acromion (approximately 20 cm). The neurovascular pedicles for both the teres major and latissimus dorsi must be identified and protected throughout the dissection. Division of these pedicles will devitalize the transfer.

Figure 21-3. The latissimus has been released, and the tendon edges have been tagged. Care is taken to free the neurovascular bundle in order to provide adequate distance for the transfer without putting excessive pressure on the neurovascular bundle.

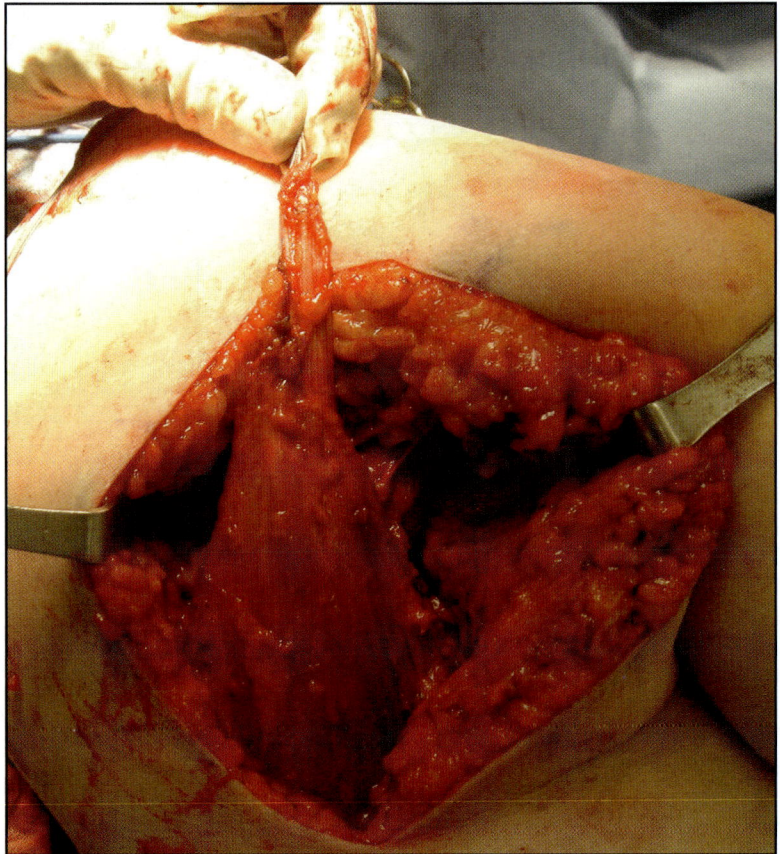

Tunneling

Next, the plane between the posterior part of the deltoid and the rotator cuff muscles is identified. The posterior deltoid is gently retracted laterally. A curved clamp is used to tunnel from the anterior incision, under the deltoid and subacromial space, and out through the posterior incision (Figure 21-4). The plane between the deep deltoid fascia and the posterior part of the rotator cuff must be carefully identified to prevent deviation into the deltoid fascia during tunneling or tendon passage, as this places the posterior branch of the axillary nerve and its divisions at risk.

Completion of the Transfer

The tagging sutures on the tendons are grasped with a clamp and passed anteriorly. The transferred tendons are fixed to the rotator cuff footprint on its lateral edge with suture anchors. If cuff tissue is adequately mobile, native rotator cuff tendon is repaired in a side-to-side manner with the transferred tendons.

An attempt is made to have the transferred tendons reach the subscapularis superiorly, to close the defect. Anteriorly, the leading edge of the latissimus dorsi is sutured to the superior border of the subscapularis muscle, and the teres major is placed laterally. Once the repair is complete, the shoulder is gently ranged to assess the degree of tension on the repair (Figure 21-5).

A drain is placed under the deltoid fascia, and the wound is closed after reattaching the anterior portion of the deltoid through drill holes into the acromion. A sterile dressing is applied, and the limb is placed in an abduction brace.

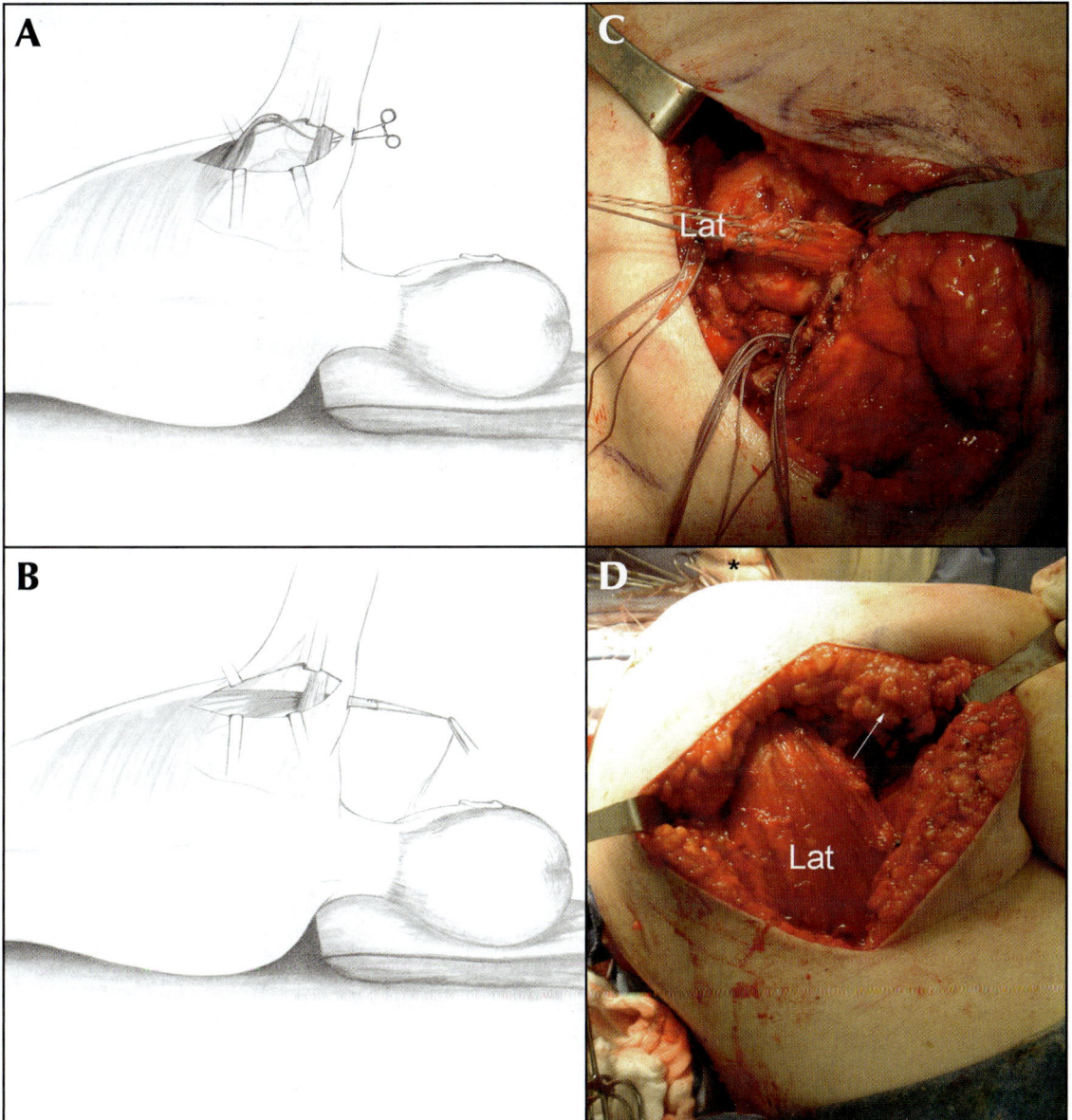

Figure 21-4. (A, B) Tunneling of the graft under the deltoid. A long grasper is passed through the anterior incision and deep to the deltoid through the posterior incision. The latissimus should be able to be passed freely under the deltoid without tension on the tendon. (Reprinted with permission of Julianne Ho.) (C) Intraoperative photo of the latissimus tagged and pulled through the superior incision prior to attachment on the humeral head. (D) After the tendon has been passed to the anterior incision (*), the latissimus will have a different orientation compared to its original insertion (arrow).

Postoperative Management and Rehabilitation

Postoperatively, the limb is immobilized in a sling with an abduction pillow for 6 weeks. For this initial 6-week period only, gentle pendulum/Codman exercises are allowed.

After 6 weeks, passive and active-assist supine forward elevation and rotation movements are begun. Excessive scapulothoracic compensatory motion (ie, shrug) must be avoided.

At 8 weeks postoperatively, the patient may begin active supine range-of-motion exercises and progress with active motion and strengthening under therapist supervision.

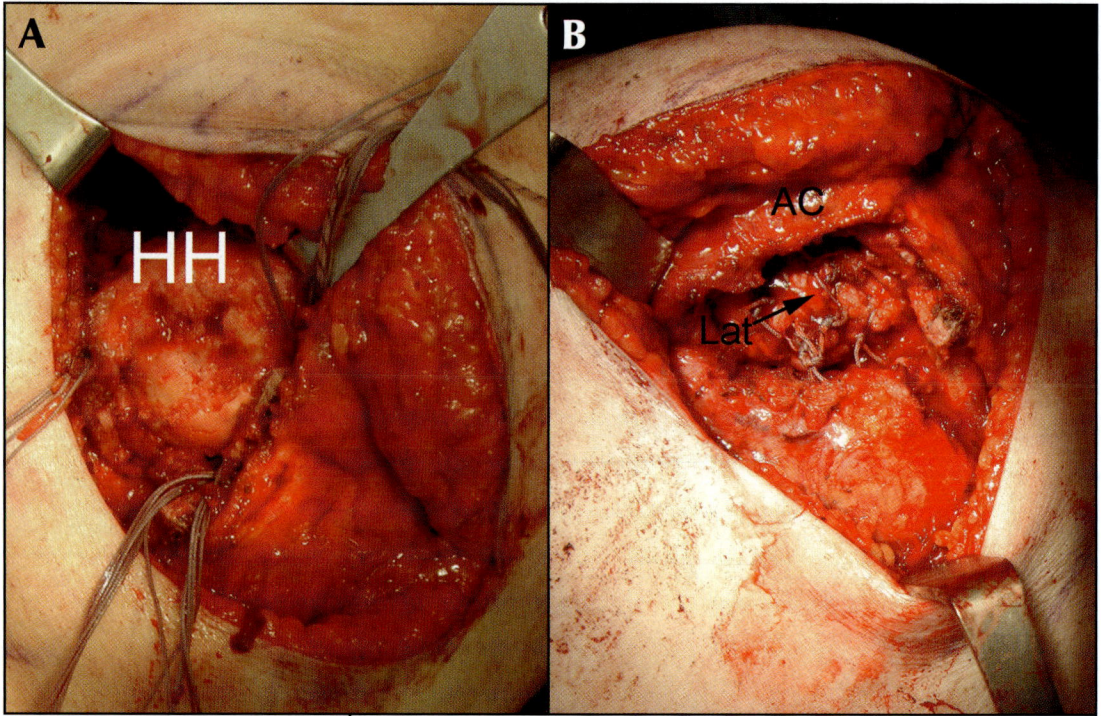

Figure 21-5. Completion of the transfer. (A) Prior to the transfer, the latissimus sutures can be seen to the right of the humeral head (HH), which is bare. (B) After repair of the latissimus. (C) Repair of the latissimus to the superior border of the subscapularis, the lateral border of the supraspinatus and/or the infraspinatus (if possible), and the articular margin of the greater tuberosity. (Figure C reprinted with permission of Julianne Ho.)

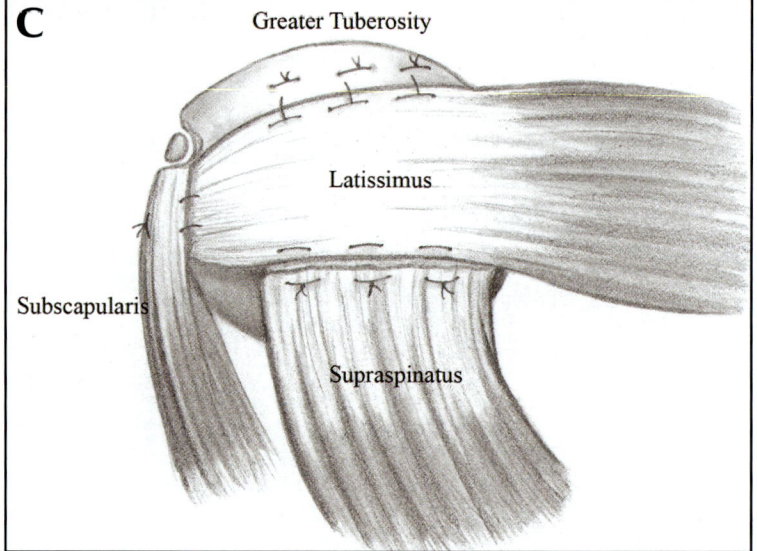

Potential Complications

In one of the largest series to date, Gerber and colleagues[29] reported no infections or permanent nerve lesions in 67 patients treated with latissimus transfer. Three patients developed postoperative dysesthesia involving the ulnar nerve, brachial plexus, or axillary nerve with spontaneous resolution by 6 months in all. Partial deltoid detachment occurred in one patient, who was then successfully revised (Table 21-1).

TABLE 21-1. OUTCOMES OF SELECT LATISSIMUS DORSI TRANSFER SERIES

AUTHORS	NUMBER OF PATIENTS	AVG DURATION OF FOLLOW-UP	PREOPERATIVE DATA	POSTOPERATIVE DATA	COMMENTS
Gerber; CORR, 1992[30]	16	33 months	Mean forward flexion: 83 degrees	Mean forward flexion: 135 degrees; Pain relief satisfactory in 94% at rest, 81% in exertion	Improved functional outcomes in those with intact subscapularis
Aoki et al; JBJS (Br), 1996[27]	10 (12 shoulders)	35.6 months	Mean forward flexion: 99 degrees	Mean forward flexion: 135 degrees	Osteoarthritic changes in 5 shoulders, proximal migration of humeral head progressed in 6
Gerber et al; JBJS (Am), 2006[29]	67 (69 shoulders)	53 months	Subjective shoulder value score: 28% Pain score 6 (of 15) Mean forward flexion: 104 degrees Mean abduction: 101 degrees Mean external rotation: 22 degrees	Subjective shoulder value score: 66% Pain score 12 (of 15) Mean forward flexion: 123 degrees Mean abduction: 119 degrees Mean external rotation: 29 degrees	Slight but significant increase in osteoarthritic changes over time
Nove-Josserand et al; OTSR, 2009[31]	26	34 months	Mean pain score: 4.8 ± 3 Mean Constant: 50 ± 12	Mean pain score: 12.2 ± 2; Mean Constant: 74 ± 9	Mean active external rotation gain of 7 degrees
Lehmann et al; Int Orth, 2010[32]	26	24 months	Mean Constant: 20 Mean acromiohumeral distance: 4.7 mm Hamada classification: 1.7	Mean Constant: 56 Mean acromiohumeral distance: 4.8 mm Hamada classification: 1.8	

PEARLS AND PITFALLS

- Careful patient selection is necessary for successful outcomes, and expectations must be reasonable. We advise patients that active shoulder motion gains can be significant, but motor strength is usually limited, with weakness persisting in elevation above shoulder level. External rotation will improve, particularly if the graft is placed laterally on the tuberosity.
- It is critical that the surgeon possess a thorough understanding of the anatomy of the approach to minimize any risk of damage to the nearby neurovascular structures as well as the pedicles.
- Safe musculotendinous axial mobilization requires knowledge of the distance between tendon insertions and the neurovascular pedicle.
  - The distance between the tendon insertion at the humerus and the neurovascular pedicle to the latissimus dorsi is 13.1 cm.
  - The distance between the tendon insertion at the humerus and the neurovascular pedicle to the teres major is 7.4 cm.
- Maximal internal rotation of the humerus at the time of tendon release can limit the risk of injury to the axillary and radial nerves by delivering the latissimus dorsi and teres major tendons into the field, thereby also increasing the length of the tendon; we do not recommend "lengthening" the transferred tendon with allograft tissue.
- Superficial deviation into the deltoid fascia during tunnel creation of passage of the tendons can place the posterior branch of the axillary nerve and its divisions at risk.
- Postoperative rehabilitation is slow and deliberate. Only gentle pendulum exercises are allowed for the first 6 weeks. Active supine range of motion with deltoid strengthening can start 6 to 8 weeks after surgery with more vigorous strengthening only after week 12.

REFERENCES

1. Gerber C, Fuchs B, Hodler J. The results of repair of massive tears of the rotator cuff. *J Bone Joint Surg Am.* 2000;82(4):505-515.
2. DeOrio JK, Cofield RH. Results of a second attempt at surgical repair of a failed initial rotator-cuff repair. *J Bone Joint Surg Am.* 1984;66(4):563-567.
3. Tauro JC. Stiffness and rotator cuff tears: incidence, arthroscopic findings, and treatment results. *Arthroscopy.* 2006;22(6):581-586.
4. Gerber C, Krushell RJ. Isolated rupture of the tendon of the subscapularis muscle. Clinical features in 16 cases. *J Bone Joint Surg Br.* 1991;73(3):389-394.
5. Galatz LM, Connor PM, Calfee RP, Hsu JC, Yamaguchi K. Pectoralis major transfer for anterior-superior subluxation in massive rotator cuff insufficiency. *J Shoulder Elbow Surg.* 2003;12(1):1-5.
6. Apreleva M, Ozbaydar M, Fitzgibbons PG, Warner JJ. Rotator cuff tears: the effect of the reconstruction method on three-dimensional repair site area. *Arthroscopy.* 2002;18(5):519-526.
7. Burkhart SS. Arthroscopic treatment of massive rotator cuff tears. Clinical results and biomechanical rationale. *Clin Orthop Relat Res.* 1991;267:45-56.
8. Ahmad CS, Kleweno C, Jacir AM, et al. Biomechanical performance of rotator cuff repairs with humeral rotation: a new rotator cuff repair failure model. *Am J Sports Med.* 2008;36(5):888-892.
9. Su WR, Budoff JE, Luo ZP. The effect of anterosuperior rotator cuff tears on glenohumeral translation. *Arthroscopy.* 2009;25(3):282-289.
10. Su WR, Budoff JE, Luo ZP. The effect of posterosuperior rotator cuff tears and biceps loading on glenohumeral translation. *Arthroscopy.* 2010;26(5):578-586.
11. Burkhart SS. Fluoroscopic comparison of kinematic patterns in massive rotator cuff tears. A suspension bridge model. *Clin Orthop Relat Res.* 1992;284:144-152.
12. Parsons IM, Apreleva M, Fu FH, Woo SL. The effect of rotator cuff tears on reaction forces at the glenohumeral joint. *J Orthop Res.* 2002;20(3):439-446.
13. Thompson WO, Debski RE, Boardman ND 3rd, et al. A biomechanical analysis of rotator cuff deficiency in a cadaveric model. *Am J Sports Med.* 1996;24(3):286-292.
14. Boes MT, McCann PD, Dines DM. Diagnosis and management of massive rotator cuff tears: the surgeon's dilemma. *Instr Course Lect.* 2006;55:45-57.

15. Walch G, Boulahia A, Calderone S, Robinson AH. The "dropping" and "hornblower's" signs in evaluation of rotator-cuff tears. *J Bone Joint Surg Br.* 1998;80(4):624-628.

16. Goutallier D, Postel JM, Gleyze P, Leguilloux P, Van Driessche S. Influence of cuff muscle fatty degeneration on anatomic and functional outcomes after simple suture of full-thickness tears. *J Shoulder Elbow Surg.* 2003;12(6):550-554.

17. Ellman H, Hanker G, Bayer M. Repair of the rotator cuff. End-result study of factors influencing reconstruction. *J Bone Joint Surg Am.* 1986;68(8):1136-1144.

18. Saupe N, Pfirrmann CW, Schmid MR, Jost B, Werner CM, Zanetti M. Association between rotator cuff abnormalities and reduced acromiohumeral distance. *AJR Am J Roentgenol.* 2006;187(2):376-382.

19. Gerber C, Vinh TS, Hertel R, Hess CW. Latissimus dorsi transfer for the treatment of massive tears of the rotator cuff. A preliminary report. *Clin Orthop Relat Res.* 1988;232:51-61.

20. Pearle AD, Kelly BT, Voos JE, Chehab EL, Warren RF. Surgical technique and anatomic study of latissimus dorsi and teres major transfers. *J Bone Joint Surg Am.* 2006;88(7):1524-1531.

21. Pearle AD, Voos JE, Kelly BT, Chehab EL, Warren RF. Surgical technique and anatomic study of latissimus dorsi and teres major transfers. Surgical technique. *J Bone Joint Surg Am.* 2007;89 Suppl 2 Pt.2:284-296.

22. Edwards TB, Baghian S, Faust DC, Willis RB. Results of latissimus dorsi and teres major transfer to the rotator cuff in the treatment of Erb's palsy. *J Pediatr Orthop.* 2000;20(3):375-379.

23. Magermans DJ, Chadwick EK, Veeger HE, Rozing PM, van der Helm FC. Effectiveness of tendon transfers for massive rotator cuff tears: a simulation study. *Clin Biomech (Bristol, Avon).* 2004;19(2):116-122.

24. Phipps GJ, Hoffer MM. Latissimus dorsi and teres major transfer to rotator cuff for Erb's palsy. *J Shoulder Elbow Surg.* 1995;4(2):124-129.

25. Herzberg G, Urien JP, Dimnet J. Potential excursion and relative tension of muscles in the shoulder girdle: relevance to tendon transfers. *J Shoulder Elbow Surg.* 1999;8(5):430-437.

26. Iannotti JP, Hennigan S, Herzog R, et al. Latissimus dorsi tendon transfer for irreparable posterosuperior rotator cuff tears. Factors affecting outcome. *J Bone Joint Surg Am.* 2006;88(2):342-348.

27. Aoki M, Okamura K, Fukushima S, Takahashi T, Ogino T. Transfer of latissimus dorsi for irreparable rotator-cuff tears. *J Bone Joint Surg Br.* 1996;78(5):761-766.

28. Bartlett SP, May JW Jr, Yaremchuk MJ. The latissimus dorsi muscle: a fresh cadaver study of the primary neurovascular pedicle. *Plast Reconstr Surg.* 1981;67(5):631-636.

29. Gerber C, Maquieira G, Espinosa N. Latissimus dorsi transfer for the treatment of irreparable rotator cuff tears. *J Bone Joint Surg Am.* 2006;88(1):113-120.

30. Gerber C. Latissimus dorsi transfer for the treatment of irreparable tears of the rotator cuff. *Clin Orthop Relat Res.* 1992;275:152-160.

31. Nove-Josserand L, Costa P, Liotard JP, Safar JF, Walch G, Zilber S. Results of latissimus dorsi tendon transfer for irreparable cuff tears. *Orthop Traumatol Surg Res.* 2009;95(2):108-113.

32. Lehmann LJ, Mauerman E, Strube T, Laibacher K, Scharf HP. Modified minimally invasive latissimus dorsi transfer in the treatment of massive rotator cuff tears: a two-year follow-up of 26 consecutive patients. *Int Orthop.* 2010;34(3):377-383.

CHAPTER 22

PECTORALIS TRANSFER FOR ANTERIOR ROTATOR CUFF (SUBSCAPULARIS) TEARS

Carolyn M. Hettrich, MD, MPH and John E. Kuhn, MD

The subscapularis has been deemed the "most important" rotator cuff muscle for function and stability of the glenohumeral joint.[1] Subscapularis ruptures, while only accounting for 3.5% to 8% of rotator cuff tears,[2,3] are associated with pain, decreased internal rotation strength, and instability. Subscapularis tears are frequently seen in patients with glenohumeral joint instability. Wirth and Rockwood reported on 221 patients who underwent surgery for recurrent anterior subluxation—13 (5.9%) of these had irreparable injury to the subscapularis.[4]

Smith first reported a rupture of the subscapularis in 1835 in a cadaveric dissection.[5] Codman reported that the subscapularis was torn only in 3.5% of 200 rotator cuff tears in 1934.[2] McAuliffe and Dowd published a case report of an acute subscapularis repair after a traumatic avulsion, which led to restoration of preoperative function by 3 months.[6] In 1991, Gerber and Krushell reported on 16 patients with isolated subscapularis tears with anterior shoulder pain and instability.[7] They described the lift-off test, as well as other clinical and surgical findings. They commented that the one patient who could not be repaired did not have a change in symptoms, and the other patients had progress similar to that seen after a supraspinatus repair.

In 1996, Gerber et al[8] reported on 16 patients with isolated, traumatic subscapularis rupture that underwent direct repair. After 24 to 48 months of follow-up, patients reported their result was good or excellent in 13, fair in one, and poor in one. Using a visual analog scale, patients reported that the function of their shoulder was 82% of normal (range, 20 to 100). The results for patients with long-standing ruptures (greater than 36 months) were significantly worse than patients who underwent repair less than 20 months from the date of rupture.[8] Other authors have reported that delayed repair is less effective due to considerable retraction of the tendon, as well as fatty infiltration.[4,9,10] Chronic tears with fatty degeneration greater than Goutallier Grade 2[11] may not be possible to repair, and the repair is more likely to fail.[12]

Many operative techniques have been described for chronic subscapularis insufficiency, including transfer of the trapezius, pectoralis minor, and pectoralis major. According to the literature,

Ma CB, Feeley BT.
*Basic Principles and Operative Management
of the Rotator Cuff (pp 323-330)*

pectoralis major transfer has provided the most reliable results and is now the accepted salvage treatment. Pectoralis major is a large triangular muscle consisting of 2 heads. The clavicular head originates on the medial one-third of the clavicle and inserts on the humerus via the anterior lamina. The clavicular head makes up 19% of the total muscle volume of the pectoralis major. The sternal head makes up 81% of the muscle volume, originates from the manubrium, superior two-thirds of the sternum, and first through sixth ribs. The sternal head of the muscle then forms the posterior lamina. The tendon insertion for both the anterior and posterior lamina is 5.4 cm in length.[13]

Transfer of the entire pectoralis muscle has been described.[4,14,15] The large bulk of the muscle may put the musculocutaneous nerve at risk if the tendon is passed deep to the conjoined tendon. This has led some authors to recommend using a portion of the pectoralis major muscle, with variations that include using the superior 2.5 to 3 cm of the tendon,[16] using the clavicular head,[17] or using the sternal head.[18]

The tendon has been passed both superficial and deep to the conjoined tendon. Wirth and Rockwood described transferring pectoralis major, minor, or both superficial to the conjoined tendon to the greater tuberosity.[4] Resch et al transferred 2.5 to 3 cm of the tendon deep to the conjoined tendon and superficial to the musculocutaneous nerve.[16] To study both of these techniques, Konrad and colleagues studied the kinematics of glenohumeral abduction, comparing pectoralis major tendon transfers deep to or superficial to the conjoined tendon in a biomechanical model.[19] Transferring the tendon deep to the conjoined tendon led to better restoration of glenohumeral kinematics. The authors suspected this was because the line of action of the transferred tendon was closer to the native subscapularis.[19]

Instead of nonanatomically dividing the tendon and taking the superior half as described by Resch et al,[16] transfer of the clavicular or sternal heads has also been described. Warner transferred the sternal head under the clavicular head and over to the greater tuberosity. The clavicular portion was passed under the sternal head to attempt to replicate the inferior pull of the subscapularis. The clavicular head then acts as a pulley or fulcrum when both muscles contract.[17] In a cadaveric study by Jennings et al, the authors found that it was possible to split the anterior and posterior lamina in all specimens by blunt dissection and transfer the sternal head (posterior lamina) to the greater tuberosity. The pectoralis could be mobilized as far as 8.5 cm medially and still avoid injuring the medial pectoral nerve.[18] This replicated the inferior action arm of the subscapularis and avoided having to reroute the tendon.[18]

SURGICAL MANAGEMENT—INDICATIONS

Any acute tear of the subscapularis with minimal fatty infiltration (Goutallier Grade 1 or 2) should undergo acute primary repair to the lesser tuberosity.

Transfer of the pectoralis is most commonly indicated for retracted and chronic irreparable tears of the subscapularis with Goutallier Grade 3 or 4 fatty infiltration with resultant pain and/or instability that has not responded to conservative management.

On occasion, a chronic subscapularis tear can be repaired anatomically, but the tissue quality may be poor, or the muscle belly may have extensive fatty infiltration. In this circumstance, the pectoralis major may be transferred to augment the repair of the subscapularis.

Finally, this transfer has also been used for patients with combined anterior supraspinatus and superior subscapularis irreparable rotator cuff tears.

Because primary repair should be performed when possible, the final decision for transfer of the pectoralis major tendon is often made intraoperatively.

PATIENT POSITIONING FOR SURGERY

This procedure is performed in the modified beach chair position. The waist of the patient is flexed to 45 degrees, with the knees flexed to 15 to 30 degrees. The back of the table is elevated to 45 to 60 degrees. A small towel rolled and placed under the thoracic spine will help open the chest by allowing the scapulae to retract toward the spine. All bony prominences are padded, and the patient is secured to the table using a safety belt across the waist.

SURGICAL TECHNIQUE

An anterolateral, deltopectoral approach is used with a 4- to 8-inch incision that is started just lateral to the coracoid process at the level of the clavicle and extended down toward the deltoid insertion. Self-retaining retractors are placed, and the subcutaneous tissues are divided using electrocautery to minimize bleeding. The cephalic vein is identified and mobilized laterally with the deltoid with care to cauterize the medial branches to the pectoralis major. If the cephalic vein is no longer intact from previous surgeries or is small/absent, the deltopectoral interval can be identified by identifying the coracoid and then developing tissue planes either superiorly or inferiorly. Once the deltopectoral interval is identified, it can then be bluntly divided. The subdeltoid space is then freed of adhesions, and the deltoid retractor is placed. The conjoined tendon is identified, and the lateral extension (falx) may be released to the lateral coracoid. A retractor is then placed under the conjoined tendon, which is retracted medially. The subacromial space is then bluntly freed of adhesions, and the capsule of the shoulder and any remnants of the subscapularis are carefully inspected. The axillary nerve should then be identified, either through palpation or direct visualization, and protected throughout the case.

Any remaining portions of the subscapularis should then be identified, and an attempt should be made to mobilize these through extensive releases. The capsule can be released along the labrum and along the anterior glenoid neck. Adhesions can be released from the coracoid. Care must be taken to avoid medial dissection here, which could compromise the suprascapular nerve or the upper and lower subscapular nerves. Adhesions between the subscapularis and the conjoined tendon may also be released with care to identify and protect the axillary and musculocutaneous nerves. Before the subscapularis has been mobilized, the musculocutaneous nerve and the branch that reflects back to the conjoined tendon is identified and protected. There exists a fair amount of anatomic variation in the musculocutaneous nerve.[20,21] The average distance is 55.7 mm between the coracoid and the musculocutaneous nerve; however, substantially shorter distances (36 mm) have been reported.[22] This distance defines the space for a potential subcoracoid transfer of the pectoralis major, and if the space is too small, adjustments in the surgical technique may be required (see below).

A repair of the subscapularis should be attempted, and the decision to proceed with the pectoralis transfer is made intraoperatively if this cannot be performed. If the repair is tenuous, the pectoralis may be transferred to augment the repair.

Attention is then turned to the pectoralis major tendon. The anterior and posterior lamina of the 2 heads of the pectoralis major are then identified (Figure 22-1). The authors prefer to use the sternal head of the pectoralis major (posterior lamina) as it provides an inferior vector and better replicates the native subscapularis function, while respecting the anatomic divisions of the muscle. The anterior lamina can be retracted inferiorly using right-angled retractor, and posterior lamina can then be released subperiosteally using a #15 blade scalpel. The tendon lamina lies adjacent to the tendon of the long head of the biceps, which should be protected during dissection. The tendon edge is then tagged with number 2 Ethibond sutures (Ethicon, Somerville, NJ). The tendon can then be mobilized up to 8.5 cm from humeral insertion and lateral to the pectoralis minor without damaging the medial or lateral pectoral nerves.

Figure 22-1. Two heads of the pectoralis major tendon. The pectoralis major has 2 heads that insert as 2 distinct lamina on the humerus. The clavicular head is superficial, the sternal head is deep. The authors prefer to isolate and use the sternal head for transfers as its line of action is closer to that of the subscapularis and leaving the clavicular head may produce less deformity compared to taking the entire muscle.

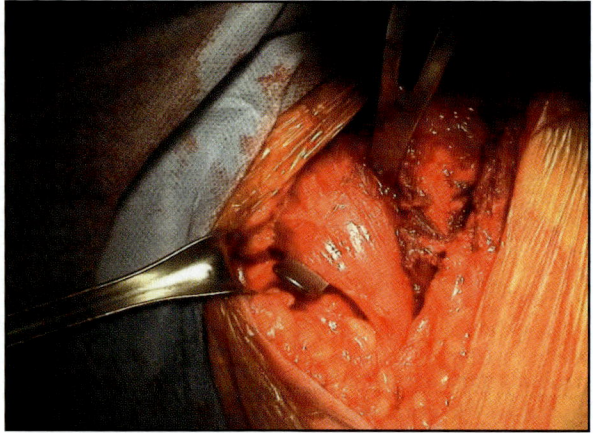

Figure 22-2. Development of the medial conjoined tendon and space deep to the tendon. The sternal head will be passed anterior to the musculocutaneous nerve and deep to the conjoined tendon. The superior border of this space is the coracoid. The inferior border is the reflected branch of the musculocutaneous nerve to the conjoined tendon. If this space is narrow, the muscle of the pectoralis may be debulked, or the muscle may be transferred superficial to the conjoined tendon.

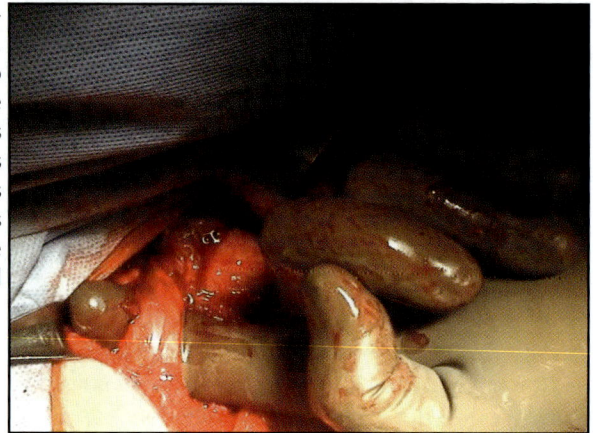

At this point, the medial edge of the conjoined tendon is identified, and a plane under the conjoined tendon is developed (Figure 22-2). The tagging sutures are then passed from medial to lateral behind the conjoined tendon, but anterior to the musculocutaneous nerve. Carefully pass the tendon through this space, checking to ensure that there is not excess tension on the nerve due to the bulk of the tendon. If there is tension on the reflected branch of musculocutaneous nerve to the conjoined tendon, the muscle may need to be debulked, or the proximal branch of the musculocutaneous nerve can be released.[15] Alternatively, if the space is extremely small, the tendon can be passed superficial to the conjoined tendon.

The attachment site on the anterior/medial aspect of the greater tuberosity is then prepared using a burr to decorticate to bleeding bone. Three or 4 suture anchors are then placed into the prepared bed, and these are then passed through the tendon and secured into place (Figure 22-3). Once secured, the musculocutaneous nerve is again palpated to ensure there is still no tension on the nerve.

After the transfer has been performed, any concomitant pathology, such as biceps instability/tendinosis, subacromial spurs, and other ruptured cuff muscles, should be addressed.

The wound is then copiously irrigated. The deltopectoral interval is loosely reapproximated using 0 colored polyester suture. The subcutaneous tissues are closed with 2-0 Vicryl (Ethicon), and the skin is closed using a buried 3-0 Monocryl (Ethicon). After a sterile dressing is applied to the wound, the arm is placed in a sling and swathe.

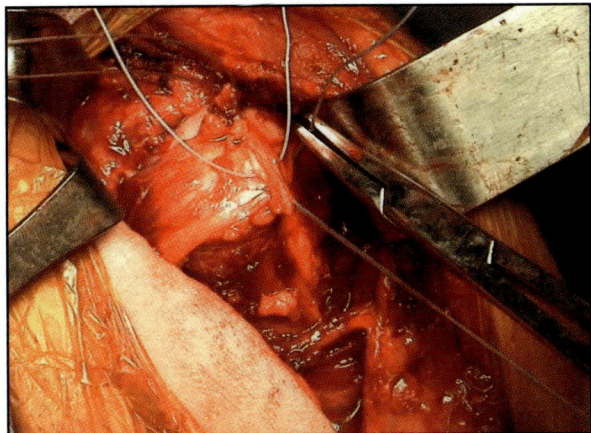

Figure 22-3. Repair of the transferred sternal head of the pectoralis major to the lesser tuberosity.

POSTOPERATIVE MANAGEMENT AND REHABILITATION

Postoperatively, a sling is used to prevent external rotation for 6 weeks. In the first 2 weeks of therapy, we allow passive and active external rotation to neutral, forward elevation to 90 degrees, with no resisted internal rotation. Over the next 4 weeks, active external rotation and forward elevation are gradually increased, aiming for full motion 6 to 8 weeks after surgery. At 8 weeks, light internal rotation-resisted exercises are permitted. At 12 weeks, more aggressive strengthening is permitted.

POTENTIAL COMPLICATIONS

Potential complications include injury to the musculocutaneous or axillary nerve, failure of the repair to heal, infection, recurrent dislocation, need for revision surgery, and no improvement in pain or function.

Elhassan et al[17] passed the sternal head under the clavicular head to the greater tuberosity. They reported that 4 of 11 in the instability group had no relief of pain and did not report subjective improvement. Of the 3 patients who had anterior subluxation preoperatively, there was no improvement in the patient's pain, Constant scores, or subjective outcome scores. In these 3 patients, postoperative computed tomography scans confirmed rupture of the transfer. One of these patients underwent revision with improvement in pain, but not function. Another underwent a glenohumeral joint fusion, and the last patient was offered a fusion. In the post-total shoulder arthroplasty group, the majority of the patients (75%) reported no significant improvement in pain, Constant, or outcome scores. These patients also all had confirmed failures of their repair postoperatively. In the massive rotator cuff tear group, 4 of 11 patients had rupture of their transfer.

Jost et al,[23] who transferred the entire tendon over the conjoined tendon to the greater tuberosity, reported 6 complications: 2 avulsions of transferred pectoralis tendon, 1 failure of the supraspinatus and infraspinatus repair, 1 infection, 1 "mechanical conflict of the coracoid process with the humeral head" requiring corrective osteotomy of the coracoid, and 1 deep thrombosis of the axillary vein. However, 18 of the 30 shoulders were still mildly painful at last follow-up, 11 of which had tenderness at the insertion site of the transfer.[23]

Wirth and Rockwood transferred the superior 2.5 to 3 cm of the tendon to the greater tuberosity. He had 3 unsatisfactory results (out of 13). Two of these patients had recurrent dislocations with pain and numbness. All of the patients with unsatisfactory results had at least 2 prior operations.[4]

Resch and colleagues, who described passing the superior half to two-thirds of the tendon above the musculocutaneous nerve but below the conjoined tendon, reported that they did not have any complications, but did note that very thin patients had a slightly more prominent anterior bulging of the deltoid in comparison to the contralateral side.[16]

Gavriilidis et al, who transferred the superior two-thirds of the clavicular head under the conjoined tendon to the lesser tuberosity and anterior greater tuberosity, only had 2 postoperative hematomas and one patient with advanced cuff tear arthropathy of the 15 patients in his series.[24]

OUTCOMES

As this operation is performed relatively infrequently, the literature has only Level IV case series. Outcomes and the techniques used by the authors are reported in Table 22-1.

PEARLS AND PITFALLS

- Dissect and release the subscapularis, as a successful primary repair will have better results than a pectoralis transfer.
- Assess space between the musculocutaneous nerve and conjoined tendon to prevent tension on the nerve.
- Do not dissect more than 8.5 cm lateral to the insertion of the pectoralis to avoid iatrogenic injury to the medial pectoral nerve.
- The sternal head (posterior lamina) of the pectoralis major most closely replicates the line of pull of the subscapularis.
- The anterior lamina can be retracted inferiorly with a right-angled retractor, and the posterior lamina can be released subperiosteally using a scalpel.
- Prepare the anterior/medial aspect of the greater tuberosity using a burr to create bleeding bone prior to placing suture anchors.

REFERENCES

1. McMahon PJ, Debski RE, Thompson WO, Warner JJ, Fu FH, Woo SL. Shoulder muscle forces and tendon excursions during glenohumeral abduction in the scapular plane. *J Shoulder Elbow Surg.* 1995;4(3):199-208.
2. Codman EA. Rupture of the supraspinatus tendon and other lesions in or about the shoulder. In: Codman EA. *The Shoulder.* Boston, MA: Norman Publishing; 1934.
3. Frankle M, Cofield R. Rotator cuff tears involving the subscapularis tendon. Paper presented at: Proceedings of the Fifth International Conference on Surgery of the Shoulder; July 12-15, 1992; Paris, France.
4. Wirth MA, Rockwood CA. Operative treatment of irreparable rupture of the subscapularis. *J Bone Joint Surg Am.* 1997;79(5):722-731.
5. Smith JG. Pathological appearances of seven cases of injury of the shoulder joint with rem. *Am J Med Sci.* 1835;16:219-224.
6. McAuliffe TB, Dowd GS. Avulsion of the subscapularis tendon. A case report. *J Bone Joint Surg Am.* 1987;69(9):1454-1455.
7. Gerber C, Krushell RJ. Isolated rupture of the tendon of the subscapularis muscle. Clinical features in 16 cases. *J Bone Joint Surg Br.* 1991;73(3):389-394.
8. Gerber C, Hersche O, Farron A. Isolated rupture of the subscapularis tendon. *J Bone Joint Surg Am.* 1996;78(7):1015-1023.
9. Warner JJ. Management of massive irreparable rotator cuff tears: the role of tendon transfer. *Instr Course Lect.* 2001;50:63-71.
10. Warner JJ, Higgins L, Parsons IM, Dowdy P. Diagnosis and treatment of anterosuperior rotator cuff tears. *J Shoulder Elbow Surg Am.* 2001;10(1):37-46.
11. Goutallier D, Postel JM, Bernageau J, Lavau L, Voisin MC. Fatty muscle degeneration in cuff ruptures. Pre- and postoperative evaluation by CT scan. *Clin Orthop Rel Res.* 1994;304(July):78-83.

TABLE 22-1. Outcomes

Author	Patients	Study	Technique	Level of Outcomes
Elhassan et al, *JBJS (Br)*, 2008[17]	N = 30 Group 1—Failed instability repair; 11 patients, average age 37 Group 2—Post TSA; 8 patients, average age 55 Group 3—Massive rotator cuff tear; 11 patients, average age 58	Minimum 2-year follow-up, retrospective (LOE 4)	Sternal head, passed under clavicular head to GT	Failure of tendon transfer highest in Group 2, for which only 1/8 had improvement in pain scores Constant from 40.9 to 60.8 in Group 1, and 28.7 to 52.3 in Group 3
Resch et al, *JBJS (Am)*, 2000[16]	12 patients, 8 with isolated subscapularis, 4 with supraspinatus; average age 65	Minimum 2 year follow-up, retrospective (LOE 4)	Superior 1/2 to 2/3 of tendon, passed above nerve, below conjoined to LT	9/12 G/E, 3 fair Constant from 26.9 to 67.1 All shoulders stable
Jost et al, *JBJS (Am)*, 2003[23]	28 patients, 12 isolated, 16 combined; average age 53	Minimum 2 year follow-up, retrospective, consecutive (LOE 4)	Entire tendon, over conjoined to GT, with anchors	23 G/E, 2 Fair, 3 poor Constant from 47% to 70% Isolated better than massive tears; 2 ruptures of transfer
Gavriilidis et al, *Int Orthop*, 2010[24]	15 patients, all subscapularis and supraspinatus tears; average age 61.9	Average follow-up of 37 months, retrospective (LOE 4)	Superior 2/3 of clavicular head to LT and anterior GT, under conjoined	Constant score from 51.7 to 68.2 70% intact, 15% "thin," and 15% ruptured on MRI follow up
Wirth & Rockwood, *JBJS (Am)*, 1997[4]	13 patients, pectoralis major in 7, minor in 5, both in 1; average age 49	Mean of 5 years follow-up, minimum 2, retrospective (LOE 4)	Superior 2.5 to 3 cm of tendon, transferred to GT and attached via bone troughs	Satisfactory 10, unsatisfactory 3 Two patients recurrent anterior dislocation

LOE = level of evidence; GT = greater tuberosity; LT = lesser tuberosity; G/E = good to excellent

12. Neviaser RJ, Neviaser TJ, Neviaser JS. Concurrent rupture of the rotator cuff and anterior dislocation of the shoulder in the older patient. *J Bone Joint Surg Am.* 1988;70(9):1308-1311.

13. Fung L, Wong B, Ravichandiran K, Agur A, Rindlisbacher T, Elmaraghy A. Three-dimensional study of pectoralis major muscle and tendon architecture. *Clin Anat.* 2009;22(4):500-508.

14. Galatz LM, Connor PM, Calfee RP, Hsu JC, Yamaguchi K. Pectoralis major transfer for anterior-superior subluxation in massive rotator cuff insufficiency. *J Shoulder Elbow Surg Am.* 2003;12(1):1-5.

15. Klepps SJ, Goldfarb C, Flatow E, Galatz LM, Yamaguchi K. Anatomic evaluation of the subcoracoid pectoralis major transfer in human cadavers. *J Shoulder Elbow Surg Am.* 2001;10(5):453-459.

16. Resch H, Povacz P, Ritter E, Matschi W. Transfer of the pectoralis major muscle for the treatment of irreparable rupture of the subscapularis tendon. *J Bone Joint Surg Am.* 2000;82(3):372-382.

17.   Elhassan B, Ozbaydar M, Massimini D, Diller D, Higgins L, Warner JJP. Transfer of pectoralis major for the treatment of irreparable tears of subscapularis: does it work? *J Bone Joint Surg Br.* 2008;90(8):1059-1065.

18.   Jennings GJ, Keereweer S, Buijze GA, De Beer J, DuToit D. Transfer of segmentally split pectoralis major for the treatment of irreparable rupture of the subscapularis tendon. *J Shoulder Elbow Surg Am.* 2007;16(6):837-842.

19.   Konrad GG, Sudkamp NP, Kreuz PC, Jolly JT, McMahon PJ, Debski RE. Pectoralis major tendon transfers above or underneath the conjoint tendon in subscapularis-deficient shoulders. An in vitro biomechanical analysis. *J Bone Joint Surg Am.* 2007;89(11):2477-2484.

20.   Yang ZX, Pho RW, Kour AK, Pereira BP. The musculocutaneous nerve and its branches to the biceps and brachialis muscles. *J Hand Surg.* 1995;20(4):671-675.

21.   Lo IKY, Lind CC, Burkhart SS. Glenohumeral arthroscopy portals established using an outside-in technique: neurovascular anatomy at risk. *Arthroscopy.* 2004;20(6):596-602.

22.   Clavert P, Lutz J-C, Wolfram-Gabel R, Kempf JF, Kahn JL. Relationships of the musculocutaneous nerve and the coracobrachialis during coracoid abutment procedure (Latarjet procedure). *Surg Radiologic Anatomy: SRA.* 2009;31(1):49-53.

23.   Jost B, Puskas GJ, Lustenberger A, Gerber C. Outcome of pectoralis major transfer for the treatment of irreparable subscapularis tears. *J Bone Joint Surg Am.* 2003;85-A(10):1944-1951.

24.   Gavriilidis I, Kircher J, Magosch P, Lichtenberg S, Habermeyer P. Pectoralis major transfer for the treatment of irreparable anterosuperior rotator cuff tears. *Int Orthop.* 2010;34(5):689-694.

***Please see video on the accompanying Web site at
http://www.slackbooks.com/rotatorcuffvideos***

CHAPTER 23

ROTATOR CUFF ARTHROPATHY

Elisan Tabarace, MD and Brian T. Feeley, MD

The increasingly aging population will undoubtedly present orthopedic surgeons with the challenges of addressing the functional limitations of shoulder arthritis. Our understanding of the pathogenesis and treatment options for rotator cuff tear arthropathy (CTA) is continuing to evolve, especially with better surgical treatment options. Several methods have been proposed to solve the bony and soft-tissue deficiencies in CTA, but most efforts have had difficulty balancing stability without limiting range of motion and therefore function. This chapter will discuss the basic understanding of CTA with a detailed overview of conservative and operative treatment options. It will end with a detailed discussion regarding a promising prosthesis for CTA, the reverse total shoulder.

NATURAL HISTORY AND ETIOLOGY

The earliest reported cases of glenohumeral arthritis and cuff arthropathy were documented by Adams and Smith in the 1850s with numerous subsequent case reports and descriptions following over the next 125 years. However, most recognize Neer et al's report in 1983 as the first to accurately define the disease process known as CTA.[1] In that report, the distinct radiographic morphology of CTA were identified: superior migration and femoralization of the proximal humerus, collapse of the proximal aspect of the humeral articular surface, and acetabularization of the acromion.

There is a lack of data regarding the long-term outcomes of nonoperative care for massive rotator cuff tears. Without intervention, the shoulder in massive rotator cuff tears is thought to progress with a final picture that includes atrophy and fatty infiltration of the rotator cuff complex, degeneration of the glenohumeral cartilage, and superior migration of the humeral head. Despite these distinct features, there is a lack of data correlating radiographic findings with the functional state of the patient.[2] Overall, further study is necessary to elucidate the long-term natural history of massive rotator cuff tears and CTA.

Ma CB, Feeley BT.
*Basic Principles and Operative Management
of the Rotator Cuff (pp 331-344)*
© 2012 SLACK Incorporated

Etiology

The evolution from massive rotator cuff tear to CTA continues to be an area of scientific interest. Not all patients who sustain small cuff tears progress to massive cuff tears, and not all patients with massive cuff tears develop CTA. Zingg and colleagues evaluated 19 patients with massive cuff tears treated nonoperatively.[2] There was progression of glenohumeral osteoarthritis, superior migration of the humeral head, increasing tear size, and progression of fatty infiltration over a 4-year period. Ironically, most patients maintained adequate shoulder function despite deteriorating radiographic studies.

The rheumatology literature has consistently advocated a biological pathway for the development of CTA.[3-6] One of the etiologies proposed for CTA is based on a similar disease process described as the "Milwaukee shoulder." The basis of this theory is that development of CTA is secondary to an inflammatory process that has developed within the shoulder that causes the destruction of cartilage and soft tissue around the glenohumeral joint. Their theory is based on several studies that observed an accumulation of calcium phosphate crystals within joints that developed CTA.[3,4] The authors proposed that calcium phosphate crystals initiate a cascade of events that trigger the release of collagenases and proteases, which cause degradation of cartilaginous tissue.[5,6]

A second theory, termed the *nutritional theory*, suggests that the underlying cause behind articular cartilage degradation is the lack of nutrition provided to the cartilage within the glenohumeral joint. In this theory, a torn rotator cuff allows the escape of nourishing synovial fluid and decreases the joint pressures required for the distribution of nutrients.[1] These changes lead to a functional decline. With disuse of that joint, atrophy of the muscles and articular cartilage follow.

The mechanical theory behind the development of CTA focuses on the pathologic distributions of physical stresses placed on the humeral head after anterosuperior migration through the cuff tear. The deterioration of the articular cartilage is a result of repetitive trauma between the undersurface of the acromion and the superior aspect of the humeral head.

As with many diseases, a complex combination of these factors most likely contributes to the development of CTA. Neer and colleagues proposed a theory that included both nutritional and mechanical factors (Figure 23-1).[1] Collins and Harryman proposed a logical pathway for the development of CTA using a combination of these previous theories.[7] In their theory, CTA is initiated by the escape of the humeral head through a torn cuff. Repetitive mechanical wear between the humerus and acromion leads to inflammatory-inducing debris. This inflammation introduces an enzymatic milieu that exacerbates the damaged cartilage and leads to a clinical picture that consists of acute-on-chronic shoulder pain and immobility. Finally, the disuse of the joint only advances the deterioration of the articular surface and surrounding musculature, leading to atrophy and weakness of the rotator cuff muscles.

DEMOGRAPHICS

Neer et al's original description of the CTA patient still holds today.[1] The typical patient with CTA is a patient in their 60s (or older) with a long history of pain in their dominant shoulder. It is more common in women than in men. It is relatively rare for involvement of both extremities (10% to 25%) unless there is an underlying inflammatory disease, such as rheumatoid arthritis. In these situations, bilateral involvement of the shoulders is usually accompanied by polyarticular findings. Patients will consistently describe a long history (average 10 years) of progressive pain that is worse at night and weakness that leads to a major limitation of activities despite multiple corticosteroid injections. Often, a traumatic event can result in a more rapid progression of the disease process.

In CTA, the physical findings are directly related to the loss of the rotator cuff tendons. On inspection, a "fluid sign" along the anterosuperior aspect of the shoulder will hint at the presence of subacromial bursal swelling. However, the hallmark features of CTA include the loss of active and

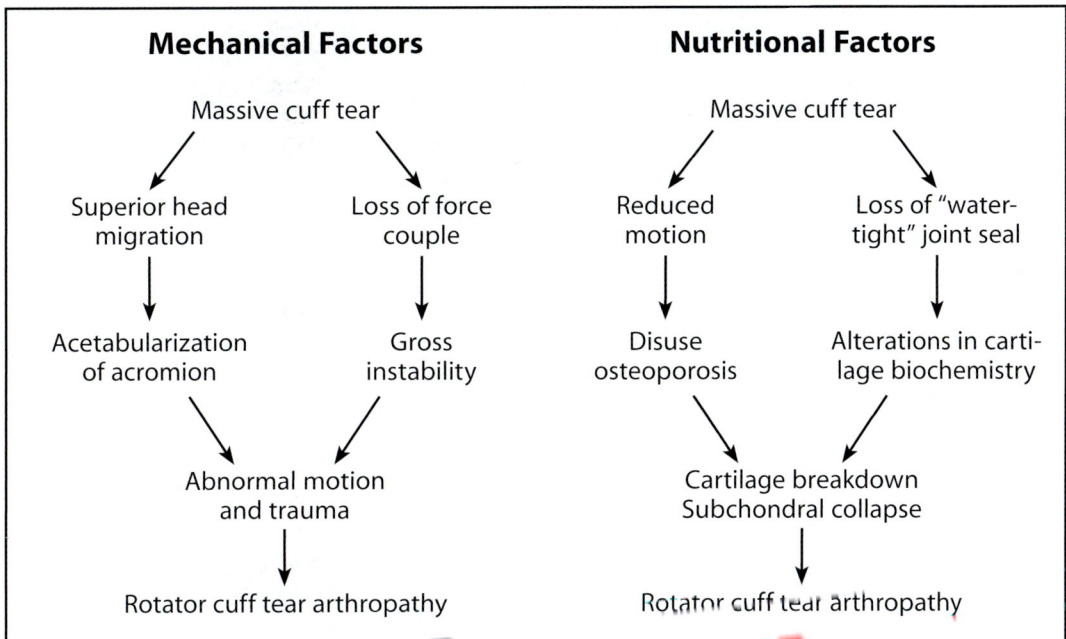

Figure 23-1, Diagram depicting the factors thought to be responsible for the development of CTA. In Neer's description, both mechanical and nutritional factors are thought to contribute to the characteristic findings seen in patients with CTA.

passive range of motion coupled with weakness. Isolated tears in the supraspinatus rarely lead to loss of active or passive motion, but tears in both the supraspinatus and infraspinatus result in a loss of the rotator cuff force couple with subsequent difficulties raising the shoulder above 70 degrees. Patients will often have weakness in external rotation as demonstrated by a positive "hornblower's sign." Tears in the subscapularis have weakness in internal rotation but a more variable change in the range of motion. Impingement syndromes with rotator cuff tears alone do not show this combination of loss of active and passive range of motion.

IMAGING

The plain radiographic findings in CTA are distinct and are thought to be secondary to the loss of the forces coupling the centers of the humeral head within the glenoid (Figure 23-2A). Overall, disuse of the shoulder leads to general osteopenia in the acromion and proximal humerus. On anteroposterior views, there is a characteristic superior migration of the humeral head in relation to the glenoid. The distance between the humeral head and underside of the acromion is often less than 7 mm but is not specific for CTA.[8] It is often helpful to obtain weight-bearing views of the affected shoulder, as this will demonstrate superior migration in the setting of a massive cuff tear that may not always be present in nonweight-bearing or supine views. CTA often leads to gradual changes in the acromion that range from a sourcil sign (inferior sclerosis) to acetabularization. Occasionally, stress fractures of the acromion can be seen.[9] Eventually, the greater tuberosity can be worn down in a process called femoralization of the humerus.[6] This is a product of chronic superior migration of the humeral head and repetitive articulations with the acromion. In early CTA, there may only be mild superior migration of the humeral head on radiographs (Figure 23-2B), but if a weight-bearing view is obtained, there is significant superior migration of the humeral head and impingement on the acromion (Figure 23-2C).

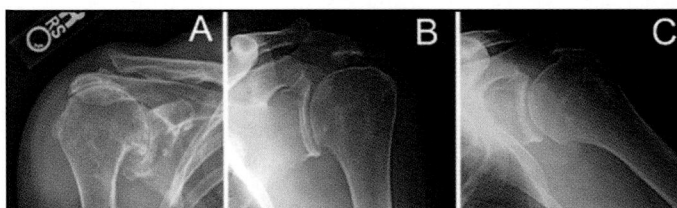

Figure 23-2. (A) Typical radiographic findings of a patient with advanced CTA. There is acetabularization of the acromion and distal clavicle, a high-riding humeral head, and femoralization of the greater tuberosity as it has rubbed against the undersurface of the acromion. There is also loss of joint space between the humeral head and the glenoid. (B, C) The same patient with a massive rotator cuff tear. (B) A nonweight-bearing view is demonstrated with mild superior subluxation; but when a weight is added (C), there is significant superior subluxation of the humeral head relative to the glenoid.

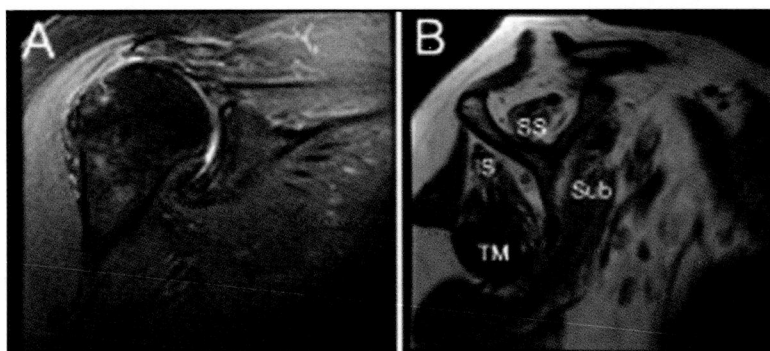

Figure 23-3. MRI of a shoulder with moderate CTA. (A) On the T2 coronal imaging, there is superior migration of the humeral head, and a significant rotator cuff tear is seen with medial retraction of the supraspinatus tendon. (B) On the T1 sagittal imaging, there is a moderate amount of muscle atrophy and fatty infiltration throughout the entire rotator cuff muscles (SS, supraspinatus; IS, infraspinatus; Sub, subscapularis; TM, teres minor).

On axillary views of the shoulder, glenohumeral joint space narrowing and peripheral osteophytes can be clearly demonstrated. Other features seen in this view include anterior or posterior migration of the humerus or wear of the coracoid process with chronic anterior subluxation of the humeral head. Humeral head erosion, flattening, and subchondral cysts can all be seen on this view as well.

Computed tomography (CT) and magnetic resonance imaging (MRI) are not necessary for diagnosis of CTA, but may aid in surgical planning in specific situations, such as revision cases and cases where the amount of bone loss in the glenoid is concerning on standard radiographs (Figure 23-3). If abnormal glenoid wear patterns raise considerations for glenoid osteotomy or bone grafting, then CT may beneficial.[10]

Patients who present with disabling pain that cannot be adequately examined may benefit from MRI to assess for the extent of rotator cuff tear, glenoid stock and orientation, and most importantly, tendon integrity. An MRI can be useful in specifically assessing teres minor and subscapularis integrity prior to planned surgical procedures in the setting of massive cuff tears without major glenohumeral arthritis.[11]

NONOPERATIVE MANAGEMENT

Many patients can function well despite a lack of rotator cuff as long as the deltoid and scapular stabilizing muscles are intact and strong. Tear size and pain do not always have a direct correlation. In these patients without distinct contraindications, pharmacologic management of symptoms includes ibuprofen, naproxen, and cyclooxygenase inhibitors.

There has been little evidence that conclusively shows that physical therapy can benefit functional outcomes in patients with massive rotator cuff tears. There are trends in the literature that suggest that exercises that focus on strengthening the deltoid and scapular musculature in select patients can lead to improved function of the involved shoulder. Ainsworth and Lewis[12] reported 10 patients who all demonstrated improved pain and functional outcome (SF 36, Oxford shoulder disability questionnaire) scores after 12 weeks of physiotherapy in patients with retracted full-thickness tears of the rotator cuff. This systematic review looked at the management of full-thickness tears of rotator cuff and concluded that, despite a lack of randomized controlled trials regarding nonoperative management of massive rotator cuff tears, a regimen of physical therapy is warranted in CTA.[12] There was significant heterogeneity among type, duration, intensity, and progression of exercises used. The included studies varied in their specific exercise routine as well as their use of additional pharmacotherapy and hydrotherapy. Nevertheless, the risks are minimal. None of the studies stated a worsening of symptoms due to the exercise programs. At a minimum, exercise may provide short-term benefits in function.

Another common treatment modality includes fluid aspiration and corticosteroid injection. There is evidence that short-term pain relief can be seen in patients with impingement and tendinosis, but the long-term benefits of steroid injections in CTA have not been demonstrated. In an unblinded and nonrandomized trial, viscosupplementation showed better Visual Analog Pain scores and Constant scores compared to a control group. However, this difference diminished after 5 months.[13] For patients with CTA who are unwilling or are unable to undergo surgical intervention, aspiration with corticosteroid or other supplemental administration may be beneficial as an adjunct to physical therapy.

Overall, patients must be counseled that nonoperative care of a torn rotator cuff will not heal the damage that is done and will not change the natural history of the disease process despite temporary improvements. Tanaka and colleagues observed certain factors that predicted success of conservative treatment.[14] An intact supraspinatus intramuscular tendon, a lack of an impingement sign, external rotation of greater than 35 degrees, and no supraspinatus atrophy were all favorable features that were consistent with successful conservative treatment in the setting of massive cuff tears. Nevertheless, only 53% of the group treated with nonoperative management showed functional improvements after 3 months. Ultimately, the treatment decision should be based on the symptoms and goals of the patient.

ARTHROSCOPY

Arthroscopy in the setting of irreparable rotator cuff damage has consistently shown limited long-term success. Irrigation of enzymes and crystals with débridement of joint surfaces can provide temporary relief of symptoms. In a study by Epis and colleagues, the effects of tidal lavage in a cohort of patients with Milwaukee shoulder were compared.[15] The 2 groups differed in that one group had radiographic changes as a result of massive cuff tears while the other did not. This second group did not need a repeat lavage, while the prior group's experience was short-lived. This difference led the authors to conclude that arthroscopic irrigation and débridement can be more effective in providing symptomatic relief if done early enough in the CTA disease process.

In the elderly with low functional demands, arthroscopic débridement with biceps tenotomy can be a safe and effective short-term procedure in the light of massive irreparable rotator cuff tears.[16]

Leim and colleagues[16] retrospectively reviewed the effect of arthroscopy and biceps tenotomy in the elderly (mean age 71). In all cases, the coracoacromial (CA) ligament was maintained. Despite the progression of arthritis in 32% of the patients, the functional outcomes scores (from 24 to 69.8 on American Shoulder and Elbow Surgeon) and pain scores (from 7.8 to 2 on Visual Analog) improved at an average of 2 years of follow-up.

A retrospective review of the effects of tenodesis and tenotomy for biceps lesion in the setting of CTA was address by Boileau and colleagues.[17] Sixty-eight patients with massive rotator cuff tears were treated with either tenodesis or tenotomy. At 3 years, 78% were satisfied, and 100% of the patients who had a painful loss of active elevation prior to the procedure had recovered. Two other points were made. First, there was no difference in outcomes between patients who underwent tenotomy versus tenodesis. Second, patients with an atrophic or absent teres minor had worse outcomes.

Klinger and colleagues compared the results of arthroscopic débridement for irreparable rotator cuff tears in 2 groups that differed only in the use of a biceps tenotomy.[18] Forty-one patients were monitored for an average of 31 months. Both groups had significant pain relief and improved function. Despite the longer duration of pain relief in the group that underwent a tenotomy, the final pain scores and functional outcomes were not statistically different.

Many elderly patients will have undergone previous arthroscopic procedures in attempts to address complete rotator cuff tears. Galatz and colleagues followed 18 patients with complete repair of massive cuff tears greater than 2 cm.[19] More than 94% (17/18) of shoulders had a recurrent tear on ultrasound at an average 12-month follow-up. Despite initial pain relief and functional gains, at an average 24-month follow-up, 12 of 18 had functional outcome scores below their maximum postoperative scores. Zumstein and colleagues[20] showed a 57% retear rate of massive rotator cuff tears 10 years after complete repair. The retear group had less strength, lower Constant scores, and higher rates of fatty infiltration.[20] These and other studies point out several conclusions about arthroscopy in elderly patients with massive cuff tears. The procedure should be done early with a thorough débridement of the bursal tissue and a tenotomy of the biceps if there is any evidence of a biceps lesion. However, if the CA arch is disrupted or if the remaining rotator cuffs are atrophic in light of advanced glenohumeral arthritis, then the patients should be counseled that they are at an increased risk for unsatisfactory outcomes.[21]

FUSION

Shoulder arthrodesis has heavily fallen out of favor as a treatment option for irreparable rotator cuff tears. Complications such as painful hardware and nonunions requiring revision are too common. During a 10-year period, Cofield and Briggs showed a 39% complication rate with 4% requiring a revision in 71 primary fused shoulders.[22] The use of shoulder arthrodesis as an option for patients with failed arthroplasty operations has not been popular either. Scalise and Ianotti found that 4 of 7 patients undergoing shoulder fusion for a failed TSA had to undergo multiple operations to achieve union.[23] One viable use for shoulder fusion can be in patients with axillary nerve palsy or deltoid dysfunction. In these patients, it has been shown that shoulder prostheses function worse than fusion.[24] Overall, up to 25% of patients present with bilateral CTA, making fusion a difficult procedure to accept as an option to help return patients to a reasonable functional level.[25]

TOTAL SHOULDER ARTHROPLASTY

Total shoulder arthroplasty (TSA) has become the standard of care for osteoarthritis and osteonecrosis of the glenohumeral joint. However, this has not been shown to be true in the setting of CTA. Early literature on the use of TSA in CTA varied in population study, design, and

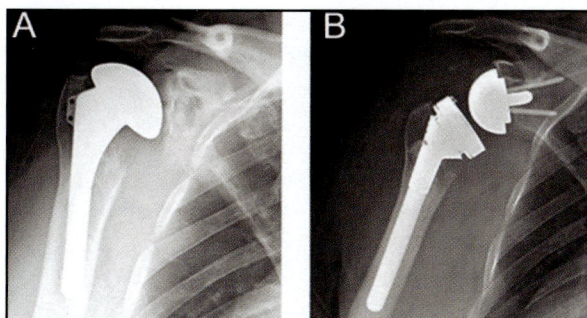

Figure 23-4. (A) Loosening of a glenoid component due to a shoulder with rotator cuff deficiency. This shoulder demonstrates the "rocking horse" effect of the humeral head migrated superiorly and placing abnormal stresses on the glenoid. The glenoid is rocked loose, requiring a conversion to a revision prosthesis, in this case a reverse shoulder arthroplasty (B).

outcomes evaluations. However, most studies suggested less-than-perfect results. In 1983, Neer et al reported 15 of 16 patients undergoing TSA for CTA were satisfied with their "limited" results, but 30% showed lucency around the glenoid component.[1] In 1991, Lohr and colleagues compared 22 patients with CTA treated with a variety of TSA implants or a hemiarthroplasty.[26] Despite the paucity of information regarding the surgeries, the group concluded that CTA was a difficult entity to treat. Their TSA group had better pain relief than the hemiarthroplasty group. However, with a mean follow-up of less than 5 years, there was a high prevalence of radiographic and clinical loosening in patients undergoing TSA for CTA. Another early comparison between TSA and hemiarthroplasty was done in 1992 by Pollack and colleauges.[27] They compared 11 shoulders with TSA to 19 shoulders with hemiarthroplasty. All patients were diagnosed with CTA, and all patients underwent reapproximation of their atrophic cuff to prevent anterosuperior migration. At an average 41-month follow-up, both groups had similar rates of satisfaction and pain relief with the only difference being that the hemiarthroplasty group had better elevation.

The primary reason for the poor clinical results in the TSA group centers on the "rocking horse" concept of glenoid component loosening (Figure 23-4). Initially, the humeral head migrates superiorly through the cuff defect. This migrated head settles and pivots at the edge of the glenoid component. Repetitive damage from unbalanced forces accumulates over time to cause glenoid loosening and finally component failure. A large series by Barrett and colleagues included 9 shoulders with TSA in the setting of rotator cuff tears.[28] Six had pain, 4 had glenoid loosening, and all had massive rotator cuff tear at average 3.5-year follow-up. Franklin and colleagues reported glenoid loosening in 7 of 14 shoulders that underwent TSA for CTA.[29] They observed that the preoperative degree of superior placement of the humeral head correlated to the amount of glenoid loosening. Nwakama and colleagues' report was an example of the severity of the "rocking horse" glenoid.[30] They followed 7 shoulders with semiconstrained TSA for CTA over an average of 69 months. Six of 7 were not satisfied: 3 were loose, 1 was completely shifted, and 2 had to be revised.[30] Sperling and colleagues looked at the clinical results of TSA in glenohumeral arthritis in the setting of a previous stabilization procedure,[31] many of which had clinical and radiographic evidence of CTA. Eleven of 18 TSA patients had radiographic signs of subluxation. Nine of 18 had signs of lucency. Overall, the revision rate for TSA was 38% (8 of 21) with survivorship diminished from 97% at 2 years to 61% at 10 years.

HEMIARTHROPLASTY

Despite variable results in the literature, humeral hemiarthroplasty has become the most common operative treatment for CTA. The percentages of shoulders that are pain-free or have mild pain vary from 47% to 86%. These are less-than-perfect results but are more consistent and effective than previously mentioned options. The aspects of hemiarthroplasty that require more development include the modest gains in range of motion as well as the concern for progressive glenoid and acromion bone loss.

Figure 23-5. Example of a large CTA head for a patient with good range of motion but poor strength. Hemiarthroplasty with a large CTA head can provide promising results in CTA patients with good range of motion, but poor strength due to a massive rotator cuff tear.

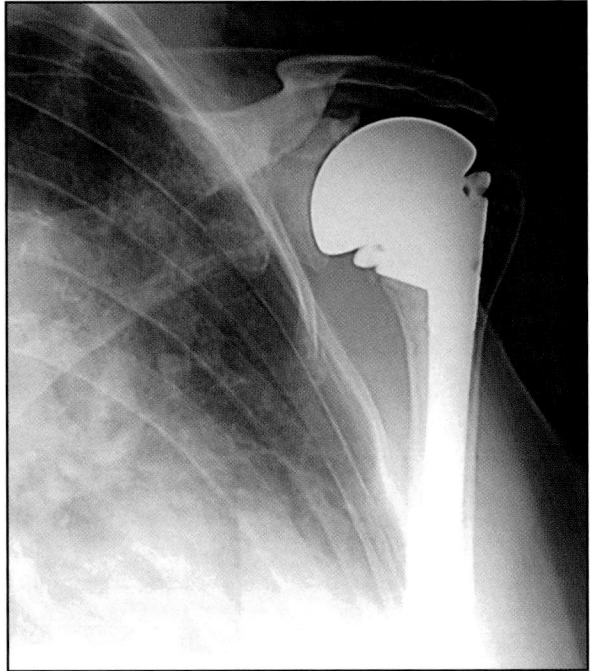

Multiple studies have shown consistent results with the use of hemiarthroplasty for CTA in outcomes of pain relief and patient satisfaction. Early short-term evidence of the success of hemiarthroplasty for CTA was found by Arntz and colleagues.[24] Eighteen shoulders with a minimum 25-month follow-up were reported. All had irreparable cuff tears, superior migration of the humerus, and an intact deltoid. Eleven of 18 had satisfactory pain relief with 4 of 18 shoulders requiring revision. Williams and Rockwood retrospectively reviewed 22 shoulders with hemiarthroplasties for CTA.[32] Seven had undergone previous procedures. The standard deltopectoral approach was used, and all CA ligaments remained intact. Eighty-six percent experienced improvements in pain, there were no cases of instability, and 86% had satisfactory results based on Neer's limited goals criteria. Sanchez-Sotelo and colleagues retrospectively reviewed the largest series of hemiarthroplasty implants for the treatment of CTA.[33] Thirty-three shoulders were followed for an average of 5 years. Overall, 67% were satisfied; however, 24% showed evidence of glenoid wear, 42% showed wear in the acromion, and 6% sustained an acromial fracture. The study did show a statistically significant association with clinical instability and superior humeral migration in shoulders that had a previous history of an acromioplasty or CA ligament reconstruction. Goldberg and colleagues reviewed 34 shoulders treated with hemiarthroplasty in CTA at a mean follow-up time of 10 years.[34] There was a mean improvement of active forward elevation from 78 to 111 degrees and active external rotation from 15 to 38 degrees. Per the Neer's limited goals criteria, 76% of shoulders were rated as successful. Complications included one patient with symptomatic anterosuperior escape and one with a symptomatic greater tuberosity osteophyte requiring reoperation.

The most recent design changes may provide better outcomes. In theory, the new extended humeral head prostheses provide increased surface area for contact and decrease impingement (Figure 23-5). Overall, hemiarthroplasty can provide satisfactory long-term outcomes for carefully selected patients with CTA. Visotsky and colleagues reported 60 shoulders using the extended humeral head prosthesis with a minimum 2-year follow-up.[35] The average range of motion in forward elevation (56 to 116 degrees) and external rotation (8 to 30 degrees) improved as well as the American Shoulder and Elbow Surgeon score (from 29 to 79) without any reported complications in the short term. More data will be required to clarify the clinical advantages of these newer designs.

There are 2 main challenges in the use of a hemiarthroplasty for CTA—the integrity of the CA ligament and glenoid bone stock. Cadaveric and clinical studies have consistently shown the importance of the CA ligament in enhancing the stability of a hemiarthroplasty implant used for CTA.[26,33,36] It has been shown that glenoid and acromion bone loss is increased after previous acromioplasty and CA resection.[8,36] Though these changes tend to happen together, there have been several attempts to address them separately. Modern surgical techniques involve biological and prosthetic reconstruction of the shoulder. Krishnan and colleagues demonstrated a technique of biologic resurfacing of the glenoid and CA ligament with an Achilles allograft.[37] The goals were to augment the glenoid and CA ligament's restraints to anterosuperior forces in hemiarthroplasty implants used for CTA. Ten of 14 were pain-free, while 3 had minimal pain with activity and 1 with moderate pain with activities. The radiographic data showed stable acromiohumeral distance and glenoid erosion at a mean 5 years of follow-up. Studies such as this highlight the major factors that play a role in the success of hemiarthroplasty procedures in CTA. However, the lack of consistent or long-term information should emphasize the importance further studies will have in evaluating the use of soft-tissue augmentation as an adjunct in shoulder reconstruction.

REVERSE TOTAL SHOULDER ARTHROPLASTY

The most recent and arguably the most successful advancement in the treatment of CTA has been the emergence of the reverse TSA (RTSA) prosthesis. The concept was proposed by Grammont over 30 years ago but was met with a lack of enthusiasm considering its early high rate of complications. Now, 6 reverse total shoulder prostheses have been approved for the treatment of CTA. Despite differences in such features as glenosphere anchoring, base plate fixation, and humeral lateralization, all systems share certain features. These similar properties include a convex glenosphere attached to a base plate drilled into the glenoid and a concave humeral polyethylene cup attached to a metallic stem.

The success of the modern RTSA in the treatment of CTA lies in the semiconstrained relationship between the convex glenosphere and concave humeral component. The hemiarthroplasty and TSA implants attempt to recreate the anatomical center of rotation that exists in the humeral head. With a deficient rotator cuff, the deltoid is unmatched, and anterosuperior migration of the humerus would alter the kinematics between the center of rotation and the center of the humeral head. This mismatch leads to a phenomenon known as pseudoparesis, where forward elevation is limited to less than 90 degrees. The RTSA overcomes this mismatch by medializing and distalizing the shoulder joint's center of rotation with its semiconstrained reverse orientation. This increases the lever arm effect of the deltoid without lateralizing the center of rotation. Overall, the prosthesis optimizes deltoid function, bypasses the need for rotator cuff restraint, and increases articulation angles.[38]

Recently, there has been an increasing amount of evidence for the use of RTSA in the setting of CTA. Clinical benefits include improved range of motion in active forward elevation and abduction with consistent pain relief. Gains in external rotation have been more variable. Clinical studies have found that 81% to 96% of their patients have experienced reduction of pain to none or minimal.[39-41] Overall, functional outcome scores have consistently been shown to improve considerably with the use of RTSA for CTA. In one of the largest multicenter series, Sirveaux and colleagues[40] reported on 80 shoulders that were followed for an average of 44 months. The average active elevation was 138 degrees, and the final average Constant score was 65.6.[40] In another recent series, Frankle and colleagues reported a short-term Constant score of 68 in 60 shoulders that underwent RTSA for CTA.[9] Boileau and colleagues observed a final average Constant score of 66 and a final average anterior elevation of 123 degrees in 21 shoulders.[39]

The widespread use of the RTSA has been limited by its relatively high reported complication rate. The main recurring issue that has yet to be overcome is instability.[42] In one of the more critical reports, Werner and colleagues[42] reported on 58 patients over an average 38-month follow-up.

Figure 23-6. Scapular notching after reverse shoulder arthroplasty. (A) There is early scapular notching (arrow) 10 months after reverse shoulder arthroplasty. Two years later, there is significantly more notching (B), as well as an acromion stress fracture (*). The patient remained asymptomatic from both findings.

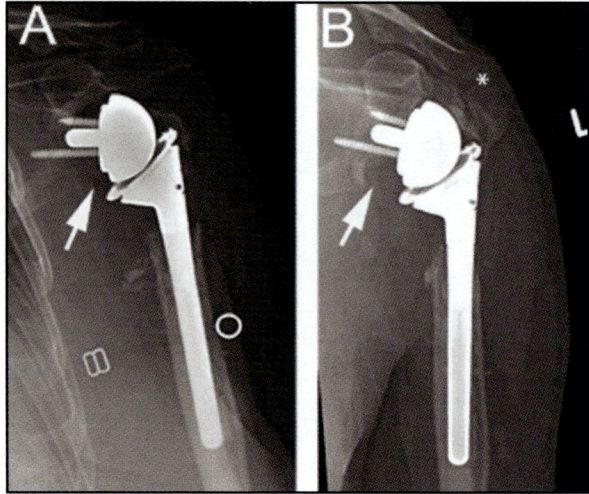

Thirty-three percent had a reoperation with an overall 50% complication rate.[42] Most studies have stated a complication rate anywhere from 15% to 20%.[9,40,42] By far the most reported concern with RTSA has been the rate of notching, wear of the inferior neck of the scapula (Figure 23-6). This wear can be a potential source of glenoid loosening or scapular neck fracture. Early series stated a 30% rate of inferior screw exposure and as much as 50% of subclinical evidence of notching in the short-term follow-up.[40] Despite the lack of clinical evidence regarding its relevance, many have attempted to address early notching by placing the glenoid component inferiorly on the rim or having the implant tilted caudad 15 degrees.[41,42]

Two considerations must be taken when interpreting complication rates for RTSA. First, these implants have been traditionally used in salvage procedures, and reported complication rates have been a heterogeneous selection of issues.[42] Second, every aspect of the RTSA is continuously evolving to optimize exposure, glenoid fixation, notching, and instability.[38,40,43,44] Surgical exposures including the deltopectoral approach as well as the anterosuperior approach have their theoretical advantages. Subtle changes in the center of rotation can help address rates of notching, but potentially alter the biomechanical advantages of the RTSA. Finally, glenoid base fixation has varied from pegs to screws.

CONCLUSION AND RECOMMENDATIONS

Optimal treatment plans for patients with CTA continue to evolve. The decision to treat with either nonoperative or operative care has to be individualized to the patient's needs and overall health. The proposed algorithm summarizes our suggestions (Figure 23-7). All patients with CTA should undergo a trial of physical therapy to specifically strengthen the scapular stabilizing muscles and deltoid muscles, as there are minimal risks to an attempt at nonoperative care. Patients must be counseled that results are not permanent nor consistent.

The overall decision to seek operative care should be based on patient goals and medical comorbidities. Due to the associated morbidity and limited functional gains, only patients with consistent pain and a defective deltoid should be considered for shoulder arthrodesis. These patients usually have a history of multiple procedures or a neurologic disease and would least likely benefit from an arthroplasty procedure. Arthroscopic débridement remains an effective option for pain relief in selected patients. This includes patients who wish to avoid a lengthy rehabilitation process or those who are high-risk surgical patients with cardiovascular or pulmonary comorbidities that preclude an extensive procedure. However, the results are variable in length and overall effectiveness.

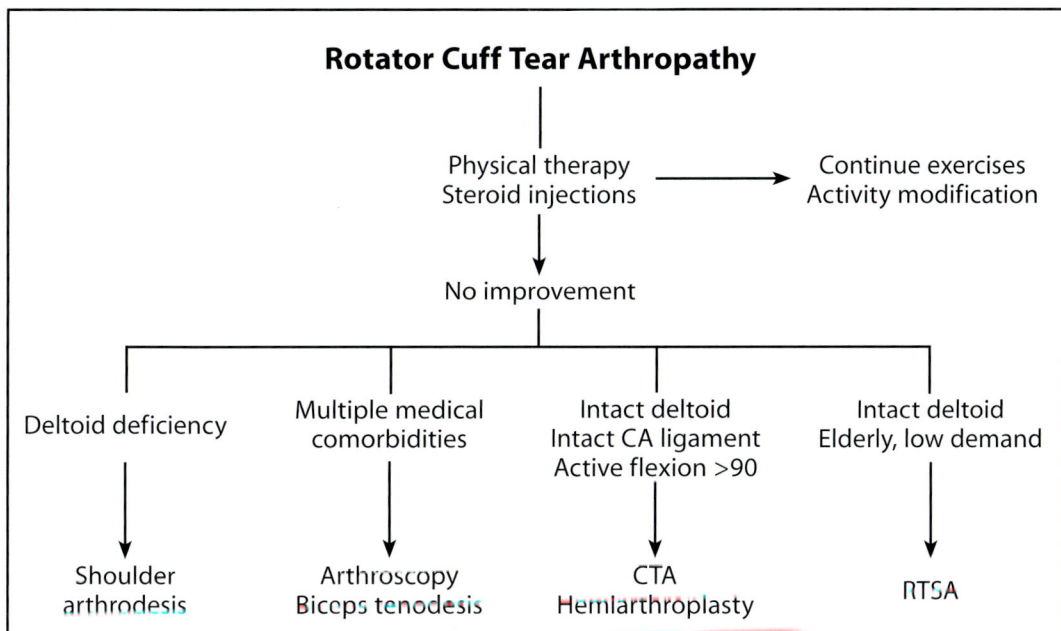

Figure 23-7. Proposed algorithm for treatment of patients with CTA. (Adapted from Feeley BT, Gallo RA, Craig EV. Cuff tear arthropathy: current trends in diagnosis and surgical management. *J Shoulder Elbow Surg.* 2009;18(3):484-494.)

When the decision to undergo shoulder arthroplasty has been made, other specific patient factors should be considered. During the preoperative planning period, clinical and radiographic evaluations should be made regarding the functional integrity of the CA ligament, rotator cuff, and deltoid. If the rotator cuff is intact or reparable, a TSA should be considered. However, in CTA, this is rarely the case, and the ultimate decision for shoulder arthroplasty has to be made between hemiarthroplasty and an RTSA. Patients with higher functional demands, preoperative range of forward motion above 90 degrees, and an intact CA ligament will have acceptable results with a hemiarthroplasty implant. The newer CTA models may provide better results. Often, patients present when CTA has become severely debilitating. An RTSA should be considered in the low-demanding elderly who have evidence of anterosuperior humeral escape or pseudoparalysis (lack of active elevation above 90 degrees). Traditionally, the complication rates are relatively high; however, RTSA technology continues to evolve, and more studies are needed to define the optimal implant design.

Despite its long history, no single nonoperative regimen or surgical treatment option has been successful in addressing the functional and structural deficits of CTA. These challenges can be better met if CTA is approached on an individual basis. With recent developments in shoulder arthroplasty, surgical options for CTA have a more promising future.

REFERENCES

1.   Neer CS 2nd, Craig EV, Fukuda H. Cuff-tear arthropathy. *J Bone Joint Surg Am.* 1983;65:1232-1244.
2.   Zingg PO, Jost B, Sukthankar A, Buhler M, Pfirrmann CW, Gerber C. Clinical and structural outcomes of nonoperative management of massive rotator cuff tears. *J Bone Joint Surg Am.* 2007;89:1928-1934.
3.   Garancis JC, Cheung HS, Halverson PB, McCarty DJ. "Milwaukee shoulder" association of microspheroids containing hydroxyapatite crystals, active collagenase, and neutral protease with rotator cuff defects. Morphologic and biochemical studies of an excised synovium showing chondromatosis. *Arthritis Rheum.* 1981;24:484-491.

4. Halverson PB, Cheung HS, McCarty DJ, Garancis J, Mandel N. "Milwaukee shoulder" association of micro-spheroids containing hydroxyapatite crystals, active collagenase, and neutral protease with rotator cuff defects. II. Synovial fluid studies. *Arthritis Rheum*. 1981;24:474-483.

5. Halverson PB, Garancis JC, McCarty DJ. Histopathological and ultrastructural studies of synovium in Milwaukee shoulder syndrome a basic calcium phosphate crystal arthropathy. *Ann Rheum Dis*. 1984;43:734-741.

6. McCarty DJ, Halverson PB, Carrera GF, Brewer BJ, Kozin F. "Milwaukee shoulder" association of microspheroids containing hydroxyapatite crystals, active collagenase, and neutral protease with rotator cuff defects. I. Clinical aspects. *Arthritis Rheum*. 1981;24:464-473.

7. Collins DN, Harryman DTI. Arthroplasty for arthritis and rotator cuff deficiency. *Orthop Clin North Am*. 1997;28:225-239.

8. Zeman CA, Arcand MA, Cantrell JS, Skedros JG, Burkhead WZ Jr. The rotator cuff deficient arthritic shoulder: diagnosis and surgical management. *J Am Acad Orthop Surg*. 1998;6:337-348.

9. Frankle M, Levy JC, Pupello D, Siegal S, Saleem A, Mighell M. The reverse shoulder prosthesis for glenohumeral arthritis associated with severe rotator cuff deficiency. A minimum two-year follow-up study of sixty patients surgical technique. *J Bone Joint Surg Am*. 2006;88(suppl 1 pt 2):178-190.

10. Klein SM, Dunning P, Mulieri P, Pupello D, Downes K, Frankle MA. Effects of acquired glenoid bone defects on surgical technique and clinical outcomes in reverse shoulder arthroplasty. *J Bone Joint Surg Am*. 2010;92(5):1144-1154.

11. Tauber M, Moursy M, Forstner R, Koller H, Resch H. Latissimus dorsi tendon transfer for irreparable rotator cuff tears: a modified technique to improve tendon transfer integrity: surgical technique. *J Bone Joint Surg Am*. 2010;92 Suppl 1 Pt 2:226-239.

12. Ainsworth R, Lewis JS. Exercise therapy for the conservative management of full thickness tears of the rotator cuff: a systematic review. *Br J Sports Med*. 2007;41:200-210.

13. Tagliafico A, Serafini G, Sconfienza LM, et al. Ultrasound-guided viscosupplementation of subacromial space in elderly patients with cuff tear arthropathy using a high weight hyaluronic acid: prospective open-label non-randomized trial. *Eur Radiol*. 2011;21(1):182-187.

14. Tanaka M, Itoi E, Sato K, et al. Factors related to successful outcome of conservative treatment for rotator cuff tears. *Ups J Med Sci*. 2010;115(3):193-200.

15. Epis O, Caporali R, Scire` CA, Bruschi E, Bonacci E, Montecucco C. Efficacy of tidal irrigation in Milwaukee shoulder syndrome. *J Rheumatol*. 2007;34:1545-1550.

16. Leim D, Lengers N, Dedy N, Poetzl W, Steinbeck J, Marquardt B. Arthroscopic débridement of massive irreparable rotator cuff tears. *Arthroscopy*. 2008;24:743-748.

17. Boileau P, Baque´ F, Valerio L, Ahrens P, Chuinard C, Trojani C. Isolated arthroscopic biceps tenotomy or tenodesis improves symptoms in patients with massive irreparable rotator cuff tears. *J Bone Joint Surg Am*. 2007;89:747-757.

18. Klinger HM, Spahn G, Baums MH, Steckel H. Arthroscopic débridement of irreparable massive rotator cuff tears: a comparison of débridement alone and combined procedure with biceps tenotomy. *Acta Chir Belg*. 2005;105:297-301.

19. Galatz LM, Ball CM, Teefey SA, Middleton WD, Yamaguchi K. The outcome and repair integrity of completely arthroscopically repaired large and massive rotator cuff tears. *J Bone Joint Surg Am*. 2004;86-A(2):219-224.

20. Zumstein MA, Jost B, Hempel J, Hodler J, Gerber C. The clinical and structural long-term results of open repair of massive tears of the rotator cuff. *J Bone Joint Surg Am*. 2008;90(11):2423-2431.

21. Hockman DE, Lucas GL, Roth CA. Role of the coracoacromial ligament as restraint after shoulder hemiarthroplasty. *Clin Orthop Relat Res*. 2004;419:80-82.

22. Cofield RH, Briggs BT. Glenohumeral arthrodesis: operative and long-term results. *J Bone Joint Surg Am*. 1979;61:668-677.

23. Scalise JJ, Ianotti JP. Glenohumeral arthrodesis after failed prosthetic shoulder arthroplasty. *J Bone Joint Surg Am*. 2008;90:70-77.

24. Arntz CT, Matsen FA 3rd, Jackins S. Surgical management of complex irreparable rotator cuff deficiency. *J Arthroplasty*. 1991;6:363-370.

25. Feeley BT, Gallo RA, Craig EV. Cuff tear arthropathy: current trends in diagnosis and surgical management. *J Shoulder Elbow Surg*. 2009;18(3):484-494.

26. Lohr JF, Cofield RH, Uhthoff HK. Glenoid component loosening in cuff tear arthropathy. *J Bone Joint Surg Am*. 1991;73(suppl 2):106.

27. Pollack RG, Deliz ED, McIlveen SJ, Flatow EL, Bigliani LU. Prosthetic replacement in rotator cuff deficient shoulders. *J Shoulder Elbow Surg*. 1992;1:173-186.

28. Barrett WP, Franklin JL, Jackins SE, Wyss CR, Matsen FA 3rd. Total shoulder arthroplasty. *J Bone Joint Surg Am*. 1987;69:865-872.

29. Franklin JL, Barrett WP, Jackins SE, Matsen FA 3rd. Glenoid loosening in total shoulder arthroplasty: association with rotator cuff deficiency. *J Arthroplasty*. 1988;3:39-46.

30. Nwakama AC, Cofield RH, Kavanagh BF, Loehr JF. Semiconstrained total shoulder arthroplasty for glenohumeral arthritis and massive rotator cuff tearing. *J Shoulder Elbow Surg*. 2000;9:302-307.

31. Sperling JW, Antuna SA, Sanchez-Sotelo J, Schleck C, Cofield RH. Shoulder arthroplasty for arthritis after instability surgery. *J Bone Joint Surg Am*. 2002;84- A(10):1775-1781.

32. Williams GR, Rockwood CA. Hemiarthroplasty in rotator cuff-deficient shoulders. *J Shoulder Elbow Surg*. 1996;5:362-367.

33. Sanchez-Sotelo J, Cofield RH, Rowland CM. Shoulder hemiarthroplasty for glenohumeral arthritis associated with severe rotator cuff deficiency. *J Bone Joint Surg Am*. 2001;83:1814-1822.

34. Goldberg SS, Bell JE, Kim HJ, Bak SF, Levine WN, Bigliani LU. Hemiarthroplasty for the rotator cuff-deficient shoulder. *J Bone Joint Surg Am*. 2008;90:554-559.

35. Visotsky JL, Basamania C, Seebauer L, Rockwood CA, Jensen KL. Cuff tear arthropathy: pathogenesis, classification, and algorithm for treatment. *J Bone Joint Surg Am*. 2004;86(suppl 2):35-60.

36. Field LD, Dines DM, Zabinski SJ, Warren RF. Hemiarthroplasty of the shoulder for rotator cuff arthropathy. *J Shoulder Elbow Surg*. 1997;6:18-23.

37. Krishnan S, Burkhead WZ, Nowinski RJ. Humeral hemiarthroplasty with biologic resurfacing of the glenoid and acromion for rotator cuff tear arthropathy. *Tech Shoulder Elbow*. 2004;5:51-59.

38. Matsen FA 3rd, Boileau P, Walch G, Gerber C, Bicknell RT. The reverse total shoulder arthroplasty. *J Bone Joint Surg Am*. 2007;89:660-667.

39. Boileau P, Watkinson DJ, Hatzidakis AM, Balg F. Grammont reverse prosthesis: design, rationale, and biomechanics. *J Shoulder Elbow Surg*. 2005;14:147S-161S.

40. Sirveaux F, Favard L, Oudet D, Huquet D, Walch G, Mole D. Grammont inverted total shoulder arthroplasty in the treatment of glenohumeral osteoarthritis with massive rupture of the cuff. Results of a multicentre study of 80 shoulders. *J Bone Joint Surg Br*. 2004;86:388-395.

41. Wall B, Nove-Josserand L, O'Connor DP, Edwards TB, Walch G. Reverse total shoulder arthroplasty: a review of results according to etiology. *J Bone Joint Surg Am*. 2007;89:1476-1485.

42. Werner CM, Steinmann PA, Gilbart M, Gerber C. Treatment of painful pseudoparesis due to irreparable rotator cuff dysfunction with the Delta III reverse-ball-and-socket total shoulder prosthesis. *J Bone Joint Surg Am*. 2005;87:1476-1486.

43. Anglin C, Tolhurst P, Wyss UP, Pichora DR. Glenoid cancellous bone strength and modulus. *J Biomech*. 1999;32:1091-1097.

44. Bufquin T, Hersan A, Hubert L, Massin P. Reverse shoulder arthroplasty for the treatment of three- and four-part fractures of the proximal humerus in the elderly: a prospective review of 43 cases with a short-term follow-up. *J Bone Joint Surg Br*. 2007;89:516-520.

CHAPTER 24

REVERSE SHOULDER ARTHROPLASTY FOR THE TREATMENT OF CUFF TEAR ARTHROPATHY

Suketu Vaishnav, MD and James D. Kelly II, MD

Multiple disease processes have been described that ultimately lead to a common pathologic pathway causing the phenomenon known as cuff tear arthropathy (CTA). A combination of biologic and mechanical dysfunction leads to disturbances in glenohumeral kinematics, causing instability and, in its end stage, producing a predictable pattern of arthritic change. Many different etiologies can lead to this shared final outcome.

Stability to the glenohumeral joint is provided through both static and dynamic stabilizers. Dynamic stability in large part is imparted by the rotator cuff complex through balanced force couples in both the coronal and transverse planes.[1-3] These balanced moments produce a model of concavity—compression of the humeral head on the glenoid articular surface.[4] This in turn creates a stable fulcrum from which active motion, specifically abduction and rotation, can be accomplished.

Due to various causative factors, instability results from the loss of these force couples. This in turn produces imbalance about the humeral head and an inability to maintain a stable fulcrum. A spectrum of instability exists and is dependent on the extent of rotator cuff pathology and the competency of accompanying static restraints. In early stages, instability may only be evident with active elevation where superior subluxation of the humeral head is present with active abduction. In these cases, the depressive effect on the humeral head is absent due to a tear of the rotator cuff. When this compressive effect is lost and a stable fulcrum is no longer present, deltoid contraction results in superior migration instead of abduction. Multiple studies have demonstrated a direct relationship between the size and location of the rotator cuff tear with the amount of instability seen in both cadaveric and in vivo models.[1,5-8]

In later stages of CTA, static instability can be visualized radiographically as fixed superior migration of the humeral head with the acromiohumeral distance decreasing to less than 6 mm.[9,10] When the humeral head is no longer contained within the glenoid, the bony morphology of the proximal humerus, glenoid, and acromion undergo progressive deterioration as a result of altered mechanics.[11] With superior migration, the humeral head articulates with the undersurface of the

Ma CB, Feeley BT.
*Basic Principles and Operative Management
of the Rotator Cuff (pp 345-364)*
© 2012 SLACK Incorporated

acromion, resulting in femoralization of the head and acetabularization of the coracoacromial (CA) arch. Eccentric glenoid wear patterns result in preferential superior glenoid wear and deficiency.[12]

Under more severe circumstances, frank anterosuperior escape of the humeral head develops with attempted active elevation. This is usually observed when there is compromise of the CA ligament or a massive anterosuperior rotator cuff tear. The CA ligament is an important secondary stabilizer, and escape in this setting is usually preceded by iatrogenic causes involving subacromial decompression and release of the ligament.[13] Anterosuperior rotator cuff tears are often seen in the setting of glenohumeral dislocations, especially in the elderly patient.[14] Patients with escape usually present with pseudoparalysis and extremely poor function.

In addition to mechanical dysfunction contributing to CTA, multiple authors have suggested that biologic factors contribute to what has been described by Neer et al as classic CTA.[15] The fact that only a small percentage of patients with massive rotator cuff tears develop this pathology directs investigators to search for other causes aside from pure mechanical failure. It is more likely that a combined biomechanical theory is responsible for this entity. Biologic theories have been based on an inflammatory model mediated by calcium pyrophosphate deposition,[16-18] leakage of synovial fluid, and nutritional malnourishment.[10,15,19]

Due to this combination of mechanical and nutritional dysfunction, glenohumeral articular degeneration results with subsequent osteoporosis and bone collapse. Bone loss is further potentiated by impaired motion and disuse atrophy.

CLASSIFICATION

Multiple classification systems have been described to diagnose the severity and stages of CTA. The most commonly used schemes include the Seebauer, Hamada-Fukuda, and Favard systems. The limitations of these systems is poor inter- and intraobserver reliability.[20]

The Seebauer system is based on a biomechanical assessment of the center of rotation of the glenohumeral joint and its functional and morphologic implications.[10,21] In Type 1, the center of rotation is maintained, whereas in Type 2, it is superiorly migrated. Type 1a is defined by acetabularization of the acromion and femoralization of the humeral head while Type 1b also includes glenoid erosion evident by medialization of the humeral head. Stability imparted by the CA arch distinguishes Type 2a from 2b. It is important to differentiate Type 1 from Type 2 deformities—an indication of rotator cuff dysfunction creating coronal plane instability.

Hamada and colleagues[9] based their classification on the severity of radiographic findings seen in patients with massive rotator cuff tears graded on the basis of the acromiohumeral interval (AHI; Figure 24-1). Grade 1 is defined as an AHI of 6 mm or more, while Grade 2 is defined as an AHI of 5 mm or less. In addition to an AHI less than 5 mm, Grade 3 represents patients with acetabularization of the acromion. Grade 4 patients have the added finding of glenohumeral space narrowing. Walch further subdivided Grade 4 into 4a, where there is eccentric superior glenoid wear without acetabularization of the acromion, and 4b, superior wear with acetabularization. This was specifically done to note that there is not necessarily a temporal relationship in this classification system and that some patients progress directly from Grade 2 to Grade 4a and then to 4b.[12] Grade 5 denotes end-stage disease with humeral collapse, indicating CTA. There are some difficulties in applying this classification scheme, however. In cases with significant subacromial effusions, the AHI can appear normal or increased. In addition, rotation of the humerus tends to decrease the AHI, which may not be present on radiographs taken in neutral rotation.[12]

The Favard classification focuses on staging glenohumeral arthritis and is divided into 5 stages (Figure 24-2). Stage E0 denotes eccentric glenoid cartilage wear without subchondral bone erosion. Stage E1 indicates concentric glenoid erosion, while stage E2 involves eccentric erosion producing a biconcave glenoid on an anteroposterior (AP) view. Stage E3 signifies advanced erosion with a

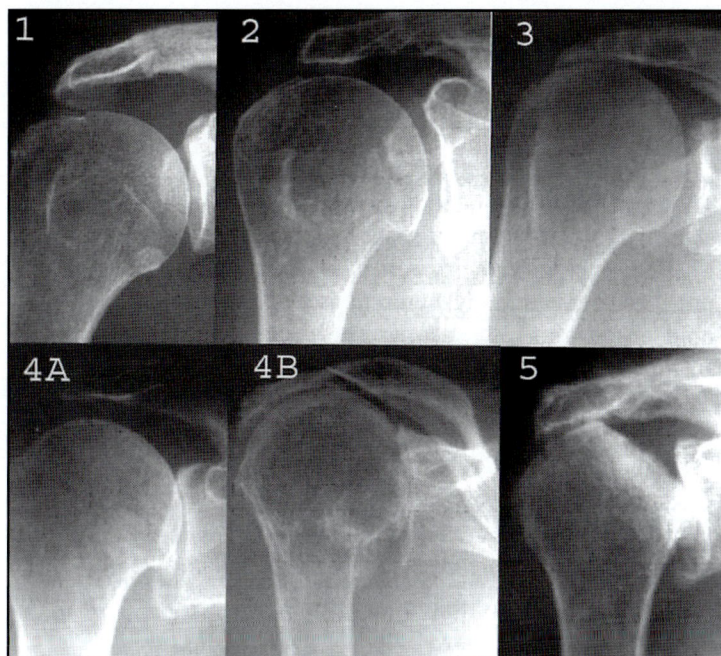

Figure 24-1. Hamada classification.[9] 1 = AHI >6 mm; 2 = AHI <5 mm; 3 = acetabularization of the acromion; 4A = glenohumeral narrowing; 4B = superior wear with narrowing; 5 = humeral collapse.

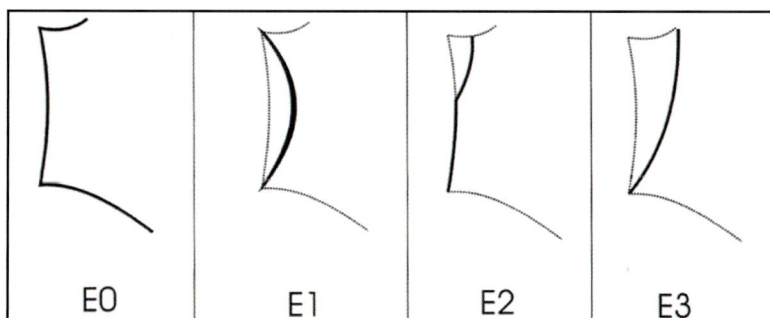

Figure 24-2. Favard classification.[12]

large, cephalad-oriented deformity. Lastly, stage E4 represents anteroinferior erosion associated with a massive rotator cuff tear. The authors point out that Stage E1 likely represents a condition where osteoarthritis precedes the rotator cuff tear, while, in all other stages, the cuff tear likely occurred prior to glenohumeral arthritic change, explaining the eccentric wear patterns.

EVALUATION

History and Physical

The clinical presentation of these patients varies and is based on the spectrum of disease present and in part the causative etiology. More commonly, patients may present with chronic deterioration of strength and function but can present with acute symptoms after recent trauma. In the earlier instance, progressive enlargement of a massive rotator cuff tear and associated fatty muscle atrophy lead to a gradual decline in function. In cases of sudden loss of function preceded by acute trauma, distinction must be made between an acute massive rotator cuff tear and instances of acute inflammatory subacromial bursitis in a pre-existing or enlarged chronic rotator cuff tear.

Patients are more commonly elderly women with the dominant extremity being preferentially affected. Bilateral involvement is seen in a little more than half of cases.[22] Symptoms of pain are more common in patients with advanced glenohumeral or acromiohumeral arthritis. Those presenting with pseudoparalysis typically present with significant loss of motion and strength with variable amounts of pain.

If the patient had prior surgery, a thorough history is obtained to rule out the possibility of infection. This includes recent or prolonged postoperative drainage, pain at rest and at night, or complaints of fever or chills. The surgical incision should be carefully inspected for erythema, warmth, fluctuance, and active drainage.

Physical exam findings include swelling, which can be substantial in the presence of a subacromial effusion. In extreme cases, a geyser sign can be seen due to the escape of a hemorrhagic effusion through a massive rotator cuff tear into the subcutaneous tissue.[23] Atrophy of the supraspinatus and infraspinatus fossae will often accompany longstanding cuff tears. Patients with advanced arthritis will show diminished active and passive range of motion. In contrast, patients with massive rotator cuff tears without significant arthritis will exhibit pseudoparalysis and the inability to actively elevate the shoulder above 90 degrees, but will retain their passive range of motion. It can be difficult to differentiate between painful loss of active motion and true pseudoparalysis. In instances of pseudoparalysis, one may be able to visualize anterosuperior subluxation of the humeral head between the acromion and coracoid process with attempted elevation.[24-26] This is often a subtle sign and may not always be obvious. The landing test can also be used to confirm the diagnosis of pseudoparalysis.[26] Here, the examiner passively elevates the arm up to 120 degrees and asks the patient to maintain this position. Those with pseudoparesis will be unable to do so, causing the arm to fall down to the side.[26] If the diagnosis of pseudoparalysis is still in doubt, we perform a diagnostic lidocaine injection, thus eliminating pain as a confounding factor. Those with a compromised CA ligament or massive anterosuperior tear may also exhibit frank escape of the humeral head with attempted elevation.

Strength testing is performed to assess the clinical integrity of the rotator cuff muscles. Supraspinatus function is absent, and the Jobe test is always weak. External rotation strength with the arm adducted is used to test the posterior cuff. In addition to measuring internal rotation strength, the subscapularis is evaluated by performing the belly-press and lift-off tests. It is also important to evaluate the integrity of the infraspinatus and teres minor tendons through the external rotation lag and hornblower's test, respectively (Figures 24-3).[25] Patients with evidence of preoperative teres minor fatty atrophy or deficiency have decreased active external rotation after reverse shoulder arthroplasty (RSA) and lower functional outcome scores, despite restoration of active elevation. These patients are less satisfied with RSA as they exhibit significant dysfunction with overhead activities and activities of daily living.[27] It is therefore imperative to identify patients with an incompetent posterior rotator cuff as they are considered for RSA with a combined latissimus dorsi/teres major transfer to restore external rotation strength.

The acromion and other deltoid origin sites should be carefully examined prior to performing an RSA. Acromial insufficiency can result from progressive erosion and thinning of the undersurface of the acromion seen in Hamada III and greater deformities. Significant tenderness to palpation about the deltoid origin should raise clinical suspicion about pre-existing or impending fracture, and further radiographic evaluation should be performed. The presence of an asymptomatic os acromiale, however, has not been shown to lead to poor results and is not a contraindication to RSA.[28] As RSA restores deltoid tension and places increased stress on the deltoid origin, any evidence of pre-existing acromial insufficiency should be carefully considered prior to proceeding with RSA.

The acromioclavicular joint and long head of the biceps tendon should be examined as possible sources of pain. If the biceps tendon is found to be major cause of a patient's symptoms, good results can be achieved simply with isolated biceps tenotomy or tenodesis even in the presence of irreparable rotator cuff tears.[26]

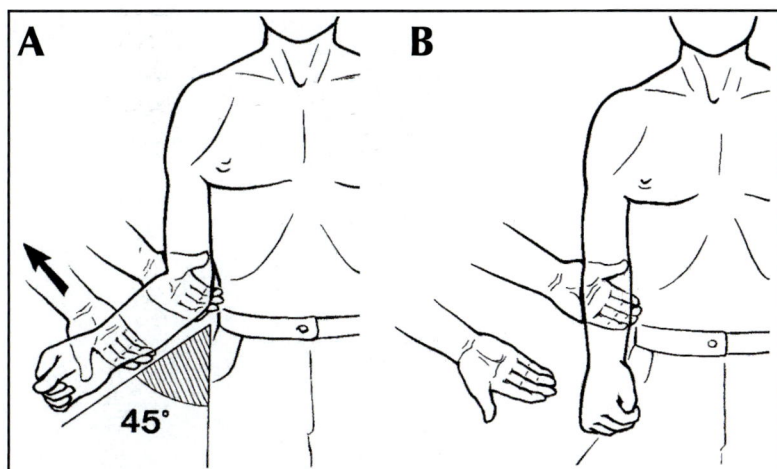

Figure 24-3. External rotation lag test for evaluation of infraspinatus function. (A) With the patient seated, the shoulder is placed in 0 degrees of abduction and 45 degrees of external rotation with the elbow flexed to 90 degrees. The examiner holds the patient's forearm in this position and instructs the patient to maintain it when he or she lets go of the forearm. (B) On releasing the forearm, a positive test is recorded when the patient's forearm drops back to 0 degrees of external rotation, despite efforts to maintain external rotation. (Reproduced with permission and copyright © of the British Editorial Society of Bone and Joint Surgery. Walch G, Boulahia A, Calderone S, Robinson AH. The "dropping" and "hornblower's" signs in evaluation of rotator-cuff tears. *J Bone Joint Surg Br.* 1998;80(4):624-628.)

A thorough neurologic and cervical spine exam is performed in every patient, which is especially important in those who have undergone previous surgical intervention. Specifically, an actively functioning anterior, middle, and posterior deltoid must be confirmed when considering RSA. A patient with extreme rotator cuff weakness, an intact or nearly intact rotator cuff, and severe atrophy may actually have cervical radiculopathy. Nerve conduction and electromyography testing should be used to further evaluate any suspicion of neurologic injury.

Radiographic Imaging

Standard AP views of the glenohumeral joint in neutral and internal rotation, axillary, and scapula-Y views are obtained. These will show characteristic findings of a decreased AHI (<6 mm). As the AHI is variable with rotation, we rely on an AP view taken in neutral rotation to assess the true amount of superior humeral head migration.

Long-term articulation of the humeral head with the acromion produces acetabularization of the acromion and CA arch with femoralization of the humeral head due to rounding off of the greater tuberosity. Glenohumeral arthrosis is variable and can present with significant medialization of the joint to the level of the coracoid process. Superior glenoid wear is often seen. Anterior and posterior instability can also be appreciated on the axillary view. If a large glenoid defect is seen, computed tomography (CT) or magnetic resonance imaging (MRI) is useful to evaluate the adequacy of glenoid bone stock for baseplate implantation.[22] Acromial adequacy should also be judged on radiographic imaging, as considerable stress is placed on the deltoid insertion when an RSA is performed. In particular, an overly thinned acromion from a previous acromioplasty can lead to acromial insufficiency and fracture. Walch and colleagues showed that preoperative lesions of the acromion, both acquired and congenital, are not a contraindication to RSA.[28] In their series, the results obtained were not different from those of patients with a normal acromion.

Figure 24-4. MRI cross-section demonstrating fatty degeneration of the supraspinatus, infraspinatus, and teres minor muscles.

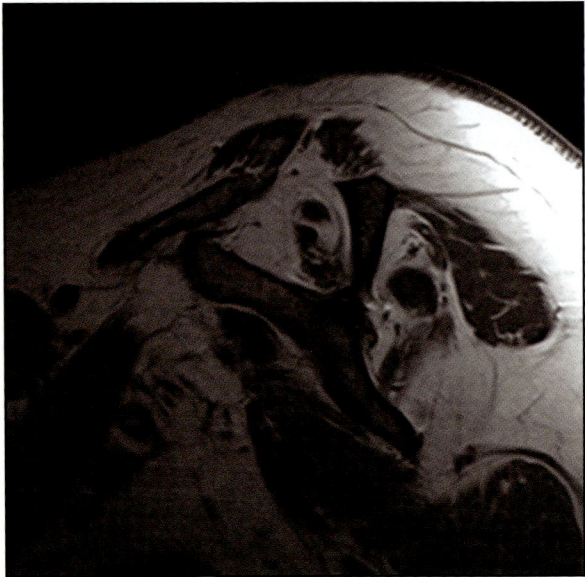

Advanced 3-dimensional imaging can provide added detail with respect to glenoid bone stock and version, evaluation of the rotator cuff tendons and muscle atrophy and fatty infiltration, and degree of osteoporosis. CT scans are preferred for the assessment of bony anatomy, but can also provide insight into the status of the rotator cuff muscles and tendons. MRI is optimal for soft-tissue evaluation while providing limited information regarding bony morphology. Muscle atrophy is characterized as the percentage of fat based on cross-sectional area with regard to overall muscle bulk, while fatty infiltration is graded using the system described by Goutallier (Figure 24-4).[29,30]

NONOPERATIVE TREATMENT

Nonoperative management is the first line of treatment and includes activity modification, nonsteroidal anti-inflammatory drug use, and a formalized physical therapy program focused on anterior deltoid strengthening. Nonsurgical treatment is especially helpful in those patients who present with acute inflammation (usually subacromial bursitis) in the setting of a chronic, pre-existing rotator cuff tear. In these patients, MRI shows evidence of a chronic tear with a significant effusion in a patient who previously was well-adjusted and had good function. These patients often respond well to corticosteroid injections and a physical therapy program. However, repeated injections should be avoided, as their efficacy is limited and can cause harm in the form of iatrogenic infection.[31] Physical therapy focused on gradual anterior deltoid strengthening has resulted in both pain and functional improvements in cases of massive, irreparable rotator cuff tears. Authors of this program feel that patients with pseudoparalysis who benefited from this program progressed from a stage of unstable fulcrum kinematics to captured fulcrum kinematics as described by Burkhart.[1,32]

OPERATIVE TREATMENT

When nonoperative treatment fails, various surgical options can be considered to provide pain relief and improve function. Surgical treatment includes arthroscopic lavage and débridement, biceps tenotomy or tenodesis, partial rotator cuff repair, tendon transfer, resurfacing arthroplasty, hemiarthroplasty, bipolar arthroplasty, total shoulder arthroplasty (TSA), and RSA.

Limited intervention in the form of arthroscopy can be helpful in patients with pain as the primary complaint who otherwise maintain good active range of motion. At times, range of motion may be limited secondary to pain, and a diagnostic lidocaine injection can assist in differentiating a lack of motion due to pain versus weakness. Subacromial bursectomy and glenohumeral débridement have been shown to provide short-term relief.[33] Acromioplasty and CA ligament release should be judiciously applied, as they can lead to anterosuperior instability.[13,34-36] Biceps tenotomy and tenodesis can improve pain in the setting of a massive, irreparable rotator cuff tear.[26] However, many patients with CTA already have a ruptured long head of the biceps in advanced stages of the disease process.[9,15] Patient education is paramount when recommending such interventions so as to ensure short- and long-term expectations are met. Patients must be aware that pain relief may be short-term and future arthroplasty may be needed for definitive treatment.

Latissimus dorsi tendon transfers have been performed for massive, irreparable posterosuperior rotator cuff tears with mixed results.[37,38] The ideal candidate is a young patient with well-maintained forward elevation but with pain and external rotation deficit. Tendon transfers do not restore the depressive function of the native rotator cuff. Therefore, once static superior migration exists indicating an uncontained humeral head, a latissimus dorsi transfer will not restore normal glenohumeral kinematics. Furthermore, a tendon transfer is not helpful in patients with painful glenohumeral arthritis secondary to a massive rotator cuff tear.

Hemiarthroplasty in the form of conventional hemiarthroplasty, extended head prosthesis,[10] and bipolar options have all been used for CTA. Hemiarthroplasty has been used with good success in regard to pain relief, but results are suboptimal in those patients with poor preoperative motion.[39] Furthermore, hemiarthroplasty is limited to earlier stages of disease without escape and an intact CA arch.[13,34-36] Despite addressing humeral head arthrosis, hemiarthroplasty options do little to correct the inherent pathology of instability present in CTA, and therefore result in only moderate improvement in function. Additionally, the pathologic process involved in CTA is not halted and can progress to worsening instability and dysfunction through progression of rotator cuff tears and further erosion of the glenoid. In order to maintain or impart stability, a large humeral head runs the risk of overstuffing the joint and further compromising motion. Despite these limitations, hemiarthroplasty does have a role in treating patients with CTA, though patient selection is imperative to success. The optimal patient is one in whom pain is the primary complaint and who has moderately good range of motion (>120 degrees). In our experience, younger, more active patients with a well-contained head and isolated humeral arthrosis without severe glenoid wear are optimal candidates.

TSA in patients with massive rotator cuff tears has resulted in early glenoid loosening and failure due to what has been described as the "rocking horse" phenomenon. Altered kinematics in the cuff-deficient patient lead to superior migration of the humeral head with edge loading and uneven glenoid component wear.[40] Therefore, TSA is contraindicated in patients without a functional rotator cuff due to eccentric wear patterns that predispose these patients to early glenoid failure.

RSA offers the shoulder surgeon a creative solution to the complex and difficult problem of rotator cuff deficiency and glenohumeral arthrosis. Unconstrained arthroplasty options have yielded suboptimal results with regard to restoration of function and long-term pain control. The biomechanical rationale for current RSA designs are founded on the principles set forth by Grammont.[41,42] These rely on a semi-constrained prosthesis to restore stability using a convex glenosphere and concave humeral articulation with similar radii of curvature. The center of rotation is medialized to the glenoid surface, thus transforming torque generated by abduction into compressive forces at the prosthesis-bone interface (Figure 24-5). This medialized center of rotation in turn lengthens the deltoid lever arm, allowing more deltoid fibers to be recruited for abduction and elevation. Additionally, lowering the humerus further increases deltoid tension.[43,44]

Figure 24-5. The effect of the center of rotation on the biomechanics of RSA components. (A) In the midrange of motion, the resultant force vector passes through the center of rotation of the glenosphere (white arrow). Because the center of rotation is at the former joint line, abduction becomes possible and creates shear forces (Fs) and compressive forces (Fc) on the interface (black arrows). (B) Lateralization of the center of rotation improves the range of motion (adduction and internal/external rotation) but also results in an additional moment (M) at the interface. (© 2009 American Academy of Orthopaedic Surgeons. Reprinted from the *Journal of the American Academy of Orthopaedic Surgeons*, Volume 17(5), pp. 284-295 with permission.)

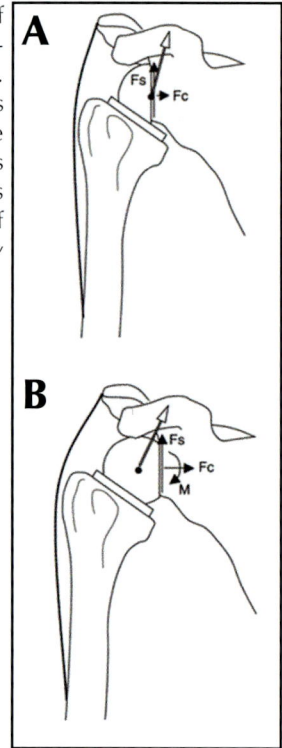

Reverse Shoulder Arthroplasty for Cuff Tear Arthropathy

Indications

The decision to perform RSA is based on a comprehensive patient assessment that takes into consideration patient complaints and functional status, history and physical examination, and radiographic findings. While we prefer to reserve this technique for the elderly patient, there are certain conditions that can only be reliably addressed with RSA. As a general outline, we use the following indications for RSA in our practice:

1. Classic CTA associated with glenohumeral arthritis
2. Pseudoparalysis due to a massive, irreparable rotator cuff tear
3. Severe pain in a patient with osteoarthritis and a massive rotator cuff tear
4. Inflammatory arthritis associated with a massive rotator cuff tear
5. Revision arthroplasty associated with rotator cuff insufficiency
6. Instability associated with revision arthroplasty or fixed primary instability
7. Glenoid deficiency precluding fixation of a glenoid component in conventional arthroplasty
8. Four-part fracture in the elderly patient
9. Fracture sequelae with irreparable tuberosities
10. Postinfection treatment
11. Tumor reconstruction

Pain unresponsive to nonoperative intervention continues to be the primary indication for RSA. In the setting of rotator cuff insufficiency, the presence or absence of glenohumeral arthritis in large part dictates treatment.

In our experience, RSA is an ideal solution for the patient with CTA and addresses both rotator cuff dysfunction and glenohumeral arthritis. The next most common primary indication should be pseudoparalysis that is refractory to an anterior deltoid strengthening program.[45]

One of the most challenging groups of patients to treat are those with massive, irreparable rotator cuff tears without arthritis but who have significant pain and possess more than 90 degrees of forward elevation. Numerous options exist, but none provide consistent or predictable results. RSA in this cohort of patients has yielded suboptimal outcomes, leaving many dissatisfied. We do not recommend RSA as the first line of treatment in this group.[27,46] In younger, high-demand patients, nonarthroplasty options include arthroscopic débridement and biceps tenodesis or tenotomy, partial rotator cuff repair, and latissimus dorsi tendon transfer.

Contraindications

In order for the RSA to successfully restore forward elevation, an intact and functional deltoid muscle must be present. Axillary nerve dysfunction and deltoid deficiency are absolute contraindications to performing an RSA. If there is any uncertainty, especially in patients who have undergone previous surgery, electromyography and nerve conduction studies are obtained. In some patients who have undergone previous open surgery, there is a deficit of the anterior deltoid fibers with preservation of the middle and posterior deltoid components. In such instances, RSA can still be performed with limited functional improvement.

As with any arthroplasty procedure, active and untreated infection is also an absolute contraindication. Patients with pain and any surrounding erythema following prior surgery should be considered infected and treated accordingly. If there is any suspicion, preoperative evaluation should be performed in the form of laboratory studies (white blood cells, erythrocyte sedimentation rate, C-reactive protein) and joint aspiration with gram stain and culture. Tagged white blood cell bone scan and indium scans are less helpful and less reliable for indolent infections.

At the time of surgery, if a question of infection remains, intraoperative gram stains and frozen section should also be obtained. Although multiple classification systems exist for the histopathologic analysis of periprosthetic tissue, we use the system advocated by Feldman et al.[47] Frozen sections of periprosthetic tissue are considered positive for active infection if there are more than 5 polymorphonuclear leukocytes per high-power field in at least 5 distinct microscopic fields. The tissue is cultured, and those cultures are held for 14 days to increase the yield of slow-growing organisms, such as *Propionibacterium acnes*. If intraoperative analysis is low for suspicion of infection and the decision was made to move forward with prosthesis implantation, we leave our patients on oral antibiotics until the final culture results are reported.

Glenoid insufficiency or bone loss and severe osteopenia are relative contraindications to RSA implantation.[11] When sufficient glenoid bone stock is not available to adequately support the baseplate, a concomitant or staged bone grafting procedure is indicated. Bone graft options include humeral head autograft, iliac crest autograft, and allograft. In our experience, allograft glenoid reconstruction results in graft resorption and implant subsidence, and therefore we do not advocate this technique.[48,49]

Reverse Shoulder Arthroplasty Technical Considerations

Scapular Notching

One of the key tenets of the Grammont prosthesis is a medialized center of rotation that is shifted to the bone-prosthesis interface. As a result of using a hemispherical glenosphere, the torque generated by actively abducting the humerus is converted to compression. Earlier RSA prosthetic designs with an excessively long lever arm that produce shear forces on the glenoid baseplate resulted in rapid loosening.[42] Consequently, the impingement-free arc of motion of the Grammont prosthesis is limited due to the absence of a scapular neck. Adduction and rotation of the shoulder result in abutment of the medial aspect of the humeral component onto the scapular neck. This is at least one contributing cause of subsequent scapular notching (Figures 24-6 and 24-7).[43,44] In addition, polyethylene wear has also been observed due to this mechanism and has the potential to cause chronic inflammation, osteolysis, and subsequent loosening.[50,51]

Figure 24-6. (A) Illustration of inferior scapular notching that occurs as a result of a medialized center of rotation seen in the Grammont design. (B) BIO-RSA (Bony-Increased Offset Reverse Shoulder Arthroplasty), which provides increased clearance of the humeral component in adduction while maintaining the center of rotation at the bone-baseplate interface. (Reprinted with permission from Walch G, Boileau P, Mole D, et al. Bony increased-offset reversed shoulder arthroplasty (BIO-RSA): the benefits of bony lateralization. In: Boileau P, Moineau G, Roussanne, O'Shea K, eds. *Shoulder Concepts 2010: The Glenoid.* Paris, France: Sauramps Medical; 2010:374.)

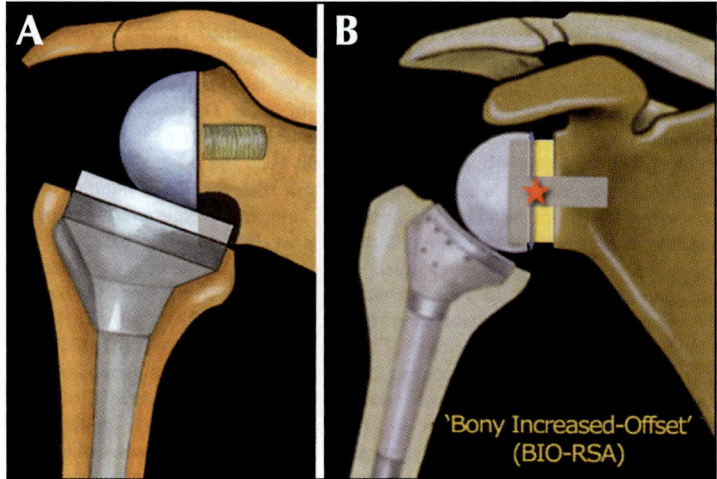

Figure 24-7. Radiograph demonstrating advanced scapular notching.

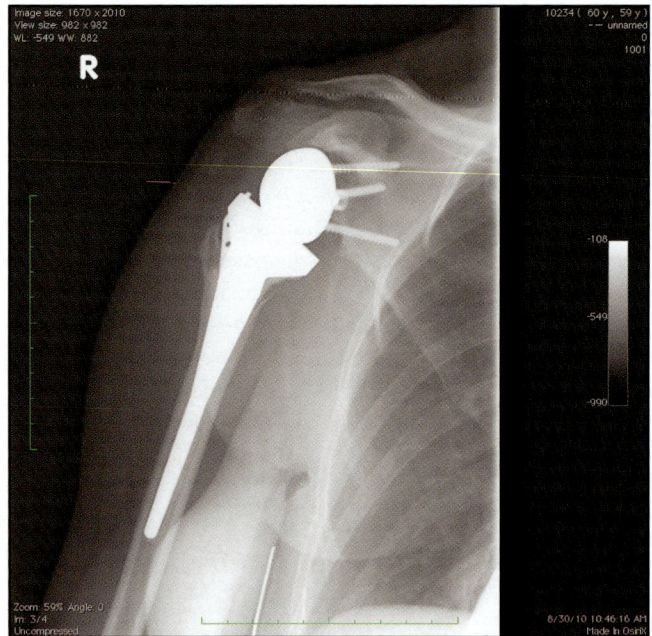

A prosthesis that uses a baseplate with a laterally offset glenosphere has a low rate of scapular notching (Figure 24-8). However, the first results of this type of glenosphere showed high baseplate loosening. More recent reports with a more robust baseplate showed no loosening of the baseplate. The tactic of using a laterally offset glenosphere reduces the notching, and newer designs may do so without concomitant increased risk of baseplate loosening.[46]

Multiple series have shown a high prevalence of inferior scapular notching seen on early postoperative radiographs. There has also been a trend toward deteriorating clinical results in patients with evidence of advanced scapular notching with an increased risk of loosening.[24,43,52-55] The significance of scapular notching is still yet to be determined.

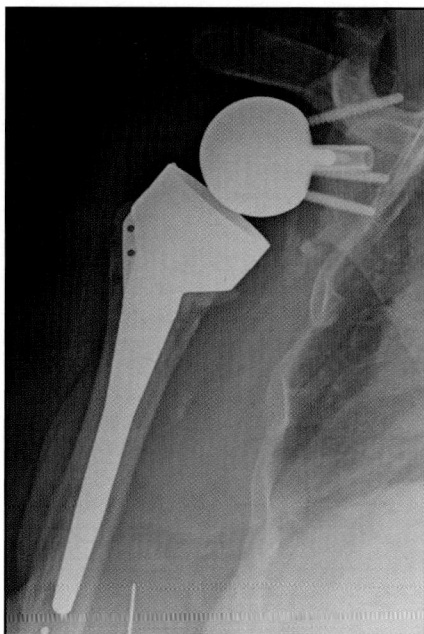

Figure 24-8. This x-ray demonstrates a laterally offset glenosphere, which was placed to correct a previously unstable RSA. Although a notch is present here, the notch is the result of the previous implant in which a glenosphere with no offset was used.

Glenoid Offset

In order to address the causes of scapular notching and loss of motion due to impingement, the center of rotation can be lateralized. This can be accomplished through 1 of 2 methods. Either an eccentric glenosphere can be used to provide prosthetic lateralization or an increased bony offset produced through bone grafting the glenoid (BIO-RSA; see Figure 24-6B).[56] Despite providing benefits of improved mobility and decreased risk of scapular notching, the lever arm on the baseplate-bone interface is lengthened with an eccentric glenosphere. This in turn increases the shear forces on the glenoid component and can place the construct at risk of failure similar to that seen in early RSA designs. However, proponents of placing the center of rotation lateral in relation to the glenoid using an eccentric glenosphere cite poor baseplate fixation and the constrained nature of early designs as the cause of failure. These authors believe improved fixation between the glenoid bone and baseplate accommodates greater loads and has resulted in success with this prosthetic design.[11,46]

The BIO-RSA technique as described by Boileau incorporates a disk of cancellous bone graft obtained from the humeral head during RSA preparation and places it between the reamed native glenoid and the glenosphere. When the bone graft ultimately heals, the scapular neck itself is essentially lateralized. This procedure therefore allows the center of rotation to remain at the baseplate-bone interface while theoretically decreasing the risks of impingement, scapular notching, and glenoid loosening.[11]

Other Considerations

In addition to lateralizing the center of rotation, other technical factors can decrease impingement and can potentially improve prosthetic longevity. This includes using a glenosphere, which has a larger radius of curvature to increase the impingement-free arc of motion.[57] In order to reduce the impingement of the humeral component onto the neck of the glenoid, the baseplate position is critical and should be placed as inferiorly as possible.[58] Modified glenospheres are also available that use an inferior offset or inferior hood extension that theoretically increases the impingement-free arc of motion as well. These tactics, however, lead to uneven loading of the inferior baseplate and can lead to early loosening. Last, the use of a varus neck shaft angle can result in the least amount of adduction deficit, but in turn can result in diminished abduction.[57]

Figure 24-9. The tug test. The axillary nerve is identified by passing a finger over the subscapularis muscle and sweeping inferiorly. This maneuver allows the nerve to be palpated as it travels into the quadrilateral space. A second finger is used to palpate the anterior branch of the nerve as it travels around the surgical neck to innervate the deep aspect of the deltoid muscle. Tension on both aspects of the nerve confirms its course and location. (© 2001 American Academy of Orthopaedic Surgeons. Reprinted from *Journal of the American Academy of Orthopaedic Surgeons*, Volume 9(5), pp. 328-335 with permission.)

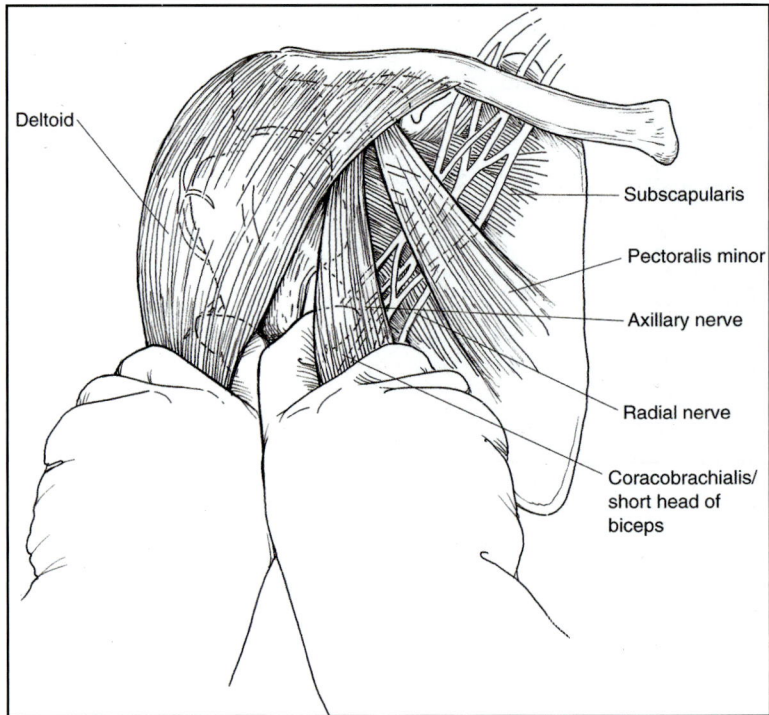

Labels on figure: Deltoid; Subscapularis; Pectoralis minor; Axillary nerve; Radial nerve; Coracobrachialis/short head of biceps

Authors' Preferred Technique

Approach

We use a standard deltopectoral incision that can easily be extended. An anterosuperior approach can also be used, but it requires the deltoid muscle to be split and elevated off the clavicle and acromion. Furthermore, the anterosuperior approach is not extensile and has limited utility in revision arthroplasty situations.

The incision begins proximally at the clavicle, extending over the lateral third of the coracoid process, and further extends distally toward the deltoid insertion for a total distance of approximately 15 cm. The incision is lateral to the axillary crease, thus minimizing the risk of axillary bacterial contamination. Full-thickness flaps are created, and the cephalic vein is usually retracted laterally with the deltoid.

To assist with humeral mobilization and ensure adequate postoperative motion, subacromial, subdeltoid, and subcoracoid adhesions are released. This is an instrumental step, which will facilitate later phases of the procedure. If no prior surgery has been performed, the bursal adhesions are released with relative ease. The axillary nerve should be located, identified, and protected during all phases of the procedure. Its position can be verified by the tug test (Figure 24-9). Adhesions from previous rotator cuff surgery should be carefully released, avoiding injury to the deltoid and axillary nerve.

If prior surgery was performed, tissue or debris including suture is sent for culture. Cultures are held for 14 days to maximize detection of slow-growing organisms, especially Propionibacterium acnes. If there is any overt suspicion for infection, at least 4 distinct cultures are taken, a thorough débridement is performed, and the arthroplasty is postponed. Further treatment for infection is performed in consultation with an infectious disease specialist.

Humeral Exposure

The upper pectoralis major tendon is released for approximately 1.5 cm. This provides immediate exposure to both the anterior circumflex vessels and the biceps tendon. First, in order to avoid subsequent bleeding during the procedure, the anterior circumflex humeral vessels are ligated. They are most easily identified at the inferior border of the subscapularis tendon with the arm in external rotation. We use absorbable 2-0 sutures for ligation followed by electrocautery of the vessels as they enter the bicipital groove. Second, tenodesis of the long head of the biceps tendon is performed, when present, as it is a common source of pain. The sheath overlying the long head of the biceps tendon is incised with mayo scissors. Using a number 2 nonabsorbable suture and a locking stitch, the tendon is secured to the lateral pectoralis tendon stump, and the tendon above the attachment point is excised.

The rotator interval is then opened using a curved mayo scissors. The most reliable method of locating it is by following the bicipital groove proximally with scissors and curving medially at the superior, rolled edge of the subscapularis tendon. Scissors directed toward the undersurface of the coracoid are used to divide the interval completely.

If present, the subscapularis is divided. A subscapularis tenotomy is usually used, but a lesser tuberosity osteotomy may be used. The superolateral border of the subscapularis tendon as it inserts onto the lesser tuberosity is tagged with a number 2 nonabsorbable suture. This serves to identify the anatomic position of the subscapularis tendon for later repair, provides a handle for retraction of the tendon, and allows easy localization of the tendon after the glenosphere is placed. A Hohmann retractor is placed intra-articularly at the neck of the humerus to provide traction and protect the inferiorly traversing axillary nerve, while the inferior capsule is released with cautery off of the neck of the humerus. A Cobb elevator can similarly be added to depress and protect the soft tissues. The arm is placed into continued extension and external rotation to place tension on the capsule and dislocate the humeral head. This must be performed with care in the elderly patient with osteoporosis to avoid a humerus fracture. Complete release of the inferior capsule and glenohumeral ligaments will improve visualization of the entire humeral articular surface.

Humeral Preparation

Humeral preparation is guided by specific manufacturer instruments. However, exposure and proper placement of retractors is necessary for all systems. Extension and external rotation of the humerus is required for adequate visualization.

A Hohmann or Fukuda retractor is placed over the greater tuberosity. A large flat retractor such as a Darrach retractor is placed between the posterior head and coracoid. This pushes the humerus into the operating surgeon's view and out from underneath the deltoid. A third retractor may be necessary for inferior exposure of marginal osteophytes, which should be removed. Once exposed, the instrumentation system directions for the humerus preparation are followed. We prefer to place the implant in 20 degrees of retroversion relative to the epicondylar axis. Both cemented and press-fit humeral components are available. Reaming and broaching proceeds according to technique guides. Correct humeral prosthesis height is judged in relation to the greater tuberosity. In general, the summit of the greater tuberosity should be between 5- and 10-mm below the summit of the prosthetic head.[59]

Aggressive reaming should be avoided, as an iatrogenic fracture can result in osteopenic bone. A trial component is impacted into place, taking care to maintain the selected retroversion. A humeral head protector can be placed on the cut surface of the proximal humerus to prevent fracture or impaction of the metaphysis during retraction for glenoid exposure.

Glenoid Exposure and Preparation

Adequate glenoid exposure is imperative to ensuring appropriate baseplate position and may ultimately determine functional outcome and the longevity of the implant. We begin by placing Hohmann retractors, one posterior and one anterior, just outside of the labrum. Placing the shoulder in slight external rotation and extension to shift the humerus away from the glenoid facilitates this. The labrum is then circumferentially resected using a scalpel. As long as the blade is kept inside the capsule, the axillary nerve should not be endangered.

Next, the anterior Hohmann retractor is placed deep to the capsule in a subperiosteal manner along the anterior glenoid neck. Using electrocautery, the superior, middle, and inferior glenohumeral capsuloligamentous complexes are released from their glenoid attachments. This retractor is then replaced with a Buxton retractor along the anterior glenoid, deep to the subscapularis. At the inferior aspect of the glenoid, the long head of the triceps tendon is released and the lateral scapular pillar identified. A 2-pronged retractor may be placed on either side of the lateral pillar and is positioned inferiorly. Due to the semi-constrained nature of the RSA prosthesis, the posterior capsule can be further released to improve exposure without risking significant postoperative instability. The capsule is left attached to the subscapularis during these maneuvers. In some cases, the humerus is still difficult to retract posteriorly. In these instances, while protecting the axillary nerve, the inferior capsule is transected. This will free the subscapularis and its attached anterior capsule from the posterior capsule.

Attention is now turned to glenoid preparation for baseplate implantation. If using a Grammont-style implant, the baseplate should be placed as low as possible. Based on previous CT studies, we use the 12-mm rule to optimize an inferior position (Figure 24-10A).[58] A guide pin is placed 12 mm from the inferior glenoid rim with a 10-degree inferior tilt. By placing the post in this spot, the resulting baseplate position is low on the glenoid surface. The glenoid is modestly reamed. The inferior glenoid is more completely reamed, leaving a crescent shape of exposed subchondral and sometimes cancellous bone (Figure 24-10B). This appearance generally corresponds with a neutral or slight inferiorly (10 degrees) tilted reamed surface. Reaming deep into subchondral bone should be avoided so as to maintain adequate bony support and prevent component subsidence. Any remaining cartilage superiorly should be removed using curettes and drill holes placed to stimulate bony ingrowth. When using power reamers, they should be started prior to making contact with the glenoid surface to minimize the risk of fracture. If difficulty is encountered when attempting to introduce the reamers, the retractors should be removed or repositioned.

If necessary for certain implant systems, the central hole for the baseplate is further enlarged to accept the central post. The baseplate is then impacted into position.

To maximize screw purchase, we use the 3-column concept of the scapula when determining screw trajectory.[60] The 3 major columns of bone in the scapula are the base of the coracoid process, scapular spine, and the lateral pillar (Figure 24-11). To increase screw length for the inferior locking screw, this screw hole is rotationally aligned with the lateral scapular pillar. Aim points for the screws have been analyzed in cadaveric studies.

Proper screw placement and security are critical to initial implant stability. The operating surgeon should carefully and completely review the scapular anatomy relative to available bone and potential screw position before proceeding to the operating room.

If present, the anterior and posterior compression screws are first drilled to compress the baseplate to the glenoid. The anterior screw is usually aimed upward and centrally, and the posterior screw is aimed downward and centrally. We avoid multiple passes with the drill bit so that bone is preserved. Usually, the superior and inferior screws are locking screws. The inferior screw is placed into the lateral scapular pillar. Last, the superior screw is placed into the base of the coracoid process. The exit point for this screw is just anterior and inferior to the scapular notch and away from the course of the suprascapular neurovascular bundle. The baseplate should be cleared of all soft tissue circumferentially prior to inserting the glenosphere.

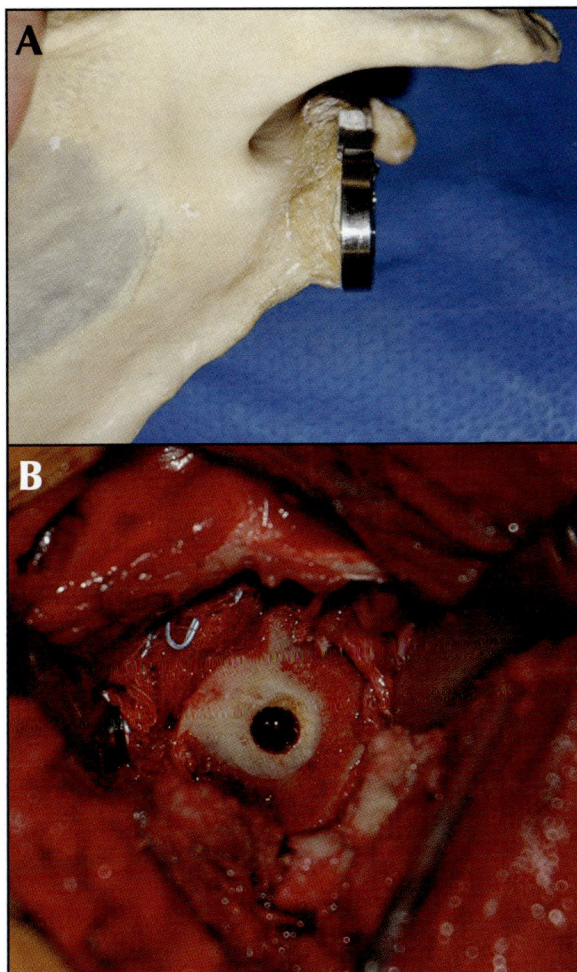

Figure 24-10. (A) Model demonstrating inferior baseplate position using the 12-mm rule. (B) Intraoperative photograph demonstrating preferential inferior reaming of glenoid face obtained when the glenoid component is placed with a slight inferior tilt.

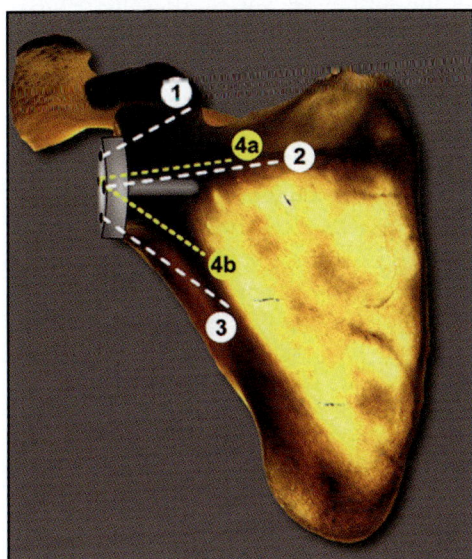

Figure 24-11. A transilluminated scapula shows the authors' preferred method of baseplate screw fixation into the 3 bony columns: the superior screw is placed into the base of the coracoid (1), the anterior screw is placed into the spine of the scapula (2), and the inferior screw is placed into the pillar (3). The posterior screw hole of the baseplate may be filled in 1 of 2 ways. The drill may be aimed anteriorly and superiorly toward the base of the scapular spine (4a), or it may be aimed anteriorly and inferiorly into the pillar (4b).[60]

Implantation and Reduction

Next, the humeral component may be trialed. In most cases of primary arthroplasty, the thinnest polyethylene is used. In general, the top of the polyethylene should reach the top of the greater tuberosity. The quality of the final reduction can also be estimated by comparing the proximal medial edge of the humeral trial component to the equator of the glenosphere. In our experience, adequate deltoid tension is established when the medial edge of the polyethylene component is within 1 to 2 mm of the center of the glenosphere.

If the deltoid is overtensioned, additional resection of the metaphysis can be performed to place the humeral component at a more distal level. Conversely, if tension is lacking, a thicker polyethylene component or spacer can be used. Most primary CTA cases require a 6-mm polyethylene component with the technique described here.

The trial component is removed, and the canal is prepared with thorough irrigation and drying. At this time, 3 sets of drill holes are placed on either side of the bicipital groove for later subscapularis repair. A looped nonabsorbable number 2 suture is placed with the 2 free ends exiting medially and the loop laterally.

When performed, cementing is performed with standard third-generation technique after a cement restrictor is inserted. During insertion of the final components, version must continually be checked. The shoulder is then reduced through a combination of flexion, distraction, and internal rotation.

Appropriate deltoid tensioning is ensured by making certain there is no pistoning of the construct when the humerus is distracted. Complete separation of the humerus from the glenosphere indicates a lack of tensioning and should be addressed with a thicker polyethylene component. The conjoined tendon can also be evaluated to confirm deltoid tensioning.

Intraoperative range of motion is now checked. Restoration of abduction and forward flexion is confirmed. There should be no impingement of the humeral component onto the lateral pillar with adduction. Internal and external rotation with the arm at the side are checked to make certain there is no subluxation.

Closure

The subscapularis tendon is now repaired. The 2 free ends from each suture are passed through the subscapularis tendon in mattress fashion. Once all of the sutures are passed, they are secured using a racking half hitch knot. This knot allows sequential tightening of each of the other 2 knots after the first is cinched down with the base knot and a half hitch. Placement of the first half hitch prevents the knot from slipping, but continues to allow subsequent tightening. This can be repeated multiple times amongst the 3 knots until they are completely seated. Placing a second reverse half hitch will lock the knot permanently.

To avoid complications associated with postoperative hematoma, a drain is placed in the deep layers. The deltopectoral interval is next approximated and marked with a nonabsorbable number 2 suture, which can serve to identify tissue planes in cases of revision surgery. Closure is completed in standard layered fashion with absorbable suture and dermal adhesive. The patient is placed in an abduction sling orthosis prior to awakening. In cases requiring a latissimus dorsi/teres major tendon transfer, an orthosis that allows the shoulder to be placed in 15 degrees of external rotation is used.

Postoperative Rehabilitation Protocol

Patients are instructed to wear the orthosis for 4 weeks at all times and to only wear it outside the home for an additional 2 weeks. Initial rehabilitation is focused on pendulum exercises and elbow, wrist, and hand range of motion. Formal physical therapy begins at 6 weeks postoperatively and is directed toward passive stretching without forced external rotation and active-assist motion. Strengthening begins at the 12-week point. In our experience, a gradual and delayed protocol allows adequate time for tissue healing without resulting in range of motion deficit.

TABLE 24-1. FUNCTIONAL RESULTS OF REVERSE SHOULDER ARTHROPLASTY

	MEAN AGE	NUMBER	MEAN FOLLOW-UP (MONTHS)	PREOPERATIVE FUNCTIONAL SCORE
Sirveaux, *JBJS (Br)*, 2004[55]	72.8	80	44.5 (24 to 97)	22.6 (Constant)
Werner, *JBJS (Am)*, 2005[24]	68	58	38	29 (Constant)
Boileau, *JSES*, 2006[27]	77	21	40 (24 to 72)	18 (Constant)
Wall, *JBJS (Am)*, 2007[61]	72.7	74	40 (26 to 86)	21.7 (Constant)
Mulieri, *JBJS (Am)*, 2010[46]	NR	60	52 (24 to 101)	33.3 (ASES)

	POSTOPERATIVE FUNCTIONAL SCORE	PREOPERATIVE FORWARD ELEVATION	POSTOPERATIVE FORWARD ELEVATION	COMPLICATION RATE
Sirveaux, *JBJS (Br)*, 2004[55]	65.6	73	138	NR
Werner, *JBJS (Am)*, 2005[24]	64	42	100	50%
Boileau, *JSES*, 2006[27]	66	55	123	19%
Wall, *JBJS (Am)*, 2007[61]	65.1	76	142	19%
Mulieri, *JBJS (Am)*, 2010[46]	75.4	53	134	20%

NR = not reported

RESULTS

In the appropriately selected patient, functional results and pain reduction for CTA have been promising (Table 24-1). Most patients can expect improved range of motion to 120 degrees of forward elevation with substantial pain relief. However, those patients with teres minor insufficiency tend to have decreased external rotation, decreased outcome scores, and a higher rate of dissatisfaction. These patients should carefully be evaluated for latissimus tendon transfer. Complication rates in primary procedures have been reported to be around 20%. Complications in revision arthroplasty cases are significantly higher, with Boileau and colleagues[27] reporting a revision surgery rate of 42% over an average of 40 months of follow-up in their series.

COMPLICATIONS

Complications associated with RSA have been reported to be 4 times those seen in anatomic shoulder arthroplasty.[62] However, due to inconsistencies in the literature in regard to technique, prosthesis type, and follow-up, complication rates vary considerably.

Scapular notching is the most common complication seen with an incidence varying between 5% and 100%.[24,63,64] Currently, the long-term implications are not completely understood. Some studies reveal a trend toward deteriorating clinical results with advanced scapular notching, while others do not.[22,24,53-55] Risk factors for notching include CTA, grade 3 and 4 fatty infiltration of the infraspinatus, a narrowed AHI, and a superiorly oriented glenoid preoperatively.[53] Operative factors that increase the risk of notching have been described to be an anterosuperior surgical approach and a superiorly positioned or tilted baseplate.

Glenoid side complications have been reported to occur in 0% to 16% of cases and include loosening, dissociation, and scapular fracture. Instability (including dislocation) after RSA has been documented in 0% to 14% of cases. This is usually in the anterior/anterolateral direction and is often associated with infection.[62,65] Humeral complications occur with low incidence but include periprosthetic fractures and stem loosening. Loosening is usually seen in the setting of either osteolysis or infection.

The incidence of infection after RSA is reported to be around 5% and is often due to *Propionibacterium acnes* and other skin flora. It is attributed to large dead space creation and lack of soft tissue coverage after RSA.[62] The incidence of infection is noted to be higher in revision versus primary cases.[61]

Patients with CTA often have acromial insufficiency due to articulation of the undersurface of the acromion with the humeral head. This, in association with increased deltoid tension seen after RSA, can result in acromial fractures (0% to 15%).[64,66] Neurologic complications such as axillary nerve neuropathy and brachial plexopathy are rare and usually temporary as a result of traction injury.[62]

REFERENCES

1. Burkhart SS. Fluoroscopic comparison of kinematic patterns in massive rotator cuff tears. A suspension bridge model. *Clin Orthop Relat Res.* 1992;284:144-152.
2. Burkhart SS. Arthroscopic débridement and decompression for selected rotator cuff tears. Clinical results, pathomechanics, and patient selection based on biomechanical parameters. *Orthop Clin North Am.* 1993;24(1):111-123.
3. Burkhart SS. Reconciling the paradox of rotator cuff repair versus débridement: a unified biomechanical rationale for the treatment of rotator cuff tears. *Arthroscopy.* 1994;10(1):4-19.
4. Matsen FA 3rd, Harryman DT 2nd, Sidles JA. Mechanics of glenohumeral instability. *Clin Sports Med.* 1991;10(4):783-788.
5. Mura N, O'Driscoll SW, Zobitz ME, et al. The effect of infraspinatus disruption on glenohumeral torque and superior migration of the humeral head: a biomechanical study. *J Shoulder Elbow Surg.* 2003;12(2):179-184.
6. Sahara W, Wugamoto K, Murai M, Tanaka H, Yoshikawa H. The three-dimensional motions of glenohumeral joint under semi-loaded condition during arm abduction using vertically open MRI. *Clin Biomech (Bristol, Avon).* 2007;22(3):304-312.
7. Paletta GA Jr, Warner JJ, Warren RF, Deutsch A, Altchek DW. Shoulder kinematics with two-plane x-ray evaluation in patients with anterior instability or rotator cuff tearing. *J Shoulder Elbow Surg.* 1997;6(6):516-527.
8. Yamaguchi K, Sher JS, Andersen WK, et al. Glenohumeral motion in patients with rotator cuff tears: a comparison of asymptomatic and symptomatic shoulders. *J Shoulder Elbow Surg.* 2000;9(1):6-11.
9. Hamada K, Fukuda H, Mikasa M, Kobayashi Y. Roentgenographic findings in massive rotator cuff tears. A long-term observation. *Clin Orthop Relat Res.* 1990;254:92-96.
10. Visotsky JL, Basamania C, Seebauer L, Rockwood CA, Jensen KL. Cuff tear arthropathy: pathogenesis, classification, and algorithm for treatment. *J Bone Joint Surg Am.* 2004;86-A Suppl 2:35-40.
11. Frankle M, Pupello D, Gutierrez S. Rationale and biomechanics of the reverse shoulder prosthesis: the American experience. In: Frankle MA, ed. *Rotator Cuff Deficiency of the Shoulder.* New York, NY: Thieme; 2008:76-104.
12. Favard L. The glenoid in the frontal plane: the Favard and Hamada classifications of cuff tear osteoarthritis. In: Walch G, Boileau P, Molé D, Favard L, Lévigne C, Sirveaux F. *Shoulder Concepts 2010: The Glenoid.* Paris, France: Sauramps Medical; 2010:53-58.
13. Hockman DE, Lucas GL, Roth CA. Role of the coracoacromial ligament as restraint after shoulder hemiarthroplasty. *Clin Orthop Relat Res.* 2004;419:80-82.
14. Simank HG, Dauer G, Schneider S, Loew M. Incidence of rotator cuff tears in shoulder dislocations and results of therapy in older patients. *Arch Orthop Trauma Surg.* 2006;126(4):235-240.
15. Neer CS 2nd, Craig EV, Fukuda H. Cuff-tear arthropathy. *J Bone Joint Surg Am.* 1983;65(9):1232-1244.
16. Garancis JC, Cheung HS, Halverson PB, McCarty DJ. "Milwaukee shoulder"—association of microspheroids containing hydroxyapatite crystals, active collagenase, ad neutral protease with rotator cuff defects. III. Morphologic and biochemical studies of an excised synovium showing chondromatosis. *Arthritis Rheum.* 1981;24(3):484-491.
17. Halverson PB, Cheung HS, McCarty DJ, Garancis J, Mandel N. "Milwaukee shoulder"—association of microspheroids containing hydroxyapatite crystals, active collagenase, and neutral protease with rotator cuff defects. II. Synovial fluid studies. *Arthritis Rheum.* 1981;24(3):474-483.
18. McCarty DJ, Halverson PB, Carrera GF, Brewer BJ, Kozin F. "Milwaukee shoulder"—association of microspheroids containing hydroxyapatite crystals, active collagenase, and neutral protease with rotator cuff defects. I. Clinical aspects. *Arthritis Rheum.* 1981;24(3):464-473.

19. Feeley BT, Gallo FA, Craig EV. Cuff tear arthropathy: current trends in diagnosis and surgical management. *J Shoulder Elbow Surg.* 2009;18(3):484-494.

20. Iannotti JP, McCarron J, Raymond CJ, et al. Agreement study of radiographic classification of rotator cuff tear arthropathy. *J Shoulder Elbow Surg.* 2010;19(8):1243-1249.

21. Seebauer L, Walter W, Keyl W. Reverse total shoulder arthroplasty for the treatment of defect arthropathy. *Oper Orthop Traumatol.* 2005;17(1):1-24.

22. Jensen KL, Williams GR Jr, Russell IJ, Rockwood CA Jr. Rotator cuff tear arthropathy. *J Bone Joint Surg Am.* 1999;81(9):1312-1324.

23. Ecklund KJ, Lee TQ, Tibone J, Gupta R. Rotator cuff tear arthropathy. *J Am Acad Orthop Surg.* 2007;15(6):340-349.

24. Werner CM, Steinmann PA, Gilbart M, Gerber C. Treatment of painful pseudoparesis due to irreparable rotator cuff dysfunction with the Delta III reverse-ball-and-socket total shoulder prosthesis. *J Bone Joint Surg Am.* 2005;87(7):1476-1486.

25. Walch G, Boulahia A, Calderone S, Robinson AH. The "dropping" and "hornblower's" signs in evaluation of rotator-cuff tears. *J Bone Joint Surg Br.* 1998;80(4):624-628.

26. Boileau P, Baque F, Valerio L, Ahrens P, Chuinard C, Trojani C. Isolated arthroscopic biceps tenotomy or tenodesis improves symptoms in patients with massive irreparable rotator cuff tears. *J Bone Joint Surg Am.* 2007;89(4):747-757.

27. Boileau P, Watkinson D, Hatzidakis AM, Hovorka I. Neer Award 2005: the Grammont reverse shoulder prosthesis: results in cuff tear arthritis, fracture sequelae, and revision arthroplasty. *J Shoulder Elbow Surg.* 2006;15(5):527-540.

28. Walch G, Mottier F, Wall B, Bioleau P, Mole D, Favard L. Acromial insufficiency in reverse shoulder arthroplasties. *J Shoulder Elbow Surg.* 2009;18(3):495-502.

29. Zanetti M, Gerber C, Hodler J. Quantitative assessment of the muscles of the rotator cuff with magnetic resonance imaging. *Invest Radiol.* 1998;33(3):163-170.

30. Goutallier D, Postel JM, Bernageau J, Lavau L, Voisin MC. Fatty muscle degeneration in cuff ruptures. Pre- and postoperative evaluation by CT scan. *Clin Orthop Relat Res.* 1994;304:78-83.

31. Williams GR Jr, Rockwood CA Jr. Hemiarthroplasty in rotator cuff-deficient shoulders. *J Shoulder Elbow Surg.* 1996;5(5):362-367.

32. Levy O, Mullett H, Roberts S, Copeland S. The role of anterior deltoid reeducation in patients with massive irreparable degenerative rotator cuff tears. *J Shoulder Elbow Surg.* 2008;17(6):863-870.

33. Verhelst L, Vandekerckhove PJ, Sergeant G, Liekens K, Van Hoonacker P, Berghs B. Reversed arthroscopic subacromial decompression for symptomatic irreparable rotator cuff tears: mid-term follow-up results in 34 shoulders. *J Shoulder Elbow Surg.* 2010;19(4):601-608.

34. Field LD, Dines DM, Zabinski SJ, Warren RF. Hemiarthroplasty of the shoulder for rotator cuff arthropathy. *J Shoulder Elbow Surg.* 1997;6(1):18-23.

35. Arntz CT, Jackins S, Matsen FA 3rd. Prosthetic replacement of the shoulder for the treatment of defects in the rotator cuff and the surface of the glenohumeral joint. *J Bone Joint Surg Am.* 1993;75(4):485-491.

36. Lippitt S, Matsen F. Mechanisms of glenohumeral joint stability. *Clin Orthop Relat Res.* 1993;291:20-28.

37. Gerber C, Maquieira G, Espinosa N. Latissimus dorsi transfer for the treatment of irreparable rotator cuff tears. *J Bone Joint Surg Am.* 2006;88(1):113-120.

38. Gerhardt C, Lehmann L, Lichtenberg S, Magosch P, Habermeyer P. Modified L'Episcopo tendon transfers for irreparable rotator cuff tears: 5-year follow-up. *Clin Orthop Relat Res.* 2010;468(6):1572-1577.

39. Goldberg SS, Bigliani LU. Hemiarthroplasty for the rotator cuff-deficient shoulder. *J Bone Joint Surg Am.* 2008;90(3):554-559.

40. Franklin JL, Barrett WP, Jackins SE, Matsen FA 3rd. Glenoid loosening in total shoulder arthroplasty. Association with rotator cuff deficiency. *J Arthroplasty.* 1988;3(1):39-46.

41. Grammont P, Laffay JP. Concept study and realization of a new total shoulder prosthesis. *Rhumatologie.* 1987;39:407-418.

42. Grammont PM, Baulot E. Delta shoulder prosthesis for rotator cuff rupture. *Orthopedics.* 1993;16(1):65-68.

43. Boileau P, Watkinson DJ, Hatzidakis AM, Balg F. Grammont reverse prosthesis: design, rationale, and biomechanics. *J Shoulder Elbow Surg.* 2005;14(1 Suppl S):147S-161S.

44. Gerber C, Pennington SD, Nyffeler RW. Reverse total shoulder arthroplasty. *J Am Acad Orthop Surg.* 2009;17(5):284-295.

45. Drake GN, O'Connor DP, Edwards TB. Indications for reverse total shoulder arthroplasty in rotator cuff disease. *Clin Orthop Relat Res.* 2010;468(6):1526-1533.

46. Mulieri P, Dunning P, Klein S, Pupello D, Frankle M. Reverse shoulder arthroplasty for the treatment of irreparable rotator cuff tear without glenohumeral arthritis. *J Bone Joint Surg Am.* 2010;92(15):2544-2556.

47. Feldman DS, Lonner JH, Desai P, Zuckerman JD. The role of intraoperative frozen sections in revision total joint arthroplasty. *J Bone Joint Surg Am.* 1995;77(12):1807-1813.

48. Hill JM, Norris TR. Long-term results of total shoulder arthroplasty following bone-grafting of the glenoid. *J Bone Joint Surg Am.* 2001;83-A(6):877-883.

49. Phipatanakul WP, Norris TR. Treatment of glenoid loosening and bone loss due to osteolysis with glenoid bone grafting. *J Shoulder Elbow Surg.* 2006;15(1):84-87.

50. Nyffeler RW, Werner CM, Simmen BR, Gerber C. Analysis of a retrieved delta III total shoulder prosthesis. *J Bone Joint Surg Br.* 2004;86(8):1187-1191.

51. Nam D, Kepler CK, Nho SJ, Craig EV, Warren RF, Wright TM. Observations on retrieved humeral polyethylene components from reverse total shoulder arthroplasty. *J Shoulder Elbow Surg.* 2010;19(7):1003-1012.

52. Favard L, Sirveaux F, Oudet D, Kerjean Y, Huquet D. Hemi arthroplasty verus reverse arthroplasty in the treatment of osteoarthritis with massive rotator cuff tear. In: Walch G, Boileau P, Mole D, eds. *2000 Shoulder Prosthesis. Two to Ten Year Follow-Up.* Montpellier, France: Sauramps; 2001:261-268.

53. Levigne C, Boileau P, Favard L, et al. Scapular notching in reverse shoulder arthroplasty. *J Shoulder Elbow Surg.* 2008;17(6):925-935.

54. Simovitch RW, Zumstein MA, Lohri E, Helmy N, Gerber C. Predictors of scapular notching in patients managed with the Delta III reverse total shoulder replacement. *J Bone Joint Surg Am.* 2007;89(3):588-600.

55. Sirveaux F, Favard L, Oudet D, Huguet D, Walch G, Mole D. Grammont inverted total shoulder arthroplasty in the treatment of glenohumeral osteoarthritis with massive rupture of the cuff. Results of a multicentre study of 80 shoulders. *J Bone Joint Surg Br.* 2004;86(3):388-395.

56. Boileau P, Youssanne Y, O'Shea K. Bony increased-offset reversed shoulder arthroplasty (BIO-RSA): the benefits of bony lateralization. In: Walch G, Mole D, Favard L, Levigne C, Sirveaux F, eds. *Shoulder Concepts 2010. The Glenoid.* Paris: Sauramps Medical; 2010.

57. Gutierrez S, Comiskey CA 4th, Luo ZP, Pupello DR, Frankle MA. Range of impingement-free abduction and adduction deficit after reverse shoulder arthroplasty. Hierarchy of surgical and implant-design-related factors. *J Bone Joint Surg Am.* 2008;90(12):2606-2615.

58. Kelly JD 2nd, Humphrey CS, Norris TR. Optimizing glenosphere position and fixation in reverse shoulder arthroplasty, Part One: the twelve-mm rule. *J Shoulder Elbow Surg.* 2008;17(4):589-594.

59. Boileau P, Krishnan SG, Tinsi L, Walch G, Coste JS, Mole D. Tuberosity malposition and migration: reasons for poor outcomes after hemiarthroplasty for displaced fractures of the proximal humerus. *J Shoulder Elbow Surg.* 2002;11(5):401-412.

60. Humphrey CS, Kelly JD 2nd, Norris TR. Optimizing glenosphere position and fixation in reverse shoulder arthroplasty, Part Two: the three-column concept. *J Shoulder Elbow Surg.* 2008;17(4):595-601.

61. Wall B, Nove-Josserand L, O'Connor DP, Edwards TB, Walch G. Reverse total shoulder arthroplasty: a review of results according to etiology. *J Bone Joint Surg Am.* 2007;89(7):1476-1485.

62. Farshad M, Gerber C. Reverse total shoulder arthroplasty-from the most to the least common complication. *Int Orthop.* 2010;34(8):1075-1082.

63. Klein M, Juschka M, Hinkenjann B, Scherger B, Ostermann PA. Treatment of comminuted fractures of the proximal humerus in elderly patients with the Delta III reverse shoulder prosthesis. *J Orthop Trauma.* 2008;22(10):698-704.

64. Levy JC, Virani N, Pupello D, Frankle M. Use of the reverse shoulder prosthesis for the treatment of failed hemiarthroplasty in patients with glenohumeral arthritis and rotator cuff deficiency. *J Bone Joint Surg Br.* 2007;89(2):189-195.

65. Gallo RA, Gamradt SC, Mattern CJ, et al. Instability after reverse total shoulder replacement. *J Shoulder Elbow Surg.* 2011;20(4):584-590.

66. Grassi FA, Murena L, Valli F, Alberio R. Six-year experience with the Delta III reverse shoulder prosthesis. *J Orthop Surg (Hong Kong).* 2009;17(2):151-156.

Please see video on the accompanying Web site at http://www.slackbooks.com/rotatorcuffvideos

FINANCIAL DISCLOSURES

Dr. Christina Allen has no financial or proprietary interest in the materials presented herein.

Dr. Asheesh Bedi is an education and research consultant for Smith and Nephew Endoscopy and BioMimetics Therapeutics.

Dr. Fernando Contreras has no financial or proprietary interest in the materials presented herein.

Dr. Edward V. Craig has no financial or proprietary interest in the materials presented herein.

Dr. Ryan Dellamaggiora has no financial or proprietary interest in the materials presented herein.

Dr. Demetris Delos has no financial or proprietary interest in the materials presented herein.

Dr. Jonathan F. Dickens has no financial or proprietary interest in the materials presented herein.

Dr. William H. Dunbar V has no financial or proprietary interest in the materials presented herein.

Dr. Warren R. Dunn has no financial or proprietary interest in the materials presented herein.

Dr. Neal S. ElAttrache receives patent royalties with Arthrex as well as research support as the primary investigator from Arthrex and Omeros Corporation.

Dr. Brian T. Feeley has no financial or proprietary interest in the materials presented herein.

Dr. Robert A. Gallo has no financial or proprietary interest in the materials presented herein.

Dr. Seth C. Gamradt is a consultant for Depuy/Mitek and Stryker. He is also on the editorial board for *Techniques in Shoulder and Elbow Surgery* and the *Journal of Bone and Joint Surgery Sports Medicine Newsletter*.

Dr. Jonathan Gelber has no financial or proprietary interest in the materials presented herein.

Dr. Carolyn M. Hettrich has no financial or proprietary interest in the materials presented herein.

Dr. Stephanie H. Hsu has no financial or proprietary interest in the materials presented herein.

Dr. Jack G. Skendzel has no financial or proprietary interest in the materials presented herein.

Dr. Alison R. I. Spouge has no financial or proprietary interest in the materials presented herein.

Dr. Ehsan Tabaraee has no financial or proprietary interest in the materials presented herein.

Dr. Suketu Vaishnav has no financial or proprietary interest in the materials presented herein.

Dr. Russell F. Warren receives royalties from Biomet. He is also on the scientific advisory board for Cayenne.

Dr. Brian R. Wolf has no financial or proprietary interest in the materials presented herein.

Dr. Bob Yin has no financial or proprietary interest in the materials presented herein.

INDEX